AF480036

Footprints of Toxicology in India

Footprints of Toxicology in India

Ankita Pandey and AB Pant [CA]
CSIR-Indian Institute of Toxicology Research, Lucknow-India

CA: Corresponding Author:
Dr. AB Pant
PhD, ATS (USA), UK-RT (London), FST, FIANs, FAsAW, FAEB, MNASc, MAMS
Senior Principal Scientist
System Toxicology & Health Risk Assessment Group
CSIR-Indian Institute of Toxicology Research
Vishvigyan Bhavan, 31, Mahatma Gandhi Marg
Lucknow, Uttar Pradesh, India

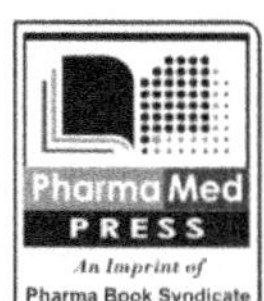

PharmaMed Press
An imprint of Pharma Book Syndicate
A unit of BSP Books Pvt. Ltd.
4-4-309/316, Giriraj Lane,
Sultan Bazar, Hyderabad - 500 095.

Footprints of Toxicology in India
by Ankita Pandey and AB Pant

© 2021, *by Publishher,* All rights reserved.

No part of this book or parts thereof may be reproduced, stored in a retrieval system or transmitted in any language or by any means, electronic, mechanical, photocopying, recording or otherwise without the prior written permission of the author.

Published by

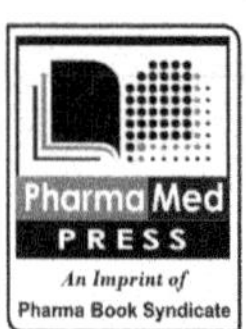

PharmaMed Press

An imprint of Pharma Book Syndicate

A unit of BSP Books Pvt. Ltd.

4-4-309/316, Giriraj Lane, Sultan Bazar, Hyderabad - 500 095.

Phone: 040-23445600, 23445688; Fax: 91+40-23445611

E-mail: info@pharmamedpress.com

www.pharmamedpress.com/pharmamedpress.net

ISBN: 978-93-89974-27-0

Preface

The book "Footprints of Toxicology in India" is a testimonial to the unsung journey of India in the field of Toxicology. Toxicology, considered to have evolved from ancient poisoners, stands as one of the historic practical sciences in India. Although toxicology has been one of the branches of Ayurveda, a health care system, historically practiced in India for more than 5000 years, it began to receive a formal recognition since the mid-1900s. Post-1947, the increasing participation of the workforce in the chemical and agricultural industries, dramatically increased opportunities for occupational exposure to hazardous substances necessitating the need to predict and evaluate the danger potential of these chemicals correctly, therefore offering stimulation for the emergence of toxicology as a freestanding entity. In parallel to these initiatives, various disasters (mass pesticide poisonings, the Bhopal Gas Tragedy and Endosulfan Disaster) also played catalytic roles. Since its inception in the 1960s, over the years, the range and interest in this area has continued to broaden and the subject, formerly a part of pharmacology, has undergone a dimensional change to build up into a fully-fledged discipline with its dedicated group of clubs, journals, regulatory agencies, research institutions and scientists.

From the 'science of poisons' to the 'science of protection', toxicology research in India, today, stands as a highly evolved, multidisciplinary endeavor that develops its conceptual frameworks while also drawing upon advances in the chemical, medical and biological sciences. Toxicology research in India has not just addressed the complex interaction between biological systems and chemicals, but also provided an appropriate basis for precautionary, protective and restrictive strategies. This book speaks about a brief overview of the earliest descriptions of toxicological phenomena in India, significant breakthroughs that underlie the emergence of this discipline and the extensive research carried out for the identification, control/mitigation of various toxicants as well as to understand their mechanistic basis. From the concept of biomarkers, omics approaches, alternatives to animal models to mathematical modelling and predictive toxicology, this book encompasses all and speaks high volumes of the substantial progress India has made in revolutionizing the understanding of human occupational and environmental diseases.

The arena of toxicology has constantly been expanding and diversifying, driven by the need to investigate and understand the human and ecological risks of exposure to newer chemicals and other toxicants. India has made great strides to keep itself abreast of this evolving discipline, which has placed the country on the pedestal of toxicology research. This book conveys a basic appreciation of the contributions made by India while also providing a thumbnail sketch of how modern toxicology evolved in recent times. The book entails a string of subtopics that are dedicated towards different facets of toxicology viz. occupational toxicology, environmental toxicology, medical toxicology, nanotoxicology, toxicogenomics, regulatory toxicology and organ-specific toxicology, that have intricately orchestrated to provide an advanced understanding of the harmful effects of chemicals for the protection of human and environmental health.

The chapter on 'History of Toxicology in India: Antiquity' provides a brief overview of the earliest descriptions of toxicological phenomena in India tracing the origin of poison to mythological Gods. The next chapter 'Milestones that Shaped Toxicology Growth in India' documents a few episodes of environmental, occupational and industrial disasters worldwide that underlie the emergence of toxicology as a scientific discipline as a whole. In addition to these, this chapter also traces the historical growth of the discipline, its origin and development since its formal inception in the 1960s along with an overview of the significant breakthroughs that have revolutionized the face of toxicology and risk assessment in the country. 'Occupational Toxicology' highlights the work that has been undertaken aiming at the recognition, identification and control/mitigation of hazards resulting from exposure to different risk factors encountered at occupational setups (various industries, mines and agricultural fields). Similarly, 'Environmental Toxicology' sheds light on several landmark activities and enactment of several pieces of legislation aimed at regulating and limiting the release of chemicals into the environment. Regular monitoring of air, water and soil quality, ecotoxicology and environmental risk assessment, biomonitoring approaches using biomarkers of exposure, susceptibility and effect have been included as well. Detection and quantification of environmental pollutants and novel strategies framed for remediation/ mitigation of hazardous and persistent chemical substances have been comprehensively discussed.

The chapter on 'Medical Toxicology' encompasses the pathophysiology, diagnosis, treatment, management and prevention of clinical problems associated with acute poisoning, adverse drug events; drug abuse, addiction and withdrawal; chemicals and hazardous materials; venomous bites and stings; and environmental and workplace exposures. The chapter on 'Nanotoxicology' speaks high volumes of the substantial progress India has made in the realm of nanotoxicology research directed towards the synthesis and detailed characterization of nanoparticles, their bioavailability, uptake, bio distribution and excretion profiles, investigation of interactions with biological systems (from the whole organism to molecular level) and understanding their important routes of exposure as well as their ecological impacts. The chapter on 'Toxicogenomics' deals with how the development in the post-genomics era has provided immense opportunities for pragmatic assessment of environmental and occupational exposure to noxious substances that have offered new insights into their mechanistic basis. It also highlights the identification and validation of various biomarkers, toxicogenomic effects and genes susceptibilities that have revolutionized the understanding of human occupational and environmental diseases.

The chapter on 'Regulatory Toxicology' is an appraisal of the fast-paced strides that India has made in the development of standard protocols and new testing methods using novel analytical and molecular tools in order to improve the scientific basis for decision-making processes continuously. This chapter provides an overview of the major legislations that have shaped the regulatory framework in India in the context of toxicology and significant contributions of the institutions that underlie the basis of various regulatory decisions in the country. The chapter on 'Organ-specific Toxicity' highlights the progress India has made in exploring the mechanistic basis of drug/chemical/xenobiotics induced toxicity on the different organs as well as identification of new organ-specific toxicants. Establishment of novel screening strategies, validation of new alternatives to animal models, *in vitro* approaches, computational modeling and microarray approaches have been subtly discussed. This section also includes therapeutic avenues that have been proposed to prevent/protect against respective organ-specific toxicity.

There are several toxicological books available, but none of them is based on Indian toxicology. This book would be the first of its kind to unravel the untold journey of this discipline along with the various developments, achievements, lessons learned and issues addressed that have ultimately shaped the current face of toxicology research in the country. Equipped with case histories, technical but applied approach, informative tables and easy to comprehend language, this book could be an unparalleled reservoir of information for graduate and postgraduate students, pre- and post-doctoral research scholars and scientists studying/working in different arenas of toxicology with a practical understanding of the discipline leaving them marveled over the outstanding efforts made by the Indian scientific fraternity to contribute to the understanding of the complexities the subject offers. Moreover, the book also aims to reach out to the common masses, the non-scientific fraternity, to advance their basic understanding of the subject with better relativity in day-to-day life.

Writing a book with such a comprehensive database of toxicological events of over 50 years in India was harder than we thought, but this was possible with the support of many personal and professional friends and well-wishers. Dr. Maqssod Ahmad Siddiqui, Associate Professor, King Saud University, Riyadh, is one among them, who constantly helped us in collecting the details of research publications from Web of Science. We pay our candid thanks to him for his immense support during the entire project of this book. Authors are also acknowledging Dr. Richa Gupta and Dr. Chetan Singh Rajpurohit and Mr. Vivek Pant for their technical support in the compilation of data and preparation of graphs. Authors are also thankful to all those individuals whose names could not be mentioned here, but they are remembered and we deeply acknowledged their support in one or the other way during the writing of this manuscript.

-Authors

Contents

Abbreviations

A

AA	Argemone alkaloid
ABT	American Board of Toxicology
ACE	Angiotensin I converting enzyme activity
AchE	Acetylcholinesterase
AD	Alzheimer's disease
ACP	Acid phosphatase
ADI	Accepted Daily Intake
ADH1B/1C	Alcohol Dehydrogenase 1B/1C
ADP	Adenosine diphosphate
ADR	Adverse drugs reaction
AIDS	Acquired immunodeficiency syndrome
ALP	Aluminium phosphide
AIIMS	All India Institute of Medical Sciences
ALA-D	Erythrocyte-aminolevulinicacid dehydratase
ALP	Alkaline phosphatase
ALS	Amyotrophic lateral sclerosis
AFLP	Amplified fragment length polymorphism
ALT	Alanine aminotransferase
AMPs	Antimicrobial peptides
AMPK 5'	AMP-activated protein kinase
ANN	Artificial neural networks
AO	Argemone oil
AQ	Anthraquinone
ARDS	Acute respiratory distress syndrome
ARV	Anti-retro viral
AST	Aspartate aminotransferase
ASV	Anti-snake venom
ATP	Adenosine triphosphate
ATPase	Adenosine triphosphatase
ATRA	All-trans retinoic acid
ATT	Antituberculosis treatment

B

BA/BZ	Benzathrone
3-BBA	Bromobenzanthrone
BchE	Butyrylcholinesterase
Bcl2	B-cell lymphoma 2

BHC	β-Hexachlorocyclohexane
BIS	Bureau of Indian Standards
BM-MSCs	Bone marrow-mesenchymal stem cells
BN	Binucleated
BOD	Biochemical oxygen demand
BP	Benzophenone
BPA	Bisphenol A
BPAD	Bipolar affective disorder
BQ	Benzoquinone
BSOF	Benzene solvent organic fraction
BT	Benzenetriol
BUN	Blood urea nitrogen

C

CA	Chromosomal aberrations
CA3/CA4	CornuAmmonis 3/4
Ca2+	Calcium ion
cAMP	Cyclic adenosine monophosphate
CAR	Constitutive androstane receptor
CAT	Catalase
CCL2	Cysteine-Cysteine motif chemokine ligand 2
CCl3	Trichloromethyl
CCl3 O2	Trichloromethylperoxyl
CCl4	Carbon tetrachloride
CCMB	Centre for Cellular and Molecular Biology
CCR5	Cysteine-cysteine motif chemokine receptor 5
CD	Conjugated diene
CDK2	Cyclin-dependent kinase 2
CDRI	Central Drug Research Institute
CDSCO	Central Drugs Standards Control Organization
CEPI	Comprehensive Environmental Pollution Index
CeO$_2$	Cerium oxide
CFTRI	Central Food Technological Research Institute
ChAT	Choline acetyltransferase
CHO	Chinese hamster ovary
CHRM2	Cholinergic receptor muscarinic 2
CINC-1	Cytokine-induced neutrophil chemoattractant 1
CIS	Cisplatin
CIT	Citrinin
CKD	Chronic Kidney disease
CL	Cardiolipin

CLI	Central Labour Institute
CML	Chronic myeloid leukaemia
CNS	Central nervous system
CO	Cassia occidentalis
COMT	Catechol-O-methyl transferase
Con A	Concanavalin A
COPD	Chronic obstructive pulmonary disease
COX2	Cyclooxygenase-2
CP	Cyclophosphamide
CPCB	Central Pollution Control Board
CPCSEA	The Committee for the Purpose of Control and Supervision of Experiments on Animals
CPF	Chlorpyrifos
CREB	cAMP response element binding
CRO	Contract research organization
CRS	Congenital rubella syndrome
CSF	Cerebrospinal fluid
CSIR	Council of Scientific and Industrial Research
CT	Catechol
CTLA-4	Cytotoxic T-lymphocyte-associated protein 4
CTN	Chronic tubulointerstitial nephritis
CYP	Cytochrome P450s

D

DA	Dopamine
DABT	Diplomat of American Board of Toxicology
DART	Development and reproductive toxicity
DAT	Dopamine transporter
DBP	Dibutyl phthalate
DBT	Department of Biotechnology
DCGI	Drug Controller General of India
DDD	dichlorodiphenyldichloroethane
DDE	dichlorodiphenyldichloroethylene
DDT	Dichlorodiphenyltrichloroethane
DEHP	Di (2-ethylhexyl) phthalate
DGHS	Directorate General of Health Services
2,5-DHBA	2,5-Dihydroxybenzoic acid
DHS	Drug hypersensitivity syndrome
DIH	Drug-induced hepatotoxicity
DIKD	Drug-induced kidney disease
DIPAS	Defence Institute of Physiology & Allied Science

DIRECT	Drug Induced Renal Injury Consortium
DLLME	Dispersive liquid-liquid microextraction
DME	Drug metabolizing enzymes
DMSA	Dimercaptosuccinic acid
DN	Diabetic nephropathy
DNA	Deoxyribonucleic acid
DNT	Developmental neurotoxicity
DOP	Dioctyl phthalate
DPMS	2,3 Dimercapto-1-propanesulfonate
DRDE	Defence Research and Development Establishment
DSB	Double-stranded break
DST	Department of Science and Technology
DT	Decision tree
DTB	Decision tree boost
DTF	Decision tree forest
DTH	Delayed type hypersensitivity
2 ¢ -dGuO	2'–Deoxyguanosine

E

ECVAM	European Centre for the Validation of Alternative Methods
EDC	Endocrine disrupting chemicals
EDTA	Ethylenediaminetetraacetic acid
EFSA	European Food Safety Agency
EIP	Eye irritation potential
ELISA	Enzyme-linked immunosorbent assay
EMCV	Encephalomyocarditis
EMEA	European Medicines Agency
ENM	Engineered nanomaterial
eNOS	Endothelial-derived nitric oxide synthase
EPA	Environment Protection Act
EPRS	Glutamyl-prolyl-tRNA-synthetase
ERK1/2	Extracellular signal-regulated kinases
EROD	Ethoxyresorufin-O-deethylase
ERR	Estrogen-related receptor
ESAT-6	6-kDa early secretory antigenic target

F

FDA	Food and Drug Administration
FDP	Fructose 1,6-diphosphate
FDTRC	Food and Drug Toxicology Research Centre
Fe-NTA	Ferric nitrilotriacetate

FEV	Forced expiratory volume
FISH	Fluorescence *in situ* hybridization
FQ	Fluoroquinolones
FSH	Follicle stimulating hormone
FSSAI	Food Safety and Standards Authority of India
FVC	Forced vital capacity

G

GABA	Gamma aminobutyric acid
GAD	Glutamic acid decarboxylase
GAP-43	Growth associated protein 43
GCLC	Glutamate—cysteine ligase catalytic subunit
GC-MS	Gas chromatography mass spectrometry
GD	Gestational day
GE	Genetically Engineered
GEVAC	Gelatin-vinyl-acetatecopolymer
GFAP	Glial fibrillary acidic protein
GFP	Green fluorescent protein
GLDH	Glutamate dehydrogenase
GLP	Good Laboratory Practices
GMO	Genetically modified organism
GPx	Glutathione peroxidase
GR	Glutathione reductase
GST	Glutathione-S-transferases
GSH	Glutathione
GSSG	Oxidized glutathione
GTS	Green tobacco sickness
GWAS	Genome-wide association study

H

HAART	Active anti-retroviral therapy
HAP	Household air pollution
HB-EGF-EGFR	Heparin-binding EGF-like growth factor-EGF receptor
HCH	Hexachlorocyclohexane
HCN	Hydrogen cyanide
HET-CAM	Hen's egg test chorioallantoic membrane
HIF-1α	Hypoxia inducible factor-1α
HIV	Human immunodeficiency virus
HK-2	Human kidney-2
HKM	Head kidney macrophages
HLA	Human leukocyte antigen

HLL	Hindustan Lever Limited
HME	Hepatomyoencephalopathy
HNE	4-hydroxy-2-nonenal
HO1	Heme oxygenase 1
H_2O_2	Hydrogen peroxide
HPV	Human papilloma vaccine
HQ	Hydroquinone
HSP	Heat shock protein
5-HT	5-hydroxytryptamine
hUCBSCs	Human umbilical cord blood-derived stem cells

I

ICA	Islet cell autoantibodies
ICAR	Indian Council of Agricultural Research
ICCVAM	Interagency Coordinating Committee on the Validation of Alternative Methods
ICE	Isolated chicken eye
ICMR	Indian Council of Medical Research
IFN	Interferon
IgA	Immunoglobulin A
IgG	Immunoglobulin G
IgM	Immunoglobulin M
IGIB	Institute of Genomics and Integrative Biology
Igf2	Insulin like growth factor 2
IICB	Indian Institute of Chemical Biology
IICT	Indian Institute of Chemical Technology
IIT	Indian Institute of Technology
IL	Interleukin
ILO	International Labour Organization
INH	Isoniazid
INMAS	Institute of Nuclear Medicine & Allied Sciences
iNOS	Inducible nitric oxide synthase
INS VNTR	Insulin gene variable number of tandem repeats
INSEARCH	Indian Study on Epidemiology of Asthma, Respiratory Symptoms and Chronic Bronchitis
iSAEC	International Serious Adverse Event Consortium
ISO	International Organization for Standardization
ISRO	Indian Space Research Organisation
ITRC	Industrial Toxicology Research Centre
IUGR	Intrauterine growth retardation
IUTOX	International Union of Toxicology

J

JAK-STAT	Janus kinase-signal transducer and activator of transcription
JNK	c-Jun N-terminal kinases

K

K+	Potassium ion
KIM-1	Kidney injury molecule-1
k-NN	k-nearest neighbour

L

LA	Lipoic acid
LC	Lethal concentration
LC-MS	LC-tandem mass spectrometry
LD	Lethal dose
LDH	Lactate dehydrogenase
LDL	Low density lipoprotein
LEL	Lowest effective level
LH	Luteinizing hormone
LLP	Light liquid paraffin
LMI	Leukocyte migration inhibition
LPO	Lipid peroxidation
LPS	Lipopolysaccharide
LVFX	Levofloxacin
β-L-ODAP	N-oxalyldiaminoproprionic acid

M

MA	Trans muconic acid
MAD	Mutual acceptance of data
MAO	Monoamine oxidases
MAP	Mitogen-activated protein
MAPK	Mitogen-activated protein kinase
MBP	Monobutyl phthalate
Mc1l	Melanocortin 1
MCHC	Mean corpuscular hemoglobin concentration
MCL	Maximum contamination level
MCP	Monocrotophos
MCP-1	Monocyte chemoattractant protein-1
MCV	Mean corpuscular volume
MDA	Malondialdehyde
MDR	Multidrug resistance

6-MFA	Sixth mycelial fraction of acetone
MFO	Mixed-function oxidase
MHC	Major histocompatibility complex
MiADMSA	Monoisoamyl 2, 3-dimercaptosuccinic acid
MIC	Methyl isocyanate
MIP-2	Macrophage-inflammatory protein 2
miRNA	Micro Ribonucleic acid
MLD	Minimum lethal dose
MLR	Multiple linear regression
MLT	Malathion
MMI	Macrophage migration inhibition
MMP	Mitochondrial membrane potential
MMP-9	Matrix metalloproteinase 9
MnSOD	Manganese superoxide dismutase
MPT	Methyl parathion
MPTP	1-methyl 4-phenyl 1,2,3,6-tetrahydropyridine
mRNA	Messenger Ribonucleic acid
MRL	Maximum residue limit
MROD	Methoxyresoruiin
MSCs	Mesenchymal stem cells
MSD	Musculoskeletal disorder
MT	Metallothionein
MTD	Maximum tolerated dose
MTHFR	Methylenetetrahydrofolate reductase
MTMR2	Myotubularin-related-proteins 2
mTOR	Mammalian target of rapamycin
MTSA-10	10-kDa M. tuberculosis secretory antigen
MYBPC3	Myosin binding protein C3
MYH7	β-cardiac myosin heavy chain

N

Na+	Sodium ion
NABL	National Accreditation Board for Testing and Calibration Laboratories
NAC	N-acetyl cysteine
NAD	Nicotinamide adenine dinucleotide
NADPH	Nicotinamide adenine dinucleotide phosphate
NAMP	National Air Monitoring Programme
NAT2	N-Acetyltransferase 2
NaTS	Sodium thiosulphate
NAAQS	National Ambient Air Quality Standard

NCE	New chemical entities
NCGMA	National GLP Compliance Monitoring Authority
NCTCF	National Coordination of Testing and Calibrating Facilities
NDG	Neurodegeneration
NEERI	National Engineering and Education Research Institute
NF-kB	Nuclear FactorkB
NHRC	National Human Rights Commission
NIPER	National Institute of Pharmaceutical Education & Research
NIHL	Noise-induced hearing loss
NIMHANS	National Institute of Mental Health and Neuro-Sciences
NIN	National Institute of Nutrition
NIOH	National Institute of Occupational Health
NM	Nanomaterial
NMDA	N-methyl-D-aspartate
NMR	Nuclear magnetic resonance
NO	Nitric oxide
NP	Nanoparticle
3-NP	3-nitropropionic acid
NPP	National Pharmacovigilance Program
NP-SH	Non-protein thiol activity
NQO1	NAD(P)H dehydrogenase (quinone) 1
NRDC	National Referral Diagnostic Centre
NSAIDs	Nonsteroidal anti-inflammatory drugs
NSC	Neural stem cell

O

$^{1}O_2$	Singlet oxygen
$O.^{-}$	Superoxide radicals
O_2^{-}	Superoxide anion radicals
OCP	Organochlorine pesticide
ODC	Ornithine decarboxylase
OEL	Occupational exposure limit
.OH	Hydroxyl radical
OECD	Organization for Economic Co-operation and Development
OFLX	Ofloxacin
OGD	Oxygen glucose deprivation
6-OHDA	6-hydroxydopamine
5-OHPA	5-hydroxy pyrazinoic acid
OIP	Overall Index of Pollution
OP	Organophosphate
OPIDN	Organophosphate delayed induced neuropathy

OS	Oxidative stress
OSHA	Occupational Safety and Health Administration
OTA	Ochratoxin A

P

P75 NTR	Neurotrophin Receptor P75
PA	Protein A
PAC	Pharmaceutical active compound
PAH	Polycyclic aromatic hydrocarbons
2-PAM	Pralidoxime
PARP	Poly (ADP-ribose) polymerase
PAWR	Pro-apoptotic WT1 regulator
PC	phosphatidylcholine
PC12 cell line	Phaeochromocytoma 12 cell line
PCB	Polychlorinated biphenyls
PCK	Plantation Corporation of Kerala
PCR	Polymerase chain reaction
PCT epithelium	Proximal convoluted tubule
PD	Parkinson's disease
PDGF-BB	Platelet-derived growth factor-BB
PE	Phosphatidylethanolamine
β-PEA	β-phenethylamine
PEA-3	Polyoma enhancer activator 3
PEFR	Peak expiratory flow rate
PFA	Prevention of Food Adulteration
pGSK3β	Phospho Glycogen synthase kinase 3 β
PHA	Phytohemagglutinins
PHLPP2	PH Domain and Leucine Rich Repeat Protein Phosphatase 2
PINK1	PTEN-induced kinase 1
PI3K	Phosphatidylinositol–3 kinase
PIL	Post implantation loss
PKA	Protein kinase A
PLGA	Polymer-poly (lactic-co-glycolic) acid
PLSR	Partial least squares regression
PM	Particulate matter
PMA	Phorbolmyristate acetate
PND	Postnatal day
PNS	Post nuclear supernatant
ppb	Parts per billion
PPD	Paraphenylenediamine
ppm	Parts per million

PON-1	Paraoxenase 1
POP	Persistent organic pollutant
PROD	Pentoxyresorufin
PS	Phosphatitylserine
PSD95	Postsynaptic density protein 95
PSH	Protein sulfhydryls
PSM	Proteasome
PXR	pregnane X receptor
PYC	Pycnogenol
PYZ	Pyrazinamide

Q

QAMP	Quality Assurance of Medicinal Plants
QSAR	Quantitative Structure-Activity Relationships
QSTR	Quantitative Structure-Toxicity Relationship

R

RAAS	Renin angiotensin-aldosterone system
RIF	Rifampicin
RNA	Ribonucleic acid
RNAse	Ribonuclease
RFLP	Restriction fragment length polymorphism
RISUG	Reversible inhibition of sperm under guidance
ROCK	Rho-associated protein kinase
ROS	Reactive oxygen species
RPTEC/TERT1	Renal proximal tubule epithelial cells
RSPM	Respirable Suspended Particulate Matter
rWEC	Rodent whole embryo culture

S

SA/SAN	Sanguinarine
SAC	Staphylococcus aureus Cowan I
SACE	Serum angiotensin converting enzyme activity
SAFAR	System of Air Quality Weather Forecasting and Research
SAH	Severe alcoholic hepatitis
SCE	Sister chromatid exchange
SCZ	Schizophrenia
SDH	Sorbitol dehydrogenase
SELEX	Systematic evolution of ligands by exponential enrichment
SEPT5	Septin 5

SEWA	Self Employed Women's Association
SGF	Simulated gastric fluid
SGOT	Serum glutamic oxaloacetic transaminase
SLA	Spontaneous locomotor activity
SMA	Styrene maleic anhydride
SNCA	Synuclein alpha
SNP	Single nucleotide polymorphism
SOD	Superoxide dismutase
SOX-2	SRY-related HMG-box 2
SPM	Suspended Particulate Matter
SRBC	Sheep red blood cell
SSA	Sarva Shiksha Abhiyan
STI	Sexually-transmitted infections
STOX	Society of Toxicology
SVIL	Supervilin
SVM	Support vector machines
SVZ	Subventricular zone
SYM	Solidarity Youth Movement

T

TB	Tuberculosis
TCA	Tricarboxylic acid
TCOP	Tri-O-cresyl phosphate
T1D	Type 1 diabetes
TGF	Transforming growth factor
TH	Tyrosine hydroxylase
TiO2	Titanium oxide
TLR	Toll-like receptor
TLV	Threshold limit value
TNF	Tumor necrosis factor
TrkA	Tropomyosin receptor kinase A
TRPM7	Transient receptor potential melastatin 7
TSA	Total sialic acid

U

UCIL	Union Carbide of India Ltd
US EPA	United States Environment Protection Agency
US FDA	Unites States Food and Drug Administration
UV	Ultraviolet

V

VOC	Volatile organic compound
VMAT-2	Vesicular monoamine transporter 2

W

WBC	White blood cell
WHO	World Health Organization

Z

ZnO	Zinc oxide
ZPP	Zinc protoporphyrin

About the Corresponding Author

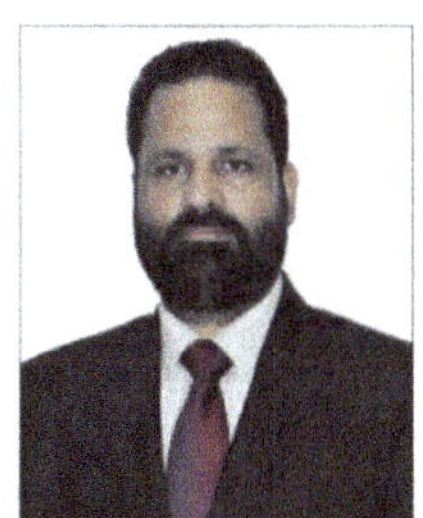

Dr AB Pant is a seasoned toxicologist with over thirty years of active research career. He started his research career at CSIR-Central Drug Research Institute, Lucknow, India, and earned his Ph.D. in Biotechnology from IIT Roorkee, Uttarakhand, India. Presently, he is serving as Senior Principal Scientist at CSIR-Indian Institute of Toxicology Research, Lucknow, India. In the scientific fraternity, Dr Pant is renowned for his elegant research on the application of human cord blood stem cells (hCBSCs) in developmental neurotoxicity (DNT) and establishing the number of *in vitro* model systems as an alternative to Laboratory animals for biomedical research. His DNT research provides profound insights into the complex processes involved in neuronal development, injury and repair mimicking to the human brain during the gestation and early stage of life. More precisely, his work discovered that how the master regulator signalling molecules/cascades are critical to converting hCBSCs into functional neurons and what exactly happens when things go wrong during the intricate process of neuronal development. In his much-acclaimed research, he has uncovered new links between the xenobiotic metabolizing capabilities and their regulators in hCBSCs derived neuronal cells all through the differentiation. His work on the developing neurons not only offers a much sought after the framework for understanding the neurodegenerative disorders and potential therapeutic interventions but also is a strong base for future studies aimed at interpreting the human brain-specific DNT. Dr Pant has handled and currently being handling numbers of research projects as Principal Investigator, awarded from National and International funding agencies, including ICMR, DBT, DST, CSIR, Indo-Brazil, UP-CST, etc.

Besides the laboratory work, he dedicated himself to fostering the science among students through public outreach talks and mentoring pre-and post-doctorates. Since 2010 he has also been associated with National GLP Compliance Monitoring Authority, Government of India as Lead GLP Inspector. The accreditation agencies of the country-BIS, CDSCO, FSSAI, NABL, and so on are also utilizing his expertise through different task forces. He was a member of the draft committee of "National SOP for Patients' Consent in India" developed by the Institute of Medicine & Law, Mumbai. As an International Advisor, he has been instrumental in establishing the WHO funded "Centre of Excellence for Nanotechnology" at Makerere University, Uganda. In the acknowledgement of his achievements in the professional career, he has been elected Fellow Several Scientific and Academies bodies, to name a few are: Academy of Toxicological Sciences, USA, Society of

Toxicology, India, Indian Academy of Neurosciences, Academy of Sciences for Animal Welfare, India, Academy of Environmental Biology India, etc. Dr Pant is a UK Registered Toxicologist of the Royal Society of Biology, London, UK. Dr Pant is a recipient several prestigious awards such as Shakuntala Amir Chand Prize-2007 (ICMR), Vigyan Ratna Award-2010 (UP-Council of Science & Technology-Uttar Pradesh), National Bioscience Award-2012 (DBT), Prof. KT Shetty Memorial Oration Award-2017 (Indian Academy of Neurosciences), Toxicology Promotion Award-2018 (National Academy of Sciences, Allahabad), etc. Dr Pant has over 150 research publications in International journals of high impact and author of 11 book chapters. Dr Pant is also rendering the Editorial services to several research journals of high repute, to mention a few are: Editorial Member: Scientific Report (Nature Publishing Group), Academic Editor: PLoS ONE (2010-2018), Advisory Member: Toxicology Research (Royal Society of Chemistry), Associate Editor: Annals of Neurosciences (Journal of Academy of Neurosciences), and so on. Dr. Pant is also serving as Chairman/Expert Members in various taskforces/ Regulatory/Scientific Bodies at the national level.

About the Co-author

Dr. Ankita Pandey is an alumnus of CSIR-Indian Institute of Toxicology Research, Lucknow, India. In her active research career, she has made dedicated and sustained efforts to decipher the signalling cascade involved in the development of neuronal cells derived from human and animal stem cells. She has further investigated the influence of organophosphate pesticides on regulatory mechanisms of these stem cell-derived neuronal cells at various stages of maturity. Her research work has been instrumental in culminating the stem cell-based high-throughput *in vitro* system for assessing the neurotoxicity and developmental neurotoxicity potential of drugs and chemicals. She has several research papers in National and International journals of high repute that are well recognized and have a good number of citations. She has been the recipient of the most prestigious **'Tulsabai Somani Education Trust Award'** conferred by the Indian Academy of Neurosciences.

CHAPTER 1

Introduction

The word 'toxicology,' originally derived from the term in Greek 'toxikon' meaning 'a bow' (for shooting poisoned arrows) or 'poison' (for dipping arrowheads) was classically connotated as the 'science of poisons'. Centuries ago Philippus Aureolus Theophrastus Bombastus von Hohenheim Paracelsus (1493-1541), regarded as the 'Father of Toxicology' fostered the emergence of this scientific discipline by establishing the importance of dose-response relationship, summarizing the concept in his well-known statement:

"All substances are poisons; there is none that is not a poison.
The right dose differentiates a poison and remedy"

Paracelsus in his time advanced several revolutionary views which are now considered as fundamental concepts in the field of toxicology. Even, an old Sanskrit adage says that nectar ('amrit' or that which removes 'mrtyu' or death) is a poison if consumed in excess. This has been proven more than correct in recent times. The response is related to the dose and the same chemical, which acts effectively as a drug in low doses, could be a poison in higher doses. However, over the past few decades this field has expanded beyond the dose-response relationship to encompass studies addressing not only the interaction between chemicals and biological systems determining their potential to cause adverse effects in living organisms, but to also assess their hazard and risk of human exposure thus providing a basis for appropriate precautionary, protective and restrictive measures.

Toxicology, considered to be a borrowed science evolved from ancient poisoners, stands as one of the historic practical sciences in India, drawing insights from the knowledge of extracts from plants and animal venom for the use in medicines, hunting, warfare, and assassination. The rapid growth of chemical and pharmaceutical industry post-liberalization era in India unleashed a spectrum of hazards potentially towards human and environmental health, underlying the need to accurately predict and assess the risk potential of these chemicals, providing a stimulus for the emergence of toxicology as a separate entity. Since its inception in the 1960s, the scope and interest in this arena has continued to broaden and the subject, formerly a part of pharmacology has undergone a dimensional change to develop into a fully-fledged discipline.

Today, toxicology research in India is positioned at the crossroad of transition from traditional studies of experimentation using animals in the late 1960s to the mechanistic understanding of toxicological endpoints using 'omics' approaches that allow better confidence in the subsequent risk assessments. Once a part of pharmacology, toxicology now stands as separate entity capitalizing in interdisciplinary areas of pharmacology, analytical chemistry, microbiology, molecular biology and biotechnology. With time, toxicology in India has evolved into a recognized discipline with its dedicated group of toxicologists, educational institutions, sub-disciplines, professional societies and reputed journals. This book aims to trace the historical growth of the subject in India, its origin and development, highlighting significant innovative breakthroughs that revolutionized the discipline in the country. This book also envisages to provide a comprehensive overview of few of the most significant contributions of India in the field of toxicology.

CHAPTER 2

History of Toxicology in India: Antiquity

Knowledge of the healing and toxic properties of several plants, animals, and minerals has moulded civilizations for millennia. It is safe to assume that toxicology's history is as old as the human race: the early man drawing insights from the knowledge of toxic properties of plants and animals gained during their hunter and gatherer existence over thousands of years. From simple discoveries through trial-and-error, the knowledge of toxic properties of noxious plants, animal venom, poisonous minerals and metals were compiled and passed on from one generation to the next.

The earliest mention of toxicological phenomena in India could be traced back to ancient books on mythology and legendary, attributing the inception of poison to mythological Gods such as Lord Brahma, Lord Vishnu and Lord Shiva. Documentary evidence reveals *Aconitum* (yielding aconitine), as the principal source of poison 'Visha'. Sanskrit literature, mentions the term 'visha-kanya' meaning 'poison girl' who gradually developed tolerance for the use of aconitine (resulting in death from her embrace). The concept of using young girls as death instruments basically originated in India, later spreading to European literature in the Middle Ages through Arabic and Greek transcripts. Few years down the time lane, some of this information was codified into the Vedas. The hymns of Rig Veda and Atharva Veda (1200-900 BC) reveal the use of poisoned arrows in war (aconitine) and the Sanskrit and Buddhist writings also find mention of the use of poisoned arrows (for warfare, hunting and covert purposes) revealing the secondary source of poison derived from decomposed snakes; the latter also confirmed through Diodorus Siculus's account of Alexander the Great's campaign (325 BC) in western parts of India (Bisset and Mazars 1984).

Numerous Indian medical writings pertaining to poisons, became rich sources of information for toxicologists worldwide, such as Charaka's (second century AD), Susruta (around 500 AD), and Shanaq which held elaborate information related to signs, symptoms and treatment for several poisons, such as aconite (Chinese poison for arrows), hemlock (poison of the Greeks), opium (used both as an antidote and a poison) and few metals such as a lead, copper and arsenic. Sushruta also mentioned agada tantra, quite parallel to modern toxicology, dealing with the diagnosis as well as treatment of a person bitten by poisonous animals or adversely affected by poisons (Aggrawal 2005).

CHAPTER 3

Milestones that Shaped Toxicology Growth in India

It is fair to state that few episodes of environmental, occupational and industrial disasters worldwide underlie the emergence of toxicology as a scientific discipline as a whole (Table 3.1). By raising participation in the chemical industries, the Industrial Revolution dramatically increased opportunities for occupational exposure to hazardous substances. Paralleling these initiatives, several disasters involving pharmaceuticals gone awry also played catalytic roles. The growth in this discipline was further spurred by awareness of the need for close monitoring to the environmental impact of the use of synthetic chemicals in modern industry and agriculture. In 1962 the author of *Silent Spring*, Rachel Carson, touched off a heated debate about the links between industrialization and pollution when she claimed that 'we have put poisonous and biologically potent chemicals indiscriminately into the hands of persons largely or wholly ignorant of their potentials for harm' (Marco 1987).

Table 3.1 An overview of the worst industrial/environmental disasters of the world

Period	Country	Environmental/ Industrial disaster	Consequences
Late 1930s	America	Sulphanilamide, disaster due to Diethylene glycol used as a solvent	Death of 105 victims due to kidney disease
1930	Southern and Midwestern states	Ginger Jake alcohol adulterated with plasticiser tri-O-cresyl phosphate (TOCP)	Delayed-onset neurotoxic syndrome inflicting around 40,000–50,000 people
1950	Germany as epicentre	Thalidomide disaster	Limb malformations in new born babies; 10,000 victims
Mid 20th century	Japan	Minamata bay disaster	Food chain contaminated with mercury due to poor management of waste water in a chemical plant area

Contd...

Period	Country	Environmental/ Industrial disaster	Consequences
1976	Serveso in Northern Italy	Dioxin disaster	Accident at chemical plant releasing tonnes of dioxin in air
1984	Bhopal, India	Bhopal Gas Tragedy	40 tons of methyl isocyanate was released from the Union Carbide plant in India which killed thousands and injured hundreds of people

The exponential growth of this discipline specifically in India dates back to the post-liberalization era (post-1947) that unleashed a spectrum of potential hazards into the environment, the uncensored use of which had repercussions, which required to be addressed. The post-1950 years found an immense boom in the chemical industry with a variety of chemicals and materials being produced for human consumption like DDT, organophosphorus pesticides, many new drugs, polymers, synthetic fibers, etc. Considering the chemical industries alone, from a small number of 98 in 1947, they grew tenfold to 964 units in 1953, and 4,364 in 1976 (Ramaswamy 1987). The increasing participation of the workforce in the chemical and agricultural industries, also increased the risk of occupational exposure towards hazardous chemicals necessitating the need for predicting and assessing the risk potential of the chemicals accurately, thus providing a stimulus for the emergence of toxicology as a separate entity. In parallel to these initiatives, various disasters involving pharmaceuticals gone awry (mass pesticide poisonings, the Bhopal Gas Tragedy and Endosulfan Disaster) also played catalytic roles.

Although toxicology has been one of the branches of Ayurveda, a healthcare system in India, historically practiced for approximately more than 5000 years, it got a formal recognition during the mid-1900s by being included in the forensic science and pharmacology course curriculum for the medical students. Toxicology research in the real sense was introduced as an individual identity with the establishment of first Plant Toxicology Research Laboratory at the Indian Veterinary Research Institute, Izatnagar (UP) in the year 1959. Subsequently, the year 1965 witnessed the establishment of Industrial Toxicology Research Centre in Lucknow (ITRC later rechristened as CSIR-Indian Institute of Toxicology Research, CSIR-IITR) with a broad scientific charter of "Safety to Environment & Health and Service to Industry" which till date stands as the only toxicology dedicated research institute in not only India but the entire South-East Asia. Later in 1966, the National Institute of Occupational Health (NIOH), Ahmedabad was established. To meet the growing challenges in the field of industrial toxicology, these institutes oriented their research efforts towards identification and control/mitigation of hazards culminating from exposure to different risk factors encountered at occupational setups. Epidemiological studies were used as a 'gold standard' in establishing strong correlations between occupational and environmental exposure to toxic compounds. These studies supplemented with animal experimentation further aided in the elucidation of the mechanistic basis to prevent risks associated with their exposure.

With the establishment of new agricultural universities, subsequently, forensic toxicology was introduced as a separate discipline in various departments of veterinary colleges/institutes and forensic toxicology soon assumed significance in medical institutes throughout India. These developments coincided with India's initiative to facilitate the exchange of ideas and knowledge among esteemed groups of scientists, practitioners and policy makers involved in various R&D areas of environment and occupational health or related fields of toxicology. To meet this goal and to bring the toxicologists at one platform, the Society of Toxicology of India (STOX) was established in 1979 with the mandate to impart scientific information to the general masses about the harmful effects of pesticides, drugs and chemicals in both targets as well as non-target species. Since 1980, STOX has served as a founder member for the International Union of Toxicology (IUTOX) with regional chapters and specialty sections to bring all the scientists involved in toxicology at one platform. The society also has its website: www.http://stoxindia.org.

Over a period from the 1950s to 1980s, with a huge rise in the consumption of pesticides and unrestricted availability of over-the-counter drugs (recreational, drugs of abuse, etc.), India became one of the central hubs for cases of acute poisonings, both accidental and suicidal. As more and more cases of overdose/adverse effects increased, the clinicians gradually began to gain interest in the specialty, as they were the one to first receive the poisoned patient and effectively manage them to help them survive thus providing stimulus for the emergence of the field of clinical toxicology (Murali, Bhalla, et al. 2009). Subsequently, in 1984, The Bhopal Gas catastrophe, hailed as the worst industrial disaster till date worldwide, taking a heavy toll on human and animal life, hit not only India but the entire medical fraternity. The subsequent awakening of the Government and the public to the unknown hazards of chemicals released indiscriminately into the environment triggered various landmark activities pertaining to environmental and human protection along with enactment of legislation directed towards limiting and regulating the release of substances and chemicals into the environment, and with these initiatives the field of regulatory toxicology received a major boost.

Since 1965, toxicity studies had a heavy reliance on animal testing to fathom the toxicity of various chemicals for risk assessment. However, post-1980s, India began to witness the emergence of *in vitro* toxicology, which increased efficiency in toxicity testing procedures by transitioning from lengthy and expensive *in vivo* testing with qualitative parameters to toxicity-pathway assays on animal or human-derived primary cultures or cell lines with mechanistic, quantitative endpoints. In the years that followed development and validation of various *in vitro* models precipitated a significant transformation in the manner toxicity testing was carried out. Cell-based assays were developed; organ-specific cell lines began to be extensively employed to unravel the complex interaction of toxicants with signal transduction systems and essential metabolic functions. Stretching over for more than four decades, *in-vitro* strategies that initiated with basic cell culture techniques using liver slices have gradually progressed towards advancing stem cell-based 3D human cultures today.

As we reflect into the last 15 years of toxicology research in India, a significant accomplishment was an advancement made into the genomics era. With the advent of omics technologies gaining popularity worldwide, India became one of the fastest users to revamp its research activities in that direction. In concert with the worldwide efforts, the field of toxicology has kept itself abreast with the advances in molecular approaches that have been extensively employed to investigate the association between environmental stress and human susceptibility to diseases; to understand the mechanism of action of toxicants, and for identifying biomarkers for prediction of onset/progression of toxicity. With these developments, the field of epidemiology also received a significant boost as molecular approaches yielded tools to identify susceptible populations, biomarkers for exposure, and a better understanding of the underlying mechanisms linking environmental/ occupational exposure to a health outcome.

Over the years an incessant rise in ethical concerns over animal testing coupled with some limitations of high costs, low throughput readouts, issues of extrapolability to humans and cases of modern drug failures (such as Opren, Practolol, Vioxx) gradually ultimately paved the way for a paradigm shift from *in-vivo* approaches to the 'science of alternatives'. The 3Rs principles described in 1959 by WMS Russel and RL Burch were the pioneer principles for animal welfare and ethics corresponding to Replacement, Reduction and Refinement clearly describing the use of alternative testing methods, reduction in the number of animals used for experimentation and refinement of the existing methods to reduce the pain and suffering of experimental animals. In addition to these, another R for 'Rehabilitation' was introduced by the CPCSEA (The Committee for the Purpose of Control and Supervision of Experiments on Animals) in India, clearly emphasizing the moral responsibility of researchers towards animals after experimentation.

During the end of the twenty-first century (post-2005), fast-paced growth in and around computer technology began transforming the face of toxicology and subsequent risk assessment in India. This era witnessed the rise of computational toxicology, which applied information from high-throughput screening, cheminformatics, and structural biology approaches for the development of virtual toxicity prediction models. These advancements took place simultaneously with continued efforts to minimize complete reliance on mammalian species by utilizing invertebrates and lower vertebrates as alternate toxicity models. With the discipline gaining popularity worldwide, a need for Board certified toxicologists was felt in the country. Subsequently, India took the need of the time initiative to convince the American Board of Toxicology (ABT) to offer Diplomate (ABT examination to award DABT) to deserving candidates in India. Undeterred efforts finally convinced the ABT and for the very first time outside USA, India got an opportunity to conduct the DABT examination in 2008. Impressed with the competence level and enthusiasm of the Indian toxicologists, ABT decided to conduct the exams each year in India since then. As of date, we have around 60 DABT qualified Indians and this figure is expected to rise further in the coming years. It is also noteworthy that in 2011, India was approved a full adherent status for Mutual Acceptance of Data (MAD) by the Organization for Economic Co-operation and Development (OECD) council. As per this provision, the OECD member and other adhering countries would accept all non-clinical studies undertaken in a Good Laboratory Practices (GLP) facility approved by the National Compliance Monitoring Authorities of India. Currently, India is equipped with around two dozen GLP certified toxicology contract research organizations (CRO's) /companies, that are providing toxicological services to the national and international clients involved in various pharmaceutical and agricultural product development. Also about two dozen NABL accredited laboratories speak of the high standards of toxicology research conducted in India. With time, India made unstinted strides in phasing out animal testing of cosmetics in 2014, in parallel to the world's concerted efforts, which was hailed as a quantum leap in an effort to diminish animal usage. Figure 3.1 provides a historical timeline view of the discipline in the country.

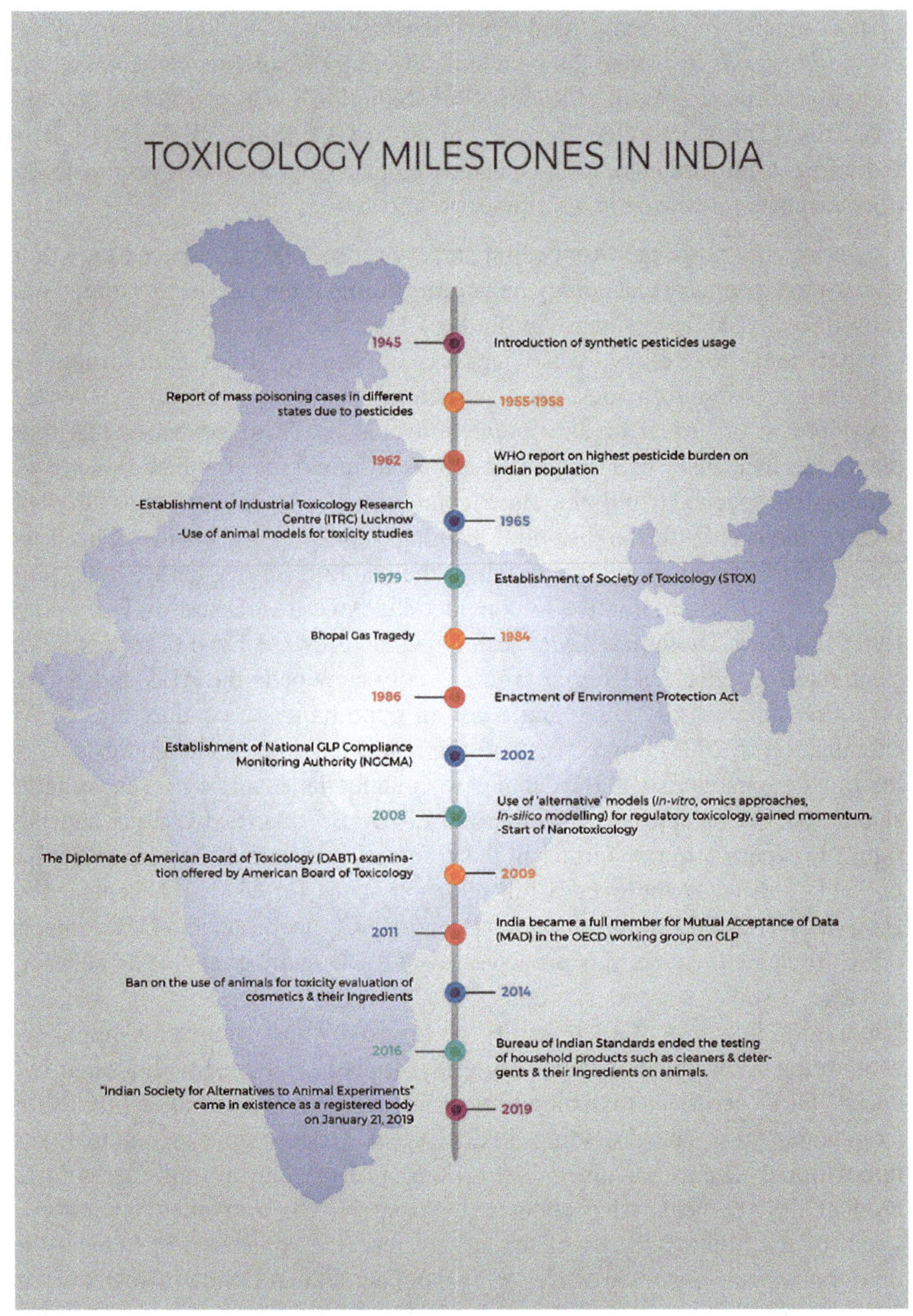

Figure 3.1 Historical timeline of major events in toxicology in India

With the growing importance of this subject, few decades in the past have also witnessed a growing focus upon degree courses in toxicology within colleges/universities, resulting in the establishment of active research centres dedicated towards toxicology. Currently more than three dozen veterinary colleges and several universities are premier organizations of toxicology research and hubs for developing skilled toxicologists in the country. Several veterinary colleges in India also offer postgraduate training in pharmacology and toxicology, which contributes to the bulk of toxicologists in the nation. The same veterinary colleges also provide postgraduate training in veterinary pathology, which ends up in toxico-pathology assessment in Biotech/Pharma companies and CROs in the country. Few of them are listed below (Table 3.2).

Table 3.2 List of the various courses in toxicology offered in India

Institutes	Courses offered
CSIR IITR, Lucknow, Uttar Pradesh	Ph.D
CSIR CDRI, Lucknow, Uttar Pradesh	Ph.D
SCMS Institute of Bioscience & Biotechnology Research & Development in Toxicology, Kerala	M.Sc Toxicology
Bhavans New Science College, Hyderabad, Andhra Pradesh	M.Sc Toxicology
University of Madras, Chennai	M.Sc (Environmental Toxicology) M.Phil (Environmental Toxicology) M.Phil (Neuro and Nanotoxicology) Ph.D Toxicology
Dr BR Ambedkar University, Agra, Uttar Pradesh	M.Sc (Environmental Toxicology)
Jamia Hamdard University, New Delhi	M.Sc (Toxicology) Ph.D Toxicology
National Institute of Pharmaceutical Education & Research (NIPER), Mohali, Punjab	Ph.D Pharmacology and Toxicology MS (Pharm)Regulatory Toxicology MS (Pharm) Pharmacology and Toxicology
Chaudhary Charan Singh University, Meerut, Uttar Pradesh	M.Sc Toxicology
Chaudhary Charan Singh Haryana Agricultural University, Hisar, Haryana	M.Sc Toxicology
All India Institute of Medical Sciences, New Delhi	M.D. Forensic Medicine and Toxicology
Baba Farid University of Health Sciences, Faridkot, Punjab	M.D. Forensic Medicine and Toxicology
Jawaharlal Nehru Medical College, Ajmer, Rajasthan	M.D. Forensic Medicine and Toxicology
IFS Education Department (Govt of India MCA & MSME Regd., SSI Government of Maharashtra Regd, ISO9001-2008 certified)-provides short term forensic courses for awareness about forensics	Forensic medicine & Toxicology (Medico-Legal)

The awareness and concerns related to the safety and health aspects of toxicology have also culminated into 51003 scientific publications (from 1950-2019, source: Web of Science database) which is a vivid reflection of the exponential growth of the subject in India. As toxicology rose and matured in India, a variety of sub-disciplines emerged which focused on specific areas. However, these various sub-disciplines have intricately orchestrated to create a scientific discipline devoted towards an advanced understanding of the harmful effects of chemicals for the protection of human and environmental health. This rapid growth provided the backdrop for the emergence of many branches of toxicology that exist today, sub-categorized into occupational toxicology, environmental toxicology, clinical toxicology, nanotoxicology, toxico-genomics, mechanistic toxicology, organ-specific toxicology and regulatory toxicology. Shedding light on some of the outstanding contributions and achievements in each sub-discipline, this book is an attempt to unravel the untold journey of this scientific discipline in India. While it is impossible to provide the minutest of details of the voluminous data that has been generated by Indian toxicologists, this book aims to cover the most significant breakthroughs in the most comprehensive manner. Mention is made of what may be considered landmark contribution and nationally relevant. Let us hasten to apologize to those whose work does not figure here even though it may be equally or even more valuable than those included. Due to space constraints, it was not feasible to cover the contribution of every single author.

CHAPTER 4

Occupational Toxicology

Participation of the workforce in the industrial sectors of India has been on a constant rise since 1947. The conventional approach to ensure the safety and health of these workers at various occupational setups in India has majorly relied on the enactment of legislation (Factory Act 1948, Mines Act 1952, Pesticide Act 1968, etc.) and regular inspections to ensure compliance with the safety standards, however, these efforts have met with little success and diseases have continued to take a heavy toll on the workers' health and safety. Being exposed to diverse occupational hazards ranging from physical, chemical and biological, workers have been reported to suffer from diseases of diverse etiology. India documents a high incidence of occupational morbidities, approximately 17 million non-fatal injuries (17% of the world) and 45,000 fatal injuries (45% of the mortality due to occupational injuries globally) occurring every year (http://www.nihfw.org/NationalHealth-Programme/NATIONAL PROGRAMMEFORCONTROL.html). Infact, high prevalence of occupational morbidities in India could be traced back to old times as mentioned by a tenth-century Tamil poet who described the symptoms of the granite sculptors in Mahabalipuram, which could later be recognized as those of silicosis (Ghosh 1964).

In view of the deteriorating conditions in occupational workplaces in India post-independence, a need for a separate discipline of occupational toxicology was foreseen to address the unrecognized occupational hazards at different workplaces. In the real sense, research in the context of occupational health gained impetus in the late 1960s with the establishment of landmark institutes like National Institute of Occupational Health (NIOH), Ahmedabad, CSIR-Indian Institute of Toxicology Research (CSIR-IITR), Lucknow and Central Labour Institute (CLI), Mumbai that have, since then, played a pivotal role in the prediction and identification of toxic effects of various physical, chemical and biological agents to which industrial workers, miners and farmers might get exposed. Occupational toxicology, a multidisciplinary arena combining occupational health with toxicological approaches, in India, has been aimed at recognition, and mitigation of hazards that could result from exposure to different risk factors encountered at occupational setups. Work-related exposures have been mostly assessed using inhalation, dermal and oral exposure monitoring as well as by employing biomarkers of exposure, susceptibility and effect. Research has been directed chiefly towards epidemiological assessment, experimental studies (*in vitro* and *in vivo* approaches) that have provided substantial evidence into the mechanistic basis as well as interventional strategies that have largely contributed towards the setting of workplace standards, and occupational exposure limits (OELs) to prevent work-related intoxications and diseases. Voluntary guidelines have been emphasized to establish a safe ambient air concentration for many chemicals found in the workplace. With time, efforts have also been channelized to develop tools for early diagnosis of health impairment. Design of appropriate measures for the prevention of workplace hazards has also been suggested to establish and maintain a safe and healthy working environment (Figure 4.1).

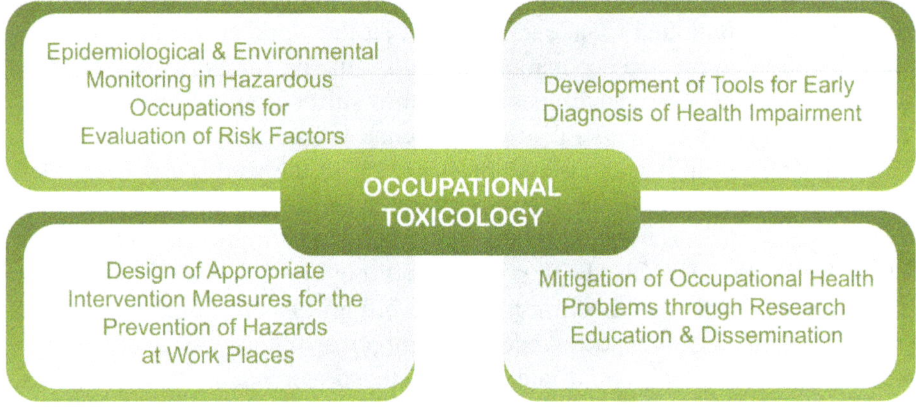

Figure 4.1 Approaches of occupational toxicology in India

Occupational diseases have been associated with a complex 'web of causations'. Various confounding factors such as personal factors (sex, age) and personal habits (smoking and alcohol consumption), different routes of exposure, genetic susceptibility and environmental factors have added another dimension of complexity in interpreting data from different health surveillance programs in these setups. However, with the progress in molecular approaches, it has been very much possible to identify genotypes that may underlie the susceptibility towards different occupational diseases. Further, with the advent of omics approaches, exposure assessments have significantly improved with the advancement in molecular epidemiology and exposure biomarkers. These biomarkers have been mainly employed as diagnostic tools for the early detection in the case of progressive diseases that may manifest their symptoms long after exposure to the initiating factor.

One of the earliest works on hazards encountered at workplaces has been put together by Ramaswamy 1987 who has concisely reviewed the health hazards attributed to toxic exposure to numerous chemicals such as benzene, asbestos, carcinogenic dye intermediates, carbon disulphide, manganese, lead, organophosphorus pesticides, phosgene, vinyl chloride, etc. in the work environment of India from 1960s to 1980s (Ramaswamy 1987). However, over the years, most of the toxicity studies in the context of occupational health have focused around few issues like pesticide toxicity, silica and asbestos induced pneumoconiosis, musculoskeletal disorders and noise-induced hearing loss.

Agriculture, employing around 58% of the workforce of the country, has exposed a major proportion of the population to the risks of pesticide exposure. In India, use of pesticides commenced in 1948 with the import of DDT and BHC for malaria and locust control respectively. India began its production of pesticides with the manufacturing plant for DDT and BHC in 1952, producing more than 5000 metric tonnes by 1958 (Gupta 2004). Production of pesticides, their formulation, packaging, distribution as well as their application in the fields have involved potential risks and various magnitudes and forms of toxicity have been observed with their indiscriminate usage. Indian history has witnessed well-recognized episodes of acute poisoning due to such exposure of pesticides. Some of the earliest cases of poisoning in 1958 in Cochin and Kerala due to parathion (Karunakaran 1958), in Uttar Pradesh in 1977 due to HCH (Nag, Singh, et al. 1977) and the "Handigodu syndrome" of Karnataka (Report of National Institute of Nutrition, Hyderabad, 1977) have been documented.

In light of the existing information on the toxic effects elicited due to exposure of these pesticides several epidemiologic investigations by CSIR-IITR and NIOH were triggered, in an attempt to identify the possible impact of pesticide exposure on human health concerning occupational exposure (especially low dose long-term exposures). The high-risk groups have been identified to include pesticide production workers, formulators, mixers, loaders and farm sprayers. Depending on the inherent toxicity of the pesticide, its route of exposure, exposure period and its formulation, workers engaged in different operations have shown to exhibit a myriad of ill effects ranging from short term poisoning effects like nausea, vomiting, chest pain, headache, eye, skin and throat irritation, etc. to long term adverse effects like allergies, liver impairments, respiratory dysfunctions, nervous system damage, genotoxicity, cancer, reproductive problems and birth defects. Table 4.1 provides a comprehensive overview of the most representative studies that have been carried out on pesticide toxicity that (along with experimental studies) have helped in understanding the underlying basis of pesticide toxicity.

Table 4.1 Pesticide toxicity associated with different operations in India

Operations	Pesticide (Single/Mixture)	Clinical manifestations	References
Manufacture and Formulation	Mixture of DDT, BHC, malathion, aldrin, chloropyrifos, parathion, carbaryl	Loss of appetite, headache, nausea, breathlessness, increased levels of serum cholesterol and SGOT activity	(Bhatnagar, Saigal, et al. 1982)
	Hexachlorocyclohexane	Higher levels of total blood HCH and ß isomers, alterations in liver enzymes (leucine aminopeptidase, ornithine carbamyl transaminase) and IgM levels	(Chattopadhyay, Karnik, et al. 1988)
	OPs and OC s	Hematoxic effects, leucocytosis and variations in differential count	(Khan and Ali 1993)
	Chloropyriphos, acephate, phorate, cypermethrin, fenvalerate, monocrotophos, carbendazim and dimethoate	Increased frequency of chromosomal aberrations in peripheral blood lymphocytes and formation of micronuclei in buccal epithelial cells	(Sailaja, Chandrasekhar, et al. 2006)
	Quinalphos, endosulfan, Monocrotophos, chlorpyriphos, lindane, phorate and parathion	Decreased levels of serum ChE activity, increased levels of serum total BHC residue positively correlated with elevated IgM levels, elevated levels of serum IgG and IgA	(Bhatnagar, Karnik, et al. 2002)
Distributers and retailers	Mixture	Gastrointestinal problems in 70% of workers, slow nerve conduction velocity and low peak expiratory flow rate	(Kesavachandran, Pathak, et al. 2009)
Farmers and field sprayers	Mixture of OP, OC and carbamates	Decrease in cholinesterase activity, elevated serum alkaline phosphatase, pulmonary tuberculosis (11.8%), pneumonitis (8.8%), paraesthesia (8.8%), skin disease (5.9%), anemia (2.9%) and conjunctivitis (2.9%)	(Srivastava, Gupta, et al. 1991)
	Mixture	2.5% decreased RBCs and HB, increase in WBCs diagnosed as Chronic Myeloid Leukaemia (CML) cases, 3% of the exposed children revealed signs of mental retardation and delayed milestones	(Jamil, Das, et al. 2007)

Contd...

Operations	Pesticide (Single/Mixture)	Clinical manifestations	References
	OPs	Muscarinic symptoms (chronic effects): Salivation 18.22% Lacrimation 17.32% Diarrhea 9.3% Nicotinic clinical manifestations (acute effects): Excessive sweating 13.78% Tremors 9.3% Mydriasis 8.9%	(Rastogi, Tripathi, et al. 2010)
	Mixture of OP, OC and carbamates	Higher mean values of hexachlorohexane (HCH), -HCH, -HCH, total HCH, op-DDT, Acetylcholinesterase (AChE) and butyrylcholinesterase (BChE) activites were reduced, risk of motor nerve conduction observed	(Pathak, Fareed, et al. 2011)
	Mixture	Prevalence of ocular morbidity 40% with symptoms of blurred vision, lacrimation, pain and irritation	(Fareed, Kesavachandran, et al. 2012)
	Mixture of OP, OC and carbamates	Higher chromatid breaks and gaps in chromosomes of peripheral blood, increased incidence of abortions 26% Stillbirths 8.7%, Neonatal deaths 9.2% Congenital deficits 3%	(Rupa, Reddy, et al. 1991)
	Methomyl	Cardiotoxic effect, significant changes in electrocardiographs	(Saiyed, Sadhu, et al. 1992)
	Mixture of pesticides	Detection of organochlorine residues (α–HCH, γ–HCH, β–HCH, total HCH, *p,p*-DDE *o,p*-DDT, *p,p*-DDD, *p,p*-DDT, total DDT, total OC in blood, decreased acetyl-cholinesterase activity in the blood, higher MDA levels, prevalence of bronchial obstruction and airway narrowing	(Kesavachandran, Singh, et al. 2006)
	OPs	AChE, BChE activities were inhibited and higher MDA levels, Respiratory morbidity (32.4%), ocular problems (8.8%), gastrointestinal (17.6%) and skin problems (23.5%), strong correlation between MDA, GSH and AcHE	(Singh, Reddy, et al. 2007)

Contd...

Operations	Pesticide (Single/Mixture)	Clinical manifestations	References
	OPs	Respiratory morbidity in 36.75% of exposed workers, respiratory illness such as wheezing, irritation of throat, dry cough and blood stained sputum that correlated with duration of exposure, activities of acetylcholinesterase and butyrylcholinesterase depleted, hematological profile viz. RBC, WBC, neutrophils, monocytes, MCH, MCV, MCHC and platelet count was altered	(Fareed, Pathak, et al. 2013)
	OPs, OCs, carbamates, pyrethroids	WBC count was decreased; uric acid and MDA level was increased, increased micronuclei in buccal mucosal cells	(Gaikwad, Karunamoorthy, et al. 2015)
	OPs and carbamates	Serum C reactive protein elevated, increase in liver function marker enzymes (AST, ALT, and ALP), creatinine, bilirubin, blood glucose, and blood urea; decline in acetyl cholinesterase activity and the level of serum cholesterol, alterations in hematologic parameters	(Jamal, Haque, et al. 2016)
	OPs, OCs, carbamates, pyrethroids	Adverse health effects in farm workers including tingling (32.3%), muscle pain (51.6%), headache (56.5%), skin disease (19%), blurred vision (35.5%), tremor (23%), stress (24.2%), depression (15.3%), anxiety (44.7%), altered taste (21.4%), altered smell (31.4%), sleep disorder (39.5%), dizziness (66.1%), memory problems (29.4%), trouble in walking (8%), and cardiac problems (16.9%) were reported, the effects were more prominent in farmers who are smokers, residing at farm and stored pesticide at home	(Kori, Thakur, et al. 2018)

Pesticide exposure has been known to elicit biochemical alterations even before clinical toxic health effects are manifested, making it imperative to identify the susceptible groups who are at a high magnitude of risk. Based on the epidemiological data a link between clinical manifestations and hematological, biochemical and enzymatic parameters have been attempted to establish biomarkers of exposure, susceptibility and effect. Biological indicators of exposure such as quantification of pesticides and/or metabolites in saliva, urine, exhaled air, tissues, or any combination of these have been routinely employed. Enzymatic biomarkers such as acetylcholinesterase (AChE) activity in the red blood cells and butyrylcholinesterase (BChE) activity in the plasma have been routinely applied to evaluate the extent of exposure to organophosphates (OP). Such studies have also triggered experimental evaluation of many pesticides to understand their accumulation and effects on long term chronic effects employing different routes of exposure (Dikshith, Gupta, et al. 1976; Dikshith, Datta, et al. 1976; Dikshith, Raizada, et al. 1980). Experimental studies have also suggested that such alterations in AChE activity could be restored on withdrawal of pesticide exposure, a piece of information that could be utilized for controlling cases of OP poisoning under field conditions (Dikshith, Datta, et al. 1976, Dikshith, Raizada, et al. 1980). Similarly, malondialdehyde (MDA) load for lipid peroxidation (LPO) and oxidative stress against OP, carbamate and organochlorine pesticides employing alterations in erythrocyte-aminolevulinic acid dehydratase (ALA-D), an enzyme in the erythrocyte, has been demonstrated.

Along with using standard tests such as AChE activity (for inhibition of cholinesterase), lung functions (for deterioration of lung volumes and flow rates) and nerve conduction velocity test (for the decline of conduction velocity), chromatography and ELISA based approaches have also been employed to characterize the biochemical changes in the workers. Alterations in thyroid and liver enzymes, creatinine levels and presence of immune complexes have been well correlated with organ-specific toxicities. Scoring of cytogenetic markers such as chromosomal aberrations (CA), sister chromatid exchange (SCE), micronuclei (MN) as well as comet assay using peripheral lymphocytes has also been extensively utilized for detecting early genotoxic effects of pesticides. Apart from employing these well-validated biomarkers, new biomarkers have been established to aid in the process of risk assessment. In this direction, the use of hair as a novel, invasive and effective biomarker has been suggested for the accurate evaluation of chronic exposure to pesticides (Kesavachandran and Mudiam 2010). More recently, Ratnasekhar, et al. 2019 have established non-invasive matrices like urine and saliva as alternative diagnostic matrices to occupational exposure of pesticides revealing 13 metabolic perturbations related to altered amino acid and energy metabolism (Ch, Singh, et al. 2019).

The field of epidemiology has significantly benefitted from molecular approaches and growing attention has been diverted towards the establishment of biomarkers of susceptibility against exposure of humans to pesticides. Genotypes underlying inter-individual differences in the various enzymes involved in bio-activation and detoxification of pesticides have been identified that may impart increased susceptibility. Polymorphism in GSTM1 and GSTP1 genes involved in metabolism and detoxification are associated with an increased susceptibility to DNA damage in a population exposed to OPs. Genetic polymorphism in GSTM1 null genotypes and an association of NAT2 slow acetylation genotypes with CYP2C9*3/*3 or GSTM1 null genotypes may also modulate DNA damage in workers exposed to OPs occupationally and alterations in this enzyme activity and serum concentrations may contribute to inter-individual variations in disease susceptibility (Singh, Kumar, et al. 2011, Singh, Kumar, et al. 2012).

Biomonitoring studies and health surveys have shed ample light on the causative agents identifying a multitude of related factors underlying the toxicity elicited. The unique features of pesticide manufacturing units (such as small space to work, poor or lack of ventilation, humidity and high temperature) have contributed further to the absorption of pesticide as the use of personal protective equipment is lacking (Sailaja, Chandrasekhar, et al. 2006). Lack of required knowledge, careless attitude and inadequate safety practices in handling of these pesticides have posed a severe health risk to the sprayers in plantations (Kesavachandran, Rastogi, et al. 2008). Indiscriminate use of a mixture of pesticides coupled with lack of adequate information and safety training is one of the primary reasons for the intoxication scenario. Poor spraying technology and inadequate personal protection and basic sanitation practices such as washing hands after pesticide use or before eating are also reported in the high incidence of pesticide toxicity (Kesavachandran, Singh, et al. 2006, Fareed, Pathak, et al. 2013) (Figure 4.2).

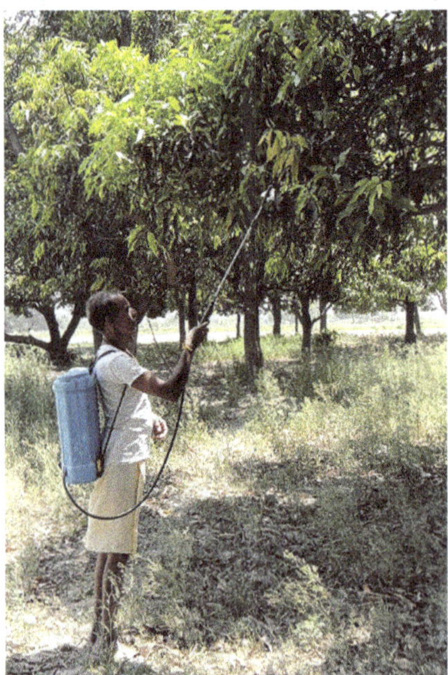

Figure 4.2 Spraying of pesticides without any personal protection procedures; Picture courtesy: Dr AB Pant, CSIR-IITR, Lucknow

Observations on how pesticides are handled have given very detailed and meaningful inputs. Applicators have been observed to mix pesticides without an appropriate protective equipment. Moreover, few application equipments were leaking and in a poor condition. A tendency to store and mix pesticides inside the house before field application also adds another dimension of risk for the high incidence of toxicity. A study revealed that less than 2% of applicators were aware of the toxicity of the pesticide formulation, only about one-third read the instructions for usage of pesticides; merely 2.5% of them took steps to follow them. Only 1.5% of applicators understand the color code system on the pesticide toxicity level, used in the region (Devi 2007). Furthermore, pesticide sprayers in India indulge in a standard practice, of chewing or smoking tobacco while spraying "to reduce the nauseating feeling", further accentuating the risk of health hazard (Kesavachandran, Fareed, et al. 2009).

In view of the plethora of these adverse effects, efforts have been directed to suggest interventional strategies and remedial measures to reduce the impact of this health hazard. Recommendations have been made to ensure the safe use of pesticides by selection of product formulations which minimize exposures (e.g., granules), using closed transfer systems for loading of spray equipments, broad-necked containers for keeping concentrates in order to prevent spillage, using personal protective equipments (PPE) such as boots, gloves, face shields and respirators and coveralls (Kesavachandran, Rastogi, et al. 2008). Redesigning of spraying equipment (use of knapsack instead of tractor mounted spraying instrument) to lower spill has been suggested as one of the possible interventional strategies to minimize occupational pesticide exposure and its adverse health effects (Pathak, Fareed, et al. 2011). Education and training in handling pesticide-contaminated clothing, introducing awareness programs on toxicity levels, trainings for safe work practices while pesticide handling and free or subsidized distribution of PPE via government/non-government organizations to the sprayers have been emphasized (Pathak, Fareed, et al. 2013).

Occupational lung diseases have also attracted attention owing to their high rate of prevalence in India with silicosis, asbestosis and byssinosis as the most common forms of pneumoconiosis. The national program for control and treatment of occupational diseases in India revealed the prevalence of silicosis in mica miners as 6.2–34%, 4.1% in manganese miners, as high as 30.4% in zinc and lead miners, 27.2% in iron foundry workers, 9.3% in deep and surface coal miners, and as much as 54.6% in slate-pencil workers (http://www.rfhha.org/images/pdf/national_health/NATIONAL_PROGRAMM E_FOR_CONTROL_of_occupational_disease.pdf). Prevalence of asbestosis has been found from 3% in the asbestos miners to 21% in the mill workers. Among textile workers, byssinosis was as common as 28–47% (National Programme for Control and Treatment of Occupational Diseases.

http://www.ndcnihfw.org/html/Programmes/NationalProgrammeForControlTre atm ent). The problems of pneumoconiosis was first described in 1933 in the Kolar Gold fields with the first case of silicosis being reported in 1947 (Jones 1933, Jindal, Aggarwal, et al. 2001), and since then, has been documented in various other industries and mines: mica, coal, lead, silver manganese mines; sand blasting; pottery and ceramics; metal grinding; rock mining; building and construction work; iron and steel industry; and many more. Silicosis gained national prominence in view of the observations made through epidemiologic studies carried out by the NIOH, CSIR-IITR and Indian Bureau of Mines. The term silicosis has been reserved for the lung disorder due to inhalation of free silica, classified as a human carcinogen (size 0.5- 5 microns in diameter). It is an untreatable progressive disorder, most widespread amongst all occupational diseases. As per estimation, in India, there are approximately more than 3 million workers exposed to silica dust with around 8.5 million more engaged in building and construction activities, exposed to quartz (Jindal 2013).

Research groups have conducted dust monitoring of work environment, including characterization and quantification of toxic substances in mines. Studies have assessed the prevalence of respiratory morbidities in such workers with respect to their age, sex, length of exposure, dust concentration in the work environment, nutritional status and smoking habits. The airborne free silica dust levels have been found to be several times higher (ranging from 1.9 mg/m^3 to 24.3 mg/m^3) as compared to the limits prescribed under the Factories Act (0.025 mg/m^3 of air). Environmental studies showed that the number of dust particles present varied from 15 to 51.5 million per cubic foot of air and 80% of them were 5 μm or less in size. Two samples of the stone contained 85.06% and 85.39% of silica respectively (Gupta, Garg et al. 1969; Gupta, Bajaj, et al. 1972). Moreover, the type of processing is shown to have an impact on the intensity of respiratory dysfunction as well as the environmental dust concentration. Another study reported a 19.6% prevalence of pneumoconiosis among the female agate stone grinders against only 8.3% in female chippers (Clerk, Gupta, et al. 1983).

Continuous inhalation of silica dust over prolonged periods has been reported to result in fibrosis of the lungs among stone cutters (Gupta, Garg, et al. 1969; Saini, Yousuf, et al. 1984) and stone crushers (Sood, Sachdeva, et al. 1984), leading to pneumoconiosis of several grades. Comorbidities such as malnutrition and co-existence of tuberculosis, inadequate ventilation facilities, excessive exposure to dust due to no protective gears, lack of knowledge of risks of silica exposure have all been documented in health and environmental surveys (Saiyed, Parikh, et al. 1985; Kulkarni 2007). The minimum time interval between first exposure to risk and appearance of silicosis was observed to be 4 years, but the disease was relatively uncommon with exposure to the risk of 10-15 years or less (Jain, Sepaho, et al. 1977).

After this length of time, the risk steadily increased and, after 25 years, all the workers developed silicosis. Based on clinical and radiological evidences, studies have reported high prevalence of silicosis ranging from 3.5% in an ordinance factory to as high as 38% and 54.6% in the agate and slate-pencil industry, respectively, based on the duration of silica exposure and silica concentration in the work environment (Table 4.2).

Table 4.2 Representative epidemiological studies conducted on silicosis

Workplaces	Environmental survey and clinical manifestations/effects	References
Ordnance factory	Rradiographic evidence of pneumoconiosis in 3.49% of exposed population, maximum prevalence of pneumoconiosis was among those who had put in more than 15 years' service whereas tuberculosis in 4.25% of all workers	(Viswanathan, Boparai, et al. 1972)
Slate pencil workers	The majority of workers had symptoms related to chest with productive cough (75%), chest pain (28%), and occasionally hemopytis (4%) with pleural thickening The average total and respirable dust concentrations in the respiratory zone of the cutters and in the general work environment were very high, with high free silica content, the dust levels in the respiratory zone of the cutters were almost twice as high as those in the general work environment, prevalence of silicosis was 54.6%. Among these, 17.7% had progressive massive fibrosis	(Jain, Sepaho, et al. 1977) (Saiyed, Parikh, et al. 1985)
Agate workers	The prevalence of pneumoconiosis was high (18 4%), other respiratory comorbidities were bronchial asthma, chronic bronchitis, tuberculosis, grinders suffered from pneumoconiosis (21.9%) than chippers (7.3%) Silicosis confirmed in 69.1% of workers, high respiratory morbidity	(Rastogi, Gupta, et al. 1991) (Chaudhury, Phatak, et al. 2010)
Sand Stone Quarry Workers	58.6% of the workers suffered from respiratory difficulties, decrease in the peak expiratory flow rate of lungs correlated with the particulate concentration and exposure duration, for duration of exposure of more than 15 years the reduction in peak expiratory flow rate was 65% for driller, 60% for dresser and 56% for labour	(Singh, Chowdhary, et al. 2006)

Studies have also reported co-existence of pulmonary abnormalities such as tuberculosis, connective tissue diseases and lung cancer in established cases of silicosis (Gupta, Bajaj, et al. 1976; Jain, Sepaha, et al. 1980; Jindal 2013). Chronic exposure to silica has been shown to increase the workers' risk of acquiring tuberculosis infection (silico-tuberculosis) and even aggravate pre-existing tuberculosis (Kulkarni 2007), suggesting the combined effect of background tubercular infection and exposure to respirable-size silica particles in causing extensive silicosis (Gupta, Bajaj et al. 1976; Jain, Sepaha et al. 1980). Infact, potential pulmonary debilitation may even occur in pneumoconiosis before, or in the absence of, any radiologic findings of silicosis (Sood, Sachdeva, et al. 1984; Rastogi, Gupta, et al. 1988).

The major challenge of elimination of silicosis in India has been in the unorganized sectors like slate pencil cutting, stone cutting and agate industry, quartz grinding industries, whose units are based in the homes of the workers, which are not under the purview of the Factory Act of India (1948) and Mines Act (1952). In addition, since the work is done at home, the workers and the families are always at risk due to respirable dust and as such report a high incidence of the disease (Rastogi, Gupta, et al. 1991). The problem has been appreciated by the NIOH that has been taking a close look at the small-scale industries, in order to identify problem areas, assign priorities, and develop low-cost engineering control measures to protect the workers. Dust control modules established on around 500 grinding machines in the agate industry in Khambhat (Gujarat) has led to a 94% reduction in the dust levels (Bhagia and Sadhu 2008).

The National Human Rights Commission (NHRC) as directed by the Supreme Court of India has enacted several recommendations pertaining to preventive, remedial and rehabilitative measures for controlling the emissions and safeguarding the health of workers in collaboration with several stakeholders such as state and central governments, individual organizations, and many other agencies. These have included installation/upgradation of air pollution control devices at dust generating sections such as stone unloading, crushing, material convening, grinding, cost-effective engineering control measures such as redesigning plant layout to prevent direct exposure, increasing the stack height to at least 2 m above roof level for proper dispersion of pollutants in the atmosphere, improvement in industrial hygiene through efficient ventilation and use of personal protection such as protective gears and good quality masks.

Other measures include regular inspections, free primary, secondary and tertiary level health facilities for diagnosis and treatment of workers exposed to toxic fibres, along with counselling of patients on ways to avoid inhalation of dust and subsequent disease progression. Awareness has also been raised through information printed on materials using the local languages (http://nhrc.nic.in/sites/default/files/NHRC_Interventions_on_Silicosis_ 2712 2016.pdf).

Considerable asbestos exposure has mainly occurred in asbestos cement factories, asbestos textile industry and asbestos mining and milling (prevalence of 3-21%). Extensive monitoring of workplace and assessment of exposure among Indian workers in asbestos-using industries in India have been performed by the NIOH, the CLI, and the Bureau of Indian Mines (reviewed by (Dave and Beckett 2005)). Studies have revealed fibre levels 2-100 times higher than the Permissible Exposure Limit (PEL) (Bhagia, Dave, et al. 1994, Dave, Ghodasara, et al. 1997). Fibre levels were revealed to be as high as 224.23 f/ml fibre concentration against a prescribed Threshold Limit Value (TLVs) of <2f/ml (Mukherjee, Rajmohan, et al. 1992, Mukherjee, Rajmohan, et al. 1996, Dave and Beckett 2005). This were despite the investigators' recommendations to lower the levels, implement process improvement, and other safety measures for exposure control following their earlier investigation in the same unit (Mukherjee, Rajmohan, et al. 1996) (Table 4.3).

Table 4.3 Representative epidemiological studies conducted on asbestosis

Workplace	Environmental survey and clinical manifestations/Effects	References
Chrysotile asbestos mines and mills	Levels were below the PEL, in areas where asbestos ore was crushed and processed, air levels were found to be in the range of 200 – 400 f/ml	(Bhagia, Dave et al. 1994)
Four asbestosis mills	In most areas, the fiber air levels were more than the prescribed PEL of 1.0 f/ml air, prevalence of asbestosis was 11.5%	(Mukherjee, Rajmohan, et al. 1992)
Slate pencil industries	Airway obstruction observed in 13 of 99 exposed workers who were non-smokers, and in higher percentage of asbestos-exposed smokers than silica-exposed smokers.	(Mohan, Dave, et al. 1993)
Asbestos cement factory	FVC on spirometry in the exposed workers was significantly lower	(Dave, Mohan Rao, et al. 1995)

Acknowledging chrysolite as an established carcinogen, according to international agencies like WHO, ILO and OSHA there are no safe exposure limits and no such "controlled use" of asbestos (LaDou, Landrigan, et al. 2001). The possible impact of asbestos mining and related adverse effects on human health in India has been extensively explored by many authors (Ramanathan and Subramanian 2001; Dave and Beckett 2005; Venkatesh and Chandramohan, 2009). In India, the observed clinical effects are pleural, parenchymal and pulmonary dysfunctions, sequelae, fibrosis, bronchogenic cancer, malignant mesothelioma and other cancer risk associated with duration of exposure and lifestyle habits like smoking (Dave, Ghodasara, et al. 1997). The latency period (length of the time from exposure to the onset of diseases) in India is estimated to be 20–37 years (Phoon 2000). However, since the latency period is 20 years or more, the asbestos-associated disease remains a significant public health issue. Indian physicians have also anticipated multiple patterns of a disease based on few characteristic features of the asbestos industries, including frequent employment of women in these industries, and an early age occupational exposure (Dave and Beckett 2005) (Figure 4.3).

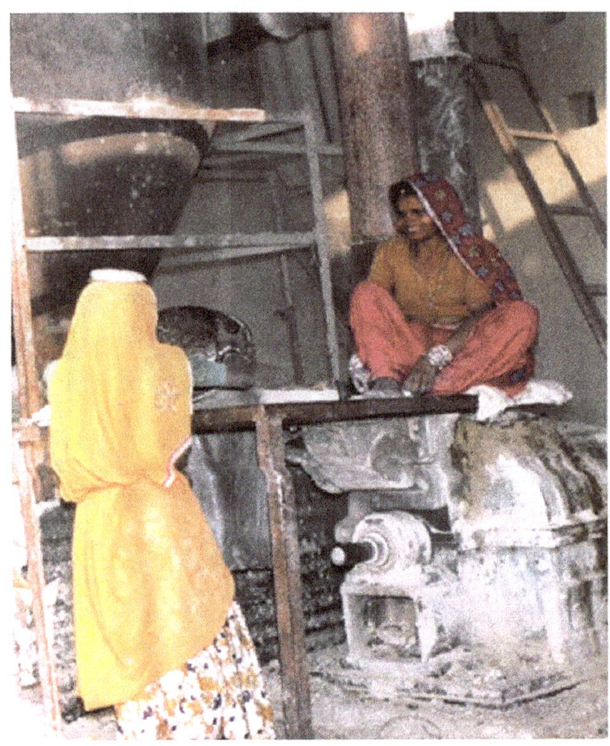

Figure 4.3 Women being exposed to asbestos dust and fibers while working in an asbestos mill in an unorganized sector. Work area heavily covered with asbestosis dust; Picture courtesy: Dr Qamar Rahman, Former Scientist, CSIR-IITR, Lucknow

It has been established that the toxicity of asbestos fibers is dependent on the number that is present in the atmosphere, type and size distribution. Apart from fiber levels estimation in the milling processes, the fiber size distribution in context of length and breadth and fiber identification have also been included (Mukherjee, Rajmohan, et al. 1992). Optical sizing of fibers with a length greater than 5 µm revealed the presence of multiple fibers of length more than 10 µm and 20 µm that are potentially more harmful. Such high levels of silica and asbestos fibers have been majorly attributed to the use of obsolete technology, direct exposure to the asbestos products without adequate precautionary measures, non-compliance to mines and safety act and lower content of the fiber in the parent rock (Ramanathan and Subramanian 2001, Dave and Beckett 2005) (Figure 4.4). Manual operations like material shifting, lump-breaking, material feeding and collection, and sorting are conducted without protective equipments.

In majority of the cases, there have been lack of monitoring platforms; inadequate maintenance of stacks and bag houses, and operations were intermittent. After recommendation of control measures and a program on health education, a follow-up investiagtion was undertaken in the same mills. The study documented a significant reduction in fiber levels (1.5-2 f/ml) as compared with the first survey, emphasizing a need for implementation of more control measures (Mukherjee, Rajmohan et al. 1996; Arif, Khan, et al. 1994).

To minimize the exposure of the workers to asbestos, housekeeping, personal protection and hygiene with shower and changing of clothes after the work shift etc., have been strongly recommended to be made mandatory. Vacuum cleaners which have a high efficiency particulate air filter have to be used instead of dry sweeping. A control device comprising of 'Hood-Filter-Fan' has been recommended for controlling emmission in the mills. In the case of a mechanized plant, the entire duct should be maintained at negative pressure to ensure that the fibers are inside the system instead of being emitted. The plant should be in a leak proof condition by effectively sealing of duct joints and elbow of the ducts etc. to control the emission (Mukherjee, Rajmohan, et al. 1996).

Pioneering studies conducted by CSIR-IITR during the initial years were associated with miners' health who inhaled dusts and fibres. Since its inception, IITR has made several contributions in the field of experimental pneumoc-oniosis identifying at a more fundamental level the cellular mechanisms of pulmonary fibrosis post exposure to a range of particulate, fibrous dusts and toxins, including carcinogens like asbestos, silica, coal fly ash, mica, wood dust, elucidating the involvement of membrane localised biochemical reactions in the molecular pathology of silicosis and asbestosis (Zaidi, Shanker, et al. 1971, Beg, Rahman, et al. 1973, Viswanathan, Rahman, et al. 1973, Rahman, Viswanathan, et al. 1976, Misra, Rahman, et al. 1978). Research has been carried out to the extent of identifying determinants that could predispose the workers to certain risk factors, these being genetic determinants, age, sex, nutritional variants or co-existence of infectious disease, and exposure to mixture of chemicals (Kaw and Zaidi 1970, Zaidi and Kaw 1970, Zaidi, Shanker, et al. 1971). For example, the effects of CYP1A1 polymorphisms on DNA damage in coal tar workers exposed to polycyclic aromatic hydrocarbons has been documented. The etiology of respiratory disease among miners has been suggested to be multifactorial in nature with studies underlying coexistence of malnutrition, smoking with pathogenesis of silicosis and asbestosis; possible synergistic effects between fuel smoke exposure and kerosene soot at home and to fibres and other contaminants at work place and coal fly ash exposure and development of pulmonary silicosis reaction (Kaw, Khanna, et al. 1990; Rahman, Dopp, et al. 2000; Lohani, Dopp, et al. 2002).

Studies have also demonstrated the role of tuberculosis infection in the causation of pulmonary massive fibrosis in coal miners and fungal infections in aggravating the fibrotic response in lungs that are exposed to many inorganic and organic dusts (Zaidi, Shanker, et al. 1973; Zaidi, Dogra, et al. 1973; Zaidi, Dogra, et al. 1977). In India majority of asbestos factory workers used kerosene as a domestic fuel due to its lower cost, creating a possibility of synergism of the two in causing serious health hazards. Experimental reports have suggested continuous derangement and alteration in metabolic activities in the pulmonary drug-metabolizing enzyme systems by asbestos that may affect the metabolism and clearance of a variety of environmental pollutants (such as kerosene) reaching the lungs resulting in a higher toxic potential (Arif, Khan, et al. 1992, Arif, Khan, et al. 1994, Arif, Khan, et al. 1997). Studies carried out using asbestos of different fiber lengths have revealed that dimension is a major factor in disease development with long fibers generally being more pathogenic than short in developing inflammatory reactions via stimulation of tumor necrosis factor (TNF) (Dogra and Donaldson 1995).

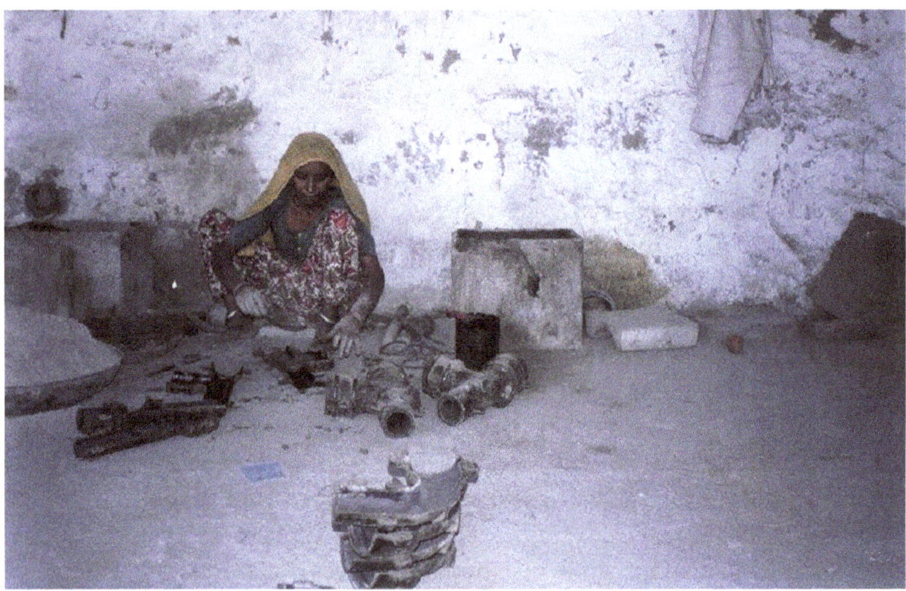

Figure 4.4 A woman making pipe joints using asbestos and cement without any personal protection measures. Picture courtesy by Dr Qamar Rahman, Former Scientist, CSIR-IITR, Lucknow

An *in vitro* study conducted in the blood lymphocytes of smokers exposed to two different types of asbestos fibers showed that crocidolite asbestos induced more micronuclei (MN) and aneuploidy in comparison to chrysotile

(Lohani, Dopp, et al. 2002). Similarly, studies are suggestive that smoking makes genetic system of the cells more vulnerable to the deleterious effects of asbestos, wherein the genetic damage in case of co-exposure to cigarette smoking was not strictly connected to chromosome 1 only, as in case of asbestos, but also involved damage to other chromosomes as well (Lohani, Dopp, et al. 2002). To get insights into the pathophysiology of silica-induced toxicity, a well-characterized murine model of silica induced lung injury has been established that has led to the identification of multiple cytokines (IL-6Rα) responsible for the inflammatory response in the airways as well as employed to identify the preventive efficacy of NAT extract (Nyctanthes arbortristis) in the early phase of pulmonary injury (Paul, Prakash, et al. 2002). Similarly, research has led to the identification of dietary components and anti-oxidants that have shown potential to reduce asbestos induced genotoxicity via different mechanisms (Afaq, Abidi, et al. 2000, Ameen, Musthapa, et al. 2003) (Lohani, Yadav, et al. 2003).

The diagnosis of occupational lung diseases has mainly been based on clinical studies of the subjects focusing on the respiratory system, pulmonary function measurement with emphasis on lung volumes and profusion grading according to the International Labour Organization classification of Pneumoconiosis. However, owing to the irreversible nature of silicosis, there has been a growing need to develop a biomarker of exposure rather than effect (Tiwari, Sathwara, et al. 2004). Two parameters viz. SACE (serum angiotensin converting enzyme activity) and serum copper levels are elevated in fibrotic diseases in lung, and as such have been suggested to be employed as a potential biomarker not only in the standard cases but also in the covert cases of silicosis to enable preventive measures (Tiwari 2005). Apart from these well-documented cases, reports of pneumoconiosis in other industries have also been reported (mentioned in Table 4.4.).

Table 4.4 Representative studies reporting pneumoconiosis in different industries

Industry	Clinical manifestations/effects	References
Cotton textile industry	Symptoms for respiratory dysfunctions were significantly more common in the cotton mill workers, an association of duration of exposure and symptoms with spirometric abnormality	(Dangi and Bhise 2017)
Jute industry	Low mean values of Forced expiratory volume (FEV1) were observed in workers exposed to high dust, links between history of smoking and productive cough on the first and last day of the week	(Chattopadhyay, Gangopadhyaya, et al. 1995)

Contd...

Industry	Clinical manifestations/effects	References
	Chest tightness and difficulty in breathing on the first day of the week in 9.18% workers, 14.28% workers complained of breathlessness and chest tightness after work on days other than Monday (atypical byssinosis)	(Chattopadhyay, Saiyed, et al. 1999)
	The areas of batching, spinning, and weaving in the mill revealed endotoxin levels of 0.22–4.42 $\mu g/m^3$, 0.04–1.47 $\mu g/m^3$, and 0.01–0.07 $\mu g/m^3$, respectively, increased exposure to bacterial endotoxin in airborne dust resulting in respiratory morbidities which included typical byssinosis symptoms, and acute changes in post shift forced expiratory volume in 1 second (FEV1.0) (31.8%)	(Mukherjee, Chattopadhyay, et al. 2004)
Glass bangle industry	Higher prevalence (16.3%) of respiratory impairment in comparison to that observed in the controls (7.9%) indicating primarily restrictive pattern of pulmonary abnormality, reduction was more marked in the smoking glass bangle workers, higher prevalence in those who worked for more than 10 years (23.0%)	(Rastogi, Gupta, et al. 1991)
Carpet industry	Dust concentration was higher (6.86 mg/m^3) in carpet finishing unit followed by 3.48 mg/m^3 in Tibbati carpet weaving unit, respiratory symptoms ranged from 20.0-41.8% that was higher in smoking workers (44.5%) as compared to that in non-smoking workers (14.0%), bronchial obstruction was almost five times higher in >10 years exposed group when compared to <10 years-exposed group (27.3% vs 5.9%)	(Rastogi, Ahmad, et al. 2003)
Coal mining industry	Coal worker pneumoconiosis was reported to be 3.03%, major category of profusion was category-I (81.09%), followed by category-II (17.84%), 3 cases of progressive massive fibrosis, round shaped opacities were predominant (89.59%), among the opacities, 'p' type was more prevalent (48.29%) followed by `q' type (40.62%)	(Parihar, Patnaik, et al. 1997)
Tobacco workers	Prevalence of green tobacco sickness was 47.0%. 55.7% in women and in men workers it was 42.66%,	(Parikh, Gokani, et al. 2005)
Bidi industry	A high respiratory morbidity (cough, sputum, and breathlessness) was observed among males than females, Age-related decrement in pulmonary function tests	(Chattopadhyay, Gangopadhyay, et al. 2014)

Agricultural workers who are engaged in cultivation of tobacco have been shown to develop characteristic symptoms, called "Green Tobacco Sickness" (GTS). Several studies have described the acute and chronic toxic health effects of nicotine amongst tobacco workers (Ghosh, Parikh, et al. 1979, Ghosh, Parikh, et al. 1980, Parikh, Gokani, et al. 2005). The airborne tobacco dust around the workplaces of bidi making units is the potential risk factor causing respiratory disorders to the bidi binders. The proximity of the tobacco and the leaves to the nostrils and the mouth as well as the microbes and airborne fungal spores added into the working atmosphere from the processed leaves have heightened the issue. Administration of bronchodilator drug could inevitably bring positive bronchodilatation and easing of airway resistance of the bidi binders indicating the obstruction in the airways might be reversible in nature (Chattopadhyay, Gangopadhyay, et al. 2014). NIOH has also carried out interventional studies against "Green Tobacco Sickness" among tobacco harvesters. The institute has developed and also popularized the use of varieties of gloves to provide protection against acute nicotine poisoning by dermal absorption among tobacco harvesters (Saiyed and Tiwari 2004). Use of the gloves revealed a considerable reduction in GTS's prevalence and absorption of nicotine as observed by cotinine and nicotine excretion rate in the urine. The application of rubber gloves provided protection among 93% of the workers, and around 78.5% with cotton gloves.

NIOH has also paid attention to the particular group of the vulnerable population, such as women workers' and child labor problems. The institute has a devoted thrust on promotion of health and safety of women workers, prevention of hazards in diverse occupational areas including both organized and unorganized areas. Nutritional status and anthropometry of women in the small scale industries, e.g., garment manufacturing, beedi industry and plastic industry have been undertaken. Safe exposure of women in a hot environment, with reference to simulated experimentation in the climatic chamber has also been given due importance. Studying the women workers' health in terms of occupational health has been a significant work area for India. Several of these occupations have been identified and studies have been initiated in collaboration with SEWA (Self Employed Women's Association). Examples are scrap cleaners, salt workers, agarbatti workers (incense stick makers), screen printing workers and agricultural workers exposed to pesticides.

Chemicals in various industries have also posed a significant occupational health hazard with studies reporting high airborne concentrations of toxic chemicals in industrial environments in India (Ramanathan and Kashyap 1975). The best example of an occupational disaster could be the massive leak of methyl isocyanate (MIC) gas stored for an extended period in the Tank 610 of the Pesticide Plant of Union Carbide of India Ltd (UCIL) leading to the notorious Bhopal Gas Tragedy in 1984. Several hypotheses were attributed for the tragedy including, bulk storage of 42 tons of MIC for prolonged periods, non-functional refrigeration system, safety measures failure and malfunctioning of neutralization facilities (Sriramachari 2004). The introduction of water apparently initiated the accident into the MIC tank which resuled in an uncontrollable reaction, liberating heat and gas. Safety systems such as the flare tower (to remove excess gas), caustic soda scrubber (for neutralization) and the refrigeration unit were either not functional or were not adequate enough to handle large volumes of escaping gas (Morehouse and Subramaniam 1986).

Table 4.5 Few representative studies conducted to characterize the effects of chemicals on industrial workers

Occupational agents	Occupation	Environmental survey and Clinical manifestations/effects	References
Metals			
Chromium (trivalent form)	Leather tannery	High levels of blood and urinary Cr, prevalence of morbidity was higher with respiratory illness (16.7%), followed by ocular illnesses (14.7%), few reported reported congestion of the nasal mucosa (3.55%)	(Rastogi, Pandey, et al. 2008)
Chromium and Nickel	Tanning industry	Higher level of blood Cr, DNA damage, MDA, SOD and lower level of GSH, oxidative stress and genotoxicity correlating with blood chromium levels and duration of exposure	(Khan, Ambreen, et al. 2012)
	Welding	Welders had higher Cr and Ni content along with a longer mean comet tail length than that of the controls in blook leucocytes, also higher induction of micronucleated cells in buccal epithelial cells indicating DNA damage	(Danadevi, Rozati, et al. 2004)
	Electroplating industry	High micronuclei frequency, karyorrhexis, karyolysis in buccal cells, binucleate and enucleated cells with a positive correlation with plasma chromium levels and duration of exposure	(Qayyum, Ara, et al. 2012)
Lead	Printing press	Lead-exposed workers had increased frequency of sister chromatid exchanges, smoking along with lead exposure inihibited mitotic activity in lymphocytes	(Rajah and Ahuja, 1995)
	Auto garage workers	Urinary N-acetyl-3-D-glucosam-inidaseactivity and beta-2-microglobulin levels were increased with blood lead levels of 30-69 µg/dl in workers (6 months-10 years), significant correlation between urinary N-acetyl-3-D-glucosam-inidase activity and level of blood lead	(Dinesh Kumar and Krishnaswamy 1995)

Contd...

Occupational agents	Occupation	Environmental survey and Clinical manifestations/effects	References
	Secondary recovery unit	Pb concentrations of 4.2 mg/m^3 was found in the air in the unit premises, mean Pb content was found to be higher in workers (248.3 mg/l vs. 27.49 mg/l) with more DNA damage (44.58% vs 21.14%)	(Danadevi, Rozati, et al. 2003)
	Three-wheeler drivers, battery workers and silver jewelery makers	Lymphocyte proliferation to phytohaemagglutinin (PHA) is inhibited, interferon-γ was elevated in T cell mitogen, PHA, stimulated PBMCs culture supernatant	(Mishra, Singh, et al. 2003)
	Pigment factory	Gross, and forward progressive motility, reduced sperm velocity with high stationary motile spermatozoa in workers (7-15 years exposure), increased seminal fructose and lower sperm ATPase activity, accessory gland dysfunctions as observed by prolonged liquefaction time, decreased semen volume, viscosity and seminal plasma protein	(Naha and Chowdhury 2005)
	Battery manufacturing units	The blood and urinary lead level were elevated in workers, urinary d-aminolevulinic acid (ALA-U), erythrocyte-zinc protoporphyrin (ZPP), and porphobilinogen (PBG-U) were elevated, decrease of hemoglobin concentration, packed cell volume, increase of total leucocytes count, increased serum MDA content and reduced activities of antioxidant enzymes	(Patil, Bhagwat, et al. 2006)
	Battery manufacturing units	High blood lead levels (53.63 vs 12.52 µg/dl), good correlation between urinary γ-amino laevulinic acid and blood lead levels	(Bhagwat, Patil, et al. 2008)
Cadmium	Electroplating	A significant increase of urine cadmium and serum amylase activity that directly correlated (with an exposure period ranging from 10 to 18 years)	(Kalahasthi, Hirehal Raghavendra Rao, et al. 2006)
	Small scale jewellery shop	10 times higher urinary Cd values than controls, 75% reported respiratory tract symptoms, a marked deficit in lung function	(Moitra, Blanc, et al. 2013)
	Jewellery manufacturing	Lower plasma antioxidant enzymes, and increased malondialdehyde and erythrocyte fragility, activities of superoxide dismutase and catalase were reduced and lipid peroxidation and erythrocyte fragility were enhanced	(Moitra, Brashier, et al. 2014)

Contd...

Occupational agents	Occupation	Environmental survey and Clinical manifestations/effects	References
Manganese and Nickel	Metal arc welders	Forced mid-expiratory flow rates were reduced in the welders, associated with both heavy metal levels and plasma MDA, higher deposition of heavy metals on the alveolar macrophages cell surface and more DNA damage in sputum cells	(Moitra, Ghosh, et al. 2018)
Copper	Mine workers	Higher contents of copper as compared to control, serum IgA and IgG were increased, decrease in serum IgM, serum IgE was more significantly increased only in miners as compared to controls	(Tumane, Nath, et al. 2019)
Gases			
Benzene	Solvent extraction units	Benzene poisoning, haemopoetic disorders dermatitis, hematological and immunological alterations	(Ramaswamy 1987)
	Gasoline station	High air benzene concentration, increase in creatinine content (563.16 μg g^{-1} vs control 266.88μg g$^{-1)}$	(Raghavan and Basavaiah 2005)
	Petroleum pump workers and automobile service station workers	Workers had 3.8 times more trans muconic acid in urine, decreased erythrocytes, haemoglobin, platelet and lymphocyte levels but elevated neutrophils, band cells, RBC anisopoikilocytosis, over expression of platelet P selectin	(Ray, Roychoudhury, et al. 2007)
Aluminium phosphide	Fumigation of stored grains	Phosphine concentration ranged from 0.17 to 2.11 ppm, headache (31.8%), dyspnoea (31.8%), tightness around the chest (27.3%), cough (18.2%), giddiness, anorexia and epigastric pain numbness and lethargy (13.6% each), abnormal physical signs included bilateral diffuse rhonchi and absent ankle reflex	(Misra, Bhargava, et al. 1988)
Carbon disulphide	Viscose rayon	Central and peripheral system impairment, digestive and ophthalmological defects	(Ramaswamy 1987)
Motor Vehicle Exhaust	Traffic police, bus drivers, auto shop workers	Increased exposure to the vehicle exhaust, as reflected by job category was associated with decreased levels of haemoglobin	(Potula and Hu 1996)

Similarly, the case of Kodaikanal mercury poisoning faced severe criticism, wherein the Unilever's subsidiary Hindustan Lever Limited (HLL) producing millions of thermometers used around 900 kg of mercury per year to mainly export to the US and Europe in 1986. The frequent way of disposing off mercury was by blowing the air contaminated with mercury outside the factory into Kodaikanal and shola forest, putting lives at risk. An investigation conducted by the Department of Atomic Energy of Government of India revealed that the free mercury level in Kodaikanal's atmosphere was around 1000 times more than under normal conditions (https://ejatlas.org/print/ hindustan-unilever-thermometer-factory-kodaikanal-tamilnadu-india). Analysis of water, sediment and fish samples collected from Kodaikanal lake revealed increased levels of mercury even four years after the mercury emissions were stopped (Karunasagar, Krishna, et al. 2006).

Over the years, the industrial workers have been regularly exposed to the dust of several potential pollutants and toxicants prevalent in the mining environment such as lead, chromium, cadmium, mercury, aluminium, manganese, arsenic, fluoride etc (Dhatrak and Nandi 2009) (Table 4.5). Apart from single chemical exposures, combined exposure (for example to dust, cyanide fumes, and solvents in electroplating shops) may cause organ-specific dysfunctions (Murti 1987). Exposure of these workers to chemicals may occur via inhalation, local action or by ingestion of salts, solutions, mists and fumes of these metals. Lack of proper awareness/education and adequate personal protective devices, has been largely responsible for these workers to be exposed to dust and fumes (Sadhu, Amin, et al. 2008).

Biological monitoring of chemicals has been undertaken by determination of residues and metabolites in biological samples such as blood/serum/urine /adipose tissue, routine hematological examinations, biochemical activities as well as enzymatic changes to quantify the magnitude of risk associated with chemical exposure. Many research institutes have been using advanced techniques for detection and/or analysis of chemicals for particular settings. New approaches such as comet assay, micronuclei, ELISA and FISH have been widely employed as a diagnostic tool alongside the classical chemical analytical monitoring to assess workplace environments and clinical/ biochemical investigations. In addition, automated sampling and validated enzymatic methods have complemented the battery of analysis to improve worker health.

Research groups have employed different biochemical indices as standard biomarkers of exposure. Urinary arsenic concentration has been employed as a key biomarker of exposure (Chatterjee, Das, et al. 1995). DNA adducts in lymphocytes, oncogene products, immunological variations and many such phenomena are used by epidemiologists to assess risk due to exposure, including heavy metals. Enzymatic antioxidants in erythrocytes may serve as diagnostic tools for early diagnosis of heavy metal poisoning. Although these RBC enzymes have been reported to change under certain pathological conditions, their use as early biomarkers of metal toxicity appear promising (Gupta and Shukla 1997). Similarly, early alterations in plasma levels of chloride, plasma sialic acid and erythrocyte acid labile phosphate (ALP) have been indicative of early manganese toxicity (Zaidi, Patel, et al. 2005). Urinary

N-acetyl-3-D-glucosaminidase activity acts as a sensitive indicator of blood lead levels and renal tubular injury (Dinesh Kumar and Krishnaswamy 1995). Identification of gene susceptibilies has further revolutionized our understanding of human occupational diseases. Delta-aminolevulinic acid dehydratase (δ-ALAD) gene polymorphism (G177C) and effects of Matrix γ-carboxy glutamic acid protein (MGP) gene promoter polymorphism (T-138C) on blood lead levels have been identified and may help in better evaluation (Shaik and Jamil 2008). Simultaneous monitoring of the biomarkers of exposure (Manganese), effect (prolactin) and susceptibility (SNPs in CYP2D6, GSTM1 and NQO1 gene) via blood proteome profiling have provided a broader view to precisely predict the miners more susceptible to manganese-related diseases in occupational settings (Vinayagamoorthy, Krishnamurthi, et al. 2010). These patterns of gene expression or 'molecular fingerprints' could be utilized as predictive or diagnostic markers of exposure which is characteristic of a specific mechanism of action of that toxic or efficacious effect. Such epidemiological studies have also triggered studies aimed at elucidating the impact of various occupational toxicants, elucidating their mechanism of actions and identifying therapeutic interventions against them. Providing an account of those would be beyond the scope of this section, but they do find a mention in the latter topics.

Taking clues from the early epidemiological studies, some of the studies at CSIR-IITR in early years of inception were also focused on elucidating the mechanistic basis of metal intoxication. Detailed studies have elucidated the mechanistic basis of manganese neurotoxicity and behavioral dysfunction (Saxena 1967, Chandra, Seth, et al. 1974, Sitaramayya, Nagar, et al. 1974). Experimental studies have highlighted neurological disturbances in the metabolism of dopamine and norepinephrine (neurotransmitters) in manganese toxicity (Mustafa and Chandra 1971). Based on these extensive investigations a clinical diagnostic test for early detection of manganese in the body prior to its neurological manifestations has been demonstrated using serum calcium, inorganic phosphates and alkaline phosphatise and ceruloplasmin as biomarkers that occurred at a much earlier stage than the development of symptoms of manganese encephalopathy (Chandra, Imam et al. 1973). Efficacy of metal chelation therapy using p-aminosalicylic acid (Tandon and Mathur 1976), polyaminocarboxylic acids (Tandon and Singh 1975), few amino acids (Khandelwal, Kachru et al. 1980) and metals (Khandelwal, Ashquin et al. 1984) in the sequestration of manganese from vital organs of poisoned animals as well as restoring certain metal induced biochemical and histological changes has been demonstrated to be useful in the management of occupational manganese poisoning (Tandon and Khandelwal 1982). Studies are also suggestive of using iron deficiency as a prophylactic measure in manganese toxicity as iron deficiency, particularly in the industrial workers, has been revealed to be the biggest metabolic factor in rendering an individual more susceptible to manganese toxicity (Chandra and Shukla 1976). Similarly, the biochemical basis of heavy metal intoxication has been elucidated with vitamin B complex supplementation diminishing the susceptibility to cadmium and lead intoxication (Tandon, Flora, et al. 1986). Other works of significance have included studies on the biochemical basis of lead intoxication, the toxicity of industrial dyes, particularly associated with benzanthrone and the effect of additives used in the plastics industry on experimental animals (Singh and Tripathi 1973, Pandya, Singh, et al. 1976).

The Central Labour Institute in Mumbai works as a national institute dealing with the scientific aspects relating to human factors in industrial development. The International Labour Organization has recognized it as a Centre of Excellence in training on Occupational Safety and Health in the Asian and Pacific Region. It also functions as a National Centre for CIS (International Occupational Safety and Health Information Centre) and the Centre for National Safety and Health Hazard Alert System. At the national level, the institute also offers services through studies, technical advice, training and dissemination of information. It also runs a National Referral Diagnostic Centre (NRDC) for the early detection and diagnosis of occupational diseases, recommending measures for effective prevention/control of occupational health problems. The Centre also established an Epidemiology Wing in 1974 which conducts surveys for identification of occupational health problems in workers involved in rural and small-scale industries. Epidemiological studies have been undertaken on workers who are engaged in processing hemp-fibre, petroleum, benzanthrone, heavy electricals, textiles, agate, nickel and chromium electroplating, and manganese welding.

Few intervention programs have been undertaken to improve the medical condition of the workers. For example, daily intake of vitamin C and vitamin B1 may prevent lead accumulation, thus reducing its toxic effects, particularly in those workers who are regularly exposed to lead (Tandon, Chatterjee, et al. 2001). Simiarly, the treatment with D-penicillamine reduced the workers' blood lead levels from 114.4, 110.0 and 120.6 mg/dL to 40 mg/dl (Sadhu, Amin, et al. 2008). Austere implementation of control measures (engineering administrative controls, use of respirators, and awareness) in lead-acid storage battery plant have shown beneficial health effects among lead-exposed workers (Kalahasthi, Tapu Barman, et al. 2016).

Musculoskeletal disorders (MSDs) represents one of the major causes of injury and disability in the occupational health setups in developing countries, including India. The primary MSDs dysfunctions include osteoarthritis, inflammatory arthritis (principally, rheumatoid arthritis), osteoporosis and back pain. Despite the enormous global impact, these disorders have not received the attention they deserve by the medical profession, policymakers or the media and are not considered national health priorities. The prevalence of musculoskeletal disorders (MSD) in different occupational settings such as agriculture, handloom industry, small scale sectors such as brick making has been well documented exploring both personal and organizational variables (Das, Ghosh, et al. 2013, Gupta and Tarique 2013, Pandit, Kumar, et al. 2013, Qutubuddin, Hebbal, et al. 2013, Bijetri and Sen 2014, Chakraborty, Das, et al. 2018). Awkward working postures, inadequate working conditions and absence of an effective work safety program has led to a high rate of MSDs with as nearly as 25% of the adult subjects suffering from chronic MSD pain (Bihari, Kesavachandran, et al. 2011). Risk factors of MSDs have included activities such as heavy load lifting, awkward working postures and repetitive tasks (Sett and Sahu 2012), long continuous hours (Singh, Lal et al. 2012), while personal factors (like Body mass index, obesity) and sociodemographic factors (Kar and Dhara 2007) have also known to be critical predictive variables in the leading causes of disability. Special focus has been given to the group of women operators engaged in physical activities in different sectors like farming, textiles, suffering from as high as 91% MSD (Metgud, Khatri, et al. 2008). The musculoskeletal complaints have been prominent in women owing to as long as 8 hours of sitting posture without any backrest. Stooping postures, excessive bending, twisting and overreaching as a result of poorly designed workstation has also lead to decreased efficiency of performance (Ikhar, Deshpande, et al. 2013).

Various studies have evaluated the impact of ergonomic interventions (engineering, administrative or behavioural) in workers in informal and agricultural sectors for the prevention of MSDs in India (Sahu, Chatopadhyaya, et al. 2010, Singh and Arora 2010, Gangopadhyay and Dev 2014, Sain and Meena 2016). Improvement of workstation design by means of low cost modifications that removes unnecessary steps (Gangopadhyay, Das, et al. 2006), implementation of better mechanical tools to relieve muscle strain and respiratory distress (Ghosh and Gangopadhyay 2012), redesign of equipments reducing physical stress and fatigue (Bhattacharyya and Chakrabarti 2012) and improving operator productivity (Chaturvedi, Kumar, et al. 2012) have been some of the few successful interventions. Administrative strategies concentrating on change of duties or job design, such as job rotation, enlargement, work cells, or policies have been recommended. Behavioral (or personal) intervention strategies with focus on increasing fitness, workshops on stress reduction, use of personal protective equipment has also been encouraged. Overall implementation of such appropriate interventions have successfully led to reduced musculoskeletal disorders, improvement in adverse physiological conditions with correction of awkward postures and ultimately, an increase in the organizational productivity.

Apart from these applied interventional strategies, general recommendations for redesigning of workstation according to ergonomic principles such as elevating the height of work tables according to the workers' anthropometric characteristics, using seats which have appropriate backrest, designing adjustable sitting-standing workstations to prevent fixation of posture, assisted lifting in case of heavy load handling specially for women and devise of an appropriate work-rest cycle have also been made (Malikraj, Senthil, et al. 2011).

Noise has been recognized as a hazardous industrial pollutant, leading to traumatic acoustic injury and noise-induced hearing loss (NIHL). Continuous exposure to high noise levels above 90 dBA can result in adverse auditory and non-auditory effects. Exposure to such noise for many years has also revealed to induce biochemical alterations affecting the pituitary-adrenocortical system in man (Rai, Singh, et al. 1981). In India, as opposed to an occupational permissible exposure limit of 8 h time, around 85% of workers actually work for more than 8 h per day with an extra overtime of 2 to 4 h per day (12 to 24 h per week) more than the Occupational Safety and Health Administration (OSHA) norms; (Singh, Bhardwaj et al. 2010), which is a major factor contributing towards high incidence of NIHL in industries such as construction, mining, crushing, printing, drop forging and, iron and steel companies (Nandi and Dhatrak 2008, Singh, Bhardwaj, et al. 2013). In India, by and large NIHL has been incorporated in the Factories Act (1976 amendment) as a notifiable disease and also made compensable but it was only in the year 1996 that the first case of NIHL got compensation.

Lately, considerable concern has also been aroused towards studying the interaction effects of other physical factors like heat and illumination with noise. The combined effect of temperature (35°C) and sound (100 dB) has been shown to cause neuromotor based dysfunctions, decreased accuracy in reasoning ability and speech interference (Singh, Bhardwaj, et al. 2010). Interaction effect of noise and illumination on motor manual and physiological parameters on performance efficiency have also been undertaken.

To contain noise below the recommended level certain safety measures have been carried out which included proper maintenance of motors, agitators, gearboxes, etc., provision of acoustically treated cabins for workers, use of ear defenders (ear plugs, ear muffs and ear canal caps) both by operatives as well as occasional visitors when work practices and engineering controls are not feasible to reduce exposure of noise to safe levels. A complete hearing conservation program, including awareness, training, job rotation and audiometry has been suggested as the most appropriate method for the protection of workers from high noise exposure in occupational setups (Singh, Bhardwaj, et al. 2012).

Lack of proper education and knowledge of the occupational hazards, poor sanitation and nutrition along with climatic proneness of the geographic region further aggravates the health hazards. Many of the developing countries like India are quite far behind in effective implementation of occupational hygiene and pollution control measures at work place. Personal protective equipments for workers are considered as luxuries rather than basic necessities. Casting and forging workers are unavoidingly exposed to a lot of noise, heat, fumes, dust, gas and chemicals among other pollutants. Exposure to these can be considerably reduced by implementation of effective pollution control methods along with use of personal protective equipments by the workers.

CHAPTER 5

Environmental Toxicology

The rapid growth of industrialization with expansion in agricultural practices post-independence has entailed the introduction of a large number of chemicals in the environment, which was relatively free from them. Every year, a huge number of chemicals and synthetic products, new chemical entities (NCEs), engineered nano-materials and GMOs are released into the environment that has resulted in the contamination of habitats at alarming levels which could potentially threaten the existence of life.

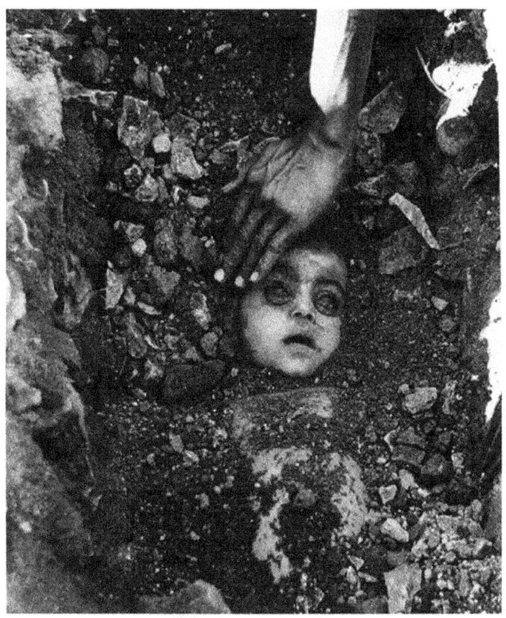

Figure 5.1 Release of 45 tons of methyl isocyanate from insecticide plant resulted in Bhopal Gas Tragedy, on December 3, 1984 taking a toll on thousands of lives and long lasting disabilities. Photograph picked up from Aajtak-daily newspaper, December 3, 1984 edition.
https://aajtak.intoday.in/education/story/main-facts-about-bhopal-gas-tragedy-1984-1-844567.html

Potential adverse impacts of the use of new chemicals on the environment were initially viewed as insignificant as compared to the benefits availed through such practices. The relevance of environmental toxicology to Indian society was specifically realized with the infamous Bhopal Gas Tragedy, a catastrophe on 3rd December 1984, having no parallel in the industry history, in which 45 tons of poisonous methyl isocyanate (MIC) gas escaped from an insecticide plant resulting in the death of thousand people, loss of pregnancy and for few people, incapacitation for life (Figure 5.1). On the basis of the chemical's quantity that released and area of spread (40 sq. km), the Central Water and Air Pollution Control Board estimated that MIC concentration was about 27 ppm, which was approximately 1,400 times than that of the OSHA's workplace standard (0.02 ppm for eight hours) (Dhara and Dhara 2002).

The estimated mortality of this accident was believed to be between 2500 and 5000 people, with up to 2,00,000 injured. Adverse effects included minor eye ailments, throat irritation and cough to pulmonary edema which were the major causes of death, with some casualties due to secondary respiratory infections (bronchitis and bronchial pneumonia and convulsions), followed by cardio-respiratory arrest (Dwivedi, Raizada et al. 1985, Kamat, Mahashur et al. 1985, Jain and Dave 1986, Pandey 1986, Dureja and Saxena 1987, Misra, Nag et al. 1988). The profound impact of the chemical was not only limited to humans but also affected flora and fauna. Moreover, the non-availability of any information pertaining to the toxicity of the parent compound, MIC, was a significant impediment to therapeutic interventions and detoxication measures for immediate effective management of the victims (Sriramachari 2004). There was an urgent need to generate authentic scientific information *de novo*.

The Indian Council of Medical Research (ICMR) acted promptly, launching over 25 research projects, including on pathology, toxicology and pathophysiology of inhalation of toxic gases in collaboration with several institutes (involving Medico-Legal Institute, Bhopal Department of Pathology, M.G.M. College, ICMR-Bhopal Institute of Pathology, S.J. Hospital, AIIMS New Delhi, G.B. Pant Hospital New Delhi, DRDE New Delhi, DIPAS New Delhi, Gwalior INMAS, IIT Madras, CSIR-IICT, Hyderabad and CSIR-IITR, Lucknow). The gas release in Bhopal was not attributed to the mere leakeage of MIC but the presence of multiple chemicals had been demonstrated (Varadarajan, Doraiswamy et al. 1985, D'Silva, Lopes, et al. 1986) revealing the presence of as much as 21 chemicals, including 9 or 10 unidentified compounds (Rao, Saraf, et al. 1991).

Soon thereafter, experimental studies were launched to recapitulate the full spectrum of lung histopathologies, as observed in the human victims, to establish MIC toxicity experimentally, understand its mechanistic basis and more importantly determine necessary antidotes on an emergency basis. As a result of these efforts, including autopsies, toxicological driven studies, management of the victims and several epidemiological investigations, quite a few positive results have been obtained that have aided in unravelling few of the mysteries underlying the disaster (Dhara 1994, Sriramachari 2004, Sriramachari 2005). These multi-disciplinary studies resolved several issues. First, the progression from pulmonary edema to chronic fibrosis was confirmed through experimental studies, subsequent to a single exposure of MIC.

Analysis of the residues in the Tank revealed around 21 chemicals. Apart from MIC and hydrogen cyanide (HCN), many of the chemicals were tracked down to the blood and viscera of the dead and living 'exposees'. The finding of 'cherry-red discoloration' of the lungs, in the preliminary autopsy studies, aroused a suspicion of cyanide toxicity. The prompt therapeutic response to sodium thiosulphate (NaTS) further substantiated this hypothesis. Apart from the cyanide, the discoloration in the lungs, was also demonstrated to result from MIC's binding to end-terminal valine residues of hemoglobin. The presence of N- carbamoylation of numerous other end-terminal amino acids of tissue proteins further confirmed MIC's distribution within the body system.

The studies also revealed that in the case of organic chemicals, not just the parent compound but also their unexpected derivatives and reaction by-products could adversely affect the human population (Sriramachari and Chandra 1997). Recalling the old adage that 'the dead teach the living' this incident was perhaps the first chemical disaster wherein the toxic chemicals were traced back into the victims' body and effective measures for detoxification were evolved. An excellent comprehensive overview of the incidents that took place, the causes behind them and the lessons learned from such occurrences have been documented (Bhardwaj, Chawla, et al 2007). Since then, a paradigm shift has been observed in the government's focus from rescue, relief and restoration-centric approach to planning, preparedness and prevention. A detailed evaluation of even small on-site accidents may be capable of providing useful clues for understanding chemical pathologies without waiting for bigger disasters to happen.

Another incident worth a mention was the Endosulfan disaster in the Kasaragod district in Kerala due to aerial spraying of the pesticide on cashew plantations from 1978. The Plantation Corporation of Kerala (PCK), aerially sprayed endosulfan on the plantations over 12000 acres in 9 villages of Kasaragod district thrice a year in order to eradicate tea mosquitoes (Mahapatro and Panigrahi 2013). Since the very beginning, there were numerous warning signals regarding the impact, including mass deaths of fishes, frogs, bees, birds, foxes and congenital deformities in animals like cows (http://files.panap.net/ resources/endosulfan_report_Kerala.pdf). By 1990s adverse health effects of critical nature among the human population started surfacing the limelight. Children with mental retardation, congenital anomalies, physical deformities, cerebral palsy, epilepsy and hydrocephalus; congenital malformations and abortions in females and dysfunctions related to the male reproductive system started surfacing (http://www.endosulfan.in/wp-content/docs/Endosulfan-KeralaStory.pdf). Between 1998 and 2002, numerous national (NIOH) and international research groups undertook toxicological and health studies; attributing the abnormalities at district Kasaragod to spraying of endosulfan.

After numerous investigations, court cases and public protest, etc., the State of Kerala banned the sale and use of the pesticide within its boundaries in 2003. Since 2007, Endosulfan Relief and Remediation Cells have been operating under the Kasaragod Jilla Panchayath (Local government at the District level) to provide financial and medical relief to the victims. Few other organizations and individuals have also been working for the welfare of the victims. Relief measures are also being provided by a non-profit organization called Solidarity Youth Movement (SYM) and an educational program by the Central Government called as Sarva Shiksha Abhiyan (SSA) that are providing food and medical support through camps and other essential provisions since 2007. The SSA has also initiated a pilot project in the district to mainstream 108 mentally and physically challenged children by conducting weekly meetings, medical and rehabilitative measures (http://www.india environmentportal.org.in/files/IndiaEndosulfan.pdf). Decades of spraying endosulfan on the village has provided an opportunity to analyze its potential impact even after the spraying has stopped. Experimental evidence also points towards academic development (Lakshmana and Raju 1994) and reproductive impairments in males (Sinha, Narayan et al. 1997, Sinha, Adhikari, et al. 2001). Despite its ban, however, endosulfan still continues to be detected in water bodies at levels much higher than the Maximum Residue Limit (MRL) (Jayaprabha and Suresh 2016).

These incidents were a clear reflection of the negligence on the part of the Government in implementing stringent laws for safe use of these chemicals. The only positive outcome was the sensitization of the Government towards the need for generating knowledge on the toxicity of compounds used in industry as well as for drugs and food additives in context of human and environmental health prior to their release in the environmental settings.

The subsequent awakening of the Government and the general public to the hazards of chemicals that were being released in the environment triggered many landmark activities pertaining to environmental protection, as well as the enactment of legislations directed at regulation and limiting the indiscriminate release of chemicals into the environment and with these initiatives the field gained a significant boost. Environmental toxicology, embracing both the disciplines of classical toxicology and ecotoxicology stands as a scientific study evaluating the potential effects of both natural and anthropogenic compounds on living organisms, populations and the ecosystem.

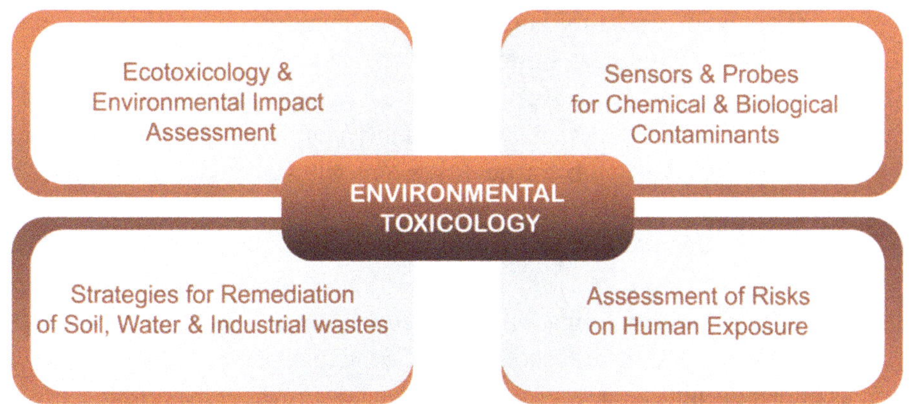

Figure 5.2 Approaches applied for Environmental Toxicology in India

In contrast, ecotoxicology revolves around the study of the potential adverse effects of toxins on a myriad of organisms that compose the ecosystems ranging from simple microorganisms to top predators. The various classes of environmental stressors have been recognized as metals, pesticides, aromatic and aliphatic hydrocarbons, radiations, particulates, volatile organic compounds, nanoparticles, cosmeceuticals (cosmetic care products), biological agents such as mycotoxins and bacterial toxins and more recently pharmaceutical agents and endocrine disruptors. Appropriate regulations pertaining to the release of chemicals into the environment has required a comprehensive knowledge of the toxic properties and potential consequences of their release into the environment. However, the main challenge in this area has been to create reliable and efficient ways to predict fate, behavior and toxic potency in the environment and exposure levels for such chemicals which lack toxicological knowledge and exposure information under environmental settings. These issues have been addressed by exploring various cellular, genetic and organismal approaches for detection and quantification of several environmental pollutants. Over the years, sensitive probes and sensors for detection of biological contaminants from multiple matrices have been developed. Protocols for ecotoxicological analysis of effluents using biological species, safety evaluation of polymers and plastics and screening of the immunotoxic, reproductive, neurotoxic, phototoxic, genotoxic, carcinogenic and mutagenic effects of chemicals have been developed. Novel strategies for remediation/mitigation of persistent hazardous chemical substances of soil, water and industrial wastes along with ecotoxicity and environmental impact assessment have been undertaken (Figure 5.2).

Several national regulatory bodies such as Central Pollution Control Board (CPCB), 1974; Environment Protection Act (EPA), 1986; Bureau of Indian Standards (BIS), 1986 have been established as apex organizations that are running nationwide air, water, and noise quality/control programs to determine the status and trends of ambient quality along with ascertaining whether the prescribed ambient quality standards are within limits. Institutes like CSIR-IITR and CSIR-National Engineering and Education Research Institute (CSIR-NEERI), Indian Institute of Technology (IITs) and other institutes are actively engaged in regular monitoring of air/water/soil quality in different cities in order to analyze the risk exposure of such contaminants on the ecosystem as well as human health.

Air pollution through the release of particulate contaminants into the ambient air through industrial effluents, burning of crude oil, coal, vehicle exhaust and household fuels (Kumari, Attri, et al. 2013, Rizwan, Nongkynrih, et al. 2013, Guttikunda, Goel, et al. 2014) etc. leading to deterioration of air quality, have raised serious concerns of potential health hazards to not only human health but also ecological health of a region (Pandey, Khan, et al. 2002, Srivastava 2004, Srivastava, Joseph, et al. 2005). Ambient air quality monitoring (based on selection of pollutants, measurement methods, sampling duration and frequency etc.) carried out at 262 towns/cities in the country, under the National Air Monitoring Programme (NAMP) initiated in 1984, provides information on air quality that forms the basis for identification of areas which have high air pollution levels and subsequently, for formulation of strategies and prioritizing actions for improving air quality. Assessment of the magnitude for air pollution risks to human health has been primarily carried out by determination of four crucial parameters which are inhalable particulates (Suspended Particulate Matter SPM and Respirable Suspended Particulate Matter (RSPM/PM_{10}/$PM_{2.5}$), metals in particulates and polycyclic aromatic hydrocarbons (PAHs) along with the gaseous pollutants and volatile organic compounds. Studies have focused on "pollution hot spots" such as traffic, industrial and commercial sites representing a holistic view of distribution, spatiotemporal variation and source apportionment of metallic species, seasonal variations and their chemical characterization along with an assessment of potential health risks to the exposed population (Gupta, Patil et al. 2004, Talapatra and Srivastava 2011, Chaudhari, Gupta, et al. 2012, Rizwan, Nongkynrih, et al. 2013, Banerjee, Murari, et al. 2015, Pant, Guttikunda, et al. 2016, Kaushik, Chel, et al. 2018, Rastogi, Singh, et al. 2019) (Table 5.1).

Table 5.1 Assessment of the magnitude of air pollution in different cities of India

City/Area	Findings	References
Kanpur	PM10 (45–589 mg/m^3), PM2.5 (25–200 mg/m^3), BSOF (1–170 mg/m^3), heavy metals were at highest concentration at commercial site followed by residential site and control site, similar to PM10 and PM2.5, heavy metals were approx 5–10 times more than the levels in European cities	(Sharma and Maloo 2005)
Kolkata	The average concentrations (24 h) of Cr, Zn, Pb, Cd, Ni, Mn and Fe from PM_{10} particulate samples were 6.9, 506.1, 79.1, 3.3, 7.4, 2.4 and 103.6 ng/m^3, respectively, 24 h average PM_{10} concentration exceeded national ambient air quality standard (NAAQS) at both residential (140.1 µg/m^3) and industrial areas (196.6 µg/m^3)	(Karar and Gupta 2006)
	PM_{10} mass concentrations found at residential site (68.2 to 280.6 µg/m$^{3)}$ due to solid waste dumping, coal combustion, vehicular emission, cooking and soil dust and at the industrial site (62.4 to 401.2 µg/m^3) due to vehicular emissions, electroplating industry, coal combustion, tyre wear and secondary aerosol	(Karar and Gupta 2007)
Hyderabad	Highest pollution was from resuspended dust (40%), then vehicular pollution (22%), combustion (12%), industrial (9%) and refuse burning (7%) in PM_{10}; while in $PM_{2.5}$ vehicular pollution was highest (31%) followed by resuspended dust (26%), combustion (9%), industrial (7%) and refuse burning (6%)	(Gummeneni, Yusup et al. 2011)
Lucknow	The concentration of PM_{10} (107.6-237.8 µg/m^3) in the air was almost double than the NAAQS, correlation with high concentrations of Fe, Mn and Mg	(Sharma, Singh, et al. 2006)
	The PM_{10} concentration in Lucknow city at 4 locations in three different seasons ranged between 148.6–210.8 µg/m^3 during summer, 111.8–187.6 µg/m^3 during monsoon and 199.3–308.8 µg/m^3 during winter while $PM_{2.5}$ ranged between 32.4–67.2 µg/m^3, 25.6–68.9 µg/m^3 and 99.3–299.3 µg/m^3 during respective seasons, mass fraction ratio of $PM_{2.5}$ ranged between 0.22–0.92 µg/m^3 and was significantly high during winter season	(Pandey, Khan, et al. 2012)
Delhi	The annual mean PM_{10} and $PM_{2.5}$ concentrations were about 219 (± 84) and 97 (±56) µgm^3 respectively, about twice the prescribed NAAQS values, the analyzed coarse fractions mainly composed of secondary inorganic aerosols species (16.0 µgm^3, 13.07%), mineral matter (12.32 µgm^3, 10.06%) and salt particles (4.92 µgm^3, 4.02%)	(Tiwari, Srivastava, et al. 2009)

Contd...

City/Area	Findings	References
	Mean annual 24–h PM_{10} levels varied from 166.5-192.3 µg m^3 at the residential sites (8–10 times of the WHO limit), identified three major sources: crustal (49–65%), vehicular (27–31%) and industrial (4–21%)	(Khillare and Sarkar 2012)
Chennai	$PM_{2.5}$ values varied between 27.2-190.2 µg/m^3, average concentration of particle-associated PAHs was from 325.7-790.8 ng/m^3 in the urban environment due to vehicular emissions as probable sources	(Mohanraj, Solaraj, et al. 2011)
Agra (Indo-gangetic plain)	$PM_{2.5}$ between 8.4-300 µg m^3 with 55% of the values exceeding the 24 h average NAAQS, particle associated total PAHs (8.9-2065 ng/m^3), benzo[a]pyrene was the dominant PAH contributor (3.64%)	(Dubey, Kumari, et al. 2015)
Raipur	The annual average concentrations for PM_{10}, $PM_{2.5-10}$, $PM_{2.5}$, and PM_1 were 270.5±105.5, 119.6±44.6, 150.9 ± 78.6, and 72.5 ± 39.0 µg/m^3, respectively which were above the annual NAAQS of 60 and 40 µg/m^3 for PM_{10} and $PM_{2.5}$, respectively, concentrations in winter were higher than summer and monsoon	(Deshmukh, Deb, et al. 2013)
Pune	The average concentration of $PM_{2.5}$ and PM_{10} were 89.7 ± 43.2 µg m^3 and 138.2 ± 68.2 µg m^3 at urban site, 197.5 ± 84.3 and 287 ± 92 µg m^3 at rural site in indoor environments, concentrations of crustal metals were greater than carcinogenic metals, among the carcinogenic metals, Ni showed highest cancer risk supported by *in-silico* studies suggestive of Ni forming co-ordination complex with histone proteins	(Satsangi, Yadav, et al. 2014)
Indian Subcontinent	1.4 billion people are exposed to pollution that exceed the World Health Organization's highest annual air quality threshold of 35 µg/m^3, while another 13% and 18% are exposed in the ranges 25–35 and 15–25 µg/m^3 respectively, in many regions, the high-levels of pollution are persistent rather than episodic, $PM_{2.5}$ concentrations in the rural areas of the Indo-Gangetic Basin are higher than many urban centers in peninsular India, five hotspots (where $PM_{2.5}$ increases by >15 µg m^3 over the ten-year period) were identified, which cover parts of the eleven Indian states	(Dey, Di Girolamo, et al. 2012)
Mumbai	High concentrations of SPM observed at traffic junctions, quantitative estimation by FA-MR model indicated that road dust contributed to 41%, vehicular emissions to 15%, marine aerosols to 15%, metal industries to 6% and coal combustion to 6% of the SPM observed at Sakinaka traffic junction	(Kumar, Patil, et al. 2001)

The extent to which airborne particles are able to penetrate the human respiratory system is majorly determined by the size of the penetrating particles (Balachandran, Meena, et al. 2000). These findings have emphasized the importance of monitoring the ambient air particulates; PM_{10} (thoracic particles) and its fractions, $PM_{2.5-10}$ (coarse particles), $PM_{2.5}$ (fine particles), and PM_1 (submicron particles). Data generated over the years reveal that these air pollutants fail to meet the guidelines for safe levels despite the implementation of fuel policies at many locations (Chaudhari, Gupta, et al. 2012). 140 out of 176 cities in 2010 were found to exceed the $PM_{2.5}$ NAAQS standard values (Gargava and Rajagopalan 2016). Critical sources of PM in India have included vehicles, industries, power plants (coal combustion), construction, dust, biomass combustion (for cooking and heating) and waste burning (Srimuruganandam and Nagendra 2012, Pant, Guttikunda, et al. 2016). Within India, few cities and the Indo-Gangetic basin have been identified as areas with the most severe air pollution (Ram and Sarin 2011, Dey, Di Girolamo, et al. 2012, Guttikunda, Goel, et al. 2014). In 2011, the CPCB had released a six-city source apportionment study, the first of its kind which included characterization of ambient PM as well as the sources (CPCB 2010, Patil, Kumar, et al. 2013). However, a majority of source apportionment studies in India have been focusing on the SPM or PM_{10} with a few number of studies on $PM_{2.5}$ and PM_1.

PM constituents' concentrations (e.g., metals, PAHs) have been documented to be very high in few cases, and many toxic metals (including Pb, Cu, Zn and Ba) have been reported to be highly water soluble (Yadav and Satsangi 2013). Studies have also reported the enrichment of elements that are associated with anthropogenic emissions in PM_{10} and $PM_{2.5}$ (Shridhar, Khillare, et al. 2010, Sudheer and Rengarajan 2012, Pant, Shukla, et al. 2015). Polyaromatic hydrocarbons (PAHs), ubiquitous constituents of airborne particulate, known to elicit lung carcinogenicity, have been identified in emissions from automobile exhaust (Yadav, Prasad, et al. 2010, Pandey, Patel, et al. 2013) and biomass fuel combustion (Kulkarni and Venkataraman 2000, Awasthi, Singh, et al. 2010) posing a potential risk to both urban and rural settings. PAHs in major cities like Delhi, Kanpur, Ahmedabad, Mumbai, and Kolkata have been reported to be 10–50 times higher than the standard limits set by regulatory agencies (Mohanraj and Azeez 2003), Further carcinogenic metals like chromium and cadmium bound to these respirable particles have been predictive of respiratory, cardiovascular mortality and high cancer risks among the exposed populations (Pandey, Patel, et al. 2013).

Indoor air pollution especially household air pollution (HAP) is one of the critical public health issues in India, specifically in the rural and semi-urban areas where the number of households that use solid fuel (wood, cow dung, kerosene) is quite high and ventilation is poor (Balakrishnan, Sambandam et al.

2004, Balakrishnan, Ghosh, et al. 2013). HAP, particularly the pollutants that are generated by the combustion of wood/biomass has been the subject of numerous studies, and detailed assessments have been conducted to analyze the profile of compounds and estimate the risk of exposure to wood/biomass smoke in causing adverse health effects (Dherani 2003, Bhargava, Khanna, et al. 2004, Sukhsohale, Narlawar, et al. 2013). HAP has been shown to be an essential contributor to ambient $PM_{2.5}$, high concentrations of PAHs, carcinogenic compounds, VOCs and metals especially in rural areas where wood/biomass and dung are utilized for cooking and heating (Pandit, Srivastava, et al. 2001, Rehman, Ahmed, et al. 2011, Satsangi, Yadav, et al. 2014). Pant, et al 2016 have concisely reviewed the pollution exposure concentrations, trends, and the associated health effects of air pollution in different cities of India providing an excellent account of the various epidemiological studies related to particulate matter exposure in different urban and rural settings, household, school and transport micro-environments (Pant, Guttikunda, et al. 2016).

Amid increasing concerns over rising air pollution, the Government of India has taken several initiatives to curb vehicular emission, adopt emission norms and fuel regulation standards, reduce dependence on biomass fuel and launch the National 'Air Quality Index'. The Comprehensive Environmental Pollution Index (CEPI) proposed by the CPCB has identified a total of 88 polluted industrial areas to monitor them centrally in order to improve their environmental components such as air and water quality data, ecological damage, and visual environmental conditions (http://cpcb.nic.in/displaypdf. php?id=Q1BBL05ld0l0ZW1fMTUyX0ZpbmFsLUJvb2tfMi5wZGY=). There have been several other significant improvements in the monitoring of ambient air pollution, and launch of few programs such as SAFAR (System of Air Quality Weather Forecasting and Research) which is helping in improving our understanding of ambient air pollution (Trivedi, Ali, et al. 2014). More recently, the India-California Air Pollution Mitigation Programme has been initiated for abatement of air pollution from the transportation sector (Ramanathan, Sundar, et al. 2014). Modelling of 10-year trends (1998-2007) for PM_{10} and toxic heavy metal concentrations in four cities (Delhi, Mumbai, Kolkata and Chennai) have shown improvement of urban air quality due to many interventions that have been conducted such as, changes in quality of fuel, improved vehicle technologies, better industrial fuel mix and shift of industries in the outer city limits. Application of face mask as a tool to diminish the particulate matter has been suggested as one of the simplest ways to prevent the deleterious effects (Singh, Singh, et al. 2010).

In India, water pollution has attained an alarming magnitude during the past few decades due to unmanaged human activities like indiscriminate disposal of sewage, untreated industrial waste and oil spills leading to disease outbreaks

(Fatima and Ahmad 2006, Dwivedi, Mishra et al. 2018, Govil and Krishna 2018, Laxmi Mohanta, Naz, et al. 2019). In India, approximately 90% of wastewater is discharged without treatment serving as major conduits for accumulations and distribution of toxic agents, thus requiring regular assessment. Monitoring and evaluation of water quality in residential, commercial and industrial areas have been mainly done for parameters of bacteriological quality (Ramteke, Bhattacharjee, et al. 1992, Grover and Thakur 2001, Pathak and Gopal 2008), physicochemical (Jameel 2002, Beg and Ali 2008, Malik, Verma, et al. 2011), heavy metals (Dixit, Verma, et al. 2003, Kaushik, Kansal, et al. 2009, Paul 2017, Giri and Singh 2019, Ravindra and Mor 2019, Siddiqui and Pandey 2019) and pesticide residue analysis (Sankararamakrishnan, Sharma, et al. 2005, Singh, Malik, et al. 2005, Mudiam, Pathak, et al. 2012, Thokchom and Thacker 2019). These contaminants have found their way into Indian rivers and soil sediments and ultimately into various food products Singh, Kapoor, et al. 1996, Raj, Patnaik, et al. 2006, Abhilash and Singh 2009). Pesticide residue analysis has been undertaken on several other food products (Dikshith, Kumar, et al. 1989, Srivastava, Budhwar, et al. 2001, Shetty 2004, Rajashekar 2005, Bhanti and Taneja 2007, Pandey, Raizada, et al. 2010, Bedi, Gill, et al. 2018, Sharma, Nagpal, et al. 2018).

Pesticide residues on the food commodities are monitored by the All India Coordinated Research Project on Pesticide Residues under the Indian Council of Agricultural Research, New Delhi, through their different centers that are located in parts of the country. In one study, 51% of food commodities were found to be contaminated with residues of pesticides and 20% of these had residues well above the MRL values, in comparison to 21% contamination with just 2% above the MRL values on a worldwide basis. High content of pesticide residues were also found in bottled water, colas, and other soft drinks (Gupta 2004). The increased popularity of herbal medicines has also brought concerns and fears over the quality, efficacy and safety of the raw materials. Such widespread use of metals and pesticides has also become a possible source of contamination of herbal ayurvedic preparations such as tonics, drugs, herbal teas, spices toiletries and cosmetics, detected above the WHO permissible limits (Srivastava, Gupta, et al. 2000, Naithani and Kakkar 2006, Naithani and Kakkar 2006, Srivastava, Kumar, et al. 2006, Rai, Kakkar, et al. 2008).

Innumerable studies have emphasized high incidence of multiple anti-microbial resistant enterotoxigenic *E. coli* (ETEC), *Enterococcus spp.* (indicator of fecal contamination) and *Salmonella spp.* in surface and drinking water (Ram, Vajpayee, et al. 2007, Lata, Ram, et al. 2009, Jyoti, Ram, et al. 2010, Patel, Vajpayee, et al. 2011, Kumar, Tripathi, et al. 2012, Mudiam, Pathak, et al. 2012, Chandra, Saxena, et al. 2016, Dheenan, Jha, et al. 2016, Rahman and Singh 2018). More recently, 'emerging contaminants' have gained importance in view of their accelerated release into the environment with limited information regarding their occurrence, fate and impact in the environment. Emerging contaminants of main concern include endocrine disrupting chemicals (EDCs: bisphenol A, polychloride biphenyls, phthalates, parabens and dioxins), pharmaceuticals active compounds (PACs) and personal care products (PCPs). Several studies on the distribution and contamination level and risk assessment of emerging contaminants such as pharmaceuticals (antiepileptic drugs, antimicrobials, anti-inflammatory drugs), estrogenic compounds (aldrin, Dialdrin), personal care products, phenolic compounds and phthalate esters in soils and rivers, some for the first time in Indian rivers, have been carried out (Shanmugam, Sampath, et al. 2014, Selvaraj, Sundaramoorthy, et al. 2015, Balakrishna, Rath et al. 2017, Philip, Aravind, et al. 2018, Vimalkumar, Arun, et al. 2018, Chakraborty, Sampath, et al. 2019, Sharma, Bečanová et al. 2019).

The impact of these pollutants on soil, water and ecosystems have been addressed by studying the transport, distribution, fate and toxicant interactions with various biotic and abiotic components that may be affected by several processes such as sorption, bioaccumulation, degradation, retention that are influenced by multiple factors such as the contaminant's physicochemical properties, environmental conditions and patterns of chemical discharge (Yadav, Patel et al. 2018). Agricultural chemicals, specifically halogenated organic compounds, are quite recalcitrant to metabolism and persist in the soil and water as contaminants. In such a scenario, they may enter the biologic food chains and gradually move to higher trophic levels or even persist in processed crops. Majority of the chlorinated pesticides, being non-degradable leave residues in living systems for extended periods of their life span leading to a variety of known and unknown toxic effects. Even when they are present in very minute quantities, they elicit adverse effects on birds, fish, and trees to which welfare of humans is inseparably bound (Gupta 2004).

Application of stringent regulations and growing public awareness on environmental issues eventually necessitated the need to monitor and quantify the more comprehensive range of analytes in air, water and soil, and to do so with higher frequency and accuracy. Although highly selective and sensitive, the traditional analysis methods (bioassays, chromatographic techniques) have been expensive, time-consuming and laborious when a high number of samples need to be screened (Bhatnagar and Minocha 2006, Verma and Bhardwaj 2015). To this end, biosensors and molecular probes have attracted much attention in the past few decades as promising bio tools, complementary and/or alternative to conventional analysis techniques, for simple, economical, fast and reliable field-portable toxicity detection and screening. Several biological recognition elements, such as cofactors, enzymes, antibodies, microorganisms have been employed in the fabrication of biosensors further classified based on the physicochemical properties of transducers applied for the toxicants' detection (e.g., optical, electrochemical, piezoelectrical, thermal or calorimetric) that offer quick and sensitive detection of toxicants in different matrices (Table 5.2). Among all the parameters used to assess the pollution load of water bodies/waste-waters, the biochemical oxygen demand (BOD) has been one of the most important and widely used benchmarks in the measurement of organic pollution. The traditional BOD measurement requires 3–5 days whereas a novel microbial based BOD sensor has been capable of sensing the load for a wide variety of synthetic and industrial wastewaters which have low to high biodegradability within few minutes with a lower detection limit of 1.0 mg/l BOD (Rastogi, Rathee et al. 2003).

Table 5.2 Different types of sensors developed and employed for detection of environmental contaminants in India

Analytes	Biosensing elements	Transducers	Samples	References
Metals				
Cadmium and Lead	Urease immobilized polypyrrole/ multi-walled carbon nanotubes	Electrochemical	Standard samples Detection limit 1-10 mM	(Meshram, Kondawar, et al. 2014)
Nickel Ions	*Bacillus sphaericus*	Potentiometer	Industrial effluents and food (Range of detection 0.03–0.68 nM (0.002–0.04 ppb) with a response time of 1.5 minutes)	(Verma and Singh 2006)
Mercury, cadmium, and arsenic	Urease enzyme	Electrochemical	Standard solutions	(Pal, Bhatta-charyay, et al. 2009)
Cadmium, lead and mercury	Pyrrole/ chitosan/ITO/Ag coated probe	Optical fiber surface plasmon resonance (SPR)	Contaminated water	(Verma and Gupta 2015)
Lead	Urea linker based tetrapodal receptor	Electrochemical	Aqueous medium limit of detection as 1.56 μM	(Mishra, Kaur, et al. 2019)
Urea	*Bacillus sp.,*	Potentiometric	milk	(Verma and Singh 2003)
Pesticides				
Methyl parathion	*Sphingomonas sp.*	Optical	Detection limit 4-80 μm. Response time 5 minutes	(Kumar and D'Souza 2010)

Contd...

Analytes	Biosensing elements	Transducers	Samples	References
Pesticides				
Lindane	*Escherichia coli.*	Electrochemical	Parts per million concentration range 2 to 45 ppm	(Anu Prathap, Chaurasia, et al. 2012)
Malathion	Aptamer conjugated with gold nanoparticle	Chemilum-insence	Detection limit as low as 0.06 ppm	(Bala, Kumar, et al. 2016)
Herbicides				
p-nitrophenol	*Pseudomonas putida*	Electrochemical	Range of concentration (10–50 µM) with varying pH (7.5–8.5) and temperature (25–40 ◦C) in short response time (7.0 min)	(Banik, Prakash, et al. 2008)
Diuron	Hapten-functionalized carbon nanotubes	Electrochemical	Water Detection limit of 0.1 pg ml^{-1}	(Sharma, Sablok, et al. 2011)
2,4-dichlorophenoxy acetic acid	Gold nanoparticles	Chemiluminescence.	Standard water samples Fast screening methodology (<30 min) with detection limit 3 ng ml^{-1}	(Boro, Kaushal, et al. 2011)
Biological contaminants				
Detection of capsular Vi polysaccharide of Salmonella enteric	Gold nanoparticles based immuno-bioprobe	Immunoassay	Water sensitivity of up to 10^2 cells ml^{-1}	(Pandey, Suri, et al. 2012)
M. tuberculosis	Nucleic acid sensor	Bio electrode based on surface plasmon-resonance	Detection of one base mismatch. Better detection limit (1.0 ng ml^{-1})	(Prabhakar, Arora, et al. 2008)

Several simple, sensitive high-throughput ultra-performance bioanalytical methods (chromatography and spectrometry-based methods) have also been developed and validated for simultaneous extraction and analysis of different categories of pollutants such as pesticides (pyrethroids), metals (arsenic, lead and mercury) and drugs (Ramesh and Ravi 2004, Srivastava, Trivedi, et al. 2011, Mudiam, Jain, et al. 2012, Srivastava, Rai, et al. 2014, Jain, Gupta, et al. 2015, Singh, Dwivedi et al. 2016, Wahajuddin, Singh, et al. 2016) in different matrices (environmental and biological materials). An economical and fast multi-residue method has been developed utilizing quick, easy, cheap, effective, rugged and safe (QuEChERS) procedure in combination with dispersive liquid-liquid microextraction (DLLME) for the quantitative determination of 36 multiclass, multi-residue pesticides (13 organochlorines, 12 synthetic pyrethroids and 11 organophosphates) in various vegetables and fruits. With a limit of detection in the range of 0.001–0.010 mg kg^{-1} this method may be more economical, time-saving replacement to the existing chemical processes, without losing its analytical efficiency (Rai, Singh, et al. 2016). Novel polymers have also been imprinted that have enabled sensitive and efficient extraction of toxic metabolites in different samples (Mudiam and Ratnasekhar 2013, Bhatia, Gupta, et al. 2016, Khan, Bhatia, et al. 2016, Tripathy, Saha, et al. 2016, Tripathy, Saha, et al. 2017). These methods are holding promising applications in the routine analysis of different environmental and biological samples in the industry.

Conventional techniques like culture-based methods routinely used for decades for identification and detection of pathogens have been replaced with more sensitive molecular, nano and bioinformatic based tools (Shanker, Singh, et al. 2014). High throughput molecular probes have aided culture free detection and enumeration of pathotypes of water and food quality 'indicator' bacteria (Patel, Vajpayee, et al. 2011, Ram, Vajpayee, et al. 2011). Keeping in view the observed surface and potable water contamination, it can be reasoned that detection and accurate identification of pathogens at an early stage to circumvent disease spread and epidemics is imperative. The development of a comprehensive database of molecular fingerprints for early accurate detection could help in unraveling the persistence. In this regard, very recently, DNA aptamers for capture and detection of very low doses of *Salmonella typhimurium* and *Salmonella enterica* (major foodborne pathogen) using a whole cell SELEX approach utilizing biofiltration strategies in designed and real-life complex matrices have also been demonstrated (Joshi, Janagama, et al. 2009, Dwivedi, Smiley, et al. 2010, Singh, Vajpayee, et al. 2012). The potential of *in-silico* amplification of target genes prior to optimization of the designed real-time PCR array for culture-independent quantitative enumeration of fecal coliforms in water has been successfully determined (Patel, Vajpayee, et al. 2011). The feasibility of "spot and read" colorimetric detection of nucleic acid signatures of Enterohemorrhagic and Enterotoxigenic *Escherichia coli* utilizing gold nanoparticles probes has also been successfully achieved (Jyoti, Singh, et al. 2011). Recently, a transgenic zebrafish model (*Danio rerio*) employing metallothionein reporter gene and DsRed2 reporter gene for detection of cadmium and zinc has been developed for preliminary monitoring toxicity in aquatic systems that may provide a response more comparable to eukaryotic systems than microbial based sensors (Pawar, Gireesh-Babu, et al. 2016).

Persistent organic pollutants (POPs) are notorious chemical substances adversely afflicting public health and the environment, owing to their persistence, recalcitrancy, bioaccumulation and biomagnification potential, thus posing a toxicological threat to environmental health. Practices to detoxify persistent pollutants pesticides have relied on chemical treatment (soil washing, vitrification, flocculation, carbon adsorption), incineration, and landfills, which are economically restrictive. Bioremediation, the removal of environmental pollutants by living organisms (such as plants and microbes), has become a viable and promising means of restoring contaminated sites. To this end, various institutes in India have made great strides in implementing bioremediation approaches using plants and microbes to mitigate/eradicate pollutants at numerous contaminated sites, the scope of bioremediation extending to inorganics viz., mercury, arsenic, fluoride, chromium, cyanide, fly ash disposed sites, abandoned mines, e-waste, developing phytotreatment technologies, construction of wetlands for wastewater treatment, biological permeable barriers; and organics viz., pesticides, petroleum hydrocarbons, explosives and nuclear power waste (Vajpayee, Rai, et al. 1995, Gupta, Srivastava, et al. 2001, Ajmal, Rao, et al. 2003, Bishnoi, Bajaj, et al. 2004, Khan and Ahmad 2006, Singh and Tripathi 2007, Bhatnagar and Kumari 2013, Singh, Kaur, et al. 2014, Banerjee, Pandey, et al. 2015, Bhattacharya and Khare 2016, Bhattacharya and Khare 2017, Bhattacharya, Naik, et al. 2018, Bhattacharya, Naik, et al. 2019). Many bacterial strains have been isolated and identified from contaminated and uncontaminated soil for their ability to transform, degrade or utilize the chemical as an energy source. Several bacterial species demonstrating biodegradative capabilities for persistent pollutants like HCH isomers (Kumari, Subudhi, et al. 2002, Manickam, Misra et al. 2007, Manickam, Reddy, et al. 2008, Manickam, Bajaj, et al. 2012), DDT residues (Kale, Murthy, et al. 1999, Bajaj, Mayilraj, et al. 2014) and endosulfan (Awasthi, Kumar, et al. 1999, Bajaj, Pathak, et al. 2010) and PAHs (Tiwari, Manickam, et al. 2016) have also been reported in literature suggestive of their utilization at contaminated sites.

Researchers have reported the concept of 'bacterial consortia' utilizing native and genetically engineered (GE) bacteria which contain a mixture of detoxification isozymes which can activate degradation of a broad range of recalcitrant compounds through natural microflora. Application of GE bacteria for bioremediation has come into the forefront due to its selective nature of transformation, detoxification and removal of toxicants and thus, posing lesser health hazards as compared to physicochemical methods (Singh, Abhilash, et al. 2011). Microbial genes have been reshuffled or tailored for creating novel metabolic routes, expansion of substrate ranges for degradation pathways, increasing the stability of catabolic activities in adverse conditions, and increasing the pollutants' bioavailability to the bacteria, etc., to enhance the biodegradation process, the ultimate concern for environmental toxicology (Kapley, Purohit, et al. 1999).

PCR based approaches have further paved the way for characterization of the catabolic genes involved in transformation such as LinC, LinB (Manickam, Misra, et al. 2007). Use of microarray technologies has aided in the detection of metabolic profiles and phylogenetic diversity of microbial communities from polluted sites based on their 16S rDNA sequence data to predict the behavior of microbial community which could be further used for generating genus-specific probes (Manickam, Pathak, et al. 2010). Pathak, et al. 2011 have described the development and application of a novel functional and 16S rRNA gene microarray which comprises of 60-mer oligonucleotide probes. This hybrid array named as "BiodegPhyloChip" consisting of 14,327 unique probes which have been derived from 1,057 biodegradative genes and 880 probes which represent 110 phylogenetic genes from diverse bacterial communities that are involved in the bio-transformation of 133 chemical contaminants has enabled the assessment of the biodegradative/functional capacities and bacterial diversity of five different contaminated ecosystems. The microarray has been validated utilizing DNAs of well-characterized pure culture strains and environmental DNA aiding in the successful application of the microarray to explore the genetic capabilities and microbial communities in real toxic environmental samples (Pathak, Shanker, et al. 2011). Homology modeling and docking studies have been further employed to analyze the active site residues of microbial enzyme biphenyl deoxygenase from *Comamonas testosteroni* B-356, involved in the degradation of chlorinated biphenyls, to identify their functions in the activity and substrate specificity, which could ultimately lead to better mutants with enhanced activity (Baig and Manickam 2010).

Based on the data collection and environmental analysis of World Bank experts, from 1995 to 2010, India has made a lot of progress, in addressing its environment related issues and improving the quality (World Bank data, https://data.worldbank.org/country/india). Biomonitoring tools (e.g., bioassays, biosensors and biomarkers) have demonstrated great potential in increasing confidence in the risk assessment of both regulated and emerging chemical pollutants in biotic and abiotic systems. Protocols for toxicity evaluation of effluents employing biological species such as bacterial and plant-based assays to the application of non-invertebrates or lower vertebrates have all been included for routine risk assessment procedures.

The aquatic system is considered to be an ultimate sink of toxicants and since aquatic plants and animals tend to accumulate pollutants from several sources such as soil sediments, erosion and runoff, air depositions of dust and aerosol, and wastewater discharges they provide ample insights into toxicity mechanisms induced by these chemicals. Bioassays have widely been undertaken on industrial effluents and other toxicants on freshwater fishes

(Kumar, Sahay, et al. 1995, Kumar, Nagpure, et al. 2010, Nwani, Lakra, et al. 2010, Awasthi, Ratn, et al. 2018) reporting a wide variety of toxicological effects in economically important fishes. To this end, the fish *C. catla* has been demonstrated to be a suitable aquatic biomonitoring species of polluted water bodies. Several cytogenetic techniques such as chromosome aberration assay, sister chromatid exchanges, erythrocyte micronucleus assay and comet assay have been routinely employed for monitoring the effects of pollutants as well as radiations in the aquatic ecosystem due to their simplicity, sensitivity and reliability for detecting DNA damage (Anbumani and Mohankumar 2012, Arunachalam, Annamalai, et al. 2013, Anbumani and Mohankumar 2015).

Plant-based bioassays have also gained popularity among the toxicological/eco-toxicological evaluation methods owing to their relative sensitivity, simplicity and cost-effectiveness and good correlation with numerous other toxicity tests (Fatima and Ahmad 2005, Fatima and Ahmad 2006). Tests using plant models have been successfully developed and standardized for monitoring of several water bodies of India, and to assess the toxicity of environmental contaminants. Indian contributions of development of plant systems to assess genotoxic effects of metals has been concisely reviewed (Patra, Bhowmik, et al. 2004). Safety evaluation of genotoxicity of plant-based drug systems has been carried out. Utilization of two plant based bioassays, i.e. *Allium cepa* test and seed germination test for monitoring of the toxicity/genotoxicity of industrial wastewater and river water and standardization with the common contaminants in Indian waters such as pesticides, heavy metals, and phenolics are being carried out. Biomarkers have been incorporated in routine monitoring of aquatic systems for screening for toxicity. EROD derived from *Allium cepa* has been routinely employed as a potential biomarker for the presence of few pesticides in water, and metallothioneins has been used as a marker of heavy metal exposure (Siddiqui, Tabrez, et al. 2011, Tabrez and Ahmad 2011, Tabrez, Shakil, et al. 2011).

Various other bioassays (Ames testing, *E. coli* survival assay, comet assay and plasmid nicking assays) have also found wide applications for mutagenicity testing data on different Indian surface waters and major rivers for pollutants heavy metals, nitrates, pesticides, phenolics that has been concisely summarized (Tabrez, Shakil et al. 2011). One study has affirmed the feasibility of using plasmid nicking assay (*in vitro* system) and two *in-vivo* assays, i.e. the survival pattern of *E. coli* K-12 repair defective mutants and the λ-prophage induction test for monitoring of water bodies of India which have shown more sensitivity as compared to already established models (Siddiqui, Tabrez et al. 2011). The efficacy of these defective mutants in estimating the genotoxicity of industrial waste and surface waters have been established by other research groups as well (Malik and Ahmad 1995, Aleem and Malik 2003, Aleem and Malik 2005, Alam, Ahmad, et al. 2010).

Majority of the toxicity testing systems for environmental pollutants have heavily relied on small mammals such as mice and rats and, which are time-consuming, expensive, and attract ethical criticism (Fatima and Ahmad 2006). The demand for high-throughput toxicity testing systems, along with ethical concerns have necessitated the pursuit of better ecotoxicological tools. Mammalian model systems have remained at the forefront of toxicity studies for predicting the adverse effects of chemicals and mechanism of action owing to their proximity to humans. In this context, use of alternative animal models like invertebrates or lower vertebrates having similarity to higher organisms, such as *Drosophila melanogaster*, Zebrafish (*Danio rerio*), and *Caenorhabditis elegans* have been proposed for risk assessment studies for information on xenobiotic-induced effects and are amenable to reduction and refinement alternatives (Table 5.3). Their evolutionarily conserved biology, well-understood genetics and development, low cost, small generation times, ease of genetic manipulation, and the potential to be used in high-throughput screening have enabled their widespread application for ecotoxicity screening. Multiple toxicity endpoints including their mortality, behavior, reproduction, courtship behavior, *in vitro* distribution and expression of heat shock proteins, stress response genes and antioxidants have been monitored. These approaches have provided useful strategies and tools for screening of ecotoxicological risks and environmental hazards of chemicals.

The European Centre for the Validation of Alternative Methods (ECVAM) has been promoting 3Rs (reduction, refinement and replacement) for the use of animals in toxicity studies. *Drosophila* has been established as a potentially useful insect model for biomonitoring environmental health with respect to the effect of toxic chemicals and pollutants on selected life cycle parameters, stress genes, etc. in India (Siddique, Chowdhuri, et al. 2005, Siddique, Gupta, et al. 2005). Studies have further revealed expression of stress response protein (hsp70, hsp26) (which assist in the adaptation of cells by transiently reprogramming cellular metabolic activity, which protects cells from further oxidative damage) and antioxidants (SOD, catalase) as early biomarkers of cellular damage in environmental risk assessments. These findings find importance since majority of the target genes in the organism have functional homologues in humans based on sequence similarity/conservation (Tiwari, Pragya, et al. 2011).

Table 5.3 Application of alternative animal models for assessment of environmental contaminants

Model Organism	Toxicant and its effects/mechanism of action	References
Drosophila melanogaster	**Hexachlorocyclohexane (HCH)** (0.5, 1.0, 1.5, 2.0, and 5.0 ng/ml, Oral, hsp70-lacZ strain): at concentration 2.0 and 5.0 ng/ml, brain ganglia, imaginal discs, proventriculus of foregut, gastric caeca (part or whole), salivary glands, midgut, and hindgut revealed galactosidase activity, the γ isomer triggered the expression of hsp70 in larval tissues followed by α isomer (proventriculus and salivary gland) and β and δ isomers which produced weak responses in the proventriculus only	(Chowdhuri, Saxena, et al. 1999)
	Argemone oil (1.0, 10.0, 50.0, and 100.0 µl/ml, 2, 4, 24, and 48 h, Oral, hsp70-lacZ strain) Bg^9: the lowest concentration also triggered hsp70 whereas maximum tissue damage was found with the higher two concentrations with maximum damage in the malpighian tubules and midgut tissue	(Mukho-padhyay, Nazir, et al. 2002)
	Effluent from the chrome plating industry (0.05, 0.1, 1.0, 10.0, and 100.0 µL/mL, 2-48 h, Oral, hsp70-lacZ strain): affected theemergence pattern of adult flies, with impaired reproductive performance at higher concentrations, effect was more pronounced in males, dose- and time-dependent expression of *hsp70*	(Mukho-padhyay, Saxena, et al. 2003)
	Phthalimides (Captan, Captafol and Folpet), 0.0002-200 ppm, 2-48 h, Oral, hsp70-lacZ strain: high hsp70 expression was observed in the Captafol-exposed larvae followed by Captan and Folpet, delay in the flies' emergence by 3 days in 200 ppm Captafol group	(Nazir, Saxena, et al. 2003)
	Endosulfan (0.02–2.0 µg mL^{-1}, 12-48 h, Oral): concentration and time dependent induction of small hsp (hsp 23 > hsp 22), ROS generation, oxidative stress and induction of xenobiotic metabolism markers, delay in the emergence, reduction in locomotor behaviour with reduced cholinesterase activity	(Sharma, Mishra, et al. 2012)
	Acephate (2, 4, 6, or 8 µg/ml, 12-24 h, Oral, Oregon R strain): concentration dependent decrease in relative proportions of plasmatocytes in hemolymph and lamellocytes, crystal cell number was found to rise with increasing pesticide concentration	(Rajak, Dutta, et al. 2014)
	Acephate (0.5, 1.5, 2.5, 3.5, 4.5, and 5.5 mg/ml, 24 h, Oral, Oregon R strain): induced shortening of developmental time and early emergence	(Rajak, Sahana, et al. 2013)

Contd...

Model Organism	Toxicant and its effects/mechanism of action	References
	Chromium (IV) (5.0–20.0 µg/ml, 24-48 h, Oral): Out of 36, 28 of the differentially expressed miRNAs were mis-regulated affecting different biological processes viz., oxidation–reduction processes, DNA damage repair, development and differentiation, decreased expression of mus309 and mus312, acon to oxidation–reduction and pyd to stress activated MAPK cascade respectively belonging to these gene ontology classes concurrent with induction of dme-miR-314-3p, dme-miR-79-3p and dme-miR-12- 5p	(Chandra, Pandey, et al. 2015)
	Industrial effluent containing toxic metal (100.0 µl/ml, Oral, Oregon R strain): drop in mean daily egg production rate, reduction in developmental time, shortening of pupation height, decreased egg-to-adult viability and a reduction in body and wing length	(Roy and Ghosh, 2018)
Zebrafish	**Malathion** (0.03-0.23 mg/l, 72-216 h, Oral): 0.09 mg/l malathion did not cause any delay in egg hatching, with increasing concentration the percent hatching gradually decreased and at 0.21 and 0.23 mg/l all the embryos died, hatchlings of zebrafish were more sensitive to malathion as compared to the embryos	(Ansari and Kumar 1986)
	Lambda-cyhalothrin and Neemgold (LC_{10}, LC_{20}, and LC_{40}, 7-21 days, Oral): protein content reduced to 38, 46, and 45% in gill, liver, and ovary, respectively, post exposure for 21 days at the LC_{40} dose, the total free amino acid content in the liver increased to 172 and 154% after exposure to LC_{40} of lambda-cyhalothrin and neemgold, respectively, DNA content decreased to 45, 41, and 41% in the gill, liver, and ovary, respectively, after 21 days of exposure to LC_{40} of lambda-cyhalothrin, the reduction in DNA content was 51, 53, and 55% in gill, liver, and ovary, respectively, from neemgold exposure at the same concentration (LC_{40})	(Ahmad, Sharma, et al. 2012)
	Titanium oxide nanoparticles (5 mg/l, 24-48 h, Oral): TiO_2 NPs was found to accumulate in gills with distorted architecture, decreased activity of AcHE and both enzymatic and nonenzymatic antioxidants, an increase in levels of protein content, ROS, protein carbonyls, and LPO products	(Purusho-thaman, Raghunath, et al. 2014)

Contd...

Model Organism	Toxicant and its effects/mechanism of action	References
	Arsenic (10–50 mg/L, 90 days, Oral): At 50 µg/l generation of ROS, MDAand conjugated diene elicited a triphasic response with peak at the end of exposure, a gradual increase in GSH level until 60 days and 90 days, a drastic reduction was recorded which increased arsenic toxicity, enhanced mRNA level of nuclear factor (erythroid-derived 2)-like 2 (Nrf2) with downregulated levels of kelch-like ECH-associated protein 1 (Keap1)	(Sarkar, Mukherjee, et al. 2014)
	Monocrotophos (10, 20, 30, 40, 50, and 60 mg/L, 96 h, Oral): moderately toxic to the embryo with a 96-h LC_{50} of 37.44±3.32 mg/L, caused developmental abnormalities such as pericardial edema, changed heart development, spinal and vertebral anomalies in a concentration-dependent manner, the whole-body AChE enzyme activity *in vivo* was downregulated with maximum inhibition of 62% at 24 h	(Pamanji, Bethu, et al. 2015)
C elegans	**Food additives** (LC_{50} concentrations, 24 h, Oral): Toxicity was in order of Tannic Acid (13±0.135 mM)>Propyl gallate (50±1.00 mM) >Thiourea (105 ±0.76 mM)>Monosodium glutamate (400±1.78 mM), the data revealed high positive correlation of toxicity in *C.elegans* with both rats and mice	(Paul and Manoj 2009)
	Dichlorvos (5, 40, and 80 µM, 4-24 h, Oral, Transgenic strain PC72): Revealed a concentration-dependent reduction in feeding with total stop in feeding beyond 4 h, dose-dependent down regulation (69%–90%) of AChE after 4 h of exposure, upregulation of Hsp after 4 h with maximum expression after 24 h which was restricted only to the pharyngeal region	(Jadhav and Rajini 2009)
	Cypermethrin (5,10 and 15 mM, 4-24 h, Oral, Transgenic strain PC72): A concentration-dependent inhibition in feeding observed (31%, 46% and 56% at 5, 10, 15 mM, respectively) after 4 h with drastic increase in hsp-16 expression after 12 h exposure, with maximum expression at 24 h	(Shashikumar and Rajini 2010)
	TiO₂ and ZnO nanoparticles (NPs) of <25 nm and <100 nm sizes (24 h, Oral):<25 nm TiO_2 and ZnO NPs revealed LC_{50} of 77 mg/L and 0.32 mg/L respectively, <100 nm TiO_2 NPs was non-toxic and LC_{50} of 2 mg/L was obtained for <100 nm ZnO NPs, in both cases, smaller particle sizes were more toxic than larger ones and ZnO NPs were more toxic than TiO_2 NPs	(Khare, Sonane, et al. 2011)

Contd...

Model Organism	Toxicant and its effects/mechanism of action	References
	ZnO NPs (35 nm, 50 nm and 100 nm) (1/2, 1/10th, 1/100th and 1/1000th of LC_{50} concentrations, 24 h, Oral): ZnO NPs affected the growth, reproduction and behavior in a size dependent manner, modulated expression/function of genes associated with Insulin/IGF-like signaling pathway and/or stress response pathway	(Khare, Sonane, et al. 2015)
	ZnO NPs (10, 50, and 100 nm ZnO-NPs) (0.1 to 2.0 g/l, 24 h, Oral): 10 nm ≥0.7 g/l adversely affected the survivability but not 50 and 100 nm ≤1.0 g/l, reproduction affected at low concentration, *mtl-1* and *sod-1* expression induced with 10 nm ≥0.7 g/l and unaffected with same concentration of 50 and 100 nm	(Gupta, Kushwaha, et al. 2015)

In view of the paucity of knowledge with respect to the toxicity of the chemicals released into the environment, the cost of procuring the information experimentally is huge in terms of time, money and animals. In such a scenario, regulatory agencies have turned towards the *in silico* models to predict toxicity, their likely behavior and fate in the environment using their structural properties. It has become important to assess in the first instance whether a pollutant would require a remedial action or not and whether a particular biological pathway would be suitable enough to remove it or break it down in the environment (Jagwani and Bhawsar 2015). This approach has enabled making accurate and robust predictions which has improved the risk assessment process while decreasing the time and economic burden of animal and/or *in vitro* testing.

Quantitative Structure-Toxicity Relationships (QSTRs) is a mathematical modeling tool that is employed for predicting the biological (pharmacological/toxic) activity associated with the chemical structure. A set of parameters known as descriptors are required for predicting the toxicity outcomes, such as reproductive toxicity, aquatic toxicity, and genotoxicity, to name a few. Several reliable QSTR models based on artificial neural networks (ANN), decision tree (DT), support vector machines (SVM), k-nearest neighbor (k-NN), multiple linear regression (MLR), and partial least squares regression (PLSR) validated by using OECD recommended procedures for screening chemicals for ecotoxicological risk have been proposed and developed. In recent years, QSTR based tools have emerged as sophisticated tools for predicting carcinogenicity of diverse substances and screening for industrial chemicals, nanoparticles as well as their endpoint toxicities.

Mathematical modeling and computer simulation activities at CSIR-IITR has been extensively focused towards water/air quality modeling, environmental exposure assessment, for source apportionment of chemicals like PAHs and bio-degradation metabolic pathway. Studies have included the integration of system biology approaches along with bioinformatics to provide a better picture of the complex biological processes such as neurodegenerative disorders/cancers due to the exposure of hazardous chemicals, drugs and environmental stressors. Research activities have also involved the use of fuzzy logic and artificial neural network models to generate decision support systems for health risk assessment for lung functional abnormalities, neurological disorders as well as cancer. Research groups have established Quantitative Structure-Activity Relationships (QSAR) models (based on decision tree forest (DTF) and decision tree boost (DTB) for prediction of developmental toxicity potential of chemicals in rodents in accordance the OECD guidelines.

The structural features of chemicals have been extracted for assessing the LEL (lowest effective level) dose of chemicals for their developmental toxicity potential followed by successful validation of its predictive power by internal and external procedures (Basant, Gupta, et al. 2016). Tree-based multispecies QSAR models have also been developed and validated for predicting avian toxicity and aquatic toxicity of a panel of structurally diverse pesticides utilizing a set of descriptors directly derived directly from chemical structures in accordance with the OECD guidelines that could have wide application in regulatory purposes (Singh, Gupta, et al. 2014, Basant, Gupta, et al. 2015).

Pharmaceutical Active Compound's (PACs) aquatic toxicity prediction models that are based on interspecies correlation estimation (ICE) have also been proposed (Kar and Roy 2010, Roy and Das 2013, Das and Roy 2014, Roy, Das, et al. 2014, Singh, Gupta, et al. 2015). Models have been established using experimentally derived toxicity data of several structurally diverse compounds including PACs in aquatic test species (daphnia, algae, fathead minnow) utilizing molecular descriptors for predicting/screening of aquatic toxicity of novel, untested compounds (Singh, Gupta et al. 2013, Singh, Gupta, et al. 2014). In recent years, QSTR based tools have also emerged as robust tools for also predicting of carcinogenicity of diverse chemicals and screening for industrial chemicals, nanoparticles and their endpoint toxicities (Singh, Gupta, et al. 2013, Singh, Gupta, et al. 2015). Though the need for animal testing cannot be ignored entirely, the proposed models can be used as effective tools for screening the chemicals for their toxicity profile prior to *in vivo* tests.

The eye irritation potential (EIP) has been a crucial toxicological endpoint for ocular toxicity of chemicals, which has faced a lot of criticism. Scientists at CSIR-IITR have developed a three-tier QSAR modeling strategy for the estimation of EIP chemicals. A qualitative (binary classification: irritating, non-irritating), semi-quantitative (four-category classification) and quantitative (regression) QSAR models employing decision tree methods have been constructed following the OECD guidelines which have been successfully validated by various procedures. These models have shown to perform much better than the previous studies in literature paving its way for the drug development process (Basant, Gupta, et al. 2016).

A web server, known as ToxinPred has been constructed, based on machine learning technique and quantitative matrix, utilizing various properties of peptides which would be useful in predicting various parameters such as toxicity/non-toxicity of peptides, the minimum mutations in peptides that could increase or decrease their toxicity. In addition, it will also be instrumental in designing the least toxic peptides and discovering new toxic regions (Gupta, Kapoor, et al. 2013). Similarly, a tool with a predictive power of molecular toxicity with aqueous permeability and solubility of any molecule/metabolite has also been constructed. Utilizing a curated panel of toxin as a training set, the different structural and chemical features have been employed for the optimization and development of the model that has been further evaluated rigorously. The tool which has been developed into ToxiM web server may be employed as a highly reliable and useful tool for predicting the toxicity, solubility, and permeability of small molecules (Sharma, Sharma, et al. 2017). Besides using these approaches, softwares (Overall Index of Pollution, OIP) for generating water quality indices in contaminated river bodies have been generated by CSIR- NEERI and CPCB Board that reflect the quality of water in terms of pollution as well as the formulation of pollution control strategies in terms of treatment required at different levels (Sargaonkar and Deshpande 2003).

As environmental ailments have continued to dominate national concerns, human biomonitoring strategies have also evolved better with regard to evaluating health risks linked with acute exposures as well as systemic uptake through chronic environmental exposures. Molecular biomonitoring of the 570,000 survivors of the notorious Bhopal gas tragedy "as a model", has provided an opportunity to elucidate the long-standing effects of acute environmental toxic exposures to MIC that extend from respiratory, immunological impairments and increased susceptibility to infections to genotoxic effects (Mishra, Bhargava et al. 2011, Mishra 2012). Increased incidence of chronic adverse effects including bronchial asthma, pulmonary fibrosis, chronic obstructive pulmonary disease (COPD), emphysema, chest infections, and corneal opacities have been documented to still persist in the MIC affected population even after 25 years (Mishra, Samarth, et al. 2009). Studies also revealed for the first time that *in utero* MIC exposure caused a persistent hyper-responsive cellular and humoral immune state in the affected individuals (Mishra, Dabadghao, et al. 2009). The cascade of events that lead to oxidative stress/inflammation, apoptosis, DNA damage response, overcoming damage repair mechanisms, genome instability, and oncogenic transformation post *in vivo* and *in vitro* exposure to MIC have also been documented (Mishra, Samarth, et al. 2009, Malla, Senthilkumar, et al. 2011, Senthilkumar, Tahir, et al. 2011, Panwar, Jain et al. 2013, Panwar, Raghuram, et al. 2014, Senthilkumar, Akhter, et al. 2015).

Human biomonitoring has highly evolved to estimate the exposure-response relationship in environmental linked diseases. Exposures encountered through accidental pesticide poisonings (Dewan, Bhatnagar, et al. 2004), cases of food intoxication (through consumption of Kesari dal) (Ganapathy and Dwivedi 1961), *Cassia occidentalis* (CO) seeds (Vashishtha, Kumar, et al. 2007), argemone contaminated mustard oil, etc.) (Sharma, Malhotra et al. 1999) poisoning through herbal medications (Dwivedi and Dey 2002, Gunturu, Nagarajan et al. 2011) and exposure to arsenic via drinking water (Mahata, Basu et al. 2003) have been well documented. In addition to acute effects, risks associated with toxic exposures have been related to Alzheimer's disease, non-familial schizophrenia, accelerated aging, congenital heart defects, diabetes, and several other life-threatening disorders including cancer. Humans are potentially exposed to these toxicants through the consumption of contaminated food, food chain, through the air, contaminated water sources, accidental exposure and hand to mouth activity in case of kids. Biological monitoring of environmental toxicants has been undertaken by determination of residues and metabolites in biological samples such as blood/serum/urine/adipose tissue, routine hematological examinations, biochemical activities as well as enzymatic changes to quantify the magnitude of risk associated with their exposure. Presence of immune complexes, alterations in liver and thyroid enzymes and creatinine levels, respiratory dysfunctions have been well correlated with organ-specific toxicities. Scoring of cytogenetic markers such as CA, SCE, MN as well as Comet assay using lymphocytes have also been extensively employed for the detection of early genotoxic effects. Studies have highlighted the underlying confounding factors like age, sex, lifestyle, nutrition, habits, genetic susceptibilities and epigenetic mechanisms that may magnify the risk to initiation/progression of environmental induced toxicities/diseases. Table 5.4 provides a comprehensive list of the few studies undertaken to assess the risk of human exposure to different categories of environmental toxicants.

Table 5.4 Few representative epidemiological studies carried out to assess the risk of human exposure to environmental contaminants

Environmental Toxicants	Effects/Clinical Manifestations	References
Metals		
Lead	Blood lead levels in the range of (2.78–15.0 µg/dL) and 29%-exceeded 10 µg/dL, influenced by area of residence, source of water supply, social status, maternal education status, and proximity to traffic density, higher MDA, lowered GSH	(Ahamed, Verma, et al. 2005)
	Level of blood lead was in the range of 1.0–27.9 µg/dl in the children, 37% had lead levels above 10 µg/dL, influenced by, proximity of home to traffic, low socioeconomic status and mother's educational status	(Ahamed, Verma, et al. 2010)
Chromium	Gastrointestinal distress documented in 39.2% males and 39.3% females; skin alterations in 24.5% males and 25% females who were residents around contaminated water sites, higher RBCs (among 30.7% males and 46.1% females), decreased MCVs (among 62.8% males) and reduced platelets (among 68% males and 72% females)	(Sharma, Bihari et al. 2012)
Arsenic	Hepatomegaly present in 76.65 % of patients with 1-15 years of consumption of arsenic contaminated water with non cirhottic portal fibrosis as the predominant lesion (91.3%), arsenic content in liver 6 mg/kg	(Santra, Das, et al. 1999)
	Incidence of shortness of breath, cough, and chest sounds (crepitations and/or rhonchi) increased with increasing concentration of arsenic, more pronounced in individuals with skin lesions	(Mazumder, Haque, et al. 2000)
	Mean arsenic concentrations in nails, hair and urine samples were 9.04 ± 0.78 (µg/g), 5.63 ± 0.38 (µg/g) and 140.52 ± 8.82 (µ g/l), respectively, higher number of aberrant cells (8.08%) and SCEs per cell (7.26%)	(Mahata, Basu, et al. 2003)
	Hyperpigmentation, keratosis, weakness, nausea, hepatomegaly, lung disease and neuropathy positively correlated with higher concentrations of arsenic in ground water	(Guha Mazumder 2003)
	Enhanced micronuclei frequency in blood lymphocytes, oral mucosa cells and urothelial cells	(Basu, Ghosh, et al. 2004)

Contd...

Environmental Toxicants	Effects/Clinical Manifestations	References
Pesticides		
Endosulfan	Development of penis, testes, pubic hair, and testosterone level in the serum was positively associated with age (10-19 years) and negatively associated with endosulfan exposure, incidence of congenital abnormalities related to testicular descent (undescended testis, congenital hydrocele, and congenital inguinal hernia) was 5.1%, may delay the sexual maturity and interfere with synthesis of sex hormone	(Saiyed, Dewan, et al. 2003)
	In 0-14 years age group 46% males and 42.5% females suffered from congenital anomalies, 0-30 year age group documented the most number mental retardation cases with 74.5% males and 74.1% females, 39.2% males had throat, lung, or prostate cancers, 35.4% females had ovarian, breast, or blood cancer	(Embrandiri, Singh, et al. 2012)
Methyl isocyanate	Chemosis, redness watering, corneal ulcers after a few weeks	(Dwivedi, Raizada, et al. 1985)
	Emphysema, pulm hypertension, pleural scars, interstitial deposits after 3 and 6 months	(Kamat, Mahashur, et al. 1985)
	Corneal opacities, chronic conjunctivitis after 2 years	(Raizada and Dwivedi 1987)
	Neurosis, anxiety states & adjustment reactions after 2-6 months	(Sethi, Sharma, et al. 1987)
	Maximum subjects had abnormalties in respiratory, gastrointestinal, cardiovascular, and musculoskeletal system, incidence of abnormalties in the gastrointestinal and respiratory system was greater in the subjects that were within 4 km, 10.1% revealed radiological alterations suggesting pulmonary tuberculosis, emphysema, pneumonitis etc, alterations in memory mainly visual perceptual and attention/response speed along with attention/vigilance	(Kumar, Kumar, et al. 1988)
	Occurrence of CA (breaks and gaps) in lymphocytes after two and a half months, reduction in the phagocytic activity of lymphocytes	(Saxena, Singh, et al. 1988)
	The frequency of CA (the form of replicating minutes and exchange configurations) was, more in individuals with higher years of exposure (post 3 years), higher prevalence in females	(Ghosh, Sengupta, et al. 1990)

Contd...

Environmental Toxicants	Effects/Clinical manifestations	References
	Exposure of pregnant women to toxic gases in Bhopal in 1984 caused greater pregnancy loss, elevated first 5-year mortality and resulted in delayed development of male progeny (from 1985-2007)	(Sarangi, Zaidi, et al. 2010)
	Higher circulating inflammatory biomarkers levels (IL-1β, IL-6, IL-8, TNF, IL-10, IL-12p70 cytokines and C-reactive protein) in the exposed population (after 20 years)	(Bhargava, Punde, et al. 2010)
	Higher prevalence of atypical lymphocytes in the peripheral blood of exposed parents and their offspring born post-exposure	(Senthilkumar, Malla, et al. 2013)
Food based toxicants		
Kesari Dal (*Lathyris savitus*)	Morphological alterations in the spinal cord, complete demyelination of posterior one-half to one-third of lateral white columns of both sides	(Sachdev, Sachdev, et al. 1969)
	Mean duration of the illness was 17.1 years (range 2-30), walking difficulty due to weakness and leg stiffness, frequency of micturition, gait abnormalities included spastic gait, toe walking	(Misra, Sharma, et al. 1993)
Argemone oil	Swelling of the lower limbs, worse on exertion, with breathlessness, and fatigue, two-thirds had an initial gastrointestinal upset, oedema associated with erythema and a raised skin temperature; blanching occurred on pressure	(Thakur and Prasad 1968)
	Blood samples contained 4.7 and 28.3 µg sanguinarine/100 ml serum	(Shenolikar, Rukmini, et al. 1974)
	The level of MDA was increased and the GSH level in erythrocytes was reduced with significant decrease in SOD and GPx activities which directly correlated with serum sanguinarine level, thus inducing oxidative stress	(Banerjee, Seth, et al. 2000)
	Total plasma protein and globulin contents were enhanced, decrease in albumin/globulin ratio in dropsy patients, total cholesterol, low density lipoprotein, triglycerides and very low density lipoprotein cholesterol were higher with a parallel reduction in high density lipoprotein cholesterol, enhanced oxidation of plasma proteins and lipids decrease in antioxidant enzymes	(Das, Babu, et al. 2005)

Contd...

Environmental Toxicants	Effects/Clinical manifestations	References
CO seeds	Vomiting preceded unconsciousness in all subjects, majority had moderate fever and abnormal behaviour/agitation, abnormal posture of trunk and limbs, blood pressure fluctuation, higher levels of creatine phosphokinase, serum aminotransferases, and lactic dehydrogenase, serum glucose was found low (<50 mg/dl) in 47.3% cases, 76.4% mortality within 72 h	(Vashishtha, Nayak, et al. 2007)
	Decreased levels of blood glucose and increased liver enzyme SGPT with collapse within 6 h with hematemesis and abrupt cardio respiratory arrest in one child, mild fever and irritability, signs of mild encephalopathy in the second one, third child of the group died on 4th day after ingestion	(Vashishtha, Kumar, et al. 2007)
Pan masala	Higher CA, SCEs and MN induction	(Dave, Trivedi, et al. 1991)
	Higher CA, SCEs and MN induction positively correlated with the duration of consumption	(Yadav and Chadha 2002)
Flouride	Consumption of fluoride contaminated water (0.25-8 ppm) led to dental fluorosis (58%), skeletal fluorosis (27%), non-skeletal fluorosis (41%) and gastrointestinal complaints (26%)	(Susheela, Kumar, et al. 1993)
	The toxic effects were more severe and complex and prevalence of metabolic bone disease (osteoporosis, rickets and PTH bone disease) and bony leg deformities (genu varum, genu valgum, bowing, rotational and wind-swept) was higher (> 90%) in children with deficiency of calcium as compared to < 25% in children with adequate calcium	(Teotia, Teotia, et al. 1998)
	89% of the children suffered from dental fluorosis and 39% had skeletal fluorosis, increased serum alanine transaminase, alkaline phosphatase and aspartate transaminase levels, lowered levels of total protein, albumin, and potassium, osteosclerosis, osteoporosis, and genu valgum was reported	(Shivashankara, Shankara, et al. 2000)
	Oxidative stress as evident via higher levels of MDA, changes in the antioxidant systems (lowered levels of uric acid and glutathione together, higher activity of ascorbic acid and glutathione peroxidase along, reduction in superoxide dismutase activity)	(Shivarajashankara, Shivashankara, et al. 2001)

Contd...

Environmental Toxicants	Effects/Clinical manifestations	References
Air pollutants		
Biomass fuel (kanda)	Increased levels of DNA damage in biomass fuel users as compared to LPG users, olive tail moment was 3.83± 0.15 vs. 2.77 ± 0.07 ; % tail DNA was 11.19± 0.35 vs. 8.29± 0.20; and comet tail length (mm) was 51.15± 1.37 vs. 40.26±0.88	(Pandey, Bajpayee, et al. 2005)
	Higher leukocyte platelet aggregates was found in women using biomass fuel, revealed higher surface expression of CD11b/CD18 in circulating polymorphonuclear leukocytes and monocytes, elevated expression of CD62P on platelets, chronic exposure may be a risk factor for thrombosis	(Ray, Mukherjee, et al. 2006)
	Incidence of hypertension (29.5 vs. 11.0% in control, higher oxLDL (170.6 vs. 45.9 U/l; $P < 0.001$), expression of platelet and P-selectin (9.1% vs. 2.4%), platelet aggregation (23.2 vs. 15.9 Ohm), raised aCL IgG (28.7% vs. 2.1%), IgM (8.6% of vs. 0.4%), and ROS (44%) but lowered (13%) SOD which positively correlated with PM_{10} and $PM_{2.5}$ in indoor air	(Dutta, Mukherjee, et al. 2011)
	Buccal epithelial cells of biomass users revealed higher DNA damage, airway cells revealed 51% rise in ROS production but 28% decrease in SOD, suggestive of oxidative stress in the airways, indoor air of biomass-using households had 3-times more PM_{10} and $PM_{2.5}$ than LPG-using households	(Mondal, Bhattacharya, et al. 2011)
	Neutrophil count in blood and sputum was increased, higher CD35 (complement receptor-1) surface expression, CD16 (FCγ receptor III), and β2 Mac-1 integrin (CD11b/CD18) expression on circulating neutrophils, 72%, 67%, and 54% increased plasma levels of the proinflammatory cytokines TNF-α, IL-6, and IL-12, respectively, and double IL-8	(Banerjee, Mondal, et al. 2012)
Diesel exhaust/ Ambient air/Particulate air pollution	Average PM_{10} concentration ranged from 184 to 295µg/m^3, residents from higher PM_{10} areas demonstrated a greater reduction in lung functions (PEFR)	(Sharma, Kumar, et al. 2004)
	Hypertension incidence was approx. 4-times higher in Delhi, upregulation in platelet P-selectin, reduced levels of CD^{4+} T-helper cells and CD^{19+} B cells but icreased number of CD^{56+} NK cells suggesting altered immunity	(Banerjee, Siddique, et al. 2012)
	Decrease in lung functions (PEFR and FEV1) due to increased (PM_1 and $PM_{2.5}$) in ambient air, reduction in airflow obstruction	(Kesavachandran, Pangtey, et al. 2013)

Contd...

Environmental Toxicants	Effects/Clinical manifestations	References
	The estimated relative death rate and hospital admissions for every rise in the PM_{10} levels of 10 $\mu g/m^3$ extended from 1.5–8% and from 3.9–8.0% respectively in persons > 65 yrs, the highest cancer risk value was estimated for chromium, 266.70 × 10^{-6}, which was related to PM_{10} and 100.92 × 10^{-6} which was associated with $PM_{2.5}$, among the PAHs, benzo(a)pyrene (51.96±19.71 ng/m^3) was maximum in the PM_{10} samples	(Pandey, Patel, et al. 2013)

While the list is endless, few environmental toxicants have received greater attention because of their prevalence or widespread application. Several epidemiological studies have established positive links between exposure to airborne particles and adverse health effects from mortality to subclinical effects such as incidences of cancer, reduced lung function, asthma and allergy, chronic respiratory diseases, pulmonary tumors, cardiovascular pathologies and birth defects. Around 100,000 premature deaths in India have been associated with air pollution exposure and in Delhi alone, in the range from 7,350 to 16,200 premature deaths have been reported due to PM exposure (Pant, Guttikunda, et al. 2016). Further carcinogenic metals like chromium and cadmium bound to these respirable particles have been predictive of respiratory, cardiovascular mortality and high cancer risks among the exposed populations (Pandey, Patel, et al. 2013). Increased levels of heavy metals in the atmospheric deposits, may eventually pollute the food chain posing health risks to humans (Sharma, Agrawal et al. 2008, Sharma, Agrawal, et al. 2008). Higher molecular weight PAHs have been linked with risks of cancer both in adults and children (Kaur, Senthilkumar et al. 2013, Singh and Gupta 2016). Peak expiratory flow rate (PEFR) has been one of the simplest and useful parameters for estimating the status of lung function in the general population as well as in areas of particulate air pollution (Malik, Jindal et al. 1982, Chowgule, Shetye et al. 1995, Raju, Prasad et al. 2005, Prasad, Verma et al. 2006, Taksande, Jain et al. 2008). Health effects of airborne particulate matter in relation to the Indian scenario has been concisely reviewed by several authors (Mohanraj and Azeez 2004, Rizwan, Nongkynrih, et al. 2013).

Studies have assessed the status of human exposure to environmental chemicals by monitoring/quantification of residue levels of pesticides, metals and xenobiotics in human adipose tissue, breast milk, semen fluid and blood. In India, IITR, NIOH and Indian Council of Agricultural Research Institute (ICAR) are primarily responsible for monitoring the health status and pesticide-residues in different samples. Pesticides and metals have been majorly criticized for their presence/residues at high levels in samples of human blood, human milk, fat samples, semen and food commodities and Indians have been documented to carry the highest body burden of organochlorine pesticides (OCP) (Dale, Copeland et al. 1965, Rathore, Bhatnagar et al. 2002, Bhatnagar, Kashyap et al. 2004, Kumar, Baroth et al. 2006, Pathak, Suke et al. 2008, Mishra and Sharma 2011).

Bio-monitoring of pesticides in human samples has been exclusively carried out for the OCPs and their metabolites (Dureja, Nair et al. 1991, Nair, Dureja et al. 1992, Jaga and Dharmani 2003, Sanghi, Pillai et al. 2003, Mustafa, Pathak et al. 2010). Since inception, attempts have been made to detect the presence of pesticides in relation to their placental transfer (Saxena, Seth, et al. 1980) wherein residue levels of DDT and its metabolites, HCH, isomers of BHC and aldrin have been detected in all the samples, indicative of their transfer from the mother to the fetus (Saxena, Siddiqui et al. 1981, Siddiqui and Saxena 1985). Mother's age has been revealed to influence OCP's accumulation in the circulating blood and its transfer to the fetus. Interestingly, increased concentrations of OCPs were found in pregnant women having non-vegetarian dietary habits as compared to those with vegetarian dietary habits. Exposure of pregnant women to OCPs has shown to increase the risk of intrauterine growth retardation (IUGR), which is a contributing factor for infant mortality in India (Siddiqui, Srivastava, et al. 2003). Knowledge of long term trends of OCPs in the placenta and accompanying fluid is of great significance for the understanding of congenial and abnormal deliveries, miscarriages etc., especially in the Indian context. Human milk has proved to be an important tool for estimating maternal contamination and for measuring the total intake of chemicals by infants during breastfeeding. Infants weighing on an average 2.8 kg and consuming 500 ml of milk/day ingested 0.065 mg endosulfan/kg/day and 0.041 mg chlorpyrifos/kg/day, which were 8.6 and 4.1 times higher than the Accepted Daily Intake (ADI) recommended by the World Health Organization (WHO). In another study malathion and lindane also exceeded the ADI recommended by WHO by 0.4 and 0.6 times, respectively (Sanghi, Pillai, et al. 2003).

Environmental lead toxicity has been an old and persistent health problem and children have been more susceptible to lead toxicity than adults due to their hand to mouth activity, higher respiratory rates and increased gastrointestinal absorption/unit body weight. In humans, particularly in children decreased dietary intakes of calcium, zinc and iron have been linked with higher blood lead levels indicating lower blood iron and copper concentrations in the presence of higher blood lead levels (Tripathi, Raghunath, et al. 2001). In addition, human studies have revealed that *in utero* exposure to reduced levels of lead may be related to deficits in fetal growth incidence of intrauterine-growth retardation (IUGR) which has the potential to induce neurobehavioral and other developmental deficits (Saxena, Singh, et al. 1994, Srivastava,

Mehrotra, et al. 2001). Arsenic has been recognized as a potent human carcinogen. The state of West Bengal has been endemic to arsenic toxicity with an estimate of about 6 million people being exposed to groundwater contaminated with arsenic and has been regarded as the biggest arsenic calamity in the world (Chatterjee, Das, et al. 1995, Chakraborti, Rahman, et al. 2002, Ghosh, Datta, et al. 2007). The groundwater of 9 out of 18 districts have been found to be contaminated with arsenic, with concentration from 50 to 800 µg/l, which was much more than the maximum contamination level (MCL), laid down by both WHO (WHO, Guidelines for Drinking Water Quality, 2nd ed., vol. 2, Health Criteria and other Supporting Information, WHO, Geneva, 1996, pp. 940–949) and US EPA (http://www.epa.gov/safewater/ars/quickguide.pdf). The term arsenicosis was coined by the group of Mazumder, et al 1988 and later used by the WHO to describe a chronic disease due to prolonged exposure of arsenic, clinically manifested as raindrop pigmentation, palmo-planter keratosis, hypo and hyper-pigmentation, conjunctivitis, peripheral vascular diseases, respiratory problems, peripheral neuropathy and various reproductive abnormalities (Mazumder, Chakraborty et al. 1988, Caussy and Organization 2005). Mazumder, et al. 2011 have summarized the toxicity studies on arsenic from population-based studies; clinical case series; and reports with various systemic manifestations (Mazumder and Dasgupta 2011).

Exposure to food-based toxicants has also been increasingly recognized as a human health hazard. Numerous outbreaks of argemone poisoning have been documented in different Indian subcontinents and other areas viz a viz Madagascar, Mauritius, Rangoon, and South Africa (Sainani, Rajkondawar et al. 1972, Das and Khanna 1997). Although, sporadic incidences of the disease have been documented for over the last 100 years, the most massive epidemic took place at New Delhi, India in 1998, affecting thousands of people out of which over 3000 people were rushed to hospitals and 65 lost their lives (Das and Khanna 1997, Babu, Ansari et al. 2008). Several studies have been conducted to uncover its underlying mechanism. Argemone oil (AO) has been shown to induce dilatation of small arterioles and capillaries, resulting in leakage of serum proteins leading to faltered osmosis, ormation of edema and higher capillary damage (Chaudhuri 1959, Kumar, Husain, et al. 1992). Clinical and experimental studies are suggestive that ROS is involved in AO's toxicity, resulting in decreased bio-antioxidant pool and antioxidant defense capacity (Das, Upreti, et al. 1991, Upreti, Das, et al. 1991, Das, Babu, et al. 2005). The toxic effects have primarily been attributed to the presence of interconvertible methylene dioxy phenyl alkaloids, sanguinarine (SA)/dihydro-sanguinarine (Sarkar 1948), which have also been shown to cause macromolecular damage (Das, Babu, et al. 2005). Several behavioral, hematological, biochemical, immunohistochemical and histopathological parameters have also been assessed to correlate the animal experimental findings with the data of HME patients during 1998–2010 to decipher the etiology of the disease. Evidence of hazardous human exposure to mycotoxins through dairy products and staple food has also been shown by several investigators (Rastogi, Dwivedi et al. 2004, Raghavender and Reddy 2008, Reddy, Abbas, et al. 2009).

The field of epidemiology has received a major boost from molecular approaches and growing attention has been directed towards the development of biomarkers of susceptibility for making better quantitative estimates of prediction of consequences of low-level chemical exposure. This has been best exemplified in arsenic-exposed population wherein genetic variations have shown to play a pivotal role in arsenic-induced toxicity through the interplay of several gene products. Association of specific p53 and p16 polymorphisms (Chanda, Dasgupta, et al. 2005, De Chaudhuri, Mahata, et al. 2006), purine nucleoside phosphorylase polymorphisms (De Chaudhuri, Ghosh, et al. 2008), epigenetic modulations such as DNA methylation have been identified on chronic arsenic exposure (Banerjee, Paul et al. 2013, Paul, Banerjee et al. 2014, Banerjee, Bandyopadhyay, et al. 2017, Bhattacharjee, Sanyal, et al. 2018). Expression profiling of few genes of toxication and detoxification pathways in peripheral blood lymphocytes (PBL) has established their potential as a sensitive and rapid tool for preliminary screening of individuals that are exposed to environmental chemicals (such as vehicular emissions, DEP and ethanol) as well as in clinical studies (Srivastava, Yadav, et al. 2012, Sharma, Saurabh, et al. 2013, Srivastava, Sharma, et al. 2014).

Epidemiological studies have not only played an important role in identifying causal relationships for different diseases/disorders but also helped in designing suitable health management programs employing chelating agents, herbal medications, antioxidants, etc. The use of d-Penicillamine has proved highly effective in treating cases of lead poisoning (Singh, Mukherjee, et al. 2009). Calcium disodium ethylene diamino tetraacetate (EDTA) along with environmental intervention and education, have also been shown to be effective strategies (Raviraja, Babu, et al. 2010). Treatment with a combination of antioxidants, riboflavin and tocopherol have shown improvement in few symptoms (pain in limbs, edema and erythema) in patients with epidemic dropsy. Clinical therapy with 2,3-dimercapto-1- propanesulfonate (DMPS), a chelating agent, in patients with chronic arsenicosis has revealed significant improvement in their condition, notably weakness, pigmentation and lung disease with enhanced excretion of arsenic in the urine (Guha Mazumder, De, et al. 2001).

Various experimental studies employing animals, isolated cells studied *in vitro, in situ* and *in vivo* methods have also been applied to investigate the toxic effects of xenobiotics. Mechanisms by which heavy metals, pesticides, industrial dust, herbal remedies, solvents, plasticizers and other plastic additives, food color and dye intermediates, and other environmental contaminants may cause deleterious effects have been elucidated. Equal importance has been given to the pursuit of novel therapeutic interventions. Several nutritional factors, chelating agents, antioxidants, phytochemicals, etc. have been screened that have shown to be important modifiers of toxicity. To avoid repetition, these have been mentioned in the following sections.

Few institutes have remained at the forefront in addressing environmental problems in India of global concern. CSIR-NEERI has been engaged in research related to arsenic in drinking water since 1973. The groundwater pollution due to arsenic in the Chowki Block of Rajnandgaon District of Chattisgarh was reported for the first time by NEERI. Therapy with DPMS (2,3 Dimercapto-1-propanesulfonate), a chelating agent known to increase excretion of arsenic in urine has shown to cause improvement in the clinical condition of chronic arsenicosis patients (Guha Mazumder, De et al. 2001, Guha Mazumder 2003). NEERI has also developed a user-friendly field kit for arsenic on behalf of the World Health Organisation (https://www.niscair.res.in/ Science Communication/RnDNewsLetters/csirnews2k7/csirnews_30july07.pdf. IITR has developed a low cost, field deployable kit which can detect arsenic up to 10 ppb in water. The technology is patented and transferred to ELICO Ltd, Hyderabad, a major player in the field of analytical instrumentation in India (http://iitrindia.org/En/pdf/techfolder.pdf). Efforts have also been made by other research groups to develop low-cost kits for arsenic detection (Baghel, Singh, et al. 2007, Das, Sarkar, et al. 2014).

Excess of fluoride ingestion has been a major clinical problem in India with few states and Union Territories being endemic for it. IITR collected different samples of fluoride contaminated water and assessed the symptoms, effects and treatments for fluorosis. NEERI has also developed a sustainable process for the mitigation of fluoride contaminated groundwater and its field application for domestic purposes. Hand pump attachable iron removal plants have been designed and installed at numerous areas in order to provide access to safe drinking water. More recently scientists at CSIR-Central Mechanical Engineering Research Institute have developed a fluorosis level detection kit utilizing a chemo-sensor liquid that indicates the level of fluorosis in the body (orange: unsafe level of more than 1.5 ppm, yellow: safe level of less than 1.5 ppm) (https://www.cmeri.res.in/technology/salivary-fluoride-detection-kit).

Purification devices like 'Bact-O-kill' and 'Amrit Kumbh' developed at IITR for water purification have increased access to safe drinking water throughout the country. IITR also has to its credit few other technologies such as argemone detection kit for rapid screening of argemone in mustard oil and CD-strip for detection of butter yellow, an adulterant in edible oils (http://iitrindia.org/En /pdf/techfolder.pdf). An economical and effective arsenic analyzer has been designed by research groups at Gujarat University, which can detect even microscopic concentration (0.5 ng/ml) of arsenic in the water (https://www.

business-standard.com/article/current-affairs/gujarat-varsity-develops-new-tech-to-remove-arsenic-from-drinking-water11510170 0224 _1. html). Using a minimal volume of the sample, the device would just cost 10-15 paise per sample. More recently, a gold nanosensor, Au–TA–DNS has been developed which is capable of detecting very low concentrations of Pb^{2+} and Cu^{2+}ions. The nanosensor produces a blue colour on paper strips and in solution, due to the formation of nanoparticle aggregates upon binding with metal ions. With a sensitive detection limit of ≤ 10.0 ppb, the method offers an added advantage of cost-effectiveness and applicability to other field-tests such as water quality monitoring (Nath, Arun, et al. 2015).

India's governance on air quality has its roots in the Air (Prevention & Control) Act of 1981. The Act focuses on the prevention and control of emissions from industrial sources and sets standards for ambient air quality for criteria contaminants. However, no indoor air quality standards exists in India to date. Balakrishnan, et al. 2011 provides an overview of the exposure and health information due to indoor air pollution due to solid fuel combustion in India (Balakrishnan, Ramaswamy, et al. 2011). Approximately 4–6% of the country's disease burden is attributed to the use of poor quality solid biomass fuel use in the rural household (Smith and Mehta 2003). Studies are suggestive of epidemiological evidence for low birth weight (Pope, Mishra, et al. 2010), COPD (Kurmi, Semple, et al. 2010), respiratory illness (Rajkumar, Pattabi et al. 2017) and lung cancer (Mondal, Bhattacharya, et al. 2011). To combat the situation, CSIR-NEERI has developed a novel, domestic natural draft multifuel improved cookstove 'NEERDHUR' inheriting innovative technological know-how for high thermal efficiency, reduced fuel consumption, reduced emissions, approved and certified by the Ministry of New and Renewable Energy (MNRE), Government of India (http://www.neeri.res.in/sites/default /files/NEER DHUR.pdf). Fifty prototypes have already been distributed in two villages in Nagpur. Numerous low-cost catalysts have been developed for controlling CO, VOCs, and PM emissions from the solid fuel combustion in rural areas.

CHAPTER 6

Medical Toxicology

The distinctive pattern of pesticide poisoning, drug abuse, natural toxicities have positioned India as a unique point for research in various aspects of medical/clinical toxicology. Medical toxicology, a clinical subspecialty encompassing the pathophysiology, diagnosis, treatment, management and prevention of clinical problems requires concerted efforts of general, and emergency physicians, intensivists, clinical pharmacologists, pediatricians, and forensic experts all put together. Even though till date medical toxicology stands as a 'neglected' subspecialty in India, it is probably the oldest sub-disciplines of toxicology in the country with its roots dating back to the agada tantra, as defined by Sushruta, dealing with the diagnosis and treatment of any person bitten by poisonous insects or affected by natural or artificial poisons (Manohar 2014). Important areas of medical toxicology in India comprise of acute poisoning, drug abuse, adverse drug events, addiction and withdrawal, environmental and workplace exposures, chemicals and hazardous materials, and venomous bites and stings.

With the availability of a vast number of chemicals and drugs, acute poisoning has become an important toxicological emergency that carries high morbidity and mortality in India. The most common agents in India are pesticides (aluminium phosphide, organophosphates, carbamates, chlorinated hydrocarbons, and pyrethroids), animal bites, sedative drugs, chemicals (corrosive acids and copper sulfate), alcohols, plant toxins (dhatura, oleander, strychnos), gastrointestinal irritants such as castor, croton, calotropis, etc.), and household poisons (mainly comprised of detergents, corrosives etc) (Srivastava, Peshin et al. 2005). The primary treatment modalities developed over the years have been stabilization (airway, breathing, circulation, and depression of the CNS), accurate diagnosis, removal of unabsorbed poison (skin/eye decontamination, gut evacuation, gastric lavage), antidote administration if available and nursing and psychiatric care.

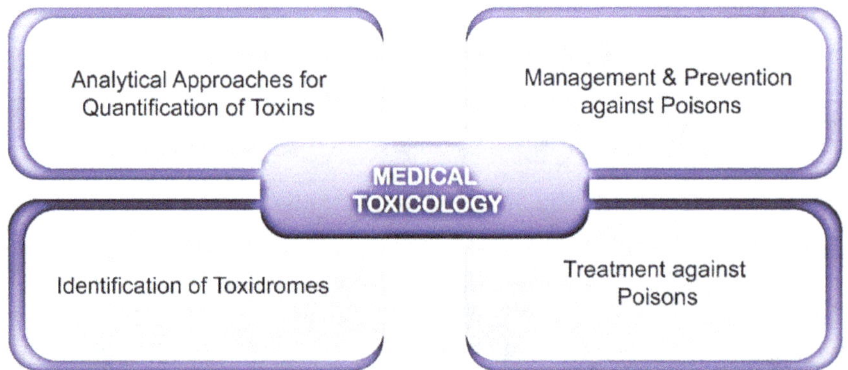

Figure 6.1 Approaches applied for Medical Toxicology in India

A toxicology laboratory was set up in 1984 at the Medicolegal Institute, Bhopal, after the Bhopal Gas Tragedy. Concerns over growing cases of poisoning in India led to the establishment of the National Poisons Information Centre at the All India Institute of Medical Sciences, New Delhi in 1994. A second center subsequently came up at NIOH, Ahmedabad. Since then, few more regional centers have opened in cities such as Cochin and Chennai that offer immediate and round the clock assessment of toxicity and disseminate diagnostic and therapeutic assistance to the doctors for management of the poisoned patient. Despite this, the spurt in the number of poisonous substances significantly increased and the effective management of toxicological emergencies has remained a challenge at every level of the health-care system. The important reasons appear to be a lack of specially trained medical and paramedical staff, specific antidotes, and life-saving drugs; wrong/ improper history given by the victim or his relatives; and unavailability of effective analytical facilities (Harish, Sharma, et al. 2002).

Proper diagnosis has been the cornerstone for the effective management of poisoned patients. Since the definitive confirmation of the toxicant's nature involved in the poisoning cannot be obtained rapidly from the majority of healthcare facilities, the diagnosis has relied mainly on the medical history and the clinical examination of patients. One of the most critical aspects that have been addressed is the analysis of body fluids for confirmation/exclusion and for assessment of the severity through quantification of toxins. To this end, the use of toxic screens have facilitated determination of type and approximate amount of drug (legal or illegal) in various fluids such as urine, blood, saliva, hair or even using stomach contents obtained through gastric lavage or after vomiting to narrow down it to a case of drug abuse, drug intoxication or overdose (commonly used for barbiturates, amphetamines, benzodiazepines, cocaine, cannabinoids, phencyclidine and opioids). The use of toxicology screens has further helped the clinicians in predicting the future toxic effects, confirmation for differential diagnosis or to guide therapy. The testing has also been imperative where there is involvement of multiple drug ingestion, as the impact of one drug may overshadow the clinical symptoms of the other drugs' effects.

Toxidromic approach to clinical diagnosis of poisoning cases has achieved much attention over the years. Characteristic clinical syndromes, called toxidromes, a portmanteau of toxic and syndrome may be linked with few poisonings and, hence, may allow valuable clues that aid in the diagnosis of an unknown poison. Grouping the different symptoms of poisoning exhibited by a patient into toxidromes has helped the clinician in rapidly identifying, evaluating and managing the patient. However, all the patients may not exhibit all features linked with a specific toxin and toxidromes have been found to overlap in patients consuming more than one agent (example - combined toxicity of snakebite and *Jatropha curcas)* (Mahajan and Shah 2016). Further improvements in the preventive and management programs has been brought about by identifying circumstances of high risk, susceptible groups, chemicals and substances involved in the poisoning cases. Toxicology laboratories such as that in AIIMS have been involved in generating baseline data on the epidemiological factors contributing to the incidence (in relation to age, sex and socioeconomic status) and mortality due to insecticide poisoning so as to highlight the problems which require planned and concerted efforts in dealing with it. Case studies have also highlighted profile and the outcome of acute toxicity cases in patients using information such as psychological analysis, patient demographics, kind of toxins involved and toxicology screens enabling the development of better preventive and management strategies (Singh, Javeri, et al. 2011). Here we would like to elaborate on the management of few toxicological emergencies with respect to India (Table 6.1).

Table 6.1 Toxidromes for various poisoning cases and their management in India

Poisoning agent	Toxidrome	Management	References
Organophosphates and carbamates	**Muscarinic features:** Urination, diarrhea, bronchorrhea, miosis, emesis, bronchoconstriction, salivation, lacrimation and sweating **Nicotinic features:** Muscle weakness, tachycardia, hypertension, fatigue, muscle cramps and muscle fasciculations **CNS features:** Restlessness, severe headache, weakness, confusion, convulsions, coma, and depression of cardio-respiratory centre.	Gastric lavage is conducted if the time between ingestion and presentation is below 4 hours, activated charcoal (30-100 g in sorbitol and water) to lower the absorption of poison, administration of antidote pralidoxime and atropine	(Singh, Dilawari, et al. 1985, Singh and Sharma, 2000, Singh, Chaudhry, et al. 2001)

Contd...

Poisoning agent	Toxidrome	Management	References
	Other features: Acute garlic odour of exhaled breath is characteristic feature of this poisoning; muscular paralysis between 24 and 96 hours		
Aluminium phosphide (ALP)	Clinical manifestations are seen within 30 minutes of ingestion with epigastric discomfort, retrosternal burning, and recurrent vomiting, fishy smell from the breath, within next few hours, hypotension and shock occur because of cardiotoxicity, respiratory features include dyspnea, cough, pulmonary edema and ARDS, severe metabolic acidosis (common), sometimes observed elevation transaminases and bilirubin levels	If the patient presents within few hours post ingestion, absorption of ALP can be decreased via conducting a gastric lavage employing potassium permanganate in 1:10000 dilution, activated charcoal is helpful since it adsorbs ALP, no antidote is available to decrease the effects of phosphine on different organs, magnesium sulphate has given different responses with ALP poisoning with variable results, supportive measures are important, shock is managed initially by infusing 2-3 litres of saline in the first 3-6 hours, low-dose dopamine (4-6 Hg/kg/min) and steroids are helpful in patients with continued hypotension, metabolic acidosis is corrected via infusion of sodium bicarbonate.	(Singh, Dilawari, et al. 1985, Chugh 1992, Chugh, Kamar, et al. 1994, Chugh 1995)
Kerosene oil (mostly children)	Sensation of immediate burning in the mouth along with nausea and vomiting, hypoxia lethargy, dizziness, headache, drowsiness, convulsions, coma, radiographic observations consist of pneumonitis, perihilar densities, atelectasis and sometimes areas of consolidation.	Maintenance of the ventilatory status of the patient	http://www.api india.org/pdf/m edicine_update _2007/58.pdf, (Gupta, Singh, et al. 1992, Sharma, Nain, et al. 1996)

Contd...

Poisoning agent	Toxidrome	Management	References
Phenol	Sensation of immediate burning in the mouth and the throat followed by abdominal pain and vomiting, hardening and whitening of the mucous membranes of lips and mouth, giddiness and drowsiness followed by coma, in severe cases, metabolic acidosis, cardiovascular depression and cardiac arrhythmias may also develop, intravascular haemolysis, methemoglobinemia, and hepatic and renal failure can occure	Support to the vital organs, cautious gastric lavage to remove the ingested phenol.	http://www.api india.org/pdf/m edicine_update _2007/58.pdf
Cannabis	In early phase, the patient has anxiety, hyperactivity and fear of death, later develops exhilarated behavior, calm euphoria and clear sense of happiness and feeling of lightness of limbs and body, after 2-4 hours, becomes lazy and drowsy, hypothermia may occur specially in children	Physical restraint may be needed in few cases, if required, diazepam may be utilized, for psychotic features, haloperidol is administered	http://www.api india.org/pdf/m edicine_update _2007/58.pdf
Benzodia-zepine	CNS depression, drowsiness, ataxic or presence of low-grade coma. complications may emerge secondary to coma particularly in elderly or patients with chronic obstructive lung disease.	Mostly supportive care, Flumazenil administration in patients with respiratory depression	(Mohan, Mohan et al. 2002)
Methanol	Initially nausea and abdominal pain, CNS features occur within the first few hours and include weakness, dizziness, and headache later, the patient may develop seizures and coma, ocular toxicity as a delayed feature, accumulation of formic acid leading to Kussmaul's breathing	Gastric lavage within 2 h of ingestion, administration of sodium bicarbonate to prevent acidosis, administration of alcohol and 4-methylpyrazole or fomepizole, hemodialysis	http://www.api india.org/pdf/m edicine_update _2007/58.pdf

Overt and indiscriminate use of pesticides has resulted in a rise in the incidences of death due to poisoning amongst the population, both accidental and deliberate. The most common pesticide poisonings in India have been due to anticholinesterases (organophosphates and carbamates) followed by aluminum phosphide (ALP). It has been anticipated that the mortality in case of

OPs has been low, as their antidotes (atropine and 2-PAM) are widely available. However, mortality due to ALP, which is the most commonly consumed pesticide, has been a matter of huge concern. Since the first case was reported in 1981, the number of incidents increasingly progressed throughout North India so much, so that the problem acquired an epidemic proportion (Siwach, Yadav, et al. 1988, Bajaj and Wasir 1990, Chugh, Ram, et al. 1991). Unfortunately, the absence of a specific antidote has lead to very high mortality and the solutions have lied majorly on immediate decontamination and resuscitative measures. A bedside test has been described enabling the diagnosis of ALP ingestion, employing gastric aspirates and paper strips that are impregnated with silver nitrate (Chugh, Ram, et al. 1989). The test revealed to be positive in all of the cases of ALP ingestion. Effective management has involved decontamination using potassium permanganate or activated charcoal and rapid excretion through the administration of magnesium sulfate. Also, some experimental studies suggest that N-acetyl cysteine (NAC), vitamin C and E, glutathione, beta-carotene, melatonin, coconut oil and atropine may play a pivotal role in reduction of the oxidative outcomes of phosphine (Moghadamnia 2012). The administration of H_2 receptor antagonists has been suggested after ALP ingestion for reducing the gastric acidity and preventing further release of phosphine gas. An important legislative preventive measure has been a better-regulated supply of ALP in the form of granulated powder in plastic sachets that could lead to a decreased severity of poisoning as ALP gets exposed to atmospheric moisture leading to escape of phosphine during the opening of these sachets (Sharma, Meena, et al. 2014).

Animal bites have been a common medical emergency in India; however, there is a lack of credible information dealing with snake bite emergencies. According to reports, India has the highest number of snake bites (81,000) and deaths (11,000) each year which is likely an underestimate due to paucity of epidemiological data (Kasturiratne, Wickremasinghe, et al. 2008). The snake venoms are majorly characterized as hemotoxic and neurotoxic. The hemotoxic venoms lead to tissue destruction on all body systems along with adverse effects on the circulatory system whereas the neurotoxic venoms affect at the molecular level, by disruption of the neuromuscular junctions, thus limiting muscle activity. Few venoms contain toxins (Russell's viper) which activate factors V, X, IX and XIII, protein C, platelet aggregation, fibrinolysis, anticoagulation and hemorrhage (Gupta and Peshin 2014). Lack of knowledge with regard to simple measures of prevention, hazard risks and shortage of anti-snake/scorpion venom all magnify the risk. Difficult transportation, inadequate access to health care services, and consequent delay in the administration of anti-snake venom (ASV) results in high fatality. In 2008, the Ministry of Health & Family Welfare, Government of India drafted the National Snake Bite Management Protocol to provide guidelines for effective management of snake bites. By implementation of these guidelines, the locally developed protocol in West Bengal has resulted in the reduction of the number of deaths and usage of ASV (Ghosh, Maisnam, et al. 2008).

ASV has been the mainstay of treatment to snake bites. In India, lyophilized polyvalent ASV is prepared by the Central Research Institute, Kasauli (Himachal Pradesh) and the Haffkine Corporation, Parel (Mumbai) which has been raised against the common species of snakes in India (Big Four: Cobra, Russell's viper, Krait, and Saw-scaled viper). The adverse effects are managed with adrenaline, antihistamines and late serum sickness with antihistamines and prednisolone. The treatment strategies used for patients against scorpion stings have included drug regimens like prazosin, angiotensin-converting enzyme inhibitors and insulin (Yugandhar, Radha Krishna Murthy, et al. 1999, Bawaskar and Bawaskar 2000, Krishnan, Sonawane, et al. 2007). The major clinical issues with ASV have been species specificity, availability, affordability and proper storage conditions. The other difficulties with ASV therapy are adverse reactions which can potentially range from early reactions (pruritus, urticaria) to fatal anaphylaxis. Several medicinal plants with accepted therapeutic values have been attracting more considerable attention. Reliance on plants has been majorly due to their effectiveness, safety, cost-effectiveness, easy availability and cultural preferences. Reviews have provided a comprehensive account of numerous Indian medicinal plants and their specific parts utilized in the treatment of snake and scorpion bite in many forms like topical application, oral formulation for relief and also for the purpose of neutralization of venom (Bahekar, Kale, et al. 2012, Gupta and Peshin 2014).

Apart from traditional substances like alcohol, tobacco, opium and its derivatives and cannabis, newer substances such as prescription drugs, injectable drugs, inhalants and others have also been posing a real threat. Effective management of these disorders, therefore, has been an important skill required by all physicians as well as health professionals. Numerous authors have reviewed the changing trends of substance use over the years (Murthy, Manjunatha et al. 2010, Basu, Aggarwal, et al. 2012, Ray and Chopra 2012). Data on drug use have been recorded through several general population surveys in the 1970s and 1980s (Ray and Chopra 2012). However, all these epidemiological surveys were regional, with difficulty in drawing references for national prevalence. The viability and effectiveness of a Drug Abuse Monitoring System in the country was examined for the first time as a ICMR-Taskforce project conducted at Delhi, Lucknow and Jodhpur in 1990 which provided one-year data on the usage trends among 10,321 persons (Mohan, Sitholey et al. 1993). The National Household Survey on Drug Abuse in the country in 2003 was the first systematic effort to record the nationwide prevalence of drug usage. Alcohol was the highest substance used (21.4%), followed by cannabis (3%) and opioids (0.7%). Follow up studies by the National Family Health Survey and Drug Abuse Monitoring System have provided further insights into the changing trends of substance use. Use of clonidine for opioid detoxification dates back to 1980 as the only choice due to its adrenergic activity (Gangadhar, Subrahmanya, et al. 1982). Sublingual buprenorphine for detoxification in patients has been reported as early as 1992. Slow release of oral morphine for opioid maintenance has also been documented (Rao, Dhawan et al. 2005). A case report of Wernicke Korsakoff syndrome (secondary to alcohol abuse) successfully treated using a combination of thiamine and magnesium sulfate (Murali, Rao, et al. 1983) and subclinical alcoholic dementia successfully managed with thiamine and Vitamin B supplementation (Mohan, Pradhan et al. 1983) has been demonstrated. Pharmacological intervention using drugs like lorazepam and chlordiazepoxide have shown effective detoxification in alcohol-dependent patients (Kumar, Andrade, et al. 2009).

Adverse drugs reactions (ADRs) are noxious, undesirable and unintended effects that result due to drug treatments at doses which are normally prescribed in man for the purpose of diagnosis, prophylaxis, and treatment. Further, concomitant administration of drug therapies possesses major challenge in the form of drug-drug interactions, cumulative drug toxicity, and high pill burden, further complicating the outcome of the treatment that have required immediate attention. The undesired effects have been categorized into types like toxic effects, side effects, adverse reactions, and adverse drug events, etc., depending upon the taxonomic classification that is used. While the exact epidemiology remains to be known in India, ADRs have gradually emerged as leading killers. Monitoring of adverse drug reactions started in India around 1982 (Dhikav, Singh, et al. 2004). Under the chairmanship of the Drug Controller of India, five centers were set up with the notion of establishing a monitoring program at the national level to generate an ADR profile which would enable the early diagnosis, prevention and effective management of ADRs and subsequently reduce the morbidity among patients. Though the pattern of such reactions may differ from country to country slightly, adverse reactions to antibiotics and analgesics (mainly, non-steroidal anti-inflammatory drugs) have constituted around half of all such reports from India. Various case studies have provided representative data on the ADR profile of the antipsychotics and antidepressants that are widely used (Sengupta, Bhowmick, et al. 2011, Lahon, Shetty, et al. 2012, Sridhar, Al-Thamer, et al. 2016). Antipsychotics have been associated with effect on the CNS and peripheral nervous system. In all cases, the suspected drugs were withheld and particular treatments like benzodiazepines, anticholinergic, and β-blockers were administered. The second most commonly documented ADR in CNS were tremors that have been managed through dose reduction and administration of central anticholinergic drug.

A simple case of drug-induced liver toxicity has been described, as it is a fairly common, but mostly unrecognized cause of liver damage which continues to fascinate and challenge clinical toxicologists. Drug-induced hepatotoxicity (DIH) is a potentially serious adverse effect of the currently used anti-tuberculosis regimens which contain isoniazid, rifampicin and pyrazinamide. Diagnosis has been inclusive of detection of five times the normal levels (upper limit) of aspartate aminotransferase (AST) and/or alanine aminotransferase (ALT), increase in serum total bilirubin levels and any rise in AST and/or ALT above the pre-treatment levels along with nausea, vomiting, anorexia, and jaundice. The underlying mechanisms of antituberculosis treatment (ATT)-induced hepatotoxicity and the several factors which predispose its development are not well understood. Idiosyncratic damage, dose-dependent toxicity, hepatic enzymes induction, drug-induced acute hepatitis and allergic reactions have all been proposed as the pathogenetic mechanisms underlying DIH. The age and sex of the patients, GSTM1 polymorphism (Roy, Chowdhury, et al. 2001), chronic alcoholism and chronic liver disease (Mukherjee, Vishnubhatla, et al. 2017), hepatitis B virus carrier status (Tandon, Acharya, et al. 1996), MHC class II alleles (Sharma, Balamurugan, et al. 2002) and slow acetylator status (Pande, Singh, et al. 1996) have also been implicated as predisposing factors in earlier studies.

Advances in analytical techniques have changed the current face of medical toxicology in the context of prognosis, diagnosis, management and prevention of poisonings. Urine toxicology screening has been utilized for providing direct evidence of intoxication, also identifying a particular toxin whose antidote may be available and quantifying a toxin through titrated therapy. LC-tandem mass spectrometry (LC/MS/MS) for toxicity screening has provided a rapid and easy technique enabling simultaneous multi-drug quantification and identification from several samples like saliva, serum or urine. LC/MS/MS quantitative methods can detect and quantify drugs of abuse at levels which are significantly lower than the current cut-off levels. Traditionally, urine has been the most widely used matrix for drug testing due to its easy collection, even in large volumes, and simple analysis. In the last decade, new matrices like oral liquids and hair have become quite prevalent at workplace drug testing and medicolegal sectors. A number of other methods, including ELISA, have been effectively developed for the detection of venoms and antibodies.

In most countries, including India, emergency medicine has not been established so well and clinical toxicology has been a low priority with respect to research and clinical management. Unfortunately, in India the idea of analysis of samples from living victims of poisoning is not yet popular, primarily due to a lack of specialized laboratories which can conduct such toxicological analysis. The only units which conduct such studies are a part of government-controlled forensic science laboratories or chemical examiner's laboratories, which carry out toxicological analysis only for forensic purposes (medico-legal cases), but not for clinical purposes. Lack of formal training in toxicology results in only a handful of doctors/scientists taking up this specialty. In such a scenario, medical toxicologists are virtually non-existent in India and hence, medical toxicology as a separate discipline has been long overdue. Only in the last decade, the importance of specialization is gaining recognition and few attempts are being made from different quarters to uplift toxicology to its rightful place in the field of medicine (Flora 2008).

CHAPTER 7

Nanotoxicology

Since Richard Feynman's popular statement that was made in 1959, "There is plenty of room at the bottom," the field of nanotechnology has rapidly expanded in the world, including India. Nanoparticles are known to exhibit significantly different physicochemical properties as compared to their bulk counterparts of the same material. These unique and improved properties have made them the most sought after for innumerable products but at the same time rendered them more biologically reactive, in the most unexpected ways, giving easy access to the distal regions of biological systems which are generally not accessible to the larger particles. Their extraordinarily small size and high surface area per unit of mass could altogether impart a different biokinetic behavior leading to unrecognized toxicological consequences. These issues have raised much apprehension regarding their safety evaluation alongside their production and application. The withdrawal of the nano drug, Albupax, (used as drug delivery system for cancer) from the Indian market in 2009, after it displayed severe side effects on the liver further sparked off debates demanding the need for a parallel risk assessment (https://www.deccanherald. com/content/66392/govt-declares-breast-cancer-drug.html).

Nanotoxicology, a nascent field concerned with the evaluation of toxicity of nanomaterials, their interactions with the living organisms as well as the environment, has been hampered mainly due to several experimental challenges faced in toxicological assessment of nanomaterials. Unlike classical toxicity studies, safety evaluation of nanomaterial (NM)/nanoparticle (NP) requires a comprehensive characterization (size, chemical composition, crystal structure, shape, surface area, charge and chemistry, solubility and state of agglomeration) that is fundamental to their toxicity. The dilemma in the selection and validation of the test methods for the NMs, their characterization coupled with dose parameters (particle mass, surface area or number) for precise dose-response relationship and suitable tools for cytotoxicity and genotoxicity assessment have further limited the progress in the field (Dhawan, Sharma, et al. 2009, Dhawan and Sharma 2010).

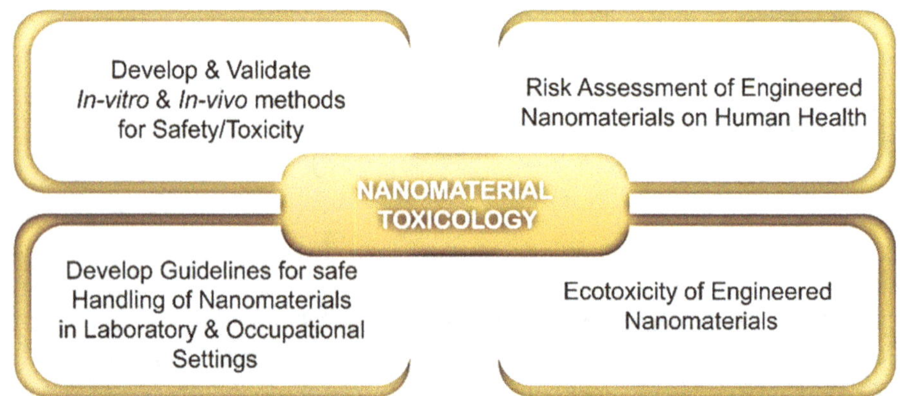

Figure 7.1 Approaches used for nanotoxicity evaluation

With the growing realization of entirely new dimensions regarding the safety of NMs, Nano-mission program was initiated under the aegis of DST in 2008, which was complemented through multi-agency involvement (CSIR, DBT, DIT, ISRO, DRDO, etc.) (Bhattacharya, Jayanthi, et al. 2012). Another major impetus in the direction of nanotoxicology research was the NanoSHE program in 2012 involving 14 CSIR laboratories that envisaged to establish impact and risk assessment of engineered NMs used in industrial application, consumer products and therapeutics in India utilizing the "Safe by Design" approach. In India, substantial progress has been made in the realm of nanotoxicology research directed towards their synthesis and detailed characterization, bioavailability, uptake, biodistribution and excretion profiles, investigation of interactions with biological systems (from the whole organism to the molecular level), understanding important routes of exposure and their ecological impact.

A plethora of studies have revealed an array of toxicological effects of NPs using different models such as prokaryotes (Kumar, Pandey, et al. 2011), plants (Kumari, Khan, et al. 2011, Vajpayee, Khatoon, et al. 2011, Burman, Saini, et al. 2013) and human cell lines (Khan, Pillai, et al. 2007, Sharma, Shukla, et al. 2009, Sharma, Singh, et al. 2011, Shukla, Kumar, et al. 2011). The risk of occupational exposure to NPs such as dolomite and granite dust has also triggered extensive research to characterize their size-dependent effects *in vitro* to ensure separate health safety standards (Ahmad, Khan, et al. 2011, Ahmad, Khan, et al. 2012, Patil, Khan, et al. 2012). Concomitantly, the risk and hazard associated with the physico-chemical characteristics is concerning, as continual research emerges to suggest the involvement of NPs in stimulating inflammatory responses, oxidative stress, promoting cell death (cytotoxicity) and DNA damage (genotoxicity) through different methods, with varying chemical compositions, size, shape, surface area, surface coatings, etc. (Sharma, Shukla et al. 2009, Sharma, Anderson, et al. 2011, Shukla, Sharma, et al. 2011, Vallabani, Mittal, et al. 2011, Sharma, Anderson, et al. 2012).

With the establishment of nanotoxicology group in 2008, CSIR-IITR began working in the area of safety evaluation of NPs with an attempt to devise new methods and validate techniques that could be applied for the toxicity assessment of engineered NPs. CSIR-IITR also added to its credit the NanoLINEN project, a consortium between CSIR-IITR and 7 European laboratories in 2010, with the goal to develop robust risk assessment methodologies to explore the potential human and environmental health risks associated with nanotechnology (Dhawan, Shanker, et al. 2011). For over a decade now, its research competencies have broadened to encompass extensive investigations of NPs biological systems interactions (using *in vitro*, *in vivo*, metabolomics approaches) to screen them for cytotoxicity, dermal toxicity, immunotoxicity, neurotoxicity, genotoxicity, reproductive toxicity and ecotoxicological impact. The institute has been actively involved in the evaluation of the mechanism-based cytotoxic potential of NPs with special focus on metal oxides like ZnO, CeO_2, TiO_2, multi-walled carbon nanotubes and C-60 fullerenes to develop surrogate biomarkers of exposure and effect.

These NPs have found usage in numerous products including cosmetics, food packaging, etc. thus increasing their chances of human exposure through multiple routes affecting the human population directly or indirectly. The experimental models for the safety/toxicity assessment of NPs have thus been based on the possible sites of contact, for example, primary cultures of human skin cells, lung cells or other organs to offer more realistic insights into the understanding of their interactions with the biological systems. To elucidate the possible mechanisms of cytotoxicity, a variety of surrogate parameters including cell viability, mitochondrial function, cell membrane damage, oxidative stress and DNA damage have also been quantitatively assessed utilizing a battery of tests like micronucleus test, comet assay (Table 7.1).

Table 7.1 Evaluation of toxic effects of various nanoparticles using *in vitro* and *in vivo* models

Type of NPs	Application	Toxic Effects/Mechanism of Action	References
Zinc Oxide (30-50 nm)	Cosmetics, sunscream, additives, packaging, fillers in orthopedic and dental implants	Cytotoxic effects, chromosomal aberrations, oxidative stress in primary human epidermal keratinocytes and human epidermal cell line (A431)	(Sharma, Shukla, et al. 2009)

Contd...

Type of NPs	Application	Toxic Effects/ Mechanism of Action	References
		Enhanced ROS generation and increase in pro-inflammatory cytokines (IFN-γ, TNF-α, IL-6, and IL-17) in murine peritoneal macrophages	(Roy, Tripathi, et al. 2011)
		Cytotoxicity, genotoxicity, oxidative stress and apoptosis in human liver cells (HepG2)	(Sharma, Anderson, et al. 2011)
		Cell shrinkage, nuclear condensation, DNA fragmentation, depletion of GSH level, elevated metallothionein gene and ROS levels in human lung epithelial cells (L-132)	(Sahu, Kannan, et al. 2013)
		Toxic effects were found to be dependent on the initial hydrodynamic particle size the concentrations, viability loss, release of LDH and ROS generation were enhanced in the water algae *Scenedesmus obliquus*	(Bhuvaneshwari, Iswarya, et al. 2015)
		Decrease in % mitotic index and higher chromosomal aberrations in a dose-dependent manner in bulbs of *Allium cepa*, increased levels of TBARS and antioxidant enzymes, ROS, disruption of mitochondrial membrane potential and DNA damage	(Ahmed, Dwivedi, et al. 2017)
		Uptake of ZnO NPs, reduction in cell viability with a concomitant induction in ROS (1-20 µg/mL) in Chinese hamster lung fibroblast cells (V-79), change of 2.84-fold in the HGPRT gene mutant frequency, manifested the cell cycle arrest, ultrastructural modifications and further cell death.	(Jain, Singh, et al. 2019)
Titanium dioxide (50 nm)	Paints and pharmaceutical preparations	Mild cytotoxic response, DNA damage, micronuclei formation, elevated levels of LPO and ROS in human epidermal cells (A431)	(Shukla, Sharma, et al. 2011)

Contd...

Type of NPs	Application	Toxic Effects/ Mechanism of Action	References
Silver (<100 nm)	Deodorants, clothing materials, bandages, cleaning solutions and sprays	Concentration (25, 20, 75, and 100 ppm) dependent reduction in the mitotic index with chromosomal abberations in *Allium cepa* root tip cells, impairment in the stages of cell division leading to stickness, chromatin bridge, multiple chromosomal breaks, disturbed metaphase, and cell disintegration	(Kumari, Mukherjee, et al. 2009)
		Caused greater extent of genotoxicity (0-80 mg/L) as compared to Ag+ ion alone in *Allium cepa* root tip cells	(Panda, Achary, et al. 2011)
Silica oxide (80 nm)	Packaging, mechanical polishing, food additive, cosmetics, optical imaging, targeted drug delivery, cancer therapy	Alterations in neurobehavioural indices, impairment in antioxidant defense system, mitochondrial and ER mediated apoptosis in corpus striatum of rat brain	(Parveen, Rizvi, et al. 2014)
Aluminium oxide (<50 nm)	Alloys, explosives, rocket fuel, wear-resistant coatings for ships, energetics, sensors, personal care products, and drug delivery systems	Dose-dependent (0.01, 0.1, 1, 10, and 100 µg/mL) reduction in the mitotic index (42 to 28%) and an increase in chromosomal aberrations in *Allium cepa* root tip cells	(Rajeshwari, Kavitha, et al. 2015)
		Chronic exposure 0.1 and 1 mM resulted in the loss of append-ages in flies resulting in five legs flies, four legs flies and absence of haltere in *Drosophila melano-gaster,* renal failure in flies as observed by swollen abdomen, 307 unique proteins were and 51 proteins were differentially expressed., alteration in striated muscle cell differentiation, digestive tract morphogenesis, photo-transduction, regulation of chromatin organization and DNA duplex unwinding	(Anand, Gahlot, et al. 2019)

Contd...

Type of NPs	Application	Toxic Effects/ Mechanism of Action	References
Chromium oxide (30 nm)	Catalyst for aromatic compound manufacture, abrading agents and as pigments	p53-mediated superoxide radical generation, leading to DNA damage, apoptosis and caspase 3-dependent apoptosis in human lung alveolar cells (A549) at concentrations 600-1000 µg/ml	(Senapati, Jain, et al. 2015)
Cerium oxide (8-20 nm)	Glass/ceramic polishing agent, television tubes, solar cells, fuel cells, ultraviolet absorbents, and gas sensors	ROS mediated DNA damage, concomitant reduction in antioxidant GSH level and cell cycle arrest in human lung cells at concentrations 25-100 µg/ml	(Mittal and Pandey, 2014)
Multi-walled carbon nanotubes (5-20 nm)	Technological and biomedical fields	Induced ROS generation and malondialdehyde with decrease in catalase acivity and glutathione associated with impaired mitochondrial activity in human lung cancer cell line-A549 at 10 and 50 µg/ml only	(Srivastava, Pant, et al. 2011)
Copper oxide (50 nm)	Catalysts, gas sensor, heat transfer fluids, microelectronics and cosmetics	Dose dependent reduction (10, 25 and 50 µg/ml, 24 h) in cell viability, decrease of glutathione and increase in lipid peroxidation, catalase and superoxide dismutase in human lung alveolar cells (A549), induction of Hsp70, up-regulated the cell cycle checkpoint protein p53 and DNA damage repair proteins Rad51 and MSH2	(Ahamed, Siddiqui, et al. 2010)
C60 Fullerenes	Technological and biomedical fields	DNA damage and genotoxic response in human lymphocytes	(Dhawan, Taurozzi, et al. 2006)
Micro and nanogranite (40-120nm)	Saw mills	Dose dependent (0.1–100 µg/ml, 6, 24 and 48 h) oxidative stress, inflammatory response and genotoxicity, increased levels of TNF-α and IL-β and increase in micronuclei formation in human lung fibroblast cell IMR-90, nano particles were more toxic	(Ahmad, Khan, et al. 2012)
Molyb-denum (40 nm)	Electron industry, cutting tools, hard alloys, textiles, microelectronic films, coatings, plastics, nano-wire, and X-ray tubes	Cytotoxicity and oxidative stress, G2/M phase arrest along with DNA damage in mouse skin fibroblast cells (L929) at 25, 50 and 100 µg/ml after 48 h	(Siddiqui, Saquib, et al. 2015)

Contd...

Type of NPs	Application	Toxic Effects/ Mechanism of Action	References
Graphite oxide (72.14 nm)	Cellular imaging and drug delivery, disease diagnosis, microbial detection, antimicrobial activity, microchips, biosensors, electrodes, conductor devices	Concentration 10-100 µg/ml, 24 and 48 h) and size dependent decrease in viability. Cytotoxicity and apoptosis induced in normal human lung Cells (BEAS-2B)	(Vallabani, Mittal, et al. 2011)
Graphene oxide/reduced graphene oxide		1–100 µg/ml for 48 h led to internalization and induced oxidative stress mediated cytotoxicity in human lung cancer (A549) and; bronchial epithelial cells (BEAS-2B)	(Mittal, Kumar, et al. 2018)
Graphene chloroquine nano-conjugate		Concentration of 25 µg/ml for 1 h induced accumulation of autophagosomes in A549 cells via blocking of autophagic flux and activation of necroptotic cell death	(Arya, Mittal, et al. 2018)

Out of all the probable routes, the skin serves as the first and most probable portal of entry for NPs either directly through the application or indirectly via breaches in the skin integrity. Human epidermal keratinocytes as an *in vitro* model have been utilized for the first time to explore biological consequences of ZnO NPs that have wide application in sunscream and cosmetics. Findings demonstrated the internalization of ZnO NPs to elicit a cytotoxic and genotoxic response. A more recent study suggested enhanced dermal penetration of ZnO NPs on exposure to environmentally relevant doses of UVB (50 mJ/cm^2) leading to pronounced inflammatory responses that could have severe implications in progression to skin cancer (Pal, Alam, et al. 2016). Studies conducted to assess the impact of ZnO nanoparticles (1µg/ml) on murine peritoneal macrophages revealed higher potency of these NPs in enhancing ROS generation as compared to bulk counterparts. The study was also indicative of the fact that the NPs owing to their small size could resist attachment and engulfment by these phagocytic cells that may enable them in escaping the macrophage immune response (Roy, Tripathi, et al. 2011). The liver has also been shown to be a susceptible target to these NPs. *In vitro* studies using human liver cells (HepG2) have established genotoxicity and oxidative stress responses against these NPs in a time and concentration dependent manner (Sharma, Anderson, et al. 2012). Biodistribution studies and excretion profiles in experimental animals further revealed access of the NPs into other organs like the kidney and liver (Srivastava, Kumar, et al. 2016). Similarly, DNA damaging potential of these NPs have also been reported in other somatic cells like lymphocytes as well as germ cells. TiO$_2$, NPs have led to DNA damage and micronucleus formation in human epidermal cells. The highest concentration of TiO$_2$ NPs was 80 µg/ml (0.080 mg/ml) which is far less than the concentrations used in sunscreens (30 mg/ml at the lowest concentration) warranting the need of monitoring the levels before incorporation in products (Shukla, Sharma, et al. 2011).

Similarly, studies have also highlighted the cytotoxic potential of other NPs, including CeO$_2$, and Cr$_2$O$_3$ on human lung cells. In view of findings reporting inhaled NPs translocating to other organs like the brain, much efforts have been diverted towards assessing the potential of these NPs in the causation of neurotoxicity. In this context, studies have highlighted impairment in neurobehavioral indices experimental rats on sub-chronic exposure of silica NPs. Such alterations were also associated with perturbed catecholamine levels and dopamine D2 receptors. This has been the very first *in vivo* study to illustrate si NPs induced apoptosis mediated responses along with mitochondrial stress signalling (Parveen, Rizvi, et al. 2014). Metabolomics has also been employed as a tool to understand the potential toxicity of nanoparticles at the molecular level and researchers have been able to identify the perturbations in the metabolism by NPs (Parveen, Rizvi, et al. 2012, Ratnasekhar, Sonane, et al. 2015).

Nanotechnology has speculated new hope in drug delivery to facilitate targeted therapy and increased efficacy of treatment strategy. Biocompatible nanoparticles, nanostructured lipid carriers, nanoemulsions, dendrimers, etc. are extensively being explored for delivery of therapeutic agents (Jain, Kumar Mehra, et al. 2015), thus demanding parallel toxicity studies to establish their safe use in medicine. In this context, noteworthy contributions have been made by NIPER which in addition to developing regulatory guidelines for approval of nanotechnology-based drugs, has directed much of its work towards synthesizing and toxicity screening of nanoparticles based drug delivery systems for therapeutic applications in cancer. These formulations have been evaluated for their release and pharmacokinetic behavior and toxicity profiling using several *in vitro* and *in vivo* models to establish their safe use. Tamoxifen has been commonly used in breast cancer oral therapy, but drawbacks like hepatic first-pass metabolism and toxic hepatitis, necrosis and cirrhosis have limited their use. PLGA-NP-mediated delivery has demonstrated better bioavailability, enhanced antitumor efficacy, and marked reduction in hepatotoxicity when compared with the marketed formulation (Jain, Swarnakar, et al. 2011). Moreover, co-encapsulation of PLGA-NPs with tamoxifen along with the flavonoid quercetin has been demonstrated to exhibit higher tumor suppression in contrast to respective free drugs with no measurable signs of hepatotoxicity and oxidative stress (Jain, Thanki, et al. 2013). Similarly, synthesis of docetaxel-loaded estradiol functionalized stealth polymeric NPs have been reported to offer efficient target delivery against cancer cells *in vitro* with reduced hepato and nephrotoxicity in comparison with the marketed formulation, Taxotere (Jain, Spandana et al. 2015). Advance strategies have been suggested to circumvent dose-dependent cardiotoxicity elicited by doxorubicin by its nanoformulation utilizing PLGA NPs prepared by a double emulsion method exhibiting enhanced therapeutic efficiency (Kalaria, Sharma, et al. 2009). Further studies have been undertaken to apprehend the effect of surface modifications like the degree of surface functionalization on biodistribution, toxicity, and biocompatibility of carbon nanotubes (Jain, Thakare, et al. 2011).

Several research groups in CSIR- Institute of Genomics and Integrative Biology (CSIR-IGIB), New Delhi, are involved in synthesizing and *in vitro* and *in vivo* activity studies of new, effective and non-toxic nano-delivery systems that are based on cationic polymers and peptides (Nimesh, Aggarwal, et al. 2007, Bansal, Tripathi, et al. 2012, Arif, Tripathi, et al. 2013, Mahato, Sharma, et al. 2013, Tripathi, Gupta, et al. 2014). The cationic surfactants' structure for controlling DNA condensation has also been studied utilizing a broad range of biophysical techniques (Sur, Tiwari et al. 2017, Vij, Alam, et al. 2017). Moreover, the mechanistic aspects on the packaging processes of several peptide and polymer DNA nanocarriers via Atomic Force Microscopy and correlating their efficiency of intracellular delivery with packaging is also being carried out (Vij, Grover, et al. 2016, Vij, Natarajan, et al. 2016). These approaches may potentially result in designing of new materials for targeted delivery with minimal toxicity. IGIB in addition to its ongoing research on drug delivery has also been applying a toxicogenomic based approach in order to observe and rationalize the toxic effects of gold, silica and other NPs in both cultured cells and zebrafish model systems. Notable contributions have also been made by CSIR-Indian Institute of Chemical Technology (CSIR-IICT), Kolkata, that has also conducted toxicity evaluation of iron oxide, aluminium oxide and gold NPs. More recently, the institute also has to its credit a novel design for delivery of doxorubicin using biosynthesized gold NPs from the extract of *Peltophorum pterocarpum* leaves. This gold NP-based drug delivery system has demonstrated to inhibit cancer cell proliferation *in vitro* and reduce tumor growth *in vivo* without showing any toxicity *in vivo*, suggestive of its application in safe cancer therapy (Mukherjee, Sau, et al. 2016).

Other institutes also working in the realm of nanotoxicological research include Jamia Hamdard University and AIIMS. Hamdard University has explored the safety of nanoformulations and nanoemulsions. Research on the effect of NPs on macrophages has been a topic of interest at AIIMS and studies are being undertaken on the toxicity and biocompatibility of few nanomedicines. The Amrita Centre for Nanoscience, a private research organization and an established Centre of Excellence, is also pursuing toxicity based research for bio-material based nanomedicines along with examination of the toxicity of NPs for cancer applications.

NP-containing products owing to their wide application have enhanced the likelihood of their inadvertent release into the ecosystem, making it critical to identify their toxicity potential on the environment and environmentally relevant organisms. Studies have explored the versatility of using microorganisms and non-vertebrate *in vivo* system as models for ecotoxicology assessment. Their short doubling time and possibilities to manipulate using recombinant techniques have given additional benefits to express different proteins in a shorter period. ZnO and TiO_2 silver nanoparticles have been demonstrated to be internalized by non-targeted ecologically beneficial microorganisms like *S. typhimurium*, *E.coli* and *Pseudomonas sp* and induce significant oxidative, metabolic stress at molecular level resulting in DNA damage (Khatoon, Vajpayee, et al. 2011, Kumar, Pandey, et al. 2011). Similarly, the soil nematode *Caenorhabditis elegans*, an alternative to animal model has offered itself as an excellent *in vivo* model to investigate the ecotoxicological effects of nano-material exposures to identify molecular signatures of size-related nanotoxicity, useful for future toxicological screening of nanomaterials. Active uptake of NPs by *C. elegans* has been documented to be a vital cause for decrease in reproduction, inhibition of growth and behavioural deficits (Khare, Sonane, et al. 2015). Further, gas chromatography-mass spectrometry (GC–MS) based metabolomics approach has been employed as a novel tool to understand the toxicity to provide valuable information regarding perturbations in metabolites of various biochemical pathways (tricarboxylic acid (TCA) cycle, arachidonic acid metabolism and glyoxalate dicarboxylate metabolism) against TiO_2 nanoparticles (Ratnasekhar, Sonane et al. 2015). Studies have also highlighted dose and size-dependent toxicity against these microorganisms that mandates the size inclusion as an additional parameter for the careful monitoring of ZnO NPs disposal in the environment.

While accumulating strong evidence for the conclusive ecological safety of engineered NMs (ENMs), it is also imperative to evaluate their environmental movement and fate within and across trophic levels of the food chains. In this regard, progress has been made to understand the trophic transfer of ENMs in the aquatic food chain. A laboratory level two trophic level food chain has been established using *Paramecium caudatum* as a predator and *E. coli* as a prey species to investigate the bioaccumulation and biomagnification potential of cadmium telluride quantum dots. *P. caudatum* a ciliated protozoan can easily ingest and digest bacteria as compared to the other free-living model ciliates, forming an important ecological association between microbes and multicellular organisms in the aquatic ecosystem. The study also proposed for the very first time that *P. caudatum* can be employed as an aquatic model to explore the impact of NMs in the food chain. Studies demonstrated a higher risk to *P. caudatum* via bioaccumulation of quantum dots in the predator model affecting its grazing potential (bacterivory) and growth rate indicative of severe implications for recycling of nutrients in the aquatic ecosystem (Gupta, Kumar, et al. 2017). These studies have substantiated the need for impact assessment of such novel materials in environmental settings that hold the potential to disrupt ecological balance.

Taking into consideration the growing number of NMs entering the market, risk assessment of every variant of NMs and their possible derivatives would be a Herculean task. Therefore, the requirement for hazard ranking and grouping according to their risk has been widely acknowledged. The Centre for Cellular and Molecular Biology (CCMB) is a participating laboratory in an International project NANOVALID that has been undertaken to generate toxicity data for 7 physicochemically well-characterized NMs utilizing a suite of 15 *in vitro* bioassays, to screen out the most sensitive bioassays (on the basis of a decision-tree) for ecotoxicity screening and initial hazard ranking of NMs. Altogether 15 different cell lines and test organisms involving a wide variety of cells and ecologically relevant organisms (3 mammalian cell lines *in vitro*, 6 medically important bacterial species, algae, yeast protozoan, 2 crustacean species and zebrafish) have bee used. The selected ecotoxicological organisms represented both, particle-ingesting (protozoa, crustaceans) and presumably non-ingesting (bacteria, algae, fish embryos) species from different trophic levels from consumers to decomposers (Bondarenko, Heinlaan, et al. 2016). This has allowed for hazard ranking of the various NMs.

Though there have been extensive studies undertaken to characterize dose and size dependent toxic effects of various NMs, unfortunately only limited studies have been directed towards the pursuit of protective/preventive agents. One study has evaluated the efficacy of curcumin and β-caryophyllene to reduce cadmium quantum dots induced oxidative stress and toxicity in the same model system (Srivastava, Pant, et al. 2016). Similarly, studies have demonstrated the efficacy of a natural triterpene ursolic acid (3β-hydroxy-urs-12-en-28-oic acid; UA) for attenuating the cytotoxicity of ZnO NPs using *C. elegans* (Negi, Saikia et al. 2017). These studies hint at the possibility of avoiding the toxic aspects of NPs via supplementation of phytochemical(s) in the biological system.

CHAPTER 8

Toxicogenomics

Conventional toxicology in India for a long stretch of the time relied upon classical toxicity testing and biochemical assessments to estimate the adverse health effects of xenobiotics on various species, at different organs, doses and time points. However, biological variations in toxicity elicited at specific endpoints could also be attributed to variations in gene expression products as a result of mRNA transcription, RNA splicing, post-translational modifications, etc. Moreover, many genes may exhibit a higher influence on vulnerability to environmental contaminants. Therefore, their identification as well as characterization of polymorphism for determining the early, late, or no response of the individual for the toxicant-induced diseases stands imperative. Toxicogenomics, a combinatorial approach of conventional toxicity testing methods and molecular toxicology (differential gene expression profiling (microarray), cell/ tissue-wide protein profiling (proteomics), genetic susceptibility (single nucleotide polymorphism) and bioinformatics) has collectively offered better strategies for toxicity prediction and identification of toxic compounds to facilitate understanding of the role of gene-environment interactions.

Despite of being a developing country, India has been at the forefront in the application of omics technologies. The fast evolution of genome-based techniques has accelerated the wide application of gene expression profiling studies in toxicology giving rise to a number of benefits, including assistance with more rapid screens for assessing compound toxicity, enabling decisions for compound selection based on safety and efficacy, facilitating novel research leads; in-depth appreciation of mechanisms of toxicity, and an improved ability to accurately extrapolate between experimental animals and humans. With the state of the art omics approaches gaining popularity worldwide, India took the need of the hour initiative wherein CSIR, Government of India in 2003 initiated a program on 'toxicogenomics of genetic polymorphism in Indian population to industrial chemicals for development of biomarkers' with CSIR-IITR as the nodal laboratory. The primary objective was to identify the individuals genetically predisposed towards higher risk for toxicant-induced diseases and elucidation of how the genome interacts with the toxicants. The program envisaged at developing a comprehensive database on the gene and protein expression profiles of exposed and unexposed human beings against various classes of chemicals including chlorinated pesticides, biomass fuels, petroleum products, and several heavy metals such as mercury, arsenic and lead and several other heavy metals with key participation of other laboratories like Centre for Cellular and Molecular Biology (CCMB), Hyderabad, National Environmental Engineering Research Institute (NEERI), Nagpur, Institute of Genomics and Integrated Biology (IGIB), Delhi, and Indian Institute of Chemical Biology (IICB), Kolkata. The goal of the Single Nucleotide Polymorphism (SNP) part of the program has been to identify sequence polymorphisms rendering an individual more or less susceptible to toxicant exposure that could enable screening of individuals for evaluations based on their susceptibilities (Patel, Parmar, et al. 2005).

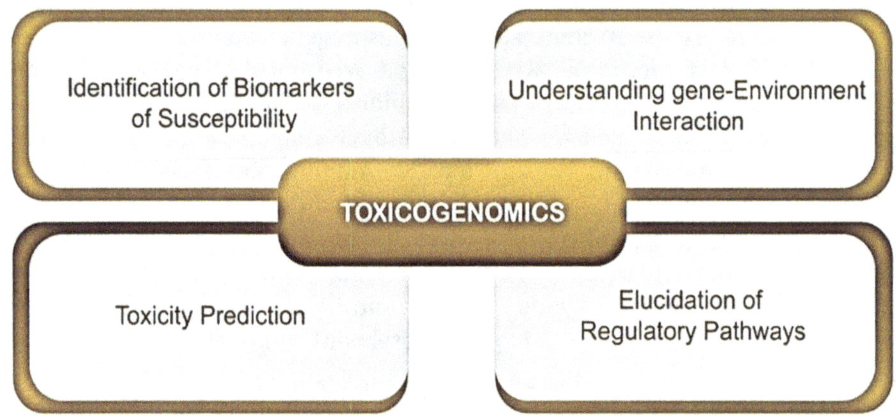

Figure 8.1 Approaches used in Toxicogenomics

The field of epidemiology has received a major boost from the molecular approaches and significant attention has been directed towards the development of biomarkers of susceptibility of human exposures to toxicants. Differential gene expression profiling and proteome analysis have become a diagnostic tool for early detection in occupational, environmental exposure and drug/chemical induced toxicity, in clinical as well as environmental settings. For example, genetic polymorphism in GSTM1 null genotypes, and a link of NAT2 slow acetylation genotypes with CYP2C9*3/*3 or GSTM1 null genotypes may be capable of modulating DNA damage in workers exposed to OPs (Singh, Kumar et al. 2011, Singh, Kumar, et al. 2012). Similarly, individuals with PON1 Q/Q and M/M genotypes in the Paraoxonase gene-1 are more susceptible toward genotoxicity of OPs (Singh, Kumar, et al. 2011). Simultaneous monitoring of biomarkers of susceptibility (SNPs in CYP2D6, GSTM1 and NQO1 gene) via blood proteome profiling have provided a broader view to precisely predict the miners more susceptible to manganese-related diseases in occupational settings (Vinayagamoorthy, Krishnamurthi, et al. 2010).

The studies undertaken in Indian populations on SNP genotyping have revealed significant potential in identifying susceptible individuals, developing preventive and effective strategies and therapies, and predicting treatment outcomes. Indian population is rich in the diverse genetic pool and has thus provided an excellent model for SNP based studies. Individual genetic variation screened through PCR-restriction fragment length polymorphism (RFLP), amplified fragment length polymorphism (AFLP), DNA microarray and direct and indirect sequencings have become a routine practice revealing significant differences in the genes involved in xenobiotic metabolism, cell cycle control, DNA repair, and cell signalling that might confer greater or reduced risk to the toxicant. As the xenobiotic metabolism is mainly carried out by cytochrome P450s (CYPs) and glutathione-S-transferases (GSTs), which can enhance, reduce and abolish drug metabolisms, the polymorphisms in these genes may influence the vulnerability of an individual to environmental toxins and have been associated with several types of diseases such as cancer, liver cirrhosis and neurological disorders like Parkinson's Disease (Table 8.1).

Table 8.1 Representative studies on the effects of genetic polymorphism of toxicant responsive genes on diseases/disorders spanning the Indian population

Diseases	Genes	Genotypes	Status	References
Head and neck cancer	CYP2A6 and GSTP1	CYP 2A6*1B, CYP 2A6*4C (Var.) GSTP1 (in regular tobacco users)	Decrease in risk Decrease in risk	(Ruwali, Pant, et al. 2009)
	CYP 1A1	CYP1A1*2A (Var) and CYP1A1*2C(A2455G) (Var) with GSTM1	Increase in risk	(Singh, Singh, et al. 2009)
	GST	GSTM1 (Null) GSTT1 (Null)	Increase in risk	(Singh, Khan, et al. 2008)
Lung cancer	CYP 1B1	Ala119Ser, Leu432Val Ala119Ser, Leu432Val with GSTM1	Increase in risk	(Shah, Singh, et al. 2008)
Liver cirrhosis	GST	GSTM1 (Null) GSTP1 (Var) GSTM1 (Null) + GSTT1 (Null) GSTP1 (Var) + GSTM1 (Null) GSTT1 (Null) GSTM1 (Null) + GSTT1 (Null)+GSTP1 (Var)	Increase in risk	(Khan, Choudhuri, et al. 2009)

Contd...

Diseases	Genes	Genotypes	Status	References
Chronic obstructive pulmonary disease (COPD)	eNOS	-786C, -922G and 4A alleles	Increased risk	(Arif, Ahsan, et al. 2007)
	COX2 and p53	–765GC+CC of COX2 and Pro/Pro+Pro/Arg genotypes of p53	Increased risk	(Arif, Vibhuti, et al. 2008)
Cardiac	Myosin binding protein C3 (*MYBPC3*)	One new frame shift mutation in exon 19 at the nucleotide position 11577^11578 and one new SNP in codon 1093 of exon 31, (MYBPC3)	Increased risk	(Tanjore, Rangaraju, et al. 2008)
	Methylenetetrahydrofolate reductase (MTHFR) gene	MTHFR 677C-T polymorphism	Increased risk	(Dhar, Chatterjee, et al. 2010)
	β-cardiac myosin heavy chain (*MYH7*)	c.965C>T (p.S322F) (*MYH7*)	Increased risk	(Bashyam, Purushotham, et al. 2012)
Schizophrenia (SCZ), Bipolar Affective Disorder (BPAD)	MLC1 (putative cation-channel gene)	Val210Ile, Leu308Gln, and Arg328His, Val210Ile irs2235349 and rs2076137 with SCZ and ss16339163 with BPAD	Increased risk	(Verma, Mukerji, et al. 2005)

Genetic susceptibility has played a pivotal role in the pathogenesis of many disorders and numerous genetic approaches, including candidate gene association studies and the genome-wide association study (GWAS) have been pursued to establish the contributory role of gene polymorphisms in the development of different diseases. Higher frequency of mutant genotypes like CC (-786T [C), TT (894G [T) and AA genotypes (27VNTR) in eNOS gene, allele 59029A of CCR5 gene have been found to be associated with a greater risk of nephropathy (Prasad, Tiwari et al. 2007, Ahluwalia, Ahuja, et al. 2008). Polymorphism in cytochrome P450 2E1(CYP2E1), leading to higher generation of ROS, has been linked with a higher susceptibility to alcoholic liver cirrhosis (Khan, Ruwali et al. 2009). A much greater risk to this disease has also been observed in patients who carry a combination of wild genotypes of ADH1C (ADH1C*1/*1) and variant genotype of ADH1B (ADH1B*2/*2) or CYP2E1 (CYP2E1*5B) or null genotype of GSTM1 (Khan, Husain, et al. 2010).

Case-control studies have also revealed that polymorphisms in GST gene lead to decreased metabolizing activity which could further increase the individual's susceptibility to head and neck cancer and an interaction with several environmental factors, such as cigarette smoking and alcohol drinking have shown to further modify the associated risk (Singh, Shah, et al. 2008). Strong association of 4 SNPs of CYP1B1 to a higher risk of lung cancer among tobacco users (Shah, Singh, et al. 2008) and association of tobacco chewing, cigarette smoking, and consumption of alcohol with CYP1A1 and GSTM1 gene polymorphisms resulting in altered susceptibility to lung cancer have also been implicated (Shah, Singh, et al. 2008). The link between SNPs of CYP1A1, CYP1B1, and Catechol-O-methyl transferase (COMT) genes with breast cancer risk in Indian women have revealed that SNPs may not just play crucial roles in incidences of breast cancer, rather few SNPs may also be related with protection (Singh, Rastogi, et al. 2007, Yadav, Singhal, et al. 2009).

The impact of genetic polymorphism of proteins and enzymes associated with drug metabolism (such as CYP and GST M1 and T1 genetic polymorphism) in the alteration of DIH has been studied extensively (Roy, Chowdhury et al. 2001, Gupta, Singh, et al. 2013, Singla, Gupta, et al. 2014). In complex disorders, where several variant loci contribute towards disease susceptibility, instead of single locus polymorphisms, haplotypes are potentially more crucial as the alleles' combination in the different genes may have difference in the effects on gene expression. Gene-gene interactions in the risk alleles of GST family, has been implicated in modulating the risk of Anti Retro Viral (ARV) linked hepatotoxicity in HIV-infected individuals. Singh, et al. 2015 have documented additive effects of GSTM1-null and GSTT1-null in contributing towards greater risk of hepatotoxicity in HIV-infected individuals (Singh, Lata, et al. 2017). Singh et al 2017 have critically evaluated the role of gene-gene/gene-environment interactions in relation to metabolic susceptibility genes and established that the individuals with carriage genotype 3801CC and heterozygous 3801CT genotypes of CYP1A1m1 gene may have a higher chance to develop ARV-associated hepatotoxicity, its severity, and advancement of disease independently and in the presence of environmental factors like alcohol and nevirapine regimen (Singh, Lata et al. 2017).

Applications in toxicogenomics have also aided in the identification of populations of different ethnic groups which may elicit a differential response for toxicity for the same chemical entity. The SNP-based Y-haplotypes have enabled distinguishing South Indian populations on the basis of Y-specific short repeat tandem markers that may aid in the identification of different ethnic groups amongst Indian population (Ramana, Su et al. 2001). The SNPs are also crucial for gaining insights into the mechanism of pathogenesis of different cardiac diseases and its population-specific prevalence. A probable role of MTHFR A1298C SNP in the pathogenesis of heart diseases has also been observed in Tamilians (Angeline, Jeyaraj, et al. 2004).

Toxicant mediated epigenetic regulation of gene expression has rapidly developed into one of the most influential areas of toxicogenomics research. DNA methylation and chromatin modifications are essential components of the regulation of gene activity and epigenetic modulation may confer an increased risk of toxicity. Research groups have identified various toxicant responsive imprinted genes (Igf2 (Insulinlike growth factor 2) and H19) that play a pivotal role in embryonic development, aberrant DNA methylation of which could lead to loss of chromatin integrity resulting in intrauterine and postnatal growth retardation ultimately leading to embryo loss (Doshi, D'souza, et al. 2013). Sub-chronic exposure of methylmercury has been shown to interfere with cellular and epigenetic processes, leading to aberrant alterations in MMP9 methylation, causing cytoskeleton disruption and loss of renal functions (Khan, Singh, et al. 2017).

A research group has identified hypermethylation in the activity of two genetic loci, parkin and PINK1 (associated with PD) upon manganese exposure that may be considered risk factors for the onset of sporadic Parkinson's. DAVID analysis further indicated the involvement of these differentially methylated genes in several crucial biological pathways like regulation of neuronal development and differentiation, signal transduction, synaptic transmission, inflammation and programmed cell death (Tarale, Sivanesan, et al. 2017). Developmental exposure to toxicants like PAHs, phenobarbital, and ethanol may induce epigenetic alterations in CYPs that may eventually increase the responsiveness/vulnerability of the individual, predisposing them to the toxic effects of the chemicals at later stages in life. This epigenetic imprinting may be of toxicological significance as it may alter the response of environmental toxicants or drugs in the exposed offsprings specifically for those chemicals that require CYP-mediated metabolism in order to elicit their beneficial or adverse effects (Johri, et al. 2006, Singh, Yadav, et al. 2013, Singh, Singh, Mudawal, et al. 2015, Singh, Agrahari, et al. 2016).

Toxicogenomics has also led to the elucidation of regulatory networks for various diseases. Genetic variations have been shown to confer risk/protection towards arsenic-toxicity and research groups have identified the underlying biomarkers of susceptibility that have helped in the mechanistic elucidation of arsenic-induced keratosis and carcinogenicity (Paul, Banerjee, et al. 2014; De Chaudhuri, Ghosh, et al. 2008). Link of specific p53 polymorphisms with keratosis (De Chaudhuri, Mahata, et al. 2006), individual variability in arsenic metabolism (purine nucleoside phosphorylase) (De Chaudhuri, Ghosh, et al. 2008), deficiency in DNA repair capacity due to ERCC2 codon 751 Lys/Lys genotype/polymorphism have been demonstrated (Banerjee, Sarkar, et al. 2007). DNA methylation has also been proposed as one of the epigenetic mechanisms which potentiates cancer and perturbations of methylation status in tumor suppressor genes (p53 and p16), as well as DNA repair genes, have been identified on chronic arsenic exposure (Chanda, Dasgupta, et al. 2005, Banerjee, Paul, et al. 2013, Paul, Banerjee, et al. 2014). Moreover, the role of few genes such as GSTM1 null (Ghosh, Basu, et al. 2006), polymorphism in XRCC3 T241M (Kundu, Ghosh, et al. 2011) have also been shown to confer protection against arsenic exposure.

Genetic susceptibility to neurotoxins has been documented as one of the main causes of Parkinsons' Disease (PD). Genetic susceptibility to OP pesticide-induced parkinsonism has been suggested (Bhatt, Elias, et al. 1999). Case-control studies indicated that polymorphism in various genes (NAT, DAT, etc.) that are involved in detoxification/metabolism and dopamine regulation could be significant risk factors in the pathogenesis of PD (Chaudhary, Behari, et al. 2005, Singh, Khan, et al. 2008, Punia, Das, et al. 2010). The contribution of genomics, proteomics and molecular biology approaches have made it possible to understand the modifying factors in the onset/progression of PD and given a better insight into detection of new biomarkers in brain proteome and the underlying mechanisms; those that were not feasible with conventional biochemical procedures. The involvement of toxicant responsive genes (CYP2E1 and GSTA4-4 expression), metallothionein genes (MT-I, MT-II) and transporter genes (VMAT-2, DAT) have been verified in the animals exposed to combined exposures to maneb+paraquat and zinc+paraquat (Patel, Singh, et al. 2006, Kumar, Ahmad, et al. 2010). Alterations in the transcript levels of 61 genes that are involved in DNA replication and repair, genomic surveillance, oxidative stress, and toxicity pathways have been identified in cypermethrin (Cyp) induced neurotoxicity (Singh, Tiwari, et al. 2011). Differential expression of several transcripts employing high-density microarray approach has revealed exposure-dependent modification in the expression of various genes in the mouse striatum that were not reported previously in many other animal models of PD, thus identifying the potential biomarkers that may aid in the understanding of putative mechanisms and etiology of PD phenotype that could be well extrapolated in humans (Patel, Sinha, et al. 2007, Patel, Singh, et al. 2008, Tiwari, Singh, et al. 2012).

Employing *ex vivo* approaches, IITR has established the involvement of toxicant responsive genes, such as CYP1A1, CYP1A2, CYP2E1, CYP2D22, and GST, in 1-methyl 4-phenyl 1,2,3,6-tetrahydropyridine (MPTP)-induced PD phenotype or nicotine- and caffeine-mediated neuroprotection in experimental settings (Singh, Singh, et al. 2008; 2009). *Ex vivo* approaches have been extensively utilized for elucidation of regulatory networks that are involved in diverse biological phenomena. For example, pyrogallol which causes liver damage and the release of specific serum protein biomarkers have been reported to elevate oxidative stress, lower reduced glutathione levels, glutathione peroxidize and glutathione reductase, and reduce the expression of some xenobiotic metabolizing genes (Upadhyay, Singh, et al. 2008). Resveratrol and silymarin, two naturally-occurring herbal antioxidants, alter pyrogallol-induced modifications in markers of hepatotoxicity, xenobiotic metabolizing enzymes, and oxidative stress (Upadhyay, Kumar, et al. 2007, Upadhyay, Singh, et al. 2008). Multiple approaches have been employed to assess the toxicity of the biomass fuel cow dung (kanda) smoke that has revealed differential expression of CYP1A1, GST-ya, GST-yc in 12 week exposed lung tissues (Lal, Mani, et al. 2011). Such specific patterns of gene expression or 'molecular fingerprints' could be utilized as predictive/diagnostic markers of exposure that would be characteristic of a particular mechanism of induction of that beneficial or adverse effect. The gene-toxicant interaction of different toxicants has been further mentioned in the following topics as well.

CHAPTER 9

Regulatory Toxicology

In the rapid developing era, new products such as NCE (new chemical entities), genetically engineered/modified organisms, finished or semi-finished products, drugs, pesticides, NMs, etc. are being daily introduced into the market. According to the guidelines laid down by the regulatory agencies, it is mandated for industries to get their raw materials and finished products assessed for safety and efficacy as they are liable to come in human and environmental contact. Regulatory Toxicology encompassing the collection, processing and evaluation of scientific data to permit toxicologically based decisions has been directed towards the protection of human and environmental health against a legacy of these products. The transformation of scientific evaluations based on experimental and epidemiological data into regulatory decisions such as recommendations, directives, regulations, laws and bans form the basis of regulatory toxicology. India has managed to make fast-paced strides in the development of standard protocols and new testing methods using novel analytical and molecular tools to improve the scientific basis for decision-making processes continuously. This section provides an overview of the major legislations that shaped the regulatory framework in India in the context of toxicology and significant contributions by institutes that underlie the basis of various regulatory decisions in India.

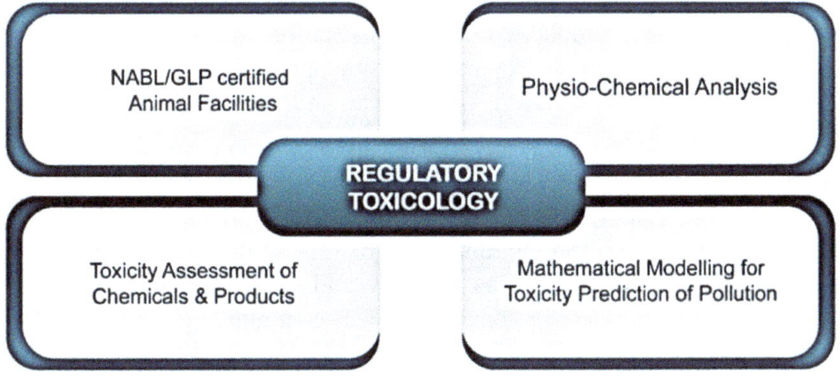

Figure 9.1 Approaches used in Regulatory Toxicology

Prior to India's independence in 1947, British misrule-offered inadequate healthcare system to Indians based on the observations made by the Drugs Enquiry Committee, Indian Medical Association as reported in the Indian Medical Gazette during 1920-30. The need for careful vigilance was felt as early as in the 1940's with the enactment of the Drugs and Cosmetics Act 1940 with the primary objective to regulate the "import, manufacture, distribution and sale of drugs and cosmetics". The Central Drugs Standards Control Organization (CDSCO) was established as the apex central regulatory authority for discharging duties assigned to the Central Government under the Act, such as new drugs approval (including medical devices), regulating clinical trials, laying down standards for quality control for imported drugs. Further, it also gives expert advice to the state authorities that are entrusted with overseeing the regulation for manufacture, sale and distribution of drugs. CDSCO, though a separate organization, functions within the structure of Directorate General of Health Services (DGHS), an agency which looks into the functioning and implementation of several health schemes including drug regulation and standard setting.

The drive for industrialization post-independence had several economic as well as social implications. As such, gradual changes in regulatory frameworks ushered in from a period extending from the country's independence to the 1980s. The Factories Act (1948) and Mines Act (1952) were formulated post-independence for the enactment of a safe working environment of the industrial workforce. Before 1968, 4 insecticides used majorly in health programs were regulated under the Drugs and Cosmetics Act, 1940. The period from 1955-1968 witnessed outbreaks of mass poisonings to various pesticides like parathion, malathion, aldrin and HCH in multiple states (Gupta 2004). Extensive epidemiological investigations undertaken by CSIR-IITR, NIOH and few agricultural universities highlighted the magnitude of pesticide risks in terms of occupational and environmental exposures. Post these outbreaks, the Insecticides Act was promulgated in 1968 and enforced in 1971 that envisaged regulating the import, manufacture, sale, transport, distribution, and use of insecticides, in order to prevent risks to human and environmental health.

At the same time, with the growing awareness of environmental pollution, the Water (Prevention and Control of Pollution) Act, 1974 and Air (Prevention and Control of Pollution) Act in 1981 were formulated. The resulting awakening of the general public to the hazards of chemicals in the environment through the notorious Bhopal Gas Tragedy and endosulfan disaster triggered the enactment of legislations directed towards regulating and limiting the indiscriminate release of chemicals into the environment such as Environment Protection Act (EPA) 1986. These have laid down standards for emissions and discharge; regulating the location of industries; managing hazardous wastes, and protection of human health. The Bureau of Indian Standards (BIS) established under the Bureau of Indian Standards Act, 1986, on the other hand, has been laying down safety and quality standards for several products. The existence of authorities such as BIS has helped in setting rules, particularly in situations of low consumer awareness regarding quality.

In the late 1980s, the Department of Science and Technology, Government of India, established the National Coordination of Testing and Calibrating Facilities (NCTCF). Consequently, in 1992, a need was felt to align the Indian Laboratory Accreditation program with the international standards. During the same year, the National Accreditation Board for Testing and Calibration Laboratories (NABL) in place of NCTCF was also established, that is in accordance with ISO/IEC Guide 25 (1990) and aims at bringing the criteria in lines with the European standards as in EN 45001 (1989).

In the case of agro-biotechnology, the regulations for manufacture, import, export, storage and use of hazardous microorganisms/genetically modified (GM) organisms or cells were developed and enforced in 1989. At that time point, domestic pressure was absent and moreover India did not possess any indigenous pharmaceutical or agro-biotechnology sector. It was a clear case of regulatory foresight, when the government acknowledged the necessity of developing regulations in response to GM related health disasters which backlashed European regulatory structures in the 1980s.

With time, India has forged ahead in the development of generic drugs, new biopharmaceuticals, biosimilars, diagnostics and agro-biotechnology products and managing contract services from R&D to complete manufacture. In the last couple of years, there has been a growing interest in the pharmaceutical industries towards outsourcing of drug and clinical development programs to Asia, specifically India owing to cost effectiveness and speed as well as productivity of R&D phases that are needed to bring an effective and safe drug into the market. India is equipped with a huge patient pool, well-trained investigators, premier medical institutes, low per-patient trial cost and a favorable regulatory scenario. Till 2004, India lacked a formal pharmacovigilance program wherein the regulatory bodies and drug companies based their efficacy and safety assessments on the data that was derived from chronic drug use in European, US and Japanese markets. However, it was realized that the Indian population is different both in physiological and genetic composition and therefore information generated by other countries would not be a correct parameter to monitor the ADRs on the Indian populace. It was on November 23, 2004 that CDSCO launched a formal National Pharmacovigilance Program (NPP) with a nationwide network of peripheral, regional and zonal centres to monitor the ADRs of medicines, explore the regulatory information submitted by drug companies with regard to safety, efficacy and toxicity of all novel chemicals and drugs as well as to provide information to the end-users through ADR news bulletins, drug alerts and seminars. The major aim of the program has been to develop and manage a database of ADRs reports which would be the basis for making regulatory decisions for market authorizations of drugs in India (Kumar 2011, Kalaiselvan, Thota, et al. 2016).

With the growing production of indigenous drugs, pharmaceuticals, etc., the non-hazardous nature of chemicals, drugs, NCEs have been required to be established via experimental studies, that would be assessed by the regulatory authorities. Thus in India, the concept of GLP was initiated in 1983 and was published in the official gazette. Apart from the establishment of few GLP facilities by the private sector, no significant progress had been made towards implementation of this concept. National GLP Compliance Monitoring Authority (NGCMA) was established by the Department of Science & Technology, Government of India in 2002. India became a full-member for Mutual Acceptance of Data (MAD) in the OECD's Working Group on GLP w.e.f. March 3, 2011. Consequently, the data generated by GLP certified laboratories in India is acceptable in all the OECD member countries facilitating the export of drugs, chemicals, pesticides, etc. to these countries. To meet the increasing demand of monitoring GLP compliance in the country, NGCMA trained around 60 GLP Inspectors from different public funded institutes to assess the technical competency of the applicant laboratories for its compliance to OECD Principles of GLP and OECD Test Guidelines. A list of GLP certified Test Facilities in National GLP Programme can be found here at http://www.dst.gov.in/sites/default/files/Certified-Test-Facilities-14122018.pdf.

The CDSCO is discharged with the role of administering the Drugs and Cosmetics Act, 1940, which prescribes, in depth, the requirements that needs to be fulfilled by a drug under Schedule Y of the Drugs and Cosmetics Rule, 2005. Schedule Y includes protocols and rules with respect to pre-clinical and clinical testing for the import and manufacture of a drug. An extensive revision of schedule Y has been launched on March 19, 2019, by DCGI Office in Delhi. Appendix III of Schedule Y describes the type of tests that need to be conducted, the timelines, number of animals to be employed, etc. These guidelines have to be complied with by Indian companies or other drug manufacturers in order to manufacture and market their products in this country. Currently, Schedule Y specifies the following tests for pre-clinical animal toxicology for approval to Phase I clinical trials: Single-dose toxicity studies – Minimum lethal dose (MLD) and Maximum tolerated dose (MTD), repeated dose systemic toxicity studies, female reproduction and development study, male fertility study, teratogenic study, perinatal study, local toxicity, genotoxicity and carcinogenicity (http://cdsco.nic.in/html/D&C_Rules_Schedule _Y.pdf).

Table 9.1 List of various regulatory agencies in context with toxicology in India

Product	Regulating Act	Regulating Authority	Regulatory Ministry
Drugs and Pharmaceuticals	Drugs & Cosmetics Act, 1940 Schedule Y	Central Drugs Standard Control Organization	Ministry of Health & Family Welfare
Cosmetics	Drugs & Cosmetics Act, 1940 Schedule S	Central Drugs Standard Control Organization	Ministry of Health & Family Welfare
Vaccines	Drugs & Cosmetics Act, 1940	Central Drugs Standard Control Organization	Ministry of Science and Technology
Biosimilars and Biologicals	Department of Biotechnology guidelines	Department of Biotechnology Genetic Engineering Appraisal Committee	Ministry of Environment & Forests
Food and food products	Food standard & Safety Act, 2006	Food Standard and Safety Authority of India	Ministry of Health & Family Welfare
Genetically Modified Crops	Revised Guidelines for Research in Transgenic Plants, 1998, 1989 Rule	Department of Biotechnology, Genetic Engineering Appraisal Committee	Ministry of Science & Technology, Ministry of Environment & Forests
Pesticide and Agricultural Chemicals	Central Insecticides Act, 1968	Central Insecticides Board and Registration Committee	Ministry of Agriculture and Farmers Welfare
Medical Devices	Drugs & Cosmetics Act, 1940	Central Drugs Standard Control Organization	Ministry of Health & Family Welfare
Household chemicals, detergents and other surface active agents	Chemical Council Division Committee (Voluntary)	Bureau of Indian Standards (Voluntary)	

Many authors have comprehensively compiled the history, growth and evolution of the regulatory aspects in toxicology; clinical research (Imran, Najmi, et al. 2013), traditional herbal medicines (Kumar and Dua 2016), similar biologics (Ramkishan and Khan 2017) and GM crops (Sheelendra 2015) which have provided a comprehensive look of various regulatory requirements existing for clinical trial and toxicity data in India.

Over the years India has enacted numerous laws and regulations (with suitable amendments) to regulate the marketing, labelling (in few cases), and transportation and use of pesticides, chemicals, medical products, consumer products, food additives, and other substances that can be of potential safety concerns. In India, apart from the above mentioned regulations, few international standards have also been important players in toxicity testing such as U.S Food and Drug Administration (USFDA) guidelines for pre-clinical testing, OECD guidelines for estimating the toxic effects of chemicals for the purpose of risk assessment. The International Conference on Harmonisation and ISO standards are also extensively used by Indian pharmaceutical and chemical companies in order to standardize their products at the international level.

We would like to mention some few significant contributions made by research organizations over the years that have laid the groundwork for the establishment of various regulatory guidelines in toxicology. Few Government institutes (NIPER, Mohali, CSIR-IITR, CSIR-CDRI, CSIR-NEERI, and IITs) and preclinical CROs are actively engaged in generating data on the toxicological potential thus providing a unique platform for industrialists and entrepreneurs to answer concerns on safety/toxicity of their products. This data generated has provided the basis for the formulation of guidelines for prescribing the limits of new entities or regulating the use/ban of existing chemicals. The regulatory authorities, industries and R&D organizations constantly engage in estimating the levels of risk that are acceptable to the public and elaborate on technical and scientific inputs ensuring that the risks posed by the chemicals does not exceed the contemplated risk levels. Requirements to develop robust and reliable test methods for human health and environmental safety risk assessment has led to considerable optimization of *in vitro* and *in silico* assays that have now become the undisputed choice of tools in prediction of toxicity. Institutes through their scientific expertise have provided complete facilities for toxicity studies, health and environmental risk assessment and testing services in compliance with GLP using NABL and international standards by employing latest toxicity systems, analytical instruments, biomarkers, and mathematical tools. CROs were initially set up as service outsourcing companies, but in more recent times there has been increasing participation of CROs in regulatory toxicity testing that provide both GLP toxicity services as well as non-GLP toxicity studies to aid in the lead optimization/candidate selection services for drug development.

Epidemiological monitoring studies carried out by CSIR-IITR and NIOH in their formative years sensitized the Government towards the deteriorating health effects of agricultural farmers which led to the enactment of the Pesticide Act 1981. Since then these institutes have been entrusted to carry out national level surveillance programs to regularly monitor the health status and work environment of various industries. They have been actively involved in providing recommendations for setting up Occupational Exposure Limits (OELs) for dust fibres. Based on their suggestions, the Threshold Limit Value (TLVs) of < 2 f/ml for asbestos fibres was brought down to 0.5 fibre/cc. The asbestos ban in India has been an on-going debate. The ban on mining asbestos was imposed in phases in 1986 and 1993. However, later the ban was lifted despite deteriorating conditions in both organized and unorganized sectors. Various studies have also led to a ban on the manufacture, import and use of 27 pesticides including lindane, aldrin and aldicarb whose toxicological effects are well documented http://www.indiaenvironmentportal.org.in/files/file/Use%20 of%20Banned%20Pesticides.pdf.

Institutes like CSIR-IITR and CSIR-NEERI, IITs are also actively engaged in regular monitoring of air/water/soil quality in different cities in order to estimate the risk exposure of such contaminants on the ecosystem as well as human health. Based on CPCB/IIT Kanpur research Suspended particulate matter (SPM) has been replaced by $PM_{2.5}$ which has more relevance for public health. Other parameters, such as Arsenic, Nickel, Ozone, Benzene and Benzo(a)Pyrene were also included into the NAAQS for the first time (http://pib.nic.in/newsite/erelcontent.aspx?relid=54189).

Disposal of plastic waste has become a severe concern in India. It has been estimated that approximately 15722 tonnes/day of plastic waste is generated in India (Singh and Sharma 2016). Migration of phthalic acid esters used as plasticizers and organometallic stabilizers from the packaging material into stored food material, biological fluids and from disposal waste into surrounding soil and water have been reported (Srivastava, Sharma, et al. 2010, Ma, Salama, et al. 2012, Selvaraj, Sundaramoorthy, et al. 2015). Plastic components like phthalates, bisphenol A(BPA), polychlorinated biphenyls (PCBs) recently declared to be endocrine disrupting chemicals (EDCs) have been strongly associated with reduced semen quality, specifically reduced sperm motility (Singh, Shafeeque, et al. 2015). Acknowledging rampant usage of plastics products and the threats they could impose, CSIR-IITR has offered its expertise for toxicological evaluation of plastics, polymers and polyelectrolytes to many manufacturers/exporters. Based on the R&D work, suitable specifications have been developed and updated for testing of products used in packaging and storage of food materials, drugs, life-saving fluids, cosmetics, transportation of water, etc. In order to minimize the risk of migration from the finished plastic, safer plasticizer cum stabilizer complexes have been developed that exhibit lower toxicity with the same biological properties (lightweight, flexibility and colour). Toxics Link (Indian environmental research and advocacy organization) also raised the issue of BPA in baby feeding bottles with the parliamentarians and the concerned ministry including the Consumer Ministry and Bureau of Indian Standards resulting in the ban in the use of BPA in baby feeding bottles in India since 2014 (http://toxicslink.org/docs/BPA-study-report.pdf).

There has been a growing concern on food safety either through environmental pollution or adulteration. Monitoring and surveillance data from National Institute of Nutrition (NIN), Central Food Technological Research Institute, (CFTRI) IITR, ICMR, Indian Council of Agricultural Research (ICAR) etc. were pooled together to form initial database for the establishment of the Food Safety and Standards Authority of India 2006 (FSSAI), under the Food Safety and Standards Act 2005 to suggest science-based decisions in respect of limits for contaminants and set threshold limits. With the increase in production of GM crops there has been an increasing interest in the available approaches for the assessment of allergenicity/toxicity potential of novel genes/products introduced to confer pest resistance or improve nutritional quality. Few GM crops like Chickpea, Brinjal, Cabbage, Pea, Groundnut, Potato, Maize, Rice, Sorghum and Tomato etc. are under field trial stages in India. Random inclusion of a new gene into the host crop genome to confer pest resistance/herbicide tolerance or improve nutritional quality may sometimes lead to an over expression of a previously silent gene/product. Thus, allergenicity/ safety evaluation of GM crops is required prior to its release into the marketplace. Food and Drug Toxicology Research Centre (FDTRC) is involved in premarket safety assessment of transgenic crops including screening of Bt Brinjal (cry1Fa1/Cry1Fa1), GM Mustard (bar/Bar, barstar/Barstar, barnase/Barnase), Bt Okra (cry1Ac/Cry1Ac), Bt Cotton (cry1Ac/Cry1Ac, cry1EC/Cry1EC) and Bt rice (cry1Ab/Cry1Ab). IITR has also undertaken allergenicity prediction of transgenic proteins that are expressed in several GM crops in India using computational tools. The method has been suitable for the screening of any vip3A-carrying transgenic cotton and tobacco that would facilitate rapid and efficient regulatory compliance. IITR and IGIB have also been engaged in the detection, quantification and risk assessment of biological contaminants including mycotoxins like Alfatoxin1 and Ptaulin that have not yet been included under Prevention of Food Adulteration (PFA) Act of India but pose a high risk of carcinogenicity.

With the rapid development of industries for food processing, the trend of using several food additives and preservatives for many different technological purposes has also grown. The utilization of non-permitted colours has been a topic of concern for food regulators in the country (Biswas, Sarkar, et al. 1994, Babu and Shenolikar 1995, Dixit, Pandey, et al. 1995, Bhat and Mathur 1998, Mishra, Dixit, et al. 2007, Tripathi, Khanna, et al. 2007, Dixit, Purshottam, et al. 2009). Experimental studies conducted by CSIR-IITR revealing the enhanced health risk due to the use of these colors has prompted the regulatory authorities to increase control, limiting them to selective use (Yadav, Kumar, et al. 2012, Yadav, Kumar, et al. 2013). Surveillance programs have been undertaken to assess the exposure level of various food colors in order to develop a scientific yardstick for fixing the level of colors in commodities on the basis of safety and technological requirements. The FSSAI permits the use of only 8 synthetic colors in particular food commodities at 100 mg/kg or per litre (Dixit, Khanna, et al. 2013). The acceptable daily intakes (ADI) of the food colors currently approved in India range from 0.1 to 25 mg/kg body weight/day, i.e., a difference of 250-fold. IITR put forward the fact that fixing a uniform permissible limit of 100 ppm for all the food colors in various foods, irrespective of the technological requirement for particular preparation, seemed unrealistic. This was because children were generally attracted more to food colors. Owing to their low body weights as compared to adults they were likely to be exposed more than the adults. Thus, it was suggested that the prescribed limit of food colors be reviewed and regulated in light of consumption profiles of the commodities in order to control the unnecessary exposure to the vulnerable groups (Dixit, Purshottam, et al. 2011). Interestingly, the FSSAI admitted that the list and regulations on food colors had not been revised in the new Food Safety and Standards Act, 2006, and simply copied and pasted from the old Prevention of Food Adulteration Act, 1954 and that it needed to be re-looked with a scientific angle. Recently, the European Food Safety Agency (EFSA) has also included an IITR study in its 2014 report "Reconsideration of the temporary ADI and refined exposure assessment for Sunset Yellow FCF (E110)".

IITR has also been instrumental in developing a novel Quality Assurance of Medicinal Plants (QAMP) database on persistent pesticide contaminants and heavy metals in more than 1900 therapeutically important samples of medicinal plants collected from several ecological zones of India. IITR also developed Pharmacopoeial standards for 24 Ayurvedic herbal drugs of single plant origin, 17 of which were poisonous medicinal plants. Seven monographs have been published in The Ayurvedic Pharmacopoeia of India, Part-1, Vol.V (2006). NIPER has also laid down standards and adequate quality controls on the Herbal Medicinal Products and their formulations through chemo and bio profiling. For the first time, studies have been conducted by FDTRC on preclinical safety assessment of indigenously developed recombinant-DNA anti-rabies, human papilloma vaccine (HPV), therapies (human adult mesenchymal stem cells (MSCS), which do not have defined regulatory guidelines.

Several manufacturers of cosmetic products, which contain herbal ingredients, try to bypass evaluation standards by different regulatory agencies like BIS by labelling their products as "Ayurvedic medicine". Many of the tooth powders (Dant Manjans) come under this category. They have also been reported to fail in many tests prescribed in IS 5383-1978 (Toothpowders) of the BIS). Maharashtra FDA hauled up Johnson & Johnson Ltd. after a consumer complaint regarding blisters on baby skin after using baby oil. The company was instructed to avoid misbranding and mention safety warnings regarding the side effects due to the presence of chemicals like light liquid paraffin (LLP), isopropyl myristate, etc. (http://www.consumer education.in/monograms /8_cosmeticsand_consumers.pdf).

Nanotechnology has been a promising advancement, but all the major initiatives have primarily revolved around developing R&D activities and regulatory studies for risk assessment have been relatively ignored. To this end, IITR had released a guidance document for safe handling of NMs that has been incorporated in the framework of Nanomission. NIPER, on the other hand, developed regulatory guidelines for nanotechnology-based drugs and standards for toxicity tests in nano-based drug delivery systems (Dhawan, Shanker, et al. 2011).

CHAPTER 10

Organ Specific Toxicology

10.1   Neurotoxicity

Neurotoxicology has been a burgeoning area of research in the country. Its growth over the years has been attributed, primarily, to growing awareness and concerns about the increasing number of agents with a potential of neurotoxicity, including heavy metals, pesticides, and industrial chemicals, that are released into the environment. Neurotoxicity has assumed a significant concern as a large number of drugs, substances of abuse, chemicals, natural constituents of plants, heavy metals, pesticides, endocrine disruptors, etc. have shown to affect the nervous system.

The earliest studies in India could be traced back to early 1960s regarding the clinical human syndrome 'neurolathyrism' (crippling disease) attributed to the prolonged consumption of seed pulses *Lathyrus sativus* (Kesari dal) which resulted in acute and subacute onset of spastic paraplegia as mentioned in the ancient Bhav Prakash (Sleeman 1915, Ganapathy and Dwivedi 1961). Many explanations were advanced and extensive clinical, epidemiological and biochemical work was carried out to characterize the causative factor (Ganapathy and Dwivedi 1961, Roy, Nagarajan et al. 1962, Rao, Ramachandran et al. 1963, Dwivedi and Prasad 1964). The identification of β-form of N-oxalyldiaminoproprionic acid (β-L-ODAP) as the neurotoxic principle implicated in neurolathyrism by Rao, et al in 1964 was a major milestone leading to further work by other research groups in institutes around the country (Murti, Seshadri, et al. 1964, Rao, Adiga, et al. 1964, Rao, Sarma et al. 1967, Prakash, Misra et al. 1977, Rao 1978, Vardhan, Rudra, et al. 1997). Over the years, β-L-ODAP has been shown to cross the blood-brain barrier and accumulate in the central nervous system (CNS), leading to severe convulsions and neurological deficits in animals (Rao 1978). Molecular mechanisms proposed for neurotoxicity of L-ODAP have generally emphasized its binding to NMDA and non-NMDA receptors along with pharmacological and structural analogies to the excitatory amino acid glutamate (Lakshmanan and Padmanaban 1974, Lakshmanan and Padmanaban 1974, Lakshmanan and Padmanaban 1977, Amba, Seth, et al. 2002). Furthermore, the species difference in metabolism and susceptibility to β-L-ODAP has been a unique feature associated with the neurotoxin (Jyothi, Rudra, et al. 1998).

For the next few years, extensive work was undertaken by CSIR-IITR on the neurotoxicity potential of heavy metals (lead, manganese) and plastic monomers (acrylamide, styrene) that found widespread usage owing to the industrial revolution in the country. The growing number of cases of manganese poisonings reported from India (Niyogi 1958, Balani, Umarji, et al. 1967) prompted a number of investigators to develop an experimental model of manganese encephalopathy in rodents to investigate the pathological and biochemical alterations on metal exposure (Mustafa and Chandra 1971, Chandra, Seth, et al. 1974, Chandra and Shukla 1978, Chandra, Shukla, et al. 1979, Murthy, Srivastava, et al. 1980). Such studies led to the identification of early biomarkers of exposure such as alterations in serum calcium, inorganic phosphates, alkaline phosphatase, adenosine deaminase that were found to occur much earlier than the pathological changes in the brain of rabbits (Chandra, Seth, et al. 1974, Sitaramayya, Nagar, et al. 1974). Research groups also provided preliminary evidence on the interaction of acrylamide, associated with the 'dying back' type of neuropathy and behavioral disorders. Numerous studies demonstrated the ability of acrylamide to interfere with disposition of catecholamines and form glutathione conjugates on biotransformation (Dixit, Husain, et al. 1981, Dixit, Mukhtar, et al. 1981). It was considered that an alteration in the steady-state concentration of cellular glutathione might influence the cellular biotransformation of acrylamide, subsequently resulting in altered neurotoxicity (Dixit, Mukhtar, et al. 1981, Das, Mukhtar, et al. 1982).

The complexity of the brain and its needs for normal functioning has rendered the system vulnerable to different toxic insults. The physiological and behavioral manifestations of such toxic insults have been shown to be influenced by numerous variables. Apart from dose, and duration of exposure, other confounding factors such as age, region and species specificity, stress, nutritional status, interaction with other confounding factors have been emphasized. As an example, toxicity of lead is highly dose and age dependent (Nehru and Sidhu 2001, Nehru and Sidhu 2002) and the effects are highly region specific, due to differential accumulation of lead in the brain (Kala and Jadhav 1995). Moreover, there is also a species relative difference in the sensitivity of acute intoxication to chemicals such as anticholinesterase compounds (example monocrotophos) (Siddiqui, Rahman et al. 1988, Qadri, Swamy, et al. 1994). Similarly, stress is an important contributor in lambacyalothrin induced cholinergic deficits (Shukla, Gupta, et al. 2016).

Synergism between alcohol consumption and metal poisoning (Flora and Tandon 1987, Flora, Pant, et al. 1997), neurotoxicity of metals (cadmium, arsenic, lead, copper and mercury) modulated through their interactions with few essential elements (Malhotra, Shukla, et al. 1982, Malhotra, Murthy, et al. 1984), higher neurotoxicity of *Lathyrus sativus* by manganese (Mishra, Shukla, et al. 2009), are some of the other examples. These studies have been of importance for understanding the neurochemical and functional implications of combined exposure to neurotoxic metals through a contaminated environment. These observations were studied in more detail and confirmed in a number of experimental studies (Flora, Kumar, et al. 1991, Dhawan, Flora, et al. 1992, Flora, Dhawan, et al. 1999, Gupta and Gill 2000). Prevalence of protein malnutrition in developing countries like India has been another crucial factor for consideration in the neurotoxicity evaluation of chemicals and environmental contaminants. Protein malnutrition is known to affect the neurotoxicity of chemicals in a way different from that observed in a nutritionally adequate condition (Murthy, Lal, et al. 1981, Ali, Murthy, et al. 1983, Ali, Lal et al. 1991, Flora, Dhawan, et al. 1999). Animals receiving lesser protein diet have been shown to be more vulnerable to the effects of chemicals in experimental animals (Khanna, Husain, et al. 1988, Khanna, Husain, et al. 1991, Khanna, Husain, et al. 1994). Similarly, levels of dietary iron have been shown to be an important predisposing factor against the effects of manganese on the brain (Chandra and Shukla 1976). Further, dietary habits, such as excessive intake of sugars during developmental stages could potentially alter the pharmacological and toxicological outcome of numerous xenobiotics (Salim and Rajini 2014).

Considerable clinical/experimental evidence, from the published literature, confirms the fact that various environmental contaminants are potent neurotoxins and act at multiple targets within the adult mammalian central nervous system (CNS). Industrial chemicals like lead, manganese, methyl mercury, pesticides, drugs and several others have caused several acute, subacute and chronic neurotoxic effects implicated in impairments in learning, memory and even onset/progression of neurodegenerative diseases. Over the years increasing evidence of neurologic dysfunction on acute exposure to OP pesticides resulting in organophosphate induced delayed neuropathy (OPIDN) (Masoud, Kiran, et al. 2009, Rastogi, Tripathi, et al. 2010, Masoud, Kiran, et al. 2011), peripheral neuropathy due to arsenic and lead exposure occurring occupationally/environmentally have been reported (Mukherjee, Rahman, et al. 2003, Shobha, Taly, et al. 2009). However, over the years, concerns regarding the neurotoxicity of chemicals has grown, with more and more evidence associating chemicals and drug exposure with not just acute effects but long-term changes in the nervous system producing biochemical and behavioral disturbances in humans and animal models. In view of the risks of different CNS disturbances, experimental studies have been undertaken to identify and assess the toxicity potential and understand the underlying mechanisms of neurotoxicity and neurodegeneration. Studies of neurotoxic effects have been extended towards various biochemical, histopathological, and motor behavioral indices. Pathological and neurochemical alterations correlated with the accumulation of xenobiotics, disruptions of cholinergic, dopaminergic serotonergic pathways, impaired mitochondrial functions, disrupted ubiquitin pathways, interference with xenobiotic metabolism, neurotransmitter metabolism, imbalance of antioxidant system, cellular events of apoptosis, etc. have all been manifested in neurotoxic mechanisms (Table 10.1).

Table 10.1 Representative studies on the neurotoxic effects/mechanisms of different classes of toxicants

Neurotoxicant	Effects/Mechanism of action	Model and Route of administration	References
Metals			
Manganese (8 mg/kg b.wt./day), 180 days	Scattered degeneration of neurons within the cerebral and cerebellar cortex at 120 days which increased in intensity up to 180 days, the manganese concentration in the brain also showed an increase, the extent of the brain lesions was directly linked to the amount of manganese in the brain tissue which increased with time	Albino rats, Intraperitoneal	(Chandra and Srivastava 1970)
Manganese (400 mg), 2 years	Rabbits became lethargic and inactive after 12-14 months, after a period of 18-24 months, they developed paralysis of hind limbs, neuronal loss and degeneration in the cerebral cortex, caudate nucleus, putamen, substantia nigra and cerebellar cortex, marked reduction of acid phosphatase and adenosine triphosphate	Rabbits, Intratracheal	(Chandra 1972)
Manganese+ Ethanol (16 mg $MnCl_2$. 4 H_2O/kg in 10% ethanol (w/v) in 10% sucrose solution + pellet diet/day, 30 days	Synergistic effect of manganese and ethanol led to increased ATPase and RNase activity, antagonistic effects on MAO activity, also affected acid phosphatase, transaminases and arginase activity	Albino rats, Oral	(Singh, Shukla, et al. 1979)
Manganese (3 mg Mn^{2+}/ml) + **Lead** (5, 8 and 12 mg/kg b.wt.) /day, 14 days	Higher disruptions in the behavioral pattern, in the biogenic amines content, lead accumulation on simultaneous exposure to the two metals as compared to individual exposures, dose dependent increase in 5-hydroxy-tryptamine and norepinephrine levels, lead accumulation in the simultaneously exposed rats	Albino rats Manganese: Oral Lead: Intraperitoneal	(Chandra, Ali, et al. 1981)

Contd...

Neurotoxicant	Effects/Mechanism of action	Model and Route of administration	References
Lead (50 mg/kg b.wt./alternate day), 8 weeks	Stimulated the activity of calmodulin and the maximum effect was observed at 30 µM, inhibitory effect on Ca^{2+}ATPase activity in both calmodulin-rich and calmodulin-depleted synaptic plasma membranes, *in vivo* exposure of lead also reduced the activity of Ca^{2+}ATPase, leading to higher intra synaptosomal calcium and LPO	Albino rats, Intragastric	(Sandhir and Gill, 1994)
Lead (10 mg/kg b.wt.) and **ethanol** (10% v/v), 8weeks	Reduction in the activity of blood δ-aminolevulinic acid dehydratase (ALAD), increase in brain MDA levels, severe reduction in the binding of [3H] fluintrazepam in membranes prepared from the fronto-cortical region, higher spontaneous locomotor activity (SLA) and aggressive behaviour	Albino rats, Oral	(Flora, Khanna, et al. 1999)
Lead (50 mg/kg b.wt./alternate days), 8 weeks	Reduced the brain and body weight, decrease in the concentration of all neurotransmitters viz dopamine, serotonin, norepinephrine, and activity of acetylcholinesterase, affected the locomotor and cognitive functions, following a recovery period of 8 weeks, improvement was seen in locomotor as well as cognitive behavior	Sprauge-Dawley rats, Oral	(Nehru and Sidhu 2001)
Lead (10 mg/kg, 50 mg/kg, and 200 mg/kg b.wt./alternate days), 12 weeks	Dose-dependent reduction in the concentration of potassium, sodium and zinc, higher concentrations of calcium and lead, decreased activity of AchE and other neurotransmitters, lead exposure affected the locomotor and cognitive functions	Sprauge-Dawley rats, Oral	(Sidhu and Nehru 2003)
Lead (50 mg/kg b.wt./day), 8 weeks	Stimulated calmodulin, in terms of its ability to activate cAMP phosphodiesterase, enhanced calmodulin-mediated synaptic vesicle protein phosphorylation, accompanied by enhanced release of acetylcholine from synaptic vesicles	Albino rats, Intragastric	(Gill, Gupta, et al. 2003)
Lead (50 mg/kg b.wt./day), 8 weeks	Decreased concentration of all the antioxidant enzymes, degeneration of neurons in cerebrum, with disruption of normal arrangement of cell layers in cerebellum, cells were bigger in size with large vascular spaces, large spaces in between purkinje cell layer and granular layer were observed	Sprauge Dawley rats, Oral	(Sidhu and Nehru 2004)

Contd...

Neurotoxicant	Effects/Mechanism of action	Model and Route of administration	References
Cadmium (0.4 mg/kg b.wt.), 30 days	Decreased membrane in all brain regions, highest in olfactory bulb (21%), increased intracellular calcium levels in cerebellum and olfactory bulb, lower phosphatidylethanolamine and phosphatidylcholine in the olfactory bulb, Higher TBA reactivity in all parts of the brain	Albino rats, Intraperitoneal	(Kumar, Agarwal, et al. 1996)
Cadmium (100 mg/kg b.wt./day), 51 days	Exposure resulted in an overall depression in all motor behaviour aspects resulting in a reduction in gross locomotor activity	Wistar rats, Intraperitoneal	(Ali, Mathur, et al. 1990)
Arsenic (1, 1.5 and 2 mg/kg b. wt./day), 12 weeks	Reduced mean log nuclear area in the neurons of cervical motor in groups receiving 2.0 mg/kg, area reduced for lumbar motor neurons at all the doses, higher expression of cytochrome oxidase in the cervical than in lumbar spinal cord, higher reduction of succinate dehydrogenase activity in the cervical and spinal cord with doses of 1.5 and 2.0 mg/kg b.wt. in comparison with lumbar spinal cord	Wistar rats, Intragastric	(Dhar, Jaitley, et al. 2005)
Arsenic (50 ppm), 10 months	Increase in ROS levels accompanied by the depletion of GSH/GSSG ratio and activity of glucose-6-phosphate dehydrogenase in various regions of the brain (pons medulla, corpus striatum, cortex, hippocampus, and cerebellum)	Wistar rats, Oral	(Mishra and Flora 2008)
Arsenic (50 µg/l/day), 90 days	Generation of ROS, MDA and conjugated diene (CD) revealed a triphasic response obtaining a peak at the end of exposure, alteration of glutathione peroxidase (GPx) and catalase (CAT) activity, changes in NRF2 and its consequent expression of NAD(P)H dehydrogenase quinone1 and heme oxygenase1	Zebrafish	(Sarkar, Mukherjee, et al. 2014)
Chromium (2 mg/kg b.wt./day as chromium nitrate (Cr(III)) and as potassium dichromate (Cr(VI)), 6 weeks	Cr(III) 3 weeks' exposure produced degeneration of neurons in the cerebral cortex, marked chromatolysis, further 6 weeks caused neuronal degeneration along with neuronophagia, neuroglial proliferation and meningeal congestion, Cr(VI), for 3 weeks, was congested with perivascular infiltration by inflammatory cells	Rabbits, Intraperitoneal	(Mathur, Chandra, et al. 1977)

Contd...

Neurotoxicant	Effects/Mechanism of action	Model and Route of administration	References
Chromium (5.0–20.0 µg/ml) of Cr(III) or Cr(VI)-salt- mixed food), 24 and 48 h	Decreased number of neuronal cells on exposure of Cr(VI) but not Cr(III)-salt-mixed food, Cr(VI) affected both cholinergic and dopaminergic cells, altered locomotor activity via only 20.0 µg/ml Cr(VI) exposure (48 h) with higher level of ROS and oxidative stress	*Drosophila melanogaster* mutant w1118, Oral	(Singh and Chowdhuri 2017)
Zinc (20 mg/kg b.wt.) + **paraquat** (5mg/ kg b.wt.), twice/ week for 2, 4 and 8 weeks	Reduction in SLA, tyrosine hydroxylase (TH) immunoreactivity, striatal dopamine (DA) levels, catalase and glutathione reductase (GR) activity, higher LPO and glutathione peroxidase, increased gene expression of DAT, GSTA4-4, MT-I and MT-II, CYP2E1, decreased expression of VMAT-2	Wistar rats, Intraperitoneal	(Kumar, Ahmad, et al. 2010)
Thallium (5 mg/kg b.wt./day), 7 days	Decrease in dopamine concentration in the limbic areas, hypothalamus, and corpus striatum, 5-hydroxytryptamine concentration reduced in the cerebellum, corpus striatum, and brain-stem	Albino rats Charles Foster, Intraperitoneal	(Hasan, Ali et al. 1978)
Pesticides			
Malathion (150 mg/kg b.wt./day), 7 days	Hypomotor activity and hyperthermia, lipids and phospholipids were diminished in the brain stem and spinal cord, respectively, increased contents of cholesterol were found in the cerebellum and spinal cord, lipid peroxidation increased in all parts	Charles Foster rats, Intraperitoneal	(Haque, Rizvi, et al. 1987)
Endosulfan (3 mg/kg b.wt./day), 30 days	Higher binding of 3H-serotonin, higher affinity of receptor (K_D), chronic exposure of endosulfan resulted in aggressive behaviour (foot-shock-induced fighting behaviour) blocked by methysergide, a 5-HT blocker	Albino rats, Intraperitoneal	(Agrawal, Anand, et al. 1983)
Deltamethrin (7 mg/kg b.wt./day), 15 days	Increase in the activity of monoamine oxidase in frontal hippocampus, cerebellum and cortex, higher AchE activity in corpus striatum, frontal cortex, cerebellum, hippocampus, and pons medulla, decreased Na+, K+-ATPase activity in hippocampus, frontal cortex, and cerebellum, the polyamine concentration affected in all regions along with neurobehavioural dysfunctions	Albino rats, Oral	(Husain, Husain, et al. 1996)

Contd...

Neurotoxicant	Effects/Mechanism of action	Model and Route of administration	References
Deltamethrin (150 mg/kg and 15 mg/kg b.wt.), 1 h	Motor coordination decreased, reduction in the onset time and higher duration of sleeping time induced by pentobarbitone, higher duration of convulsions, reduction in the GABA levels at all regions in the brain at 150 mg/kg	Wistar rats, Oral	(Manna, Bhatta-charyya, et al. 2006)
Carbofuran (0.2, 0.4 and 0.8 mg/kg b.wt.), 24 h	Dose dependent reduction in LPO and oxidative stress, induced activities of antioxidant enzymes catalase and superoxide dismutase	Albino Wistar rats, Intraperitoneal	(Rai and Sharma 2007)
Carbofuran (1 mg/kg b.wt./day), 28 days	Decreased cell viability, acetylcholinesterase and succinate dehydrogenase activity, decrease in low molecular weight thiols, lipid peroxidation, impaired cognitive and motor functions	Wistar rats, Oral	(Kamboj, Kumar, et al. 2008)
Dichlorvos (3 mg/kg b.wt./day), 10 days	Increased number of electron-dense bodies with electron-lucid vacuoles in the perikarya of cerebeller neurons, with mitochondria aggregations. Myelin-figures in dendrites and axons of the spinal cord, oedema observed in the spinal cord	Albino rats, Intraperitoneal	(Hasan, Maitra, et al. 1979)
Dichlorvos (200 mg/kg b.wt.), 7, 15 and 21 days	Development of OPIDN, higher microtubule associated Ca^{2+}/calmodulin dependent activity and cAMP dependent protein kinases on 7th, 15th and 21st day, hyperphosphorylation of MAP-2 and tubulin which consequently destabilized microtubule assembly resulting in degeneration of axons	Wistar rats, Subcutaneous	(Choudhary, Joshi, et al. 2001)
Dichlorvos (6 mg/kg body wt/day), 8 weeks **Dichlorvos** (1 and 6 mg/kg b.wt./day), 12 weeks	Modification of intracellular calcium homeostasis, higher levels of intrasynaptosomal calcium, calpain activity and depolarization caused uptake of calcium through voltage operated calcium channels, decreased Ca^{2+} ATPase activity	Wistar Albino rats, Subcutaneous	(Raheja and Gill 2002)
Dichlorvos (2.5 mg/kg b.wt./day), 12 weeks	Defects in neurobehavioral indices viz. passive avoidance, rota rod and water maze tests, lowered AchE activity, reduction in the expression of M1, M2	Albino rats, Subcutaneous	(Verma, Raheja, et al. 2009)

Contd...

Neurotoxicant	Effects/Mechanism of action	Model and Route of administration	References
	and M3 muscarinic receptor subtypes in high dose animals, only the M2 receptor subtype decreased in low dose group animals, decreased levels of phosphorylated CREB		
	60-80% reduction of nigral dopamine neurons and 60-70% decrease in tyrosine hydroxylase and striatal dopamine levels, aggregates of α-synuclein and ubiquitin with mitochondrial defects, oxidative stress, high ROS levels, reduced MnSOD activity and higher LPO, neurobehavioural abnormalities	Albino Wistar rats, Subcutaneous	(Binukumar, Bal, et al. 2010)
Dichlorvos (2.5 mg/kg b.wt./day) and **Monocrotophos** (1.8 mg/kg b.wt./day), 4 weeks	Reduced depletion in dopamine and norepinephrine levels in co-exposure group, increased AChE activity and reduced MAO activity on co-exposure, glutathione (GSH) and oxidized glutathione (GSSG) ratio reduced on exposure to either, whereas co-exposure led to higher reduction in GSH: GSSG ratio	Wistar rats Dichlorvos: Subcutaneous; MCP: oral	(Dwivedi, Bhutia, et al. 2010)
Monocrotophos (10^{-4}-10^{-6} M), 6-24 h	Increase in ROS, LPO, and GSSG/GSH ratio, mRNA expressions and protein levels increased for caspase-3/9, Bax, cytochrome-c, p53, Puma, P21, decreased levels of Bcl2, Mc11 and Bclw, long-term exposure to 10^{-5} M resulted in less apoptotic events and more necrosis	PC12 cell line	(Kashyap, Singh, et al. 2010)
Monocrotophos (10^{-5} M), 2, 6, 12, and 24 h	Higher ROS and reduction in levels of GSH, the levels of protein and mRNA expressions of caspase-3/9, Bax, Bcl2, P^{53}, P^{21}, GSTP1-1 were significantly upregulated, whereas the levels of Bclw, Mcl1 were downregulated, induction in the expression of CYP1A1/1A2, 2B1/2B2, 2E1	PC12 cell line	(Kashyap, Singh, et al. 2011)
Monocrotophos (6.4 mg/kg b.wt.), 2.5 h, 24 h, 7 days, 14 days and 30 days	Acute exposure inhibited AChE (50–82%) after 2.5 h, lower expression of synaptic AChE mRNA after 24 h in striatum and cortex, AChE activity partially recovered 24 h after exposure	Wistar rats, Oral	(Kazi and Oommen 2012)

Contd...

Neurotoxicant	Effects/Mechanism of action	Model and Route of administration	References
Monocrotophos (10^{-5} M), 6 h	Induces downregulation of phosphorylated (Thr308/Ser493) Akt1, changed levels of downstream targets of pAkt such as., decreased pGSK3β (Ser9), higher levels of caspase-9, P_{53}, and Bad, lower mitochondrial membrane potential, MAPKs activation	Human Cord Blood Stem Cells	(Kashyap, Singh, et al. 2012)
Monocrotophos (100 μM) 10 mg/kg b.wt.	Reduced the levels of neurotrophic receptor TrkA with a parallel increase in death receptor P75 NTR, associated increase in apoptotic markers viz Bax, caspase-3, decrease in MAPK pathways and neural markers	Rat neural stem cells Wistar rats, Oral	(Tiwari, Agarwal, et al. 2015)
Lindane (2, 3, or 5 mg/kg b.wt./day), 90 days	Higher geotaxis and lowered SLA, higher GABA levels in cerebellum and benzodiazepine receptors in the cerebellar membrane in 3and 5 mg/kg groups	Adult male albino rats, Oral	(Anand, Agrawal, et al. 1998)
Lindane (25 and 100 mg/kg b.wt/day), 14 days	LPO and depletion of glutathione in all brain regions, induction in glutathione reductase, glutathione peroxidase, glutathione-S-transferase and catalase activity, superoxide dismutase activity was reduced at a higher dose in all regions	Wistar rats, Oral	(Srivastava and Shivanan-dappa 2005)
Lindane (2.5 mg/kg b.wt./day), 21 days	Higher expression of SEPT5, SNCA, 14-3-3 ε and proteasomal subunits such as PSMB4, PSMB6 and PSMA5 in substantia nigra and corpus-striatum and higher levels of APOE in the hippocampus, dysfunctions of the UPP, resulting in LPO and oxidative stress	Albino Wistar rats, Oral	(Mudawal, Singh, et al. 2015)
Cypermethrin (50 mg/kg b.wt/day), 21 days	Higher oxidative stress, LPO induction, decreased glutathione content, higher expression of genes involved in cellular defense such as thioredoxin reductases (txnrd2, txnrd3), peroxiredoxins (prdx2, prdx4, prdx6-rs1), catalase, superoxide dismutase, glutathione S-transferase kappa 1, and glutathione reductase (gsr), higher expression of cytoskeleton genes tmod1, vim, and kif9	Swiss albino mice, Intraperitoneal	(Singh, Lata, et al. 2011)

Contd...

Neurotoxicant	Effects/Mechanism of action	Model and Route of administration	References
Cypermethrin (10 mg/kg, 25 mg/kg b.wt./day), 14 days	Caused astrocyte apoptosis through disruption of the autocrine/paracrine mode of HB-EGF-EGFR signaling at two levels, irreversible loss of basal EGFR and decrease in HB-EGF	Wistar rats, Oral	(Maurya, Rai, et al. 2011)
Cypermethrin (100 µM), 72 h	Induced miR-200 family and apoptosis in differentiated PC12 cells by induction of p53 levels and down regulation of Bcl2	Differentiated PC 12 cells	(Kashyap, Kumar, et al. 2015)
Deltamethrin (7 mg/kg b.wt./day), 15 days	Higher MOA activity in hippocampus, frontal cortex, and cerebellum, higher AchE activity in corpus striatum, frontal cortex, cerebellum, hippocampus, and pons medulla, lower Na+, K+-ATPase activity in hippocampus, frontal cortex, and cerebellum, the concentration of polyamine was affected, in all areas, neurobehavioural dysfunctions	Albino rats, Oral	(Husain, Husain, et al. 1996)
Deltamethrin (150 mg/kg b.wt. and 15 mg/kg b.wt), 1 h	Inhibited motor coordination, inhibited the GABA levels in all areas of the brain at 150mg/kg	Wistar rats, Oral	(Manna, Bhatta-charyya, et al. 2006)
Rotenone (2-12 µg/1 µl)	Reduction in complex-I activity and higher generation of hydroxyl radicals, dose and time dependent decrease in level of dopamine in the ipsilateral striatum, dose-dependent decrease in nigral glutathione level till day 90, lower immunoreactivity of tyrosine hydroxylase in the substantia niagra or striatum, oxidative stress induced neurodegeneration	Sprague Dawley rats, Unilateral stereotaxic infusion	(Saravanan, Sindhu, et al. 2005)
Rotenone (10^6 to 10^4 M), 24 and 48 h	10^4 and 10^5 M concentrations were found to be cytotoxic, depletion in GSH levels and dopamine DA-D2 receptor at 24 h	PC 12 cell line	(Siddiqui, Kashyap, et al. 2010)
Plastic monomers			
Acrylamide (25 mg/kg b.wt.), 7,14, 21, 28 days	Decrease in brain mixed function oxidases (MFO) and glutathione -S-transferase (GST) by day 21 and 28	Wistar albino rats, Intraperitoneal	(Das, Mukhtar, et al. 1982)
Acrylamide or bis-acrylamide Single exposure (100 or 200 mg/kg b.wt.), 2 h	Concentration-dependent reduction in GSH content, Repeated exposure inhibited the GSH content but GST activity was reduced only by acrylamide	Albino rats, Intraperitoneal	(Srivastava, Sabri, et al. 1986)

Contd...

Neurotoxicant	Effects/Mechanism of action	Model and Route of administration	References
Repeated exposure (50 mg/kg b.wt.)/day, 10 days			
Styrene (1 ml/kg b.wt./day), 15 days	Increase in serotonin and noradrenaline, decrease in monoamine oxidase	Albino rats, Oral	(Husain, Srivastava, et al. 1980)
Styrene (270, 450 and 900 mg/kg b.wt./day), 7 days	Reduction of aryl hydrocarbon hydroxylase and glutathione-s-transferase activity followed by reduction of glutathione content at 450 and 900 mg/kg groups	Albino rats, Oral	(Dixit, Das, et al. 1982)
Styrene (100 mg and 200 mg/kg b.wt./day), 14 days	Serotonin levels in the hypothalamus, hippocampus, and mid-brain were elevated at higher dose	Albino rats, Oral	(Husain, Srivastava, et al. 1985)
Methyl methacrylate (500 mg/kg b.wt./day), 21 days	Impaired locomotor activity and learning, while aggressive behaviour significantly increased, an overall enhancement of biogenic amine levels in pons-medulla and hippocampus was noted an increase of noradrenaline in cerebral cortex and corpus striatum, an increase in 5-hydroxytryptamine in mid-brain and hypothalamus and for dopamine a slight decrease in corpus striatum	Wistar albino rats, Oral	(Husain, Srivastava, et al. 1985)
Miscellaneous			
Ethanol (0.5% v/v), 72 h	0.5% v/v for 72 h increased the expression of miR-302b and miR-497, lower BCl2and/or cyclin D2 expression, neuronal apoptosis	SH-SY-5Y cell line	(Yadav, Pandey, et al. 2011)
Valproic acid (0.1–10 mg) for 3 h	Reduction in GSH and non-protein thiol activity (NP-SH), lowered activities of GST, glutathione reductase (GR) and glutathione peroxidase (GPx), catalase (CAT) superoxide dismutase (SOD), in cerebral cortex and cerebellum, higher xanthine oxidase activity, AChE and Na+, K+-ATPase activity was decreased whereas MAO was upregulated	Isolated cortex and cerebellum preparations from Wistar rats	(Chaudhary and Parvez 2012)

Contd...

Neurotoxicant	Effects/Mechanism of action	Model and Route of administration	References
Flouride (30,60 and 120ppm), 30 days	Degenerated nerve cell bodies in CA3, CA4 and dentate gyrus, cell membrane involution, mitochondrial swelling, clumping of chromatin, neurobehavioural dysfunctions	Swiss albino mice, Oral	(Bhatnagar, Rao, et al. 2002)
Flouride (5, 10, 20, and 50 mg/b.wt./day), 15 weeks	Loss of the molecular and glial layer exposed to 10, 20, and 50 mg/kg, purkinje neurons revealed chromatolysis, perikaryon showed vacuolization, and spheroid bodies were present in the neuroplasm along with seizures, tremors and paralysis at two highest doses	Albino rabbits, Subcutaneous	(Shashi 2003)
Flouride (30, 45, and 75 mg/kg b.wt./day), 20 and 35 days	The adenomatous foci developed in the cerebral cortex which contained degenerating glial cells, the cells were vacuolated and reveled nuclei hyperchromatization in 30 mg group, chain formation of cells, senile plaque and large globose shaped neurofibillary tangle inside the perikaryon in cerebral cortex in 45 mg group, Pleomorphic, irregular glial cells had necrosis, the cerebral cortex revealed diffused haemorrhages in 75 mg group	Sprague Dawley albino rats, Subcutaneous	(Shashi and Sharma 2015)
Argemone oil (1.5 ml/kg b.wt/day), 3 days (0.2 ml/kg b.wt./day), 15 days	Increase in lipid peroxidation at 3 and 15 days in discrete areas of the brain viz. striatum, hippocampus, hypothalamusand thalamus, depletion in GSH content and metabolizing enzymes	Wistar rats, Intraperitoneal	(Siddiqui, Sayeed, et al. 2002)
Metanil Yellow (20 mg/kg b.wt./day), PND1-PND60 Adults (20mg/kg b.wt./day), 90-120	Levels of amines in the striatum, hypothalamus, and brain stem were drastically affected, iireversible alterations even after withdrawal, early inhibition of AChE activity in the striatum, delayed but persistent inhibition of AChE activity in the hippocampus, animals took more sessions to learn the operant conditioning behavior	Wistar rats, Gastric intubation	(Nagaraja and Desiraju 1993)
4-Hydroxy-trans-2 -nonenal (0.1-50 µM), 30 min-24h	Cytotoxicity at 10–50 µM, physiological stress at 2–5 Mm, lower binding of 3H-QNB, 3H-Fluinitrazepam and 3H-Ketanserin which label cholinergic, benzodiazepine and serotonin receptors respectively observed at 1 h, lower binding of 3H-Spiperone, which labels dopamine receptors at 4h	PC 12 cell line	(Siddiqui, Singh, et al. 2008)

Contd...

Neurotoxicant	Effects/Mechanism of action	Model and Route of administration	References
4-Hydroxy-trans-2 -nonenal (10, 25 and 50µM), 1 h	Dose-dependent increase in ROS and early response markers (c-Jun, c-Fos, and GAP-43), with upregulation of P[53], bax and caspase 3	PC 12 cell line	(Siddiqui, Kumar, et al. 2012)
4-Hydroxy-trans-2 -nonenal (10 µM), 6 h	Depleted phosphorylated (Thr308/Ser493) Akt1 as well as the downstream targets of pAkt, such as decreased levels of pgSK3β (Ser9), β-catenin and Bcl2, increased levels of Bax, Bad, P_{53} and caspase-3/9, ROS, nuclei degradation nuclei, apoptosis *In silico* data indicated that it interacted with Akt1 kinase domain, formed H-bond with glu234 residue like the highly potent Akt1 inhibitor imidazopiperidine analog	SH-SY-5Y cell line	(Kashyap, Singh, et al. 2015)
6-hydroxyd-opamine (6-OHDA) hydrochloride (4 µg/ml), 72h	Post 72 h, the level of malonaldialdehydes and conjugated dienes were increased in corpus striatum, and GSH, SOD, phospholipid contents and membrane fluidity was decreased, whereas the intracellular calcium concentration was elevated	Albino rats, Intraperitoneal	(Kumar, Agarwal, et al. 1995)
MPTP (0.2 µl/min for 5 min)	Dose-dependent and higher depletion of dopamine in the ipsilateral striatum, loss of tyrosine hydroxylase immunoreactive neurons in the substantia niagra, shrunken, pyknotic, distorted nuclei with condensed chromatin suggestive of dopaminergic neuronal death via apoptosis	Sprague-Dawley rats, Intranigral infusion	(Banerjee, Sreetama, et al. 2007)
3- nitropropionic acid (10–20 mg/kg b.wt./day), 4 days	Weight loss, gait abnormalities, striatal lesions with higher glial fibrillary acidic protein on day 5 and 9, higher striatal dopamine, decreased tyrosine hydroxylase immunoreactivity on day 5, dose-dependent decrease in the activity of complex-I in the cerebral cortex	Sprague–Dawley rats, Intraperitoneal	(Pandey, Varghese, et al. 2008)
Homocysteine (0.25–1 µmol)	Dose-dependent and higher depletion of dopamine in ipsilateral striatum and 3,4- dihydroxyphenylacetic acid in the striatum, homovanillic acid inhibited only at the highest dose	Sprague-Dawley rats, Unilateral intranigral infusion	(Chandra, Gangopadhyay, et al. 2006)

Contd...

Neurotoxicant	Effects/Mechanism of action	Model and Route of administration	References
Homocysteine (1 µmol)	Reduction in the activity of mitochondrial complex-I, lower striatal dopamine, loss of midbrain dopaminergic neurons, motor dysfunctions, oxidative stress in the nigrostriatal pathway, higher production of hydroxyl radicals, reduced GSH and higher antioxidant enzymes (catalase and superoxide dismutase) activity	Sprague-Dawley rats, Unilateral intranigral infusion	(Bhatta-charjee and Borah 2016)
Titanium dioxide nanoparticles (5-50 µg/ml), 1h	Increased LPO and protein carbonyl content, modulation of reduced glutathione content and major glutathione metabolizing enzymes and disruption of mitochondrial complexes	Wistar rats isolated mitochondria	(Nalika and Parvez 2015)
Noise (75-95 db, 3-4 hours/day), 5 days/week for 7-8 weeks	Lowered levels of glutamate and glutaminase activity by 15% and 24% in the cerebellum, 27% and 33% in the cortex, glutamate levels increased 28% (striatum), 10% (hippocampus), glutaminase activity 15% (striatum), higher activity of glutamine synthetase in all brain regions, higher GABA levels and glutamate alpha decarboxylase activity in the cortex and hippocampus	Wistar rats	(Kazi and Oommen 2014)

Cerebral metabolism, in particular, has assumed great significance due to the protective nature of the organ and its role as a target for a variety of drugs and foreign chemicals. Significant contributions have been made on the neurochemical mechanisms involved in xenobiotic metabolism and detoxification of drugs and toxins in the brain, elucidating the role of endogenous CYP450. Metabolism and the effects of toxicants have been well characterized in the adult as well as the developing brain. The brain has been shown to be equipped with both phase I and phase II enzymes that are involved in *in situ* metabolism of xenobiotics (Das, Seth, et al. 1981, Srivastava, Seth, et al. 1983, Dhawan, Parmar, et al. 1989). The neurobehavioral toxicity of different categories of pesticides have shown to be dependent on their metabolism, mediated by xenobiotic-metabolizing cytochrome P450s (CYPs) in the rat brain (Dayal, Parmar, et al. 2001, Dayal, Parmar, et al. 2003, Parmar, Yadav, et al. 2003). Further, EROD and PROD, like in the liver, could be used as a biochemical tool to characterize and substantiate the role of xenobiotic metabolizing CYPs and demonstrate their substrate specificity and selectivity in brain microsomes (Parmar, Dhawan, et al. 1998, Dayal, Parmar, et al. 1999, Dhawan, Parmar, et al. 1999).

Expression of constitutive and inducible CYPs have also been demonstrated in rat primary neuronal cells (Yadav, Dhawan, et al. 2006). Significant cellular and regional differences have been demonstrated in the distribution of xenobiotic metabolizing CYPs within the brain areas. The prevalence of these particular CYP isoenzymes in the brain has been shown to augment the neurotoxicity of pyrethroids by modulating the response of the brain to the insecticides via regulating their relative sensitivity, concentration or their active metabolites at the target site(s) (Anandatheerthavarada, Shankar, et al. 1990, Parmar, Dhawan, et al. 1998, Dayal, Parmar, et al. 1999, Dayal, Parmar, et al. 2001). Pre-exposure with CYP modifiers may modulate the neurotoxicity of lindane, via induction in the expression and activity of CYP2B and 1A isoforms (Parmar, Yadav, et al. 2003). Studies have further demonstrated the differential sensitivity of xenobiotic metabolizing enzymes to brain cells (neurons and glial cells) that could be used as a model to identify and distinguish the xenobiotic metabolizing potential of the cells but will also aid in providing insights into the vulnerability of these selective cell types towards specific neurotoxicants (Dhawan, Parmar, et al. 1990, Kapoor, Pant, et al. 2006).

Among all the variables influencing the effect of neurotoxic potential, age has found to be a vulnerable point, that has generated interest in characterizing the effects of neurotoxicants on the developing brain. The developing brain is quite vulnerable to even minute doses of substances which may be harmless for a developed brain. This is attributed to the inadequately developed blood-brain barrier, reduced oxygen levels and high rate of mitotis (Kumar, Jahan, et al. 2015). The earliest evidence of the susceptibility of developing brain explored the possible risks of manganese-induced behavioral alterations with respect to neurochemical changes in growing animals, in order to give clues about the early detection of manganese encephalopathy, a well-recognized chronic disabling condition in man (Chandra, Shukla, et al. 1979). Manganese resulted in enzymatic and morphological changes in growing animals' brain much before as compared to observed in adult animals, even though the dose of manganese was much lower in growing rodents as compared to adults, indicating that the developing brain was much more susceptible to the effects of the metal (Chandra and Shukla 1978). These results further set the stage for considerable work with compelling evidences suggesting that the growing nervous system may be more vulnerable and/or differentially vulnerable, to the toxic insult as compared to the adult nervous system.

Since then numerous studies have been focused on the possible role of exposure to environmental toxicants on the effects on early brain development and progression of developmental neurotoxicity, particularly with respect to prenatal and postnatal exposures. The growing fetus and neonates during the crucial periods of early development have been demonstrated to be sensitive to the effects of chemicals to which they have exposed via *utero* or via lactational exposure. Metals like cadmium and manganese have been demonstrated to penetrate the developing blood-brain barrier with more ease and its retention in neonates is higher than adults who may be responsible for its increased vulnerability (Seth, Husain, et al. 1977, Shukla, Srivastava, et al. 1988). Alternatively, xenobiotic exposure (such as quinalphos) may increase the blood-brain barrier permeability of the growing brain, resulting in an increased uptake of quinalphos and its metabolites in the neonates (Gupta, Agarwal, et al. 1999). Prenatal, postnatal as well as developmental exposure to neurotoxic chemicals such as pesticides, heavy metals, nanoparticles, endocrine disruptors etc have been shown to elicit deleterious effects on the structural and functional aspects of the growing nervous system that may affect signaling mechanisms, alter expression of receptors, impair learning and memory, delay functional maturation of the brain and cause behavioural anomalies. Such developmental exposure may also interfere with the crucial processe of development, i.e., cellular proliferation, migration, differentiation, synaptogenesis, myelination, and apoptosis. The restricted potential of the growing CNS to compensate for cell disruptions and loss in neuronal networking may lead to compromised neural functions and higher risk of neurodegeneration.

Numerous studies have been undertaken to characterize the effects of developmental exposure on early brain development. Pesticides (particularly OPs and new generation type II synthetic pyrethroids) and heavy metals have evoked maximum interest among researchers owing to their widespread applications. Behavioral deficits linked with perturbations in the normal ontogeny of neurotransmitter systems and regional brain polyamines have also been documented in the offsprings on *in utero* exposure to deltamethrin and other synthetic pyrethroids (Husain, Malaviya, et al. 1992). Pesticides like monocrotophos have shown to affect the cholinergic and non-cholinergic targets associated with motor dysfunctions in the developing brain, which might have long-standing implications even after withdrawal of its exposure (Sankhwar, Yadav, et al. 2012, Sankhwar, Yadav, et al. 2016). Developmental exposure may also impair learning and memory in developing rats, with alterations persisting in adulthood (Dhuriya, Srivastava, et al. 2017). Neonatal exposure to quinalphos may result in cerebral oxidative stress, which appears to be time dependent, leading to adverse effects on CNS function immediately and in also in later life (Gupta, Gupta, et al. 1998). Studies have exhibited the vulnerability of NMDA receptors to prenatal exposure to lambda-cyhalothrin, which may alter postsynaptic signaling, linked with defective memory and learning in the growing rats (Ansari, Shukla, et al. 2012). Early life exposure to metals at low doses may cause cholinergic alterations both in the frontal cortex and hippocampus and impede learning and memory (Ali, Mathur, et al. 1990, Chandravanshi, Yadav, et al. 2014).

Studies have not just focused on characterizing the neurotoxic effects of single chemicals but have also extended towards chemical mixtures. An important concern in the risk assessment of mixtures of chemicals is the probable interactions that impede predicting the toxicity of the mixture on the basis of known toxic effects of individual components of the mixture. To address this issue, Jadhav, et al 2007 have designed a study by employing metal mixture (MM) of the most frequently occurring heavy metals (cadmium, arsenic, mercury, lead, manganese, chromium, nickel and iron) using a relative concentration (similar to what is found in the groundwater sources of India), that were assessed as a single compound to estimate the net combined effects of all the components in the mixture (Jadhav, Sarkar, et al. 2007). Similar efforts have been made towards an understanding of the mechanisms resulting in pathological dysfunctions in the growing rat brain by a mixture of heavy metals (arsenic, cadmium and lead MM). MM may manifest its toxicity by compromising blood-brain communication in developing rats (Rai, Maurya, et al. 2010). Moreover, gestation followed by postnatal exposure to MM at ground-water relevant doses of India may induce synergistic toxicity in neuroglia of developing rats (Rai, Maurya, et al. 2010, Rai, Ashok, et al. 2013). Table 10.2 provides a comprehensive overview of the most representative studies carried out to characterize the effects of a few developing neurotoxicants.

Table 10.2 Few representative studies on the effects/mechanism of different developing neurotoxicants

Developing neurotoxicants	Effects/Mechanism of action	Model and Route of administration	References
Metals			
Arsenic (0.03, 0.30 and 3.00 ppm) Culture: 0.30 ppm, 18 days	Induced changes in brain cell membrane function indicated by generation and release of reactive oxygen–nitrogen intermediates in both the models, the explants' growth was reduced, ground matrix was lost and neural networking was inhibited along with evidence of apoptotic changes	Wistar rats, Oral Human fetal brain explants	(Chattopadhyay, Bhaumik, et al. 2002)
Manganese (Prenatal exposure 5 mg/ml and total 30 ml/day) PND 3 mg/ml, 10, 12 and 25 ml/day up to 60, 90 and 120 days, respectively; 30ml/day/animal till 180 days	Motor activity of offspring revealed increase at day 60 and 90, elevation in dopamine and norepinephrine levels in the corpus striatum, higher levels of manganese, striatal tyrosine and homovanillic acid	Mice, Oral	(Chandra, Shukla, et al. 1979)

Contd...

Developing neurotoxicants	Effects/Mechanism of action	Model and Route of administration	References
Zinc (2.3 mg/kg, 3.4 mg/kg and 4.5 mg/kg b.wt., twice/week) for 2, 4, 8 and 12 weeks	Reduced SLA, rotarod performance, lowered striatal dopamine, its metabolites and TH protein expression, SOD, SOD1 and SOD2 activities and LPO were higher, catalase and GST were lowered in a time and dose dependent manner	Wistar rats, Intraperitoneal	(Singh, Kumar, et al. 2011)
Zinc (20 mg/kg b.wt.) twice a week, for 2–12 weeks	Catalytic activity, GST-π protein expression, total GST activity, neurobehavioral parameters, striatal dopamine and its metabolites, nigral tyrosine hydroxylase positive neurons, TH expression and Bcl-2 proteins decreased, incraesed JNK, phosphorylation of c-jun, apoptosis	Wistar rats, Intraperitoneal	(Chauhan, Mittra, et al. 2019)
Pesticides			
Endosulfan (6 mg/kg b.wt/daily), post natal day (PND) 2-25	Noadrenanine levels increased in olfactory bulb and brain stem on day 10 and in the cerebellum and hippocampus on day 25, lower levels of dopamine levels in hippocampus on both day 10 and 25, increased serotonin levels in olfactory bulb, hippocampus and brainstem at 10 days of age	Wistar rats, Gastric intubation	(Lakshmana and Raju 1994)
Monocrotophos (0.5-1.0 mg/kg b.wt./daily), PND 22-49	Disrupted motor coordination and activity on PND50, lower binding of 3H-spiperone to striatal membrane in both the doses and higher binding of 3H-ketanserin to the frontocortical membrane in those exposed at a higher dose, respectively along with increased oxidative stress, these changes lasted even after 15 days of withdrawal (i.e PND 65)	Wistar rats, Perorally	(Sankhwar, Yadav, et al. 2012)
Quinalphos (0.5 mg/kg b.wt./daily), PND 11 – 21/45	AcHE decreased in the brain and blood but on withdrawal it recovered, higher superoxide radical generation up to PND 21 and 45, higher hydroxyl radical production at PND 45, increased activities of catalase and superoxide dismutase at PND 21 (on withdrawal of exposure at PND 22 partially or completely recovered at PND 45)	Albino rats, Oral	(Gupta, Gupta, et al. 1998)

Contd…

Developing neurotoxicants	Effects/Mechanism of action	Model and Route of administration	References
Lamda-cyhalothrin (1.0 mg/kg or 3.0 mg/kgb.wt.), PND 22-49)	Impaired motor activity and rota-rod performance on PND 50, decrease in motor activity with changes persisting even 15 days after the withdrawal, lower expression of tyrosine hydroxylase-immunoreactivity on PND50 and PND65, increase in expression of serotonin-2A receptors in frontal cortex	Wistar rats, Oral	(Ansari, Shukla, et al. 2012)
Lamda-cyhalothrin (1.0 or 3.0 mg/kg b.wt.) (PND 22-49)	Affected grip strength and impaired learning activity on PND50, impairment persisted in the grip strength and learning at PND65 even after wuthdrawal, low binding of muscarinic–cholinergic receptors in hippocampal, frontocortical, and cerebellar membranes with downregulated expression of ChAT and AChE in the hippocampus on PND50 and PND65, higher expression of GAP-43 in hippocampus on PND50 and PND65, LPO generation and higher levels of protein carbonyl, low levels of GSH and catalase, superoxide dismutase, and glutathione peroxidase activity	Wistar rats, Oral	(Ansari, Shukla, et al. 2012)
Lamda-cyhalothrin (1 and 3 mg/kg b.wt.), gestational day (GD) 6-21	Prenatal exposure resulted in reduced binding of 3H-MK 801 (labels NMDA receptors) in hippocampus of developing rats on PD22, downregulated mRNA and protein expression of NR1 and NR2B subunits of NMDA receptors, reduced expression of positive regulators (pERK1/2, PSD95, CaMKIIα and pCREB), higher expression of negative regulators (SynGAP and Cdk5) related to NMDA receptor, neurobehavioral alterations persisted in rats exposed to 3 mg/kg but recovery observed at 1 mg/kg on PD45	Wistar rats, Oral	(Dhuriya, Srivastava, et al. 2017)

Contd...

Developing neurotoxicants	Effects/Mechanism of action	Model and Route of administration	References
Cypermethrin (25, 50, 100 and 200 µM), 48 h	Induced injury in the astrocyte through Ca++ modulation, ROS, P38 and JNK pathways, which may potentially modify expression of MMP and reelin dependent astrocyte migration during brain development, attenuated extracellular matrix molecule and claudin-5 expression, α3β1integrin, and cytosolic protein Disabled1 were increased	Astrocyte culture	(Maurya, Mishra, et al. 2014)
Carbofuran (1 mg/kg b.wt./daily), GD7-GD21	Decreased NSC proliferation and survival in the hippocampus but not in cerebellum, downregulated SOX-2 and GFAP, lowered expression of nestin messenger RNA, and lowered histone-H3 phosphorylation suggestive of less neural progenitor cells and neuronal differentiation, elevated differentiation of glial cells, decrease in the expression of neurogenic genes/transcription factors such as neurogenin, neuregulin, and neuroD1 and elevation of gliogenic gene Stat3 expression	Albino rats, Oral	(Mishra, Tiwari, et al. 2012)
Carbofuran (1, 10, 20, 50, 100, 200 and 400 µM) 1 mg/kg b.wt./daily (gestational day 7 to PND 21)	Carbofuran significantly decreased NSC viability post 24 h above 50 µM, inhibits NSC proliferation and differentiation. Induced TGF-β signaling (higher phosphorylated SMAD-2/3 and decreased SMAD-7) in the hippocampus, which decreased proliferation of NSCs due to higher levels of p21 and decreased levels of cyclin-D1, disrupted neuronal differentiation, triggered apoptosis and neurodegeneration in hippocampus	Hippocampal Neural Stem Cells Wistar rats, Oral	(Seth, Yadav, et al. 2017)
Carbofuran (1 mg/kg b.wt.) GD7-PND21 PND 21-90	Inhibited proliferation of oligodendrocyte progenitor cells and oligodendroglial differentiation in the hippocampus region at both the time points, decreased expression of key genes and proteins involved in the regulation of oligodendrocyte development and functional myelination, altered the survival of oligodendrocytes by induction of apoptosis	Wistar rats, Oral	(Seth, Yadav, et al. 2019)

Contd...

Developing neurotoxicants	Effects/Mechanism of action	Model and Route of administration	References
	Miscellaneous		
Bisphenol A (4, 40, 400 µg/kg b.wt./day), GD 6-21 *In-vitro* (2, 10, 50, 100, 200, and 400 µM), 24 h	Disrupted proliferation of NSCs and neuronal differentiation in the SVZ and hippocampus and also *in vitro*, modified expression/protein levels of neurogenic genes and the Wnt pathway genes in the hippocampus, decreased levels of p-GSK-3β and β-catenin	Wistar rats, Oral Neural stem cells	(Tiwari, Agarwal, et al. 2015)
Bisphenol A (40 µg/kg b.wt./day), GD6–PND21 *In-vitro* (1, 10, 50, 100, 200, and 400 µM), 24 h	Decreased proliferation of BrdU-positive cells and reduced number and size of oligospheres, lowered BrdU co-localization with myelination markers CNPase and platelet-derived growth factor receptor-α	Wistar rats, Oral Neural stem cells	(Tiwari, Agarwal, et al. 2015)
Bisphenol A (40 and 400 µg/kg b.wt./day), PND14-PND21	BPA exposure during early postnatal period enhanced apoptosis, loss of mitochondria, bioenergetic deficits, higher mitochondrial translocation of Parkin, elevated levels of autophagy genes/proteins, activation of intracellular energy sensor AMPK, elevated raptor and ACC phosphorylation, reduced phosphorylation of ULK1 (Ser757)	Wistar rats, Oral	(Tiwari, Agarwal, et al. 2015)
Acrylamide (25 mg/kg b.wt.), daily for 5 days	Region specific effects on the brain with lowered levels of noradrenaline in the pons medulla, basal ganglia, and mid brain regions and of dopamine in mid brain, cerebellum, hypothalamus and pons medulla in age groups (12, 15 and 21 days), the 15 and 21 days aged rats revealed a drastic decrease in 5 hydroxytryptamine in the pons medulla, cerebral cortex and hypothalamus, exposure at 2, 4, 8 and 15 days aged rats led to higher activity of MOA and lowered activity of AchE, reduction in catecholamines associated with progressive development of neurobehavioural dysfunctions resulting in complete paralysis of the hind limb	Wista albino growing rats, Oral	(Husain, Dixit, et al. 1987)

Contd...

Developing neurotoxicants	Effects/Mechanism of action	Model and Route of administration	References
Silver nanoparticles (20 nm) (0.5, 1 (lower), 10 and 15 mg/kg b.wt/day), 10 days	Toxicity in fetuses manifested as mitochondrial autophagy, dysfunction of organelles, neuronal cell vacuolization, inflammation of blood brain barrier, swelling of astrocytes, reduction in the number of dendrite arborisation and unipolar neuron along with degeneration of basket cells	Swiss albino mice, Oral	(Prakash, Royana, et al. 2017)

Manifestations of neurotoxic effects during critical periods such developmental stages either *in utero*, during lactation periods, or in early childhood, may cause some neurochemical, developmental or behavioral defects that may appear shortly. Yet, growing evidence suggests that adverse effects of toxicants may not be evident clinically after several months, or even years of exposure but may manifest in adulthood. The importance of epigenetic mechanisms in explaining the critical role of early exposures in life in causing late life dysfunctions in the nervous system has received major attention. Environmental agents may epigenetically alter the genes to remain silent for long periods and later result in pathological abnormalities.

Damage to fetus by chemicals has been demonstrated to alter the ontogeny of the enzymes that are involved in the detoxification of such xenobiotics such as CYPs. Since the biotransformation enzymes' organ-specific profiles still continue to develop and undergo prominent changes, even after the organs are morphologically distinct, these enzymes are quite vulnerable to chemical insults. Environmental agents that are known CYP inducers such as PAHs, phenobarbital, and ethanol have been demonstrated to transplacentally trigger the expression of particular CYP isoforms. Ample studies have established that the CYPs identified as functional enzymes in the brain may not just be only involved in complex metabolic pathways involving detoxification/ biotransformation, but also serve as a vulnerable target where xenobiotics could act and affect brain physiological functions. Brain CYPs have been shown to be receptive to transplacental induction by environmental agents and that their increase is regulated transcriptionally. Prenatal exposure to low doses of pesticides have demonstrated the potential to alter the ontogenic profile and catalytic activities of xenobiotic metabolizing CYPs in the brain of the offspring, such alterations even persisting up to adulthood indicating the role of epigenetic reprogramming to persistently express those CYP isoforms (Johri, Dhawan, et al. 2007, Singh, Yadav, et al. 2013). These persistent changes have been associated with alterations in circulating levels of growth hormone, neurotransmitter genes, cognitive functions, neurotransmission synthesis

(Singh, Mudawal, et al. 2016). Moreover, when the offsprings are rechallenged at adulthood, higher magnitude of changes is induced in the xenobiotic CYPs suggesting that exposure of pesticides prenatally may result in higher responsiveness of the CYPs in the brain of the offsprings at an adult stage (Johri, Yadav, et al. 2006, Singh, Yadav, et al. 2013, Singh, Mudawal, et al. 2015, Singh, Mudawal, et al. 2016, Agrahari, Singh, et al. 2019).

Mechanistic insights have further highlighted alterations in promoter regions of CYP1A- and 2B- isoenzymes in the exposed offsprings. Such epigenetic modifications in CYPs may eventually potentiate the responsiveness of the individual and render them more susceptible to the toxic effects of drugs and chemicals at later stages in life. This epigenetic imprinting may be of toxicological significance as it may alter the response to environmental exposures in the offsprings specifically for those that require CYP-mediated metabolism to elicit their beneficial or adverse effects (Singh, Agrahari, et al. 2016). Computational sequence analysis has also identified the absence of short interspersed repeat elements (SINE) in the upstream, coding and downstream sequences of metabolizing CYPs which suggests the possibility of imprinting of these CYPs in the offsprings that are exposed to cypermethrin or other similar pesticides during gestational periods (Singh, Yadav et al. 2013).

The traditional approach towards assessment of neurotoxicity has involved delivering of toxins and drugs to discrete neuroanatomical loci in different experimental animals, with the perfused brains sectioned for morphological and histopathological as well as microsomes and mitochondrial fractions, etc. that have provided us sufficient insights into the different toxicological aspects of the CNS. There has been a growing interest in using *in vitro* models for neurotoxicity and developmental neurotoxicity (DNT). Immortalized cell lines and neuronal primary culture, astrocytes and glial cells have proved to be excellent *in-vitro* models for neurotoxicity. The rat pheochromocytoma derived cell line PC12 and the human neuroblastoma cell line SH-SY5Y are few of the popular *in-vitro* models of neurotoxicity. Advancement in our understanding of the stem cell biology have opened up fresh avenues for neurotoxicity research. The availability of stem cell cultures, such as rat and human neural stem cells with their pluripotent nature and capacity for proliferation, has provided us with a simple, valuable *in vitro* tool for evaluating the potential adverse effects and molecular mechanisms that may be linked with toxicant-induced damage (Kumar, Gupta, et al. 2015, Tiwari, Agarwal, et al. 2015, Seth, Yadav, et al. 2017).

The field of neurotoxicity/DNT has so far been best represented via *in vivo* and few *in vitro* model systems which have managed to provide limited information on the effect of developing neurotoxicants. The restricted availability of live human fetal brain tissue is not just ethically restraining but also practically unfeasible too, limiting our understanding of DNT. To address this issue, research groups at CSIR-IITR have successfully established stem cell-based high throughput *in vitro* model systems for assessing different aspects of DNT and have proven that human umbilical cord blood-derived stem cells (hUCBSCs) on differentiation into neurons serve as excellent tool for the same. The studies have provided rich insights into the complexity of the processes involved in the development, injury and repair mimicking of the human brain during the gestational and early periods in response to developing neurotoxicants like MCP and 3-methylcholanthrene (Kashyap, Singh, et al. 2012, Kashyap, Kumar, et al. 2015). Their work has uncovered the master regulator signaling molecules/cascades that are critical for converting hUCBSCs into functional neurons. Establishing new links between the expression and activities of xenobiotic metabolizing enzymes and their regulators in the hUCBSCs derived neuronal cells all throughout the differentiation process, the group has established the xenobiotic metabolizing capacity of developing neurons derived from a human source. Their work has shown that early differentiating neurons are more metabolically active and more susceptible to xenobiotic compounds as compared with the mature fully differentiated neuronal cells (Singh, Kashyap, et al. 2012, Singh, Kashyap, et al. 2013). This model has been further utilized for not just understanding the mechanistic basis of developmental neurotoxicants like MCP, but also screen for therapeutic agents against the neurotoxicant (Jahan, Kumar, et al. 2017, Jahan, Singh, et al. 2018). The same group has taken the work ahead towards the development of a complete 3D tissue niche of neuronal cells derived from hUCBSCs utilizing scaffolds with an aim to establish a more efficient predictive tool for DNT by closely recapitulating the *in-vivo* 3D microenvironment (unpublished data). The results have been encouraging and hopefully, shortly, they shall come up with a novel 3D human stem cell-based model that would open fresh avenues for studying developmental neurotoxicity *in-vitro*.

Govil et al 2012 have validated Post Nuclear Supernatant (PNS) as an *in vitro* model for assessing cadmium induced neurotoxicity using enzymatic and non-enzymatic antioxidants as biomarkers of exposure (Govil, Chaudhary, et al. 2012). Similarly, other efforts have included preparation of cerebellum and cerebral cortex of young rats as an *in vitro* model to evaluate the neurotoxic potential of valproic acid (Chaudhary and Parvez 2012). The utility of sagittal slices of mouse brain as an *in vitro* model for the mechanistic evaluation of acrylamide induced neurotoxicity has been successfully demonstrated (Ravindranath and Pai 1991). Alternative models capable of genetic manipulation like *Drosophila* and *C. elegans* have also been employed as suitable models for neurotoxicity evaluation (Jadhav and Rajini 2009, Salim and Rajini 2014, Singh and Chowdhuri 2017).

Various epidemiological studies have substantiated the role of environmental exposure of metals and pesticides in the onset of neurodegenerative disorders. Numerous factors have been suspected in participating in the onset/progression of neurodegeneration (NGD) that include age, genetic susceptibility and environmental exposure to xenobiotics. In the last few decades, the environmental theory on the etiology of NGD has acquired significant importance. Among environmental factors implicated in neurodegenerative diseases exposure to pesticides, heavy metals, drinking well water and rural habitat has been strongly documented (Priyadarshi, Khuder, et al. 2001, Das, Ghosh, et al. 2011, Gourie-Devi 2014, Surathi, Jhunjhunwala, et al. 2016, Verma, Keshari, et al. 2016). This is particularly true with Parkinsons' Disease (PD) and Alzheimer's Disease (AD), where there is a wealth of information linking environmental exposures to the disease. Studies associate exposure to pesticides (b-HCH, dieldrin and DDE) and metals (iron, copper, manganese and lead) with increased risk of AD and PD in the Indian population (Chhillar, Singh, et al. 2013, Kumudini, Uma, et al. 2014). Acute exposure to OPs has been implicated and few cases of acute and reversible parkinsonism due to OP intoxication have been documented (Bhatt, Elias, et al. 1999, Kumar and Subrahmanyam 2013). Understanding the NGD mechanisms, developing biomarkers for early diagnosis and the assessment of the efficacy of anti-NGD drugs have been a matter of growing concern among scientists.

Several experimental studies have demonstrated early signs of PD and AD like pathology upon exposure to different pesticides and metals. Pesticide exposure has been associated with the enhanced progressive and irreversible nigrostriatal dopaminergic neurodegeneration and dopamine depletion leading to PD (Patel, Singh, et al. 2006). Chronic dichlorvos exposure may result in nigrostriatal NGD and severe behavioral dysfunctions (Binukumar, Bal, et al. 2010). OPs such as MCP have the potential to cause pathological alterations in the dopaminergic neurons and potentiate the NGD in a vulnerable nigrostriatal system such as in PD (Jafri Ali and Sharda Rajini 2012, Ali and Rajini 2016). Similarly, metals like zinc have shown to induce oxidative stress through NADPH oxidase activation and GSH depletion, which may consequently activate the apoptotic machinery resulting in dopaminergic NGD similar to paraquat (PQ) (Singh, Kumar, et al. 2011). A list of few representative studies on xenobiotic neurodegeneration has already been enlisted in Table 10.1.

Few studies have also hinted at the involvement of exposure to neurotoxicants during developmental phases in the induction of NGD. It is strongly believed that environmental factors may interact with the specific loci during childhood, subsequently altering their expression and leading to the onset of diseases. Studies have, therefore, focused on the critical role of environmental exposures in the progression of such diseases, specifically in the context of prenatal and postnatal exposures. A variety of other agents including heavy metals, altered intake/metabolism of maternal nutrients (Dhobale and Joshi 2012, Roy, Kale, et al. 2012) also affect early life and modulate gene expression regulation which could lead to neurological disorders. Similarly, the effects of early life exposure to cypermethrin on markers of AD have been demonstrated (Maurya, Mishra, et al. 2016). Early gestational carbofuran exposure impairs postnatal neurogenesis, produces NGD in the hippocampus, and induce cognitive impairments in rat offspring (Mishra, Tiwari, et al. 2012). Studies have shown that post-natal exposure to pesticides modulates toxicant responsive genes and induces nigrostriatal dopaminergic NGD in adult rats and its pre-exposure during the important periods of brain development may enhance its susceptibility during adult life (Tiwari, Singh, et al. 2010, Singh, Tiwari, et al. 2012).

Similarly, a low dose of early life exposure may result in neurobehavioral alterations and such modifications may continue to persist in cases of continuous exposure to lambda-cyhalothrin (Ansari, Shukla, et al. 2012). The brain's antioxidant defense system may also be susceptible to programming by an imbalance in the maternal micronutrients (especially folic acid and vitamin B12). Imbalance in micronutrients like folate, vitamin B12 may trigger oxidative stress causing epigenetic alterations which may trigger apoptosis, inducing NGD. Maternal vitamin B12 deficiency during gestational and lactational periods may result in decreased neurotrophins level (BDNF and NGF), critical for brain development of the pups which may have implications in cognitive deficits/psychiatric disorders in later life (Sable, Dangat, et al. 2011, Roy, Sable, et al. 2014, Sable, Kale, et al. 2014).

The discovery of 1-methyl-4-phenyl-1, 2,3,6-tetrahydropyridine (MPTP) induced parkinsonism created much interest in finding an environmental risk factor for the pathogenesis of PD (Langston 2017). MPTP, causing dopaminergic NGD has been widely employed for unravelling the pathophysiology of the disease and designing of therapeutic interventions. Apart from MPTP, rotenone and 6-Hydroxydopamine (6-OHDA) have been common neurotoxins for development of experimental PD. Similarly, 3-nitropropionic acid (3-NP), as an animal model of Huntington Disease which closely reproduced behavioral and neuropathological features of the disease in rodents and primates has also been widely employed (Bové, Prou, et al. 2005). Apart from these, there has been a constant endeavor among toxicologists to develop more efficient neurodegenerative models. Both apomorphine and d-amphetamine induced stereotypic rotations have been suggested as important behavioral assays to assess the efficacy of novel drugs against PD, but apomorphine-induced contralateral bias has been demonstrated to be a better indicator of specific destruction in nigrostriatal pathway and development of postsynaptic dopamine receptor supersensitivity (Sindhu, Saravanan, et al. 2005, Sindhu, Banerjee, et al. 2006). A recent study by Bhattacharjee and

Borah 2016 has established the homocysteine (Hcy) induced rat model as a valuable rodent model of PD which is capable of causing equivalent pathologies via oxidative stress (OS) (Bhattacharjee and Borah 2016).

There has been an extensive geographical overlap of several metals and pesticides and therefore, humans are always exposed to multiple toxicants. As such, combined exposure of several metals/pesticides might be a relevant area of research, mimicking the real-life situation more, which could unravel novel mechanisms through which environmental exposures modulate neurodegenerative diseases. The role of metal ions such as zinc in potentiating/aggravating the toxicity of MPTP and paraquat has been successfully demonstrated (Hussain and Ali 2002, Kumar, Ahmad, et al. 2010). Numerous studies have demonstrated higher incidences of PD in the rural areas and have hypothesized the involvement of pesticides such as paraquat and maneb in NGD. These studies have encouraged research groups to develop models to assess the effect of co-exposure of maneb and paraquat for PD phenotype in young and adult mice. Unlike most of the toxin models where acute neurotoxicity results in chronic progression of cell death in PD, in the maneb and paraquat mouse model, only long-term exposures lead to subchronic progression of neuronal death in PD.

Several other environmental pesticides, such as cypermethrin (Cyp) have also been used to develop rodent models to understand the biochemical and molecular mechanisms of PD pathogenesis. Cyp-induced nigrostriatal NGD does not only provide additional evidence to the environmental theory of PD, but may also be a relevant model to study the aspects of sporadic PD, as it triggers NGD after prolonged exposure, even more than that of maneb and paraquat co-exposures (Patel, Singh, et al. 2006, Tiwari, Singh, et al. 2010, Singh, Tiwari, et al. 2012). Ashok, et al 2014 have developed a rat model of human exposure to chronic heavy metals co-exposure (arsenic, cadmium, lead) and characterized early manifestations of AD-like pathology which has been found to be synergistic, oxidative stress and inflammation-dependent. These findings are important because they demonstrate that the metals at their environmentally relevant water doses invoked greater-than additive up-regulation of the pro-amyloidogenic proteins at an early age and could contribute to the onset of NGD (Ashok, Rai, et al. 2014).

Neurological manifestations of HIV infection have also been recognized with a frequency that parallels the increasing number of AIDS cases which is being studied under the umbrella of neuroAIDS (Pant, Garg, et al. 2012). After sub-Saharan Africa, India has the second largest burden of HIV associated pathology, caused by HIV-1 clade C and lesser by HIV-2 (Gupta, Satishchandra, et al. 2007). Various subtypes of HIV-1 have been reported including subtype C, A/C, B, E and B/C (Siddappa, Dash, et al. 2005, Tripathy, Kulkarni, et al. 2005). Neurotuberculosis (Lanjewar, Jain, et al. 1998), followed by cryptococcosis (Wadia, Pujari, et al. 2001) and toxoplasmosis (Lanjewar, Surve, et al. 1998) in many combinations are the major neuropathologies clinically manifesting via reactivation of latent infection. HIV-1 affects the nervous system directly and induces neurological deficits which cause loss of cortical functions and compromised cognitive and motor abilities (Clifford and Ances 2013). Subtype C, the predominant clade of HIV-1 prevalent in India, also renders a risk of developing severe HIV associated dementia (HAD) and other neurological complication like Alzheimers, Parkinson and Amyotrophic lateral sclerosis (ALS). At NIMHANS, Bangalore, a single case of ALS like disorder with HIV clade-C has also been detected (Sinha, Mathews, et al. 2004).

Recapitulating neuroAIDS in animal models has not been experimentally possible. To address this issue, cellular and molecular approaches have been adopted using human neural precursor cells to study the effect of HIV-1B transactivating protein on the neuropathology of AIDS. Adding a new dimension to the understanding of HIV-1 neuropathogenesis, studies have provided novel insights into cellular and molecular mechanisms such as cell cycle disruptions and alterations in MAPK pathway that may modulate the cell properties in HIV/AIDS individuals (Nath 2002, Mishra, Taneja, et al. 2010). The behavioral and neuropathological differences between HIV-1 clades have been attributed to their genotypic variations. One of the viral regulatory protein-Tat contributes to the clade-specific differences in HIV neuropathogenesis with clade-C Tat causing reduced neurodegeneration (Ranga, Shankarappa, et al. 2004). C-Tat is comparatively less neurotoxic than B-Tat, due to modification in the dicysteine motif in the neurotoxic region of B-Tat (Mishra, Vetrivel, et al. 2008). The neuropathological defects of HIV-1 in patients using illicit drugs have hinted towards extensive interactions between the two agents, leading to a higher rate of NGD progression. Cocaine-mediated alterations in the expression of several tight junction proteins, thus altering the permeability of the blood-brain barrier, has shown to facilitate virus entry into the brain (Gandhi, Saiyed, et al. 2010, Dahal, Chitti, et al. 2015). The mechanisms of enhanced toxicity due to co-exposure of HIV protein Tat and morphine have been demonstrated (involving MAPK and JNK pathway), emphasizing its significance in HIV positive drug abusers, where brain damage is reported to be more severe as compared to the non-drug abusers (Malik, Saha, et al. 2014). Moreover, neuroprotective effects of PDGF-BB against HIV-Tat and morphine induced combined toxicity have also been demonstrated that are mediated via the phosphatidylinositol–3 kinase (PI3K)/Akt pathway (Malik, Khalique et al. 2011).

Apart from environmental factors, numerous endogenous molecules have also been implicated in the development of NGD. Homocysteine (Hcy), non-proteogenic sulfur-containing amino acid synthesized during the metabolism of methionine, has been identified to be an independent risk factor for NGD (Paul and Borah 2015, Paul and Borah 2016). Hcy has been shown to decrease the levels of striatal dopamine and induce midbrain dopaminergic NGD (Chandra, Gangopadhyay, et al. 2006). L-3,4-dihydroxyphenylalanine (L- DOPA), the standard drug for PD, has shown to elevate the levels of Hcy in the plasma and in the dopamine-rich regions of the brain (Bhattacharjee, Mazumder, et al. 2016). These studies have provided strong evidence in the favour of the neurotoxic nature of Hyc, further suggesting that a higher concentration in parkinsonian patients may potentiate the disease progression. β-phenethylamine (β-PEA), a component of several food products including wine and chocolate, is an endogenous molecule produced in the brain from phenylalanine and may contribute towards the progression of PD. It has been documented that chronic exposure to β-PEA causes neurochemical and behavioral disruptions in rodents similar to the parkinsonian neurotoxins. The toxicity of β-PEA has also been linked to hydroxyl radical (.OH) production and oxidative stress generation in the dopaminergic areas of the brain, which may be mediated through inhibition of mitochondrial complex-I. Thus, over long periods, over-consumption of food products containing β-PEA may be a potential neurological risk factor (Sengupta and Mohanakumar 2010, Borah, Paul, et al. 2013).

Numerous biochemical and molecular mechanisms have been emphasized to elucidate the mechanism of onset/progression of neurodegenerative disorders. Amongst these oxidative stress (OS), proteasomal dysfunction, mitochondrial dysfunction, apoptosis, microglial activation and inflammation have been proposed as the major contributing factors. The formation of ROS and the resulting OS has been postulated as the underlying event in the pathogenesis of NDG. Infact, OS has been established to precede PQ-induced neurodegeneration (Kumar, Ahmad, et al. 2010). These studies have been supported by increased levels of endogenous 6-OHDA and basal nitrite level content in peripheral mononuclear cells in PD patients indicating involvement of early response genes in OS mediated dopaminergic cell death and increased neuronal nitric oxide synthase activity respectively (Barthwal, Srivastava, et al. 2001, Seth, Agrawal et al. 2002). Increased LPO and oxidative stress to DNA and proteins have been reported in the substantia niagra of PD patients. A positive correlation has been found between OS-induced neurological disorder and enhanced blood lead levels in children (Ahamed, Fareed, et al. 2008).

The CNS is extensively vulnerable to free radical damage by xenobiotics owing to its high metabolic rate and increased levels of unsaturated lipids and such vulnerability has been found to be region-specific (Verma and Srivastava 2001, Mehta, Verma, et al. 2005, Srivastava and Shivanandappa 2005). The brain exhibits distinct variation in the regional distribution of the antioxidant biochemical defenses and metabolic rates that could be responsible for such differential oxidative damage in the brain regions (Shukla, Srivastava, et al.

1988). Supplemental antioxidant treatment may boost the system to protect against the oxidative stress in different experimental models of neurodegeneration Zafar, Siddiqui, et al. 2003, Ahmad, Ansari, et al. 2005, Khan, Hoda, et al. 2006, Khan, Ahmad, et al. 2010). Natural antioxidants have shown a remarkable reduction in OS due to excess formation of ROS by enhancing antioxidant mechanism in the neurodegenerative disorders (Table 10.3).

Genetic susceptibility to neurotoxins has been shown to be one of the major causes of PD. Genetic susceptibility to OP pesticide-induced parkinsonism has been suggested (Bhatt, Elias, et al. 1999). Case-control studies suggest that polymorphism in various genes (CYP, NAT, DAT etc) are involved in detoxification/metabolism and dopamine regulation that may alter vulnerability to PD and could be significant risk factors for the development of PD (Chaudhary, Behari, et al. 2005, Singh, Khan, et al. 2008, Punia, Das, et al. 2010, Singh, Khanna, et al. 2010, Punia, Das, et al. 2011). The contribution of genomics, proteomics and molecular biology approaches have made it possible to understand the modifying factors in the onset/progression of PD and give a better insight into the detection of new biomarkers in brain proteome and the underlying mechanisms; those that were not feasible with conventional biochemical procedures. Gene expression profiling has been widely employed to elucidate the molecular and cellular mechanisms of NGD both in chemicals-induced PD and sporadic disease (Patel, Singh, et al. 2008, Singh, Tiwari, et al. 2011). SNP based studies have given important clues to verify the involvement of toxicant responsive genes (CYP2E1 and GSTA4-4 expression), metallothionein genes (MT-I, MT-II) and transporter genes (VMAT-2, DAT) in the animals exposed to combined exposures to maneb+paraquat and zinc+paraquat (Patel, Singh, et al. 2006, Kumar, Ahmad et al. 2010). More importantly, the role of these genes has been characterized in modulating MPTP neurotoxicity to confer protection against caffeine and nicotine (Singh, Singh, et al. 2009, Tiwari, Agarwal, et al. 2013). Studies suggest that polymorphism in the genes involved in the process of detoxification and dopamine regulation may alter the susceptibility to PD and could also be important significant risk factors (Singh, Khan et al. 2008). Modulation in the transcript levels of 61 genes that are ainvolved in DNA replication and repair, genomic surveillance, and OS have been identified in Cyp induced neurotoxicity (Singh, Lata, et al. 2011). Similarly, 65 transcripts related to several biological pathways starting from skeletal transcripts to ions channels, signaling to apoptosis pathway and transcription regulators to growth regulators have been found to be differentially regulated on Cyp exposure in the post-natal preexposed and adulthood rechallenged rats indicating that it may exert its neurodegenerative effects via involvement of several biological pathways, such as oxidative stress, cellular energy, xenobiotic metabolism, inflammation, and microglial activation (Tiwari, Singh, et al. 2012). Identifying and characterizing the macromolecules involved in nigrostriatal dopaminergic NGD may aid in unraveling the putative cellular mechanisms and offer novel clues to understand the etiology of PD phenotype and its association with sporadic PD.

NGD studies have also largely benefitted from proteomic profiling for identification of CNS markers of injury on exposure to xenobiotics. Proteomic strategies employing post-mortem human brain, blood, cerebrospinal fluid (CSF) and in animal models have enabled identification of several differentially displayed proteins (associated with oxidative stress, energy metabolism, electron transport, signal transduction, and detoxification pathways) which have offered a clearer picture of the pathological alterations, biochemical and molecular events leading to PD phenotype as well as in developing biomarkers for an early diagnosis (Patel, Sinha, et al. 2007, Sinha, Srivastava, et al. 2009, Srivastava, Singh, et al. 2010). Studies have provided a direct link between lindane induced oxidative stress and the ubiquitination/de-ubiquitination pathways with the pathogenesis of sporadic AD and PD (Mudawal, Singh, et al. 2015). Proteome profiles of maneb and paraquat-exposed striatum have revealed the differential expression of α-enolase, complexin-I and glia maturation factor-β (Patel, Sinha, et al. 2007). Differential expression of nigrostriatal proteins has been identified in Cyp induced neurodegeneration, highlighting the role of microglial and mitochondrial dysfunctions (Singh, Tiwari et al. 2011, Agrawal, Singh, et al. 2015).

Environmental agents mediating epigenetic modifications have also been implicated in the increased susceptibility and progression of environmentally induced chronic diseases (Baccarelli and Bollati 2009, Kanthasamy, Jin, et al. 2012). A research group has identified hypermethylation in the activity of two genetic loci, parkin and PINK1 (associated with PD) upon manganese exposure that may be considerable risk factors for the onset of sporadic PD. DAVID analysis further suggested the involvement of these differentially methylated genes in several crucial biological pathways such as neuronal development and differentiation, signal transduction, synaptic transmission, inflammation and apoptosis (Tarale, Sivanesan et al. 2017).

For NGD studies, animal models have immensely contributed towards a better understanding of the disease pathogenesis and designing of therapeutic strategies. Rat models have provided an easy characterization of the progressive development of tremors, rigidity, spasticity, bradykinesia and postural instability, which closely mimics several neurodegenerative diseases. However, in the past several years, the importance of developing more acceptable alternatives to traditional animal testing has been gradually recognized by toxicologists. Transgenic alternative animals such as *Drosophila, C.elegans* and Zebrafish (exhibiting a high degree conservation of physiological processes and signaling pathways with humans) have been usefully exploited for elucidating the toxicological mechanism and gene-environment interactions as well as screening for therapeutic options in association with exposure to pesticides and metals and neurodegenerative chemicals (Jadiya and Nazir 2012, Jagota and Rajadas 2012, Jagota and Rajadas 2013, Makhija and Jagtap 2014, Khatri and Juvekar 2016, Mohanty, Das, et al. 2017). Using *C. elegans* as a model, studies have established that PD associated effects of environmental chemicals (such as pesticides viz herbicides, botanicals, OPs, fungicides, pyrethroids and carbamates) have been found to be class and structure specific and stress-responsive genes (sod-1, sod-2, sod-3, hsp-16.2, hsp-60, hsp-70) may not follow a generalized pattern to these different toxicants (Pooja Jadiya and Nazir 2012). Jagota and Rajadas 2013 have employed the transgenic strain of *C. elegans* expressing 'human' alpha-synuclein as a robust model to screen out novel peptides based on their ability to inhibit Aβ oligomerization (Jagota and Rajadas 2013). Shukla, et al. 2014 have identified a mutation in *Drosophila methuselah* (mth), which is linked with aging, conferring higher resistance to PQ-induced PD phenotypes as observed via decreased NGD and reduced disruption of locomotor activity, primarily via modulation of oxidstive stress (Shukla, Pragya, et al. 2014).

Research groups have also remained at the forefront in screening out various protective/therapeutic agents. Medicinal plants and their extracts, natural compounds, vitamins, antioxidants, etc. have shown neuroprotective potential using different chemical/drug models of neurotoxicity and neurodegeneration. Research groups have identified many drugs and antioxidants that prevent neurotoxicity via their direct •OH scavenging action (Table 10.3). The inverse relationship between cigarette smoking/coffee drinking and PD risk has been reported in several studies (Powers, Kay, et al. 2008, Kandinov, Giladi, et al. 2009), which has prompted research groups to identify the mechanistic aspects of nicotine/caffeine mediated protection in neurodegenerative conditions (Singh, Singh, et al. 2010, Yadav, Gupta, et al. 2012). Co-grafting of olfactory ensheathing cells have shown to elevate the survival and functioning of transplanted NSCs in 6-OHDA lesioned parkinsonian rats (Shukla, Chaturvedi, et al. 2009). Table 10.3 provides a few of the representative studies conducted in an endeavor to identify interventional strategies against neurotoxicants/developing neurotoxicants.

Table 10.3 Few representative studies carried out to screen for preventive/therapeutic interventions against neurotoxicants

Neurotoxicants/ Developing Neurotoxicants	Effect/Mechanism of action of preventive/protective agent	Model and route of administration (toxicant)	References
Arsenic (0.3 mg/l in culture/drinking water), 24 h	**Vitamin C** (2.5 mg/kg b.wt./day), **vitamin E** (148 mg/kg b.wt./day) during gestation and **DMSA (**50 mg/kgb.wt.) for 2 days after the end of gestation: Administration showed partial reversal of increased production of NO, ROS, decrease in DNA and 54% synthesis that led to necrosis and apoptosis in human fetal brain explants Prevented higher generation of NO, ROS and loss of glutathione content on rat neonatal brain explants	Human fetal brain explants Rat neonatal brain explants	Chattopadhyay, Bhaumik, et al. 2002
Lead (20 mg/kg b.wt/alternate day), 5 weeks prior to gestation and 3 weeks during gestation (total 8 weeks)	**Selenium** (as sodium selenite): Co-exposure (0.5 ppm) for total 8 weeks led to lesser reduction in enzymes succinate dehydrogenase, AcHE and Na+/K+-activity in the cerebrum of the pups at 4 weeks of age	Sprague Dawley rats, Oral	(Sidhu and Nehru 2005)
Lead (0.2% lead acetate), 6 months in drinking water	**Calcium disodium EDTA** (50 mg/kg i.p., once daily), **DMSA** (50 mg/kg oral, once daily), **monoisoamyl meso-2,3-dimercaptosuccinic acid** (50 mg/kg oral, once daily), **DMSA** (50 mg/kg oral, once daily) + **CaNa2EDTA** (50 mg/kg i.p., once daily), **MiADMSA**(50 mg/kg oral, once daily) +**CaNa2EDTA** (50 mg/kg i.p., once daily); Post 5 days of chelation treatment, animals were left un-treated for 7 days, then given a second course of	Wistar rats, Oral	(Flora, Saxena, et al. 2007)

Contd...

Neurotoxicants/ Developing Neurotoxicants	Effect/Mechanism of action of preventive/protective agent	Model and route of administration (toxicant)	References
	5-day treatment: The combination therapy was more effective in than monotherapy in reversing lead induced ROS generation, nitric-oxide synthetase, and intracellular free calcium levels, changes in neurotransmitter level and apotosis along with behavioral defects in locomotor activity		
Lead (7.5 mg/kg b.wt./day), 14 days	**Omega-3-fatty acids**: (750 mg/kg b.wt./day, 15 days, Oral), Co-exposure decreased level of LPO, content of protein carbonyl, ROS and increased the activities of glutathione peroxidase, catalase and superoxide dismutase, content of dopamine, TH immune-reactivity, mRNA expression of VMAT 2 and p53 protein levels	Wistar rats, Oral	(Singh, Singh, et al. 2017)
Cadmium (5 mg/kg b.wt./day), 28 days	**Quercentin** (25 mg/kg b.wt./day, Oral):Co-supple-mentation protected against cadmium-induced alterations in cholinergic–muscarinic receptors, mRNA expression of genes (M1, M2, and M4), and expression of ChAT and AChE, duced ROS generation and protected mitochondrial integrity by modulating proteins involved in apoptosis and MAP kinase signaling	Wistar rats, Oral	(Gupta, Shukla, et al. 2017)
Cadmium (5 mg/kg b.wt./day), 28 days	**Quercentin** (25 mg/kg b.wt./day, Oral): Co-supple-mentation protected against cadmium-induced alterations decrease levels DOPAC and HVA in cadmium treated rats. Further, DARPP32 expression in cadmium treated rats was decreased with further increased levels of PPIa expression in rats	Wistar rats, Oral	(Gupta, Shukla, et al. 2018)

Contd...

Neurotoxicants/ Developing Neurotoxicants	Effect/Mechanism of action of preventive/protective agent	Model and route of administration (toxicant)	References
Rotenone dissolved in DMSO:PEG (1:1), infused (1 µl) (24h)	**L-deprenyl** (0.1, 1, 5 and 10 mg/kg b.wt.; i.p; one hour following rotenone infusion and thereafter twice daily for next 3 days): Elevation in the salicylate hydroxylation products, lower activity of complex-I, reduced glutathione levels in substantia niagra, tyrosine hydroxylase immunoreactivity in the substantia niagra and striatum, dose dependent reduction in the levels of striatal dopamine	Sprague Dawley rats, Unilateral stereotaxic infusion	(Saravanan, Sindhu, et al. 2006)
Rotenone (0.1-10 mg/kg b.wt.) 24 h	**Curcumin Monoglucoside** (synthesized) (24h): Pretreatment elicited antioxidant effects by restoring glutathione levels, mitochondrial complex I and IV activities and reducing reactive species by decreasing phosphorylation of JNK3 and c-jun and reduced cleavage of pro-caspase 3, attenuated up-regulation of NOS2 and down-regulation of NQO1, pretreatment revealed improved survival rate and locomotor activity, better antioxidant activity and dopamine levels	N27 dopaminergic cell line, *Drosophila* model	(Pandareesh, Shrivash, et al. 2016)
Rotenone (100 nM), 24 h	**Demethoxycurcumin** (a natural derivative of Curcumin): Pretreatment (50 nM) for 24 h reduced ROS generation, MMP disruptions, release of Cyt-c and expression of pro-apoptotic markers	SH-SY5Y neuroblastoma cell line	(Ramkumar, Rajasankar, et al. 2017)

Contd...

Neurotoxicants/ Developing Neurotoxicants	Effect/Mechanism of action of preventive/protective agent	Model and route of administration (toxicant)	References
Maneb (30 mg/kg b.wt.) and **Paraquat** (10 mg/kg b.wt.)/twice a week, 9 weeks	**Silymarin (40 mg/kg b.wt./day) or melatonin (30 mg/kg b.wt./day) for 9 weeks:** attenuated LPO generation, decrease in degenerating neurons, content of nitrite, mRNA expressions of cytochrome P-450 2E1 (CYP2E1) and GSTA4-4, CYP2E1 and GST catalytic activities, Bax, p53, and caspase 9 protein levels	Swiss albino mice, Intraperitoneal	(Singhal, Srivastava, et al. 2011)
Maneb (30 mg/kg) and **Paraquat** (10 mg/kg)/twice a week, 9 weeks	**Caffeine** (20 mg/kg b.wt.,9 weeks, i.p): Co-exposure down-regulated NO production, neuroinflammation and microglial activation by reducing levels of IL-β, p38 MAPK, NF-kB and TK	Swiss albino mice, Intraperitoneal	(Yadav, Gupta, et al. 2012)
Maneb (30 mg/kg b.wt.) and **Paraquat** (10 mg/kg b.wt.)/twice a week, 9 weeks	**Silymarin(40 mg/kg b.wt./day) or melatonin (30 mg/kg b.wt./day) for 9 weeks:** restored the disrupted expression of Bcl2, Bax, Bak1, Trp53, Fas, Casp1, Casp9 and NFjB1, downregulated inflammation markers TGF-1β, TNF-α , IL-1β and IFN-γ	Swiss albino mice, Intraperitoneal	(Singhal, Chauhan, et al. 2013)
MPTP (20 mg/kg b.wt./daily), 4 weeks	**Nicotine** (1 mg/kg) or **caffeine** (20 mg/kg) for 8 weeks: Pretreatment followed by (MPTP; 20 mg/kg) for 4 weeks restored MPTP induced attenuation of VMAT-2 and CYP1A1, elevation of CYP2E1, GST-ya, GST-yc and GSTA4-4 expression/activity	Sprague–Dawley rats, Intranigral infusion	(Singh, Singh, et al. 2008)
MPTP (30 mg/kg b.wt., twice, 16 hr apart)	**Salicyclic acid** (25–100 mg/kg b.wt., i.p.): Pretreatment led to dose-dependent generation of 2,3- and 2,5-DHBA, administration prior to or post MPTP prevented behavioural abnormalities and depletion of glutathione and dopamine on the 7th day	Albino mice, Intraperitoneal	(Mohanakumar, Muralikrishnan, et al. 2000)

Contd...

Neurotoxicants/ Developing Neurotoxicants	Effect/Mechanism of action of preventive/protective agent	Model and route of administration (toxicant)	References
MPTP (30 mg/kg b.wt., twice, 16 hr apart)	**Melatonin** (10, 20, and 30 mg/kg b.wt.; i.p 30 min prior to MPTP): dose-dependent reduction in the generation of hydroxyl radicals *in vitro, ex vivo* and *in vivo*, GSH reduction was prevented dose-dependently in the substantia niagra and NCP	Albino mice, Intraperitoneal	(Thomas and Mohanakumar, 2004)
MPTP (20 mg/kg b.wt., four times at 2-hour intervals on 1 day only	**Pycnogenol (PYC), an extract of *Pinus maritime* bark** (20 mg/kg b.wt./daily, intraperitoneal), 15 days: Pretreatment resulted in protection of antioxidant enzymes ctivity and glutathione content, replenished the levels of thiobarbituric acid reactive substances, blocked the elevation of dopaminergic D2 receptors and reduced dopamine levels and its metabolites	Albino mice, Intraperitoneal	(Khan, Hoda, et al. 2010)
6-OHDA (12.5 μg), given on day 8	**Selenium** (sodium selenite 0.1, 0.2 and 0.3 mg/kg b.wt. intraperitoneal, 7 days): Pretreatment upregulated the antioxidant status and reduced dopamine loss, functional recovery restored after 3 weeks of selenium treatment	Balb/c mice, Intraperitoneal	(Zafar, Siddiqui, et al. 2003)
6-OHDA (10 mg), on day 21	***Withania somnifera*** (100, 200 and 300 mg/kg b.wt., 3 weeks, Oral): Preexposure reversed deficiency in the activities of glutathione dependent enzyme system, catalase and superoxide in a dose dependent manner	Balb/c mice, Intraperitoneal	(Ahmad, Saleem, et al. 2005)
6-OHDA (4 μg), on day 16	**Sesame Seed Oil** (free access to 20% oil mixed in fat free diet), 15 days: Preexposure led to an improvement in glutathione reductase, glutathione-S-transferase,	Swiss albino mice, Intraperitoneal	(Ahmad, Khan, et al. 2012)

Contd...

Neurotoxicants/ Developing Neurotoxicants	Effect/Mechanism of action of preventive/protective agent	Model and route of administration (toxicant)	References
	glutathione peroxidase, catalase activities and the dopamine level, prevented activation of Nox2 and Cox2 and restored MnSOD expression		
6-OHDA (10 mg/kg b.wt.)	**Piperine (10 mg/kg b.wt/daily,15 days, Oral):** Pre exposure depleted increased inflammatory markers, TNF-α and IL-1β, blocked cytochrome-c release, caspase-3, and caspase-9, maintained the ratio of Bcl-2/Bax and prevented the overactivation of PARP	Wistar rats, Intrastriatum infusion	(Shrivastava, Vaibhav, et al. 2013)
6-OHDA (25 mM), 48 h	**Curcumin (50 μM, Oral):**Co-exposureincreased egg laying, brood size and the survival (by 3days), decreased the dopaminergic neurodegeneration with a marginal restoration of acetylcholinesterase activity among worms	*C. elegans,* Oral	(Satapathy, Salim, et al. 2016)
Aβ fragment$_{1-42}$ 0.2μg/μl), 2 weeks	**Novel triazine derivatives (20mg/kg b.wt., Oral):** Pre-treatment with TRZ-15 and TRZ-20 demonstrated neuroprotective ability as observed from better cognitive ability, lower Aβ_{1-42} burden, cytochrome-c and cleaved caspase-3 levels via Wnt/β-catenin pathway	Wistar rats, Stereotaxic injection	(Sinha, Tamboli, et al. 2015)
3-Nitropropionic Acid (10 mg/kg b.wt.), 14 days	**Cyclosporin A (2.5, 5, and 10 mg/kg b.wt.; Oral):** Co-exposure attenuated disrupted body weight, motor activity, biochemical parameters (increased LPO, nitrite concentration, reduction of catalase and super- oxide dismutase), as well as mitochondrial enzymes	Wistar rats, Intrapritoneal	(Kumar, Kalonia, et al. 2010)

Contd...

Neurotoxicants/ Developing Neurotoxicants	Effect/Mechanism of action of preventive/protective agent	Model and route of administration (toxicant)	References
3-Nitropropionic Acid (20 mg/kg b.wt.), 7 days	*Zingiber officinale* (100 mg/kg, 200 mg/kg b.wt.; peroral): Co-exposure attenuated higher LPO, nitrite and AchE levels, restored the decease in motor functions	Wistar rats, Intraperitoneal	(Sharma, Sharma, et al. 2012)
Arsenic (100 ppm), *ad litium*, 60 days	**DL- α lipoic acid** (70 mg/kg b.wt. /day, 60 days, oral): Co-treatment reduced oxidative protein damage and carbonyl residues and increased protein thiols in arsenic intoxicated rat brain regions (striatum, cortex, cerebellum, hippocampus and hypothalamus)	Wistar rats, Oral	(Shila, Subathra, et al. 2005)
Arsenic (2 mg sodium arsenite/kg b.wt.), 10 weeks	**MiADMSA**(50 mg/kg b.wt./day, 5 days, oral):Post treatment could reverse arsenic induced alterations such as elevation in malondialdehyde levels, decrease in stress marker enzymes Mn-superoxide dismutase, Cu/Zn-superoxide dismutase, catalase, glutathione reductase, glutathione peroxidase, and glutathione-S-transferase in cortex, cerebellum and hippocampus	Wistar rats, Oral	(Kumar, Flora, et al. 2013)
Arsenic (sodium arsenite, 20 mg/kg b.wt/day, 28 days)	**Curcumin** (100 mg/kg b.wt, 28 days, oral): Co-exposure increased the locomotor activity and grip strength and improved the rota-rod performance, higher binding of striatal dopamine receptors and TH expression whereas levels of arsenic and oxidative stress reduced in corpus striatum, hippocampus and frontal cortex	Wistar rats, Oral	(Yadav, Sankhwar, et al. 2009)
Arsenic (20 mg/kg b.wt)/daily , 28 days	**Curcumin** (100 mg/kg b.wt./day, 28 days, oral): Co-exposure protected against arsenic exposure by restoring	Wistar rats, Oral	(Srivastava, Yadav, et al. 2014)

Contd...

Neurotoxicants/ Developing Neurotoxicants	Effect/Mechanism of action of preventive/protective agent	Model and route of administration (toxicant)	References
	mitochondrial membrane potential, activity of mitochondrial complexes, expression of CHRM2 receptor gene and pro and anti apoptotic genes both in frontal cortex and hippocampus		
Carbofuran (1 mg/kg b.wt.), 28 days	**N-acetyl cysteine** (200 mg/kg b.wt. oral, 28 days): administration 30 min after carbofuran exposure could partially restore the activity of acetylcholinesterase, lowered LPO along with partial repletion in levels of glutathione, superoxide dismutase, glutathione peroxidase, glutathione reductase and catalase activities, restored neurobehavioural impairments	Wistar rats, Oral	(Kamboj, Kiran, et al. 2006)
Monocrotophos (0.75 mM), 24 h	Chitooligomers (0.2 mM, 24 h oral): Co-exosure led to increased lifespan, normal egg laying, higher brood size, reduced dopaminergic NGD, higher dopamine content, AChE and carboxylesterase activity increased, reduction in ROS, increased GSH and catalase and superoxide dismutase activity	*C. elegans*, Oral	(Nidheesh, Salim, et al. 2016)
Monocrotophos (10, 100, 1000 µM), 24 h	**Resveratrol (10** µM, 24 h): Co-supplementation led to significant restoration in the monocrotophos induced alterations such as ROS, MMP disruption and morphological changes by modulation of PI3K-mediated pathway	Human umbilical cord blood - Mesenchymal Stem Cells	(Jahan, Kumar, et al. 2018)
Monocrotophos (100 µM), 24-72 h	**Secretome of differentiated PC12 cells (50% conditioned medium):** restored the cell viability, oxidative stress and apoptotic cell death in both the cells through autophagy facilitated by AMPK/SIRT1/ PGC-1α signaling cascade	Human Mesenchymal Stem Cells and SHSY-5Y Cells	(Srivastava, Singh, et al. 2018)

Contd...

Neurotoxicants/ Developing Neurotoxicants	Effect/Mechanism of action of preventive/protective agent	Model and route of administration (toxicant)	References
Bisphenol A (40 µg/kg b.wt./daily), GD6 to PND28 *In-vitro* Bisphenol A(100 µM)	**Curcumin (20 mg/kg b.wt./daily,** PND7 to PND28; Intraperitoneal), *in vitro* (0.5 µM)**:** protected against reduction in NSC proliferation and differentiation and increased NGD via activation of the Wnt/β-catenin signaling pathway, prevented increased β- catenin phosphorylation, decreased GSK-3β levels, and β- catenin nuclear translocation, resulting in enhancement of neurogenesis with better learning and memory	Wistar rats, Oral Neural Stem cells	(Tiwari, Agarwal, et al. 2016)
Ischemia (oxygen-glucose deprivation (OGD)), 6 h followed by 24 h reoxygenation	*Trans*-**Reseveratrol** (5, 10, and 25 µM, 24 h prior to OGD; during 6 h of OGD; for 24 h post OGD and whole treatment group which starts from 24 h before OGD and lasted to 24 h post OGD): Restoration of LPO levels, ROS, and glutathione content, decreased caspase-3, bax, and hypoxia inducible factor-1α (HIF-1α)	PC 12 cell line	(Agrawal, Kumar, et al. 2011)
Ischemia (oxygen-glucose deprivation (OGD)), 6 h followed by 24 h reoxygenation	*Trans*-**Reseveratrol** (5, 10, and 25 µM, 24 h prior to OGD; during 6 h of OGD; for 24 h post OGD and whole treatment group which starts from 24 h before OGD and lasted to 24 h post OGD): Increased theviability of OGD-R insulted PC12 cells, significantly decreased ROS generation, levels of intracellular Ca^{2+}, and hypoxia associated transcription factors, signal transducer and activator of transcription 3 (STAT3), Cav-beta 3 (Cav β3), cationic channel transient receptor potential	PC 12 cell line	(Agrawal, Kumar, et al. 2012)

Contd...

Neurotoxicants/ Developing Neurotoxicants	Effect/Mechanism of action of preventive/protective agent	Model and route of administration (toxicant)	References
	melastatin 7 (TRPM7) and hsp-27, elevated the antioxidant defense enzymes level		
Ischemia, 1 h	L-lactate (15–30 mmol/L): Promotes neuronal survival byincreasing functional TREK1 protein expression by 1.5–3-fold via protein kinase A (PKA) dependent pathway	Rat hippocampal astrocytes	(Banerjee, Ghatak, et al. 2016)

10.2 Hepatotoxicity

The liver, referred to as the 'metabolic factory', plays a pivotal role in maintaining metabolic functions and detoxification of both endogenous and exogenous challenges such as xenobiotics, drugs, chemicals, viral infections and chronic alcoholism (Pandit, Sachdeva, et al. 2012). Its unique association and crucial link with the small intestine and systemic circulation enables it to maximize the processing of the nutrients absorbed and minimize exposure to foreign chemicals and toxins, rendering it all the more vulnerable to the persisting attack by hepatotoxicants, culminating in liver dysfunctions. Hepatotoxicity may lead to various pathological changes like fatty liver, necrosis, steatosis, hepatitis, cholestasis, vascular lesions, and granuloma, veno-occlusive diseases and hepatocellular carcinoma, which further induce portal hypertension and hepatic failure. A multitude of risk factors for hepatotoxicity have been emphasized in India and majorly include exposure to environmental toxicants, natural toxicants, herbal remedies, therapeutic drugs, viral infection, alcohol intoxication, gender, age and genetic polymorphism in enzymes of xenobiotics metabolism.

Metabolism of drugs and chemicals largely takes place in the liver, accounting for the organ's vulnerability to metabolism-dependent hepatic injury. Over the decade's studies have been streamlined to uncover the pathological and biochemical mechanisms underlying hepatotoxicity along with biochemical alterations during liver injury against a different class of hepatotoxicants. However, earliest studies can be traced back to the assessment of industrial chemicals like petroleum products and hydrocarbons like benzene and n-octane, n-hexane for their hepatotoxicity potential. Earliest studies also revolved around understanding the role of CYP450 enzymes in different steps of detoxification process of DDT, providing evidence for reductive dechlorination to DDD or dehydrochlorination to DDE (Datta 1970, Zaidi and Banerjee 1987)

The balance between the activation and detoxification processes, and thus the ultimate toxicogenic potential of xenobiotics has shown to be dependent on the activities of drug metabolizing enzymes (DMEs) that help in the maintenance of homeostasis (Upadhyay, Kumar, et al. 2007, Upadhyay, Singh, et al. 2008). Any imbalances in the enzymes' activity may ultimately lead to the shifting of equilibrium towards free radical generation that could bind to macromolecules such as DNA and induce mutation, cause membrane damage in lipids or alter activities of protein (Upadhyay, Gupta, et al. 2010). In this regard, studies have been extended to elucidate the function and role of xenobiotics metabolizing enzymes (both Phase I and Phase II; cytochrome P450s, microsomal mixed-function oxidase MFO and GSTs) in the biotransformation of xenobiotics. Innumerable studies have documented the involvement of toxicant responsive genes, for example, CYP1A2, CYP2E1, glutathione-S-transferase, glutathione peroxidase and glutathione reductase in pyrogallol and rifampicin-induced hepatotoxicity (Upadhyay, Kumar, et al. 2007, Upadhyay, Singh, et al. 2008, Upadhyay, Gupta, et al. 2010).

The toxicity of different categories of pesticides has shown to be dependent on their metabolism, catalyzed via CYPs in the liver. Liver CYPs have also been shown to be responsive to transplacental induction via environmental chemicals and that their induction is transcriptionally regulated. Pre-natal exposure to pesticides like lindane and deltamethrin produced modifications in the ontogenic profile of CYPs in the liver in adulthood upon rechallenge suggesting their capacity to imprint CYP expression in the liver of the offsprings (Johri, Dhawan, et al. 2006, Johri, Dhawan, et al. 2007, Johri, Yadav, et al. 2007).

Many chemicals have also been documented to exert their adverse effects towards hepatic cells via interfering with critical steps of metabolism or their catalytic activities. These observations are of significant concern as the alteration in biotransformation ability may alter the response of animals to drugs and other xenobiotics. Formation of glutathione-S-conjugates by acrylamide, representing the first step in its biotransformation, may inhibit GST activity (Dixit, Husain, et al. 1981). Different categories of compounds including endotoxins (Dwivedi, Verma et al. 1989), cyclophosphamide (Dohadwala and Ray 1985), carbon tetrachloride (CCl$_4$) (Rastogi, Srivastava et al. 1997), benzanthrone (BA) (DAs, Garg, et al. 1994), hydrocarbons (n-Octane and n-Nonane) (Khan and Pandya 1980) have all been shown to depress hepatic cytochrome P-450 dependent mono-oxygenase system enzymes. Interaction of acrylamide with CYP and GST enzyme may lead to their inactivation that may inhibit detoxication of several electrophilic xenobiotics or their toxic metabolites (Dixit, Husain, et al. 1981, Das, Mukhtar, et al. 1982). Metabolic activation of BA may be responsible for P450 inactivation (which revealed a type I binding spectrum of P450 with an absorbance peak at 397 nm), which catalyzes at least one or more steps of metabolic activation of BA (Das, Garg, et al. 1991).

Hepatotoxicity has been shown to manifest from not only the direct interaction of the primary compound but also from a metabolite that is reactive or an immune-mediated response adversely affecting hepatocytes, biliary epithelial cells and/or the architectural integrity of the liver. Biotransformation of exogenous compounds (by Phase I and Phase II reactions) has been demonstrated to potentially alter the properties of the hepatotoxicant via metabolic activation that may further augment its toxicity. Example, hepatotoxicity of the well established CCl_4, is majorly because of its degraded metabolites, trichloromethyl (CCl_3) and trichloromethyl peroxyl (CCl_3O_2) produced via hepatic microsomal enzyme (CYP2E1) (Nada, Omara et al. 2010). These metabolites being unstable radicals exhibit a strong affinity towards binding to lipids and protein of the cell membrane or abstracting a hydrogen atom from an unsaturated lipid, resulting in LPO generation and liver damage (Debnath, Ghosh, et al. 2013). Metanil yellow, a widely employed food color, undergoes an azo reduction in metabolic acid and p-aminodiphenylamine (Srivastava, Khanna, et al. 1982). The latter has revealed strong binding affinity towards the liver (Khanna, Tewari, et al. 1987) and is more toxic than the parent dye, metanil yellow (Khanna 1991).

The pathogenesis of hepatotoxicity mediated via reactive metabolites has been a focus of research enthusiasm. The generation of reactive intermediates has been reported to be a common process in liver damage after exposure to several agents such as hepatotoxic drugs, chemicals, and solvents. Rifampicin is a potent inducer of cytochrome P450 and elevates the covalent binding of reactive metabolites of acetyl hydrazine to the macromolecules of hepatocytes resulting in liver cell damage (Sinha 1987). Moreover, desacetylrifampicin, another reactive metabolite of rifampicin, also exerts its toxic effects by modulating the membrane permeability and causing membrane damage (Rana, Attri, et al. 2006). Its prolonged exposure drastically reduces glucose-6-phosphatase activity, which could result in higher LPO (Saraswathy and Shyamala Devi 2001).

Over the years, chemical agents such as laboratory chemicals (e.g., carbon tetrachloride), drugs (pyrogallol, paracetamol), industrial chemicals (e.g., metals and pesticides), food coloring agents, petroleum products, etc. have all been identified as potent hepatotoxicants. Carbon tetrachloride, paracetamol and alcohol induced liver damage has been lengthily used as an experimental model, to study hepatotoxicity in acute and chronic liver failure to dissect the underlying mechanisms. The various classes of hepatotoxicants have been shown to cause injury via different mechanisms like cytochrome P450 activation, LPO, higher ROS or oxidative stress, increase in the level of inflammatory markers, induction of nitric acid synthase, mitochondrial dysfunction and bile acid-induced liver cell death. Few of the representative studies have been mentioned in Table 10.4.

Table 10.4 Few representative studies undertaken on the hepatotoxicity potential of different drugs/chemicals/xenobiotics

Hepatotoxicants	Effects/Mechansim of action	Model and Route of Administration	References
Miscellaneous			
Petroleum products (Benzene, carbon tetrachloride (2 ml/kg b.wt./day), gasoline, petroleum ether/IOMEX (3 ml/kg b.wt.)/day, 3 days	The alkaline phosphatase activity of the liver was increased in all the groups, only a slight decrease in glucose- 6-phosphatase activity	Albino rats, Intraperitoneal	(Rao and Pandya 1978)
N-hexane and n-heptane (1 ml/kg b.wt/day), 2 and 7 days and twice a week for 45 days	Degenerative alterations, higher necrosis, loss in architectural integrity due to n-hexane, in n-heptane the capsule was increasingly thickened and infiltrated with lymphocytes, higher activity of alkaline phosphatase and lower activity of FDP aldolase, lower activity of serum cholinesterase activity and decreased content of albumin and cholesterol	Albino rats, Intraperitoneal	(Goel, Rao, et al. 1982)
Argemone alkaloids (5 ml/kg b.wt.)/day, 3 days	Elevation in both NADPH-supported enzymatic and non-enzymatic LPO in whole homogenate, mitochondria, and microsomes, increased vulnerability of mitochondrial membrane to peroxidative attack	Subcellular fractions of rat liver	(Upreti, Das, et al. 1988)
Metanil Yellow, Orange II (80 mg/kg b.wt./day), 3 days	Elevation in the activities of ethoxyresorufin-*O*-deethylase (40–190%), aniline hydroxylase (27–92%), aryl hydrocarbon hydroxylase (50–62%) and aminopyrine *N*-demethylase (42–49%), higher activities of cytosolic quinone reductase (34–82%) and glutathione *S*-transferase (23–43%) and reduction in glutathione levels with an increase in LPO, mixture (1:1) of Metanil yellow and Orange II revealed a synergistic or additive effect on these hepatic parameters	Albino rats, Intraperitoneal	(Ramchandani, Das, et al. 1994)

Contd...

Hepatotoxicants	Effects/Mechansim of action	Model and Route of Administration	References
CO seeds (0.5%-2%)	Oxidative stress, carbohydrate metabolism, xenobiotic metabolism, cell cycle, apoptosis at 0.5%, reduction of glutathione, LPO generation, alteration of antioxidant enzymes, lower levels of Phase 1 (EROD, MROD and PROD) and Phase 2 (QR and GST) enzymes	Wistar rats, Oral	(Panigrahi, Yadav, et al. 2014)
High glucose (50 mM), 72 h	Presence of detached and shrunken rounded cells, increased oxidative stress as revealed by higher ROS levels, LPO, formation of protein carbonyl and 3-nitrotyrosine adduct, higher intracellular antioxidant glutathione	HepG2 cell line	(Chandra-sekaran, Swaminathan, et al. 2010)
Ferric Nitrilotriacetate (Fe-NTA) (3 and 9 mg/kg b.wt.), 3, 6, 12, 24 and 48 h	Levels of GSH lowered, decrease in the activities of glutathione $-transferase, glutathione reductase, glucose 6-phosphate dehydrogenase and glutathione peroxidase, dose dependently manner, max at 12 h, enhanced the production of H_2O_2 and increased hepatic lipid peroxidation, increased transaminases	Wistar rats, Intraperitoneal	(Iqbal, Sharma, et al. 1996)
Metals			
Arsenic	Noncirrhotic portal fibrosis	Human	(Datta, Mitra, et al. 1979)
Arsenic	Out of a population of 7683 surveyed, 3467 and 4216 people consumed water which contained arsenic below and above 0.05 mg/L, respectively, hepatomegaly was found to be comparatively higher in exposed people	Human	(Guha Mazumder 2003)
Arsenic (50, 100, and 150 µg/day), 6 days a week for 3, 6, 9 and 12 months	Higher LPO and protein oxidation associated with reduced hepatic thiols (GSH, PSH), and antioxidant enzymes (GPx, Catalase), increased hepatic collagen 9 and 12 months in all the groups associated with increased in TNF-α and IL-6	BALB/c mice, Oral	(Das, Santra, et al. 2005)

Contd...

Hepatotoxicants	Effects/Mechansim of action	Model and Route of Administration	References
Cadmium (2.5 mg/kg b.wt.)/day, 6 days	Time dependent increase in cadmium tissue levels, Most of the biochemical parameters (DNA, RNA, total protein, cytochrome P450 contents, alkaline phosphatase and UDP glucuronyl transferase activities), haematological parameters (total red blood cells, total white blood cell, differential white blood cell counts, haemoglobin, serum glutamic oxaloacetic transaminase,erythrocyte sedimentation rate, serum glutamic pyruvic transaminase, plasma protein) revealed either no or less changes on the 7th day, a minimum of 21 day-exposure was required to modify the cellular architecture	Balb/c mice, Subcutaneous	(Karmakar, Bhattacharya, et al. 2000)
Chromium 3.125, 6.25, 12.5, 25, or 50 μM for 24 h	Mitochondrial damage, apoptosis, oxidative stress, and subsequently lead to a strong induction of HO1, GCLC and SOD2 via the Nrf-2 signaling pathway in hepatocytes	HepG2 cell line	(Das, Sarkar, et al. 2015)
	Pesticides		
Deltamethrin (2.56 mg/kg b.wt. and 5.12 mg/kg b.wt.)/day, 7 days	Dose-dependent dissemination of deltamethrin and its main metabolite (3-Phenoxy benzoic acid) in rat plasma, 6 liver emanated acute phase proteins (Apolipoprotein E, Apolipoprotein-AIV, Hemopexin, Haptoglobin, Vitamin D Binding protein, and Fibrinogen gamma chain) were modulated in a dose-dependent manner, toxic effects on body growth (body weight and relative organ weight), serum profile, liver functions and histology, inflammatory alterations (increased TNF-α, TGF-β and IL6 level), and oxidative stress	Wistar rats, Oral	(Arora, Siddiqui, et al. 2016)
Deltamethrin (2.56 mg/kg b.wt. and 5.12 mg/kg b.wt.)/ day, 7 days	Induced cell death was accompanied with increased ROS generation, 38 decreased mitochondrial membrane potential and G2/M arrest, resulted in a caspase-independent but non-apoptotic cell death, incites membrane disintegrity 46 and	Primary rat hepatocytes Oral	(Arora, Siddiqui, et al. 2016)

Contd...

Hepatotoxicants	Effects/Mechansim of action	Model and Route of Administration	References
	necrotic damage, increased expression 47 of inflammatory markers (TNFα, NFκB, iNOS, COX-2)		
Maneb (15 mg/kg b.wt.) **and paraquat** (5 mg/kg b.wt.), twice/week, 1, 3 and 6 weeks	Significant increase in LPO and lowered GSH content, expression and catalytic activity of CYP2E1 and GSTA4-4 were drastically elevated	Hepatic microsomes from Wistar rats (Intraperitoneal)	(Ahmad, Shukla, et al. 2010)
Fenvalerate (6500 mg/m^3, 3500 mg/m^3 and 2200 mg/m^3), 4 h/day, 5 days a week), 3 months	Hepatomegaly, increased activities of serum clinical enzymes (indicative of liver damage/dysfunction) along with pronounced histopathological damage of liver	Wistar rats, Inhalation	(Mani, Prasad, et al. 2004)
Drugs			
Isoniazid+Rifampicin (25 mg/kg b.wt. each), 11 days	Increased phospholipids in the plasma from day 5-day 11, decreased total inorganic phosphorous, cardiolipin (CL), phosphatidylcholine (PC), with elevated phosphatidylethanolamine (PE) and phosphatitylserine (PS) subfractions of phospholipids in the liver tissue	Rabbits, Intraperitoneal	(Karthikeyan 2005)
Isoniazid (50 mg/kg b.wt./day) and **Rifampicin** (100 mg/kg b.wt./day), 3 days	Co-exposure caused steatosis and increased apoptosis of the hepatocytes, hepatic oxidative stress, particularly in the mitochondrial fraction with increased mitochondrial permeability transition	Balb/c mice, Gastric intubation	(Chowdhury, Santra, et al. 2006)
Isoniazid (6.5, 13, 26, and 52 mM)	Depletion of cellular glutathione (GSH) content along with increased production of ROS mediated apoptosis	HepG2 cell line	(Bhadauria, Mishra, et al. 2010)
Isoniazid (INH) (50–200 mM), **Pyrazinamide** (PYZ) (50–200 mM), **combination drugs INH:Rifampicin (RIF)** (50 µM:200 mM) and **INH:PYZ** (100: 100 mM), 24h	Pre-exposure with non-toxic concentration of INH (5 mM), RIF (50 mM), PYZ (5 mM) for 24 h followed by respective exposures resulted in typical cubic to round shape of cells, revealed swollen morphology with membrane blebbing and necrosis	HepG2 cell line	(Singh, Sasi, et al. 2011)

Contd...

Hepatotoxicants	Effects/Mechansim of action	Model and Route of Administration	References
Paracetemol (375 and 750 mg/kg b.wt.), 24 h	Paracetamol exposure caused decrease in body weights without any alterations in the liver protein contents, however, toxic doses casued 21% reduction in the yield of mitochondrial proteins	Wistar rats, Intraperitoneal	(Katyare and Satav 1989)
Paracetemol (650 mg/kg bw.t.), 24 h	Reduction in hepatic ATP content, decreased respiratory activity, modification in respiratory enzyme complexes dysfunction in mitochondrial energy-linked functions	Rat hepatic mitochondria	(Ahmed, Khandkar, et al. 1995)
Rifampin and Isoniazid	Acute hepatitis A and B	Children	(Kumar, Misra, et al. 1991)
Rifampicin (20 mg/kg b.wt).+**Pyrogallol** (40 mg/kg b.wt.),1, 2, 3 and 4 week	Higher expression and activity of CYP1A2 and CYP2E1 and LPO levels, reduction in the activities of glutathione reductase, glutathione-S-transferase, and glutathione peroxidase	Albino mice, Intraperitoneal	(Upadhyay, Kumar, et al. 2007)
n-hexane, n-heptane (1ml/kg b.wt.), 1, 2, 7 and 45 days	Protein content in the liver reduced with n-heptane and total sulphydryl content revealed a drastic reduction in the rats exposed to either solvent, higher LPO after 24 h and 48 h exposure to n-hexane or n-heptane, reduction in drug metabolizing activity, decrease in hepatic glucose-6-phosphatase	Albino rats, Intraperitoneal	(Goel, Rao, et al. 1988)
Acrylamide (100 mg/kg b.wt.), 2 and 4 h	Reduction in contents of hepatic glutathione, lowered activities of aryl hydrocarbon hydroxylase and glutathione s-transferase	Albino mice, Topical	(Mukhtar, Dixit, et al. 1981)
Benzathrone (40 mg/kg body weight) for 3, 7, or 21 days	Decrease in ascorbic acid, content of cytochrome P-450 and phase I enzymes, addition of benzanthrone to hepatic microsomes led to spectral alterations characterized by an absorbance maximum at 397 nm (type I binding)	Wistar rats, Parenteral	(Das, Garg, et al. 1991)
Benzathrone (BA)3-bromobenzanthrone (3-BBA) (50 mg/kg b.wt./day), 10 days	Both BA and 3-BBA disrupted membrane integrity by reducing levels of endogenous glutathione and ascorbic acid and higher LPO, may lead to disruptions in hepatic P-450-dependent monooxygenase and	Guinea pigs, Oral	(Singh, Khanna, et al. 2003)

Contd...

Hepatotoxicants	Effects/Mechansim of action	Model and Route of Administration	References
	oxidative stress, 3-BBA exposure caused portal triad dilation with arterial wall thickening, hyperplasia of Kupffer cells and an influx of inflammatory cells between hepatic cords		
Cyanobacterium **Microcystis** **aeruginosa** (PCC 7806, 15.8 and 31.6 mg/kg b.wt.)	Dose dependent DNA damage and increase in liver-specific enzymes viz. plasma alkaline phosphatase, gamma-glutamyl transferase, lactate dehydrogenase, decrease in hepatic glutamic pyruvic transaminase, corresponding increase in liver body weight index and histopathological changes in liver (degeneration of hepatocytes, congestion and hemorrhage etc.)	Wistar rats, Intraperitoneal	(Rao and Bhattacharya, 1996)

Drug-Induced Hepatotoxicity (DIH), the most frequent cause of hepatic dysfunction in India, and the major reason for attrition in drug development has continued to fascinate and challenge the toxicologists (Sharma, Singla, et al. 2010). DIH extends to the entire spectrum which ranges from increased transaminases to jaundice, life-threatening acute hepatic failure to even chronic liver diseases (Devarbhavi 2012). In India antituberculosis drugs (58%) given for active disease are still a major reason for drug-induced hepatic injury followed by antiepileptic drugs (11%) (Devarbhavi 2011) Kumar, Bhatia, et al. 2010). Some medications (anti-tuberculosis, anti-retroviral) have been deeply studied in humans and animals to assess the molecular mechanisms of DIH and Isoniazid (INH), rifampicin (RMP), pyrazinamide (PZA) are the most common drugs used as components of such regimens, and all of them are potentially hepatotoxic. Both rifampicin and pyrogallol (anti-psoriasis medicine) have also been shown to induce hepatic damage, release of few serum protein biomarkers, oxidative stress, and disrupted permeability transition in the mitochondria (Gupta, Sharma, et al. 2002, Gupta, Sharma, et al. 2004, Chowdhury, Santra, et al. 2006, Rana, Attri, et al. 2006).

Currently, a combination therapy, consisting of INH, RIF and PYZ, is most commonly employed as the first line of treatment against tuberculosis. Enormous literature is available on INZ, RIF PYZ and their combinations in humans and experimental animals. Studies also suggest that the byproducts/metabolites such as hydrazine formed from isoniazid could further predispose to the development of DIH (Sarma, Immanuel, et al. 1986). The rate of hepatotoxic reactions has been comparatively more in the Indian patients as that documented in developed countries (Ramachandran 1980); with an incidence of 8-50% during rifampin and isoniazid therapy varying in different studies (Rao, Wadia, et al. 1982, Parthasarathy, Sarma, et al. 1986) and women (42%) being generally considered more at risk for DILI (Devarbhavi 2011).

Similarly, active anti-retroviral therapy (HAART), has been the cornerstone of management of patients with HIV/AIDS infection, but there has been an increasing prevalence of liver function abnormalities with a co-infection with Hepatitis B virus, Hepatitis C virus and Hepatitis E virus (Sarda, Sharma, et al. 2009, Shamanna, Naik, et al. 2016). Chronic viral hepatitis, DIH, non-alcoholic fatty liver disorder, and several opportunistic infections are the most common hepatic diseases observed in HIV-infected individuals (Rathi, Amarapurkar, et al. 1997, Puri and Kumar 2016, Puri, Sharma, et al. 2017).

There have been no conventional road maps for treating and managing TB in relation to the severity of the hepatic damage. Identification of risk factors involved in DIH has been deemed necessary as no particular treatment exists for preventing or treating hepatotoxicity. Considering such a high risk of hepatotoxic reactions in the Indian population, studies have been carried out towards a critical evaluation of various predisposing clinical and immunogenetic factors for developing DIH. This propensity is an indirect evidence supporting the idea which comes from hypoalbuminemia, a surrogate marker for malnutrition, which has been observed in patients with antituberculous DIH (Sharma, Singla, et al. 2010, Singla, Sharma, et al. 2010).

Genetic polymorphisms are thought to influence the chemical modification of drugs and its metabolites in the liver, and thus might predispose an individual to, or protect against hepatotoxicity. The impact of genetic polymorphism of proteins and enzymes associated with drug metabolism (such as CYP and GST M1 and T1 genetic polymorphism) in the modulation of DIH has been extensively studied. Individuals who have a slow acetylator status have a higher incidence and severity of INH-induced hepatitis. A recent study from New-Delhi, India revealed a slow acetylator status in 71% of their patients with TB DIH as compared to 45% without DIH. Some have found a link between CYP 2E1 genetic polymorphism and GST M1 and T1 "null" mutation with hepatotoxicity to the antituberculous drug (Roy, Chowdhury, et al. 2001, Bose, Sarma, et al. 2011). Polymorphisms at GSTM1, GSTT1, CYP, miRNA and NAT2 loci had been linked to various forms of liver injury due to drugs including hepatocellular carcinoma (Roy, Chowdhury, et al. 2001, Singh, Lata, et al. 2019, Singh, Jadhav, et al. 2019, Yadav, Kumar, et al. 2019). In complex diseases, where several variant loci contribute to the risk of disease, instead of only single-locus polymorphisms, haplotypes are more critical as differential combinations of alleles in the genes may have differential effects on the gene expression. Gene-gene interactions in the risk alleles of GST family have been observed to alter the risk to Anti Retro Viral (ARV)-associated hepatotoxicity in HIV-infected individuals. Singh, et al. 2017 have revealed additive effects of GSTM1-null and GSTT1-null in eliciting greater risk of hepatotoxicity in HIV-infected individuals by a probable reduction in cellular detoxification and higher production of metabolites in the liver which may predispose an individual to more toxic effects (Singh, Lata, et al. 2017).

Similarly, the enzymes belonging to the families CYP1, CYP2, and CYP3 catalyze biotransformation of xenobiotic, including 90% of clinically used drugs. Evidence suggested that differences in CYP enzymes metabolic capacities leads to interindividual variability in therapeutic response to medication. Singh, et al 2017 have critically evaluated the role of gene-gene/gene-environment interactions associated with metabolic susceptibility genes and established that the individuals with carriage genotype 3801CC and heterozygous 3801CT genotypes of CYP1A1m1 gene may have higher chance to develop ARV-associated hepatotoxicity, its severity, and advancement of disease independently and in the presence of environmental factors like alcohol and nevirapine regimen (Singh, Lata et al. 2017). Such studies on both phases of enzyme gene polymorphism may aid in screening the vulnerable HIV-infected population for hepatotoxicity, thus preventing chronic hepatic damage. Genotyping of inter-individual variability at the CYP and GST locus as a diagnostic tool for predicting ARV DIH and other side effects has been emerging as an additional possibility and will not only enable the determination of the suitable dosage for individual patients but also help in decreasing unnecessary outpatient visits and hospitalizations.

Convincing evidence has been presented for the association of immunogenetic factors in the development of hepatotoxicity due to antituberculosis drugs wherein the absence of HLADQA1* and presence of HLA-DQB1*0201 may be associated with the development of hepatotoxicity (Sharma, Balamurugan et al. 2002). Anti-TB DIH has been associated with a mortality of 6%–12% if the drugs are continued after the onset of symptoms. Reintroduction of anti-TB drugs following anti-TB DIH has never been studied systematically. Different predefined regimens of the re-introduction of anti-TB medicines in patients with DIH concerning safety and risk of recurrence of hepatotoxicity has been studied that could help in reducing the risk of hepatotoxicity (Sharma, Singla, et al. 2010). Similarly, research groups have explored the efficacy and safety of an ofloxacin-based antitubercular therapy for treating tuberculosis in patients with chronic liver disease. As rifampicin is known to potentiate the hepatotoxicity of isoniazid, it is postulated that an effective but safe drug substitute would be more ideal as a treatment in this subgroup of patients. In this regard, the isoniazid, pyrazinamide, and ofloxacin combination has been found to be a safer treatment in such susceptible groups (Saigal, Agarwal, et al. 2001).

Chronic heavy alcohol consumption in India has resulted in adverse health effects, including alcoholic liver diseases (Pari and Karthikesan 2007). Fatty liver disease, portal hypertension, alcoholic hepatitis with elevated transaminases and alcoholic cirrhosis have been few of its manifestations with various withdrawal symptoms most common being insomnia (37.3%) and tremors (23.3%) (Sarin, Sachdev, et al. 1988, Virukalpattigopalratnam, Singh, et al. 2013). Studies have revealed that CYP2E1 polymorphism, leading to ROS generation, has been associated with higher susceptibility to alcoholic cirrhosis (Khan, Ruwali, et al. 2009). Interaction of GSTs (GSTM1, GSTT1 (null) and GSTP1) with variant genotype of cytochrome P450 2E1 (that generates free radicals) and manganese superoxide dismutase (that detoxifies free radicals), are potential risk factors to alcoholic liver cirrhosis further demonstrating the critical role of gene-gene interactions in altering the risk to alcoholic liver cirrhosis (Khan, Choudhuri, et al. 2009). Similarly, another study reports the pivotal role of interactions among genes that are involved in metabolizing alcohol and in the generation and detoxification of free radicals with susceptibility to alcoholic liver cirrhosis. A greater risk to alcoholic liver cirrhosis has been reported in patients who carry a combination of wild genotypes of ADH1C (ADH1C*1/*1) and variant genotype of ADH1B (ADH1B*2/*2) or CYP2E1 (CYP2E1*5B) or null genotype of GSTM1 (Khan, Husain, et al. 2010).

Studies have been undertaken to correlate the utility of new clinical parameters (prior to investigations like biopsy and sonography) as a diagnostic indicator in liver functionality for differential diagnosis of alcoholic liver cirrhosis. De Ritis ratio (AST/ALT) activity of Gamma Glutamyl Transferase and Total Sialic Acid (TSA) etc. have been suggested that offer added advantages over conventional biomarkers to diagnose alcohol liver cirrhosis (https://www.ripublication.com/ijbb16/ijbbv12n2_11.pdf). CYP2E1 mRNA expression and levels of protein in the blood lymphocytes, derived from early stage alcoholic liver cirrhotic patients, can be utilized for prediction of alcohol-induced toxicity (Khan, Sharma, et al. 2011).

Randomized trials have identified drugs like Pentoxifylline for severe alcoholic hepatitis (SAH) which has shown improvement in renal and hepatic functions and reduction in short term mortality (De, Gangopadhyay, et al. 2009, Sidhu, Goyal, et al. 2012). Granulocyte-colony stimulating factor has been demonstrated to be effective and safe in the mobilization of hematopoietic stem cells, improving liver functioning and survival in patients with alcoholic hepatitis (Singh, Sharma, et al. 2014). A recent study has provided strong evidence for the potential of urinary metabolome signatures to accurately predict steroid response in patients with SAH before beginning the corticosteroids therapy. From 212 signatures that were detected in the cohort, 9 urinary metabolites associated with mitochondrial functionality have been identified and found to differentiate nonresponders to the corticosteroid treatment from responders significantly. Among these, acetyl-L-carnitine was capable of strongly predicting nonresponse and mortality in SAH with levels of >2,500 ng/mL, accurately discriminating survivors from nonsurvivors. Moreover, these metabolites closely correlated with the transcriptomic data, indicating a direct association between regulation of immune-related genes in PBMCs, metabolic genes in the liver and urine metabolic profiles in the same patients. These findings could form the basis for developing an economical dipstick screening test for limiting the steroid use in patients who have a reasonable likelihood of responding. Such a urine test could provide a practical assessment for delineating metabolic alterations, predicting mortality, and personalizing treatment approaches (Maras, Das, et al. 2018).

Apart from therapeutic and intentional exposure (alcohol), accidental consumption of toxic food may also confer risk of hepatotoxicity. This has been best exemplified by the cases of accidental poisoning of *Cassia occidentalis* (CO) seeds, which are known to contribute to hepatomyoencephalopathy (HME) in many parts of India (Vashishtha, Kumar, et al. 2007, Panigrahi, Tiwari, et al. 2014). Anthraquinones (AQs) of the *Cassia occidentalis* (CO) seeds like Rhein, Emodin, Aloe-emodin, Chrysophanol, Physcion have been identified to contribute to the etiology of HME in children (Panigrahi, Ch et al. 2015). These AQs have been detected in the serum and urine of HME patients and also in the exposed rats, linking their role in the CO seeds' toxicity. Among the above five AQs, maximum concentration of Rhein has been found in the serum, exhibiting the highest toxicity (as seen *in vitro*) and the highest affinity for protein binding as compared with other AQs clearly suggesting that Rhein is one of the major contributing factors in CO poisoning (Panigrahi, Ch et al. 2015). Studies have predicted the involvement of several pathways and associated biomolecules in CO-induced hepatotoxicity and the data may aid in the formulation of therapeutic strategies against suspected CO poisoning study cases. Involvement of oxidative stress and impairment in xenobiotic metabolism as a putative mechanism of toxicity has also been suggested (Panigrahi, Yadav, et al. 2014).

Epidemic dropsy, the food adulterant disease due to the consumption of mustard oil that is adulterated with argemone oil (AO) is quite prevalent in India (Das and Khanna 1997). Interaction of sanguinarine alkaloid which is isolated from argemone oil, with the metabolizing enzymes to understand its biotransformation and elimination has been subject to intense investigation. One of the major predetermining factors of toxicity for any compound is its retention and excretion profile in the body (DeBethizy and Hayes 1994) and SAN has been shown to eliminate from the body of rats and guinea pigs, with one of its metabolite appearing in urine post 96 h of oral administration (Tandon, Das et al. 1993). Studies have investigated the involvement of xenobiotic metabolizing enzymes in SAN metabolism, which may modify its clearance from the body vis-a-vis toxicity. It has been well documented that SAN alters some major CYP isoforms levels, causes reduction in hepatic microsomal P450 (CYP1A, 1A2, 2D1, 2E1, 3A1) and activities of phase II enzymes such as glutathione-s-transferases and even disruption of CYP activity which augments its toxicity (Upreti, Das et al. 1988, Upreti, Das et al. 1991, Eruvaram and Das 2009) The damage of hepatic microsomal membrane causes depletion of cytochrome P-450 and membrane-bound enzymes, thereby leading to delay of SAN excretion (Upreti, Das, et al. 1991, Tandon, Das, et al. 1993). More detailed studies have hinted at SAN competing with carbon monoxide to bind with the sixth ligand, heme of P450, for the formation of an enzyme-substrate complex by evaluation of binding spectra (Reddy and Das 2008).

Hepatic damage has been broadly assessed by a critical examination of biochemical 'patterns' prior to confirmation by histopathology. In view of complexity and multiplicity of liver functions, no single test could possibly establish the alterations in the liver function. Thus, an array of function tests have been utilized for its effective diagnosis, to estimate the severity of the damage, make prognosis and evaluate therapeutic strategies. Monitoring of serum hepatic leakage enzymes including alanine aminotransferase (ALT, formerly SGPT), aspartate aminotransferase (AST, formerly SGOT), sorbitol dehydrogenase (SDH) and glutamate dehydrogenase (GLDH) and changes in the blood chemistry, e.g., decreased cholinesterase and elevated serum phosphatase, have been routinely employed. Developments in molecular biology, have broadened our horizon on the understanding of toxicant-induced liver damage. With the development of novel techniques such as genomics and proteomics, there has been a growing enthusiasm to create "novel" predictive markers to detect hepatotoxicity that have enabled interpretation of the mechanism based on distinct gene expression changes. Gene expression profiling has led to the identification of differential gene patterns that may be potential biomarkers of anti-malaria therapy. It has been shown that combinatorial therapies in anti-malaria regimes result in more damages than the monotherapies (Noel, Sharma, et al. 2007, Noel, Sharma, et al. 2008). Moreover, microarray studies further suggest that current anti-malarial therapies induce inflammation and disrupted signals resulting in hepatic stress as observed via levels of expression of EPRS, SVIL, PAWR, and MTMR2 which can serve as efficient markers for anti-malarial DIH (Mishra, Singh et al. 2011).

Differential mRNA transcription profiles have deciphered involvement of various molecular events in pyrogallol-mediated hepatotoxicity. Comparative transcription pattern showed an alteration in the expression of 183 transcripts (150 up-regulated and 33 down-regulated) associated with oxidative stress, cell cycle, cytoskeletal network, cell-cell adhesion, extracellular matrix, inflammation, apoptosis, cell-signaling and intermediary metabolism in the pyrogallol-exposed liver (Upadhyay, Gupta, et al. 2010). Comprehensive approach of proteome profiling along with conventional toxico-physiological correlation analysis has enabled identification of six liver emanated plasma proteins (namely Hemopexin, Apolipoprotein A-IV, Apolipoprotein E, Haptoglobin, Fibrogen gamma chain and Vitamin D binding protein) as 'early fingerprints of toxicity' that could be employed to assess the early deltamethrin-induced hepatotoxicity in nontarget species with a minimal invasive mean. The identified target proteins are inherently coupled to various biological functions such as inflammation, immune response, antioxidant defense and oxidative stress that represent an unbiased portrait of altered liver homeostasis (Arora, Siddiqui, et al. 2016).

NMR based serum metabolic profiling have also offered mechanistic insights into erythromycin drug-induced metabolic perturbations in amino acid metabolism, energy metabolism, lipid metabolism and compromised ability of the affected liver to maintain metabolic homeostasis (Rawat, Dubey et al. 2016). Metabolomics approach has also enabled discrimination in toxicity index of pyrazinamide (PYZ) and its metabolites. It has been shown that PYZ itself is not directly responsible for hepatotoxicity; however, two of its metabolites viz. pyrazinoic acid (PA) and 5-hydroxy pyrazinoic acid (5-OHPA) are the main cause for the DIH, of which 5-OHPA has been documented to be more toxic resulting in energy deficit, inflammation, oxidative stress and muscle degradation due to hypolipidemia related with liver injury (Rawat, Chaturvedi et al. 2018). As NMR based metabolic profiling is relatively simple and rapid, therefore, the resulted NMR based serum metabolic patterns could form the basis for future preclinical studies aimed at evaluating the hepatotoxicity of a new drug regimens or as a primary screening tool to assess the therapeutic efficacy of anti-hepatotoxic agents/formulations.

Different model systems have been employed to not only study the effect of hepatotoxicants but also look for therapeutic regimes. Both small and large animals have been reliable for studying the hepatotoxicants' effects, distribution and clearance. Studies with liver microsomes have provided an affordable way to give a good indication of the CYP metabolic profile in response to various xenobiotics. Precision-cut liver slices have been the oldest hepatotoxicity models as the histology is intact, all the cells with the zonal distribution of cytochromes can be easily seen. Infact liver slices were one of the first *in vitro* models utilized in toxicity testing in India dating back to 1960s. A study showed that the liver slice model could also be successfully utilized for screening of a large number of laboratory cultures and bloom samples of cyanobacterial species for their potential hepatotoxicity. The system was sensitive enough to even detect microgram levels of toxins and any species generating 50% cytosolic LDH leakage could be positively considered as a toxic strain (Bhattacharya, Lakshmana Rao, et al. 1996).

In-vitro techniques have substantially progressed and a battery of impressive improvised models and protocols have come into the picture. Primary cultures of rat hepatocytes and immortalized cell lines all represent useful tools for assessing hepatotoxicity, metabolism of drugs and induction of liver enzymes. Apart from using whole animals and established hepatic cell lines and primary cultures, there has been a constant endeavor to develop new *in vitro* models. Various protocols have also been standardized for efficient generation of 3D spheroids from the mouse as well as human stem cells by fabricating a variety of scaffolds. It has been shown that hepatic cells (Hep G2) when seeded in the presence of 0.03% poly (N-isopropylacrylamide) (pNIPAAm) formed organoids that were much superior from their 2D and 3D *in-vitro* counterparts in exhibiting much better morphology, cytochrome CYP1A1, CYP2A6 activities and albumin secretion profiles and could successfully show dose-dependent and reproducible responses to drugs such as tamoxifen (Sarkar and Kumar 2016). Similarly, poly (L-lactic acid)-co-poly(3-caprolactone)/collagen nanofibrous scaffolds augment trans-differentiation of hMSCs towards functional hepatosphere formation with greater efficacy. Such an *in vitro* bioengineered hepatic construct might be a potential tool for future applications in hepatotoxicity testing (Bishi, Mathapati, et al. 2013).

Kulkarni and Khanna, et al. 2006 have generated high percentage of hepatocyte-like functional cells from mouse embryonic stem cells that not only showed hepatocyte-like morphology but also expressed hepatic specific genes with evidence of glycogen storage as well (Kulkarni and Khanna 2006). The research group demonstrated their utility as a suitable adjunct for *in vitro* drug metabolism and screening of hepatotoxicity by employing a well-known hepatotoxicant, carbon tetrachloride (CCl4), that revealed an increase in liver function enzymes SGPT, SGOT, ALP and LDH associated with acute liver damage thus indicating the capacity of these differentiated hepatocyte-like cells as a suitable alternative experimental system for *in vitro* drug metabolism and hepatotoxicity screening of potential drug candidates.

3D organoid culture models are also being utilized to closely mimic the *in-vivo* like organ physiology *in-vitro* and have met with success. Towards this end, hepatospheroids differentiated from human-umbilical-cord-mesenchymal stem cells (hUC-MSCs) on 3D scaffold GEVAC (Gelatin-vinyl-acetate-copolymer) as suitable *in vitro* system for assessing drug toxicity/metabolism have received much attention. These 3D biodegradable scaffolds, which supported proliferation and hepatic differentiation of hUCMSCs, employing exogenous growth factors generated metabolically active hepatospheroids of 50–80 μm. These hUC-MSCs derived hepatospheroids demonstrated better morphology and metabolic activity, including production of urea, secretion of albumin and metabolically active CYPs, employing standard LC/MS analysis approved by the FDA. These hepatospheroids efficiently responded to model inducers, namely AhR agonist omeprazole, CAR- and PXR- agonist rifampicin and revealed induction potential similar to that of HepG2 and more than hepatocyte-like cells, representing a convenient, and reproducible alternate *in vitro* system for routine hepatotoxicity testing and drug metabolism studies (Chitrangi, Nair, et al. 2017).

Due to hepatotoxicity concerns, there are no dose–response studies in children. To address this, Srivastava, et al. 2016 have developed a hollow fiber system model of disseminated intracellular tuberculosis with co-perfused 3D organotypic liver modules using HepG2 cells for pediatric dose-response studies to estimate both efficiency and toxicity simultaneously. Utilizing pediatric pharmacokinetics of pyrazinamide and acetaminophen and algorithms to determine dose-dependent pyrazinamide efficiency and hepatotoxicity, the research group has demonstrated that pyrazinamide may not give good predictive clinical outcomes in children ≤ 6 years with extrapulmonary tuberculosis. The *in-vitro* model could be utilized for identification of such new regimens which could potentially accelerate the treatment while minimizing the toxicity (Srivastava, Pasipanodya, et al. 2016).

Such as extensive database on the hepatotoxicity potential of different compounds has also accelerated the pursuit of identification of safer and better therapeutic agents. In the traditional health system, herbal treatment for a liver disorder is claimed to be most reliable and effective. In India, several medicinal plants and their formulations, such as *Solanum nigrum*, *Aegle marmelos*, and *Ficus carica* have been employed for curing hepatic disorders in traditional medicine (Saleem, Chetty, et al. 2010). Since 1950s herbal formulations, such as Liv.52 has elicited protective effects against liver injury in both clinical settings and experimental studies (Sheth, Northover, et al. 1960). Research groups have remained in the forefront in screening out various plants and their extracts that show hepatoprotective potential using different chemical/drug models of hepatotoxicity (Table 10.5). CCl_4, paracetamol, pyrogallol and tuberculosis drugs have been extensively employed as hepatotoxicants to screen out formulations for their hepatoprotective efficacy.

A lot of research interest has been fuelled on the search of herbal antioxidants for hepatoprotection. Natural products rich in flavonoids, triterpenes, polyphenols and other plant extracts, have been identified as powerful hepatoprotective agents in experimental liver-injury models (Palanivel, Rajkapoor et al. 2008, Parmar, Vashrambhai et al. 2010, Rao, Rawat et al. 2012, Sharma, Sangameswaran et al. 2012, Singh, Singh et al. 2012). The basis of protection conferred by these natural products is considered to be their antioxidant nature through which they provide protection against ROS induced damage to membrane lipids and macromolecules. Moreover, their protective capacity has also been attributed to their interaction with several CYP isoforms, their potential to elevate GSH biosynthesis, levels of Phase II/antioxidant enzymes and inhibit the toxins' entry into the cells (Gupta, Sharma, et al. 2002, Gupta, Sharma et al. 2004, Upadhyay, Kumar, et al. 2007, Upadhyay, Gupta, et al. 2010). In the last decade, numerous studies have been undertaken to explore the mechanism of action of these natural products at the biochemical, genomic and proteomic levels. Bedi et al. 2012 have concisely reviewed the chemical and biological profile as well as the application of herbal constituents in protection against a different class of hepatotoxicants along with their mechanism of action (Bedi, Bijjem, et al. 2016). The most extensively investigated products have been resveratrol, silymarin, gingko and curcumin due to their dietary nature, high efficacy, low or no toxicity and easy availability, that has provided them with an extra edge over other candidates of supplementary medication. Moreover, these herbal drugs have been employed as dietary supplements in Ayurveda owing to their hepatoprotective nature. Apart from these, new molecular targets and signalling cascades have also been identified for developing approaches to adequately manage pathological conditions induced via oxidative stress (Rizvi et al 2014).

Table 10.5 A few representative studies undertaken to screen for protective/therapeutic agents against hepatotoxicants

Hepatotoxicants	Preventive/Protective agent	Model and Route of Administration	References
Carbon tetrachloride (0.2 ml), twice a week	**LIV 52 (herbal formulations)** (0.5 ml (30 mg/rat/day, intragastric tube): Co-exposure reduced fatty change and necrosis in albino rats	Albino rats, Subcutaneous	(Part 1963)
Carbon tetrachloride (0.5 ml/kg b.wt.), 14 days	**Protein A (**60 µg/kg b.wt., Intravenous on first day, then twice a week for two weeks): Pre-exposure prevents fat accumulation, hepatic lesions and necrosis, recovery in the activities of Mixed function oxidase enzymes, glutathione-S-transferase and decrease in the activity of SGOT and SGPT	Wistar rats, Intraperitoneal	(Singh, Saxena, et al. 1988)
Carbon tetrachloride (1 ml/kg b.wt.), every 72 h for 10 days	***Solanum trilobatum*** (150, 200 and 250 mg/kg b wt/ day, 10 days): Demonstrated antioxidant and free radical scavenging	Wistar rats, Intraperiotenal	(Shahjahan, Sabitha, et al. 2004)

Contd...

Hepatotoxicants	Preventive/Protective agent	Model and Route of Administration	References
Carbon tetrachloride (1 mL/kg b.wt.) three times/weekly, 28 days	**Silymarin** (100 mL/kg b.wt., Oral)and **BM-MSCs** (9.75 million/kg b.wt., Intravenous): Post treatment combined exposure restored the plasma hepatocyte growth factor levels which were comparable with normal levels and exhibited significant antimutagenic and antiapoptotic activity by decreasing the frequency of structural chromosomal aberrations and suppressing the DNA fragmentation in liver tissue samples.	Wistar rats, Intraperitoneal	(Aithal, Bairy, et al. 2019)
Paracetemol (300 mg/kg b.wt.) for 2 days	*Cajanus indicus* **protein** (2 mg/kg b.wt., 4 days, Intraperitoneal): Pre and post exposure significantly reduced the liver enzyme level, antioxidant, free radical scavenging	Albino mice, Oral	(Ghosh and Sil 2007)
Paracetemol (750 mg/kg b.wt.), at every 72 h for 10 days	**Methanolic extract of** *Phyllanthus polyphyllus* (200 and 300 mg/kg b.wt., p.o., 10 days): Co-exposure disrupted serum marker enzymes AST, ALP, ALT levels to near normal	Wistar rats, Oral	(Rajkapoor, Venugopal, et al. 2008)
Paracetemol (2 g/kg b.wt.), 36 h	**Ethanol extract of** *Clausena dentate* (250 mg/kg b.wt./day): Pre-exposure altered serum marker enzymes AST, ALP, ALT levels to near normal	Wistar rats, Oral	(Rajesh, Rajkapoor, et al. 2009)
Paracetemol (675 μM)	**Probiotics (***Enterococcus lactis*** IITRHR1 (***EISN***) and** *Lactobacillus acidophilus* **MTCC447 (LaSN) lysate)** (20 mg/ml): inhibits activation of procaspase-3, DNA fragmentation and chromatin condensation, modulation of oxidative stress induced apoptosis	Primary rat hepatocytes	(Sharma, Singh, et al. 2011)
Paracetemol (300 mg/kg b.wt.)	**Silymarin nanoparticles** (125 mg/kg b.wt., 7 days): Pre-exposure induces rapid regeneration of hepatic GSH levels, downregulation of serum enzyme parameters and marked increase in survival against paracetemol-induced hepatic damage	Albino mice, Intraperitoneal	(Das, Roy, et al. 2011)
Ethanol (20%), 60 days	**Glycine** (0.6 g/kg b.wt./day, 60 days Intragastric tube): lowered TBARS levels and increased SOD, CAT, GSH, GPx and GR activities in the erythrocyte membrane, plasma and hepatocytes	Wistar rats, Intragastric tube	(Senthilkumar, Sengottuvelan, et al. 2004)

Contd...

Hepatotoxicants	Preventive/Protective agent	Model and Route of Administration	References
Ethanol (1.2 ml/100 gm b.wt.), 7 weeks	**Liv 52** (4.0 ml/100 gm b.wt./day, 7 weeks, Intragastric tube): Co-expoure prevents fibrosis and lobulation	Albino rats, Oral	(Kale, Kulkarni, et al. 1966)
Ethanol (5 g/kg b.wt./day), 60 days	*Emblica officinalis* **(250 mg/kg b.wt., 8 h, gastric intubation):** Pre-exposure returned the plasma enzymes towards near normal level, lowered LPO levels, protein carbonyls, replenished enzymatic and non-enzymatic antioxidants levels	Wistar rats, Gastric intubation	(Reddy, Padmavathi, et al. 2010)
D-Galact-osamine (800 mg/kg b.wt.), 6 h	**Human Wharton jelly derived mesenchymal stem cells** ($5x\ 10^5$cells/ 0.5 ml, Intravenous, 24 h after): rescues acute liver injury by reducing the levels of liver enzymes, LPO and elevating the levels of SOD	Swiss albino mice, Intraperitoneal	(Ramanathan, Rupert, et al. 2017)
Pyrogallol (100 mg/kg b.wt.), 1 h	**New Livfit® (polyherbal formulation)** (10, 25, 50 and 100 mg/kg b.wt, 1 h prior, Oral): Pre exposure results in free radical scavenging activity against pyrogallol	Wistar rats, Intraperitoneal	(Gupta, Sharma, et al. 2004)
Pyrogallol (40 mg/kg b.wt./day), 1-4 weeks	**Resveratrol** ((10 mg/kg b.wt. 2 h prior): Pre-exposure attenuated phase I enzymes, increased phase II enzymes, restored antioxidant capacity of liver, lowered levels of bilirubin, alanine aminotransaminase, aspartate aminotransaminase	Swiss albino mice, Intraperitoneal	(Upadhyay, Singh, et al. 2008)
Pyrogallol (40 mg/kg b.wt./day), 1-4 weeks	**Silymarin** (40 mg/kg b.wt/day, Intraperitoneal, 2 h prior): reduces apoptosis, diminishes complement activation, regulates extracellular matrix remodelling	Albino mice, Intraperitoneal	(Upadhyay, Tiwari, et al. 2010)
Benzene (1 ml/kg b.wt./day), 3 days	**Interferon inducer 6MFA** (10 mg/100 g b.wt., Intraperitoneal): Pre-treatment restored hepatic architecture and normalized the lipid peroxidation and iron content	Albino rats, Intraperitoneal	(Tripathi, Singh, et al. 2010)
Nimesulide (500 µM), 1 h	*Fumaria parviflora Lam.* **extract** (2 mg/ml, pre and post treatment of 30 min): Prevented LDH leake, membrane depolarization, DNA fragmentation and apoptosis	Rat primary hepatocytes	(Tripathi, Singh, et al. 2010)

Contd…

Hepatotoxicants	Preventive/Protective agent	Model and Route of Administration	References
Cyclophospha-mide (200 mg/kg), 4 and 11 days	**Protein A** (60 µg/kg, twice/week, 14 days, Intravenous): Pre treatment causes regeneration of the depleted enzyme activity (hepatic mixed function oxygenase (MFO)	Sprague Dawley rats, Intravenous	(Dohadwala and Ray 1985)
Acetaminophen (1 g/kg b.wt./day), 30 days	**Lupeol** (150 mg/kg b.wt./day, 30 days, Oral): Co-exposure lowered the levels of serum transam- inases, MDA, protein carbonyl content in Wistar rats, inhibited ROS production and depolarization of mitochondria, elevated the mitochondrial antioxidant and redox status, prevented DNA damage and cell death by inhibiting Bcl-2 downregulation, elevation of Bax, cytochrome c release and caspase 3/9 activation	Wistar rats, Oral	(Kumari and Kakkar 2012)
Acetaminophen (1 g/kg b. wt./day), 28 days	**Morin** (30 mg/kg b.wt., 28 days Oral): Co-exposure caused attenuation of APAP-mediated liver damage as observed via decrease in histological and serum markers of hepatotoxicity, reduced necroinflammation (decreased HMGB1 release, maturation of NALP3 and caspase-1), prevented oxidative stress and mitochondrial dysfunction	Wistar rats, Oral	(Rizvi, Mathur, et al. 2015)
Arsenic (13 mg/kg b.wt.), 24 h	**Nanoencapsulated Quercetin** (Single dose of 2.71 mg/kg b.wt.1 h after arsenic administration, Oral): Post exposure protected liver from decrease of antioxidant levels and oxidative stress related gene expression	Wistar rats, Oral	(Ghosh, Ghosh et al. 2010)
Maneb (15 mg/kg b.wt) **and paraquat** (5 mg/kg b.wt.), twice a week, 6 weeks	**N-acetylcyteine** (200 mg/kg b.wt.) **and silymarin** (100 mg/kg b.wt., 2 h prior): decreases oxidative stress and inflammation via modulation of xenobitic metabolizing machinery in hepatic microsomes	Wistar rats, Intraperitoneal	(Ahmad, Shukla, et al. 2013)
Isoniazid-andrifampicin (50 mg/kg b.wt.)/day, 3 weeks	**N- acetylcysteine** (100 mg/kkg b.wt., 3 weeks Intraperitoneal): Co-supplementation prevents induction of oxidative stress in Wistar rats	Wistar rats, Intraperitoneal	(Attri, Rana, et al. 2000)

Contd...

Hepatotoxicants	Preventive/Protective agent	Model and Route of Administration	References
Chloroquine (CQ) (360-2000mg/kg b.wt.), 24 h	**Quercetin** (50mg/kg b.wt., Oral): Pre exposure reverts CQ induced oxidative stress by scavenging the free radical generation	Albino mice, Oral	Mishra, Singh, et al. 2013
Cisplatin (6 mg/kg b.wt.), 4 days	**Fish oil** (15%, 10 days, Oral): Pre-exposure prevented reduction in antioxidant enzymes activities viz. catalase, superoxide dismutase and glutathione peroxidase, prevented alterations in enzymes that are involved in TCA cycle, glycolysis, gluconeogenesis and HMP shunt pathway	Wistar rats, Intraperitoneal	(Naqshbandi, Khan, et al. 2011)
Aflatoxin1 (1 mg/kg b.wt. 5% w/v acacia mucilage), four times at 12 hr intervals and a single dose of aflatoxin 1 mg/kg, 30 minutes after the administration of first dose of acacia mucilage	**Ethanolic leaf extract of *Trianthema portulacastrum l.*** (50-800 mg/kg b.wt., 4 times, 12 h interval, Oral): Pre-treatment showed dose dependent reduction in SGPT, SGOT, ALP and total bilirubin levels	Wistar rats, Oral	(Banu, Kumar, et al. 2009)
Alfatoxin 1 (0–50 µg/ml), 24 h	**Ginger Extract** (0–200 µg/ml, 24 h): Pre-exposure prevented the generation of ROS, DNA strand break in HepG2 cells, reduced LPO and elevated the antioxidant enzymes activities	HepG2 cells	(Vipin, Rao, et al. 2017)
Alfatoxin 1 (200 µg/kg), every alternative day for 28 days.	**Ginger Extract** (100 and 250 mg/kg/day, gastric tube): Reduced the induced toxicity on serum markers of liver damage, reduced LPO and enhanced antioxidant enzymes activities, elevated the Nrf2/HO-1 pathway	Wistar rats, Intraperitoneal	
Rhein (50 µM), 24 h	**Cyclosporin A** (100 nM 24 h): Co-exposure prevented generation of ROS, increase in the intracellular Ca^{2+}, decrease in the mitochondrial membrane potential and depletion of GSH, prevented DNA damage resulting in reduced expression of γ-H2AX protein, prevented apoptosis and alteration of signaling molecules such as MAPK kinases	Primary rat heptocytes	(Panigrahi, Yadav, et al. 2015)

Contd...

Hepatotoxicants	Preventive/Protective agent	Model and Route of Administration	References
High glucose (40 mM), 1.5 h	**Morin** (5 µg, pre and post treatment of 30 min, co-treatment 1.5 h): increased the cell viability and decreased ROS, maintained mitochondrial integrity, prevented release of apoptotic proteins from mitochondria, inhibited DNA fragmentation, condensation of chromatin and hypodiploid DNA	Primary rat hepatocytes	(Kapoor and Kakkar 2012)
Radiation (5 Gy), 30 days	**Flaxseed** (once daily for 15 consecutive days, Oral): Pre-treatment significantly ameliorated radiation-induced higher levels of LPO, AST, ALT and acid phosphatase	Swiss albino mice	(Bhatia, Sharma, et al. 2007)

10.3 Nephrotoxicity

Kidneys are dynamic organs representing the main control system that maintain body homeostasis. Having substantial metabolic capacity, the organ is also involved in detoxifying and eliminating several chemicals, thus becoming a potential site for xenobiotic toxicity. Since the very inception, the focus was on drug-induced nephrotoxicity in patients receiving anti-cancer drugs and acute tubular necrosis following intravesical instillation of formalin, used as a food preservative (Chugh, Singhal, et al. 1977). Since then, several environmental contaminants, chemicals and drugs including antibiotics, anticancer agents and NSAIDs have been shown to modify the structure and function of various tissues dramatically and induce several adverse effects on the kidney.

Over past several years, acute renal toxicity has been a major problem for the patients, especially those who have cancer, tuberculosis, etc., and due to the prolonged use of potent clinical compounds including NSAIDs, radiocontrast agents, antimicrobial, anesthetic agents and more recently anticancer agent like cisplatin. As such, studying drug-induced nephrotoxicity has been one of the top priorities of research groups.

To assess the rate of drug-induced nephrotoxicity innumerable single and multi-center case series and cohort studies have been carried out. High nephrotoxicity rates while on colistin A (13%) (Dewan and Shoukat 2014, Ghafur, Gohel, et al. 2017), parenteral polymyxin B in patients with the multidrug resistance (MDR) (18.1%) (Ramasubban, Majumdar et al. 2008, Nandha, Sekhri et al. 2013) have been documented. Mani, et al. 1993 has provided a comprehensive account for patterns of renal disease in indigenous populations in India attributing to diabetic neuropathy, snake bite, leptospirosis, malaria as the commonest (Mani 1993). Another study reported high rates for infection (22.4%), and drugs (14.9%). Anti-inflammatory drugs were the most commonly used drugs that resulted in the acute decline in renal function (Mittal, Kher, et al. 1997).

Acute renal failure from venomous snakes and insects together constitute approximately 3% of all cases being as high as 13% to 32% following *Echis carinatus* or Russell's viper bite (Chugh, Pal, et al. 1984, Chugh 1989, Mittal 1994). Apart from drug-induced nephrotoxicity, over the years, various other environmental factors have been identified to induce nephrotoxicity. Acute renal failure observed with systemic mucormycosis (Gupta, Radotra et al. 1989), *Falciparum* malaria (Prakash, Gupta, et al. 1996), everolimus (Evl) (management of hormone receptor-positive metastatic breast cancer) associated nephrotoxicity (Chandra, Rao, et al. 2017), urolithiasis due to fluoride (Singh, Barjatiya, et al. 2001), paraquat poisoning (Pavan 2013), exposure to lead (Kumar and Krishnaswamy 1995), microalbuminuria due to heat and PAHs emissions from indoor environment (Singh, Kamal et al. 2016), and food-based toxicants (such as oxalate nephropathy due to Starfruit (*Averrhoa carambola*) (Barman, Goel, et al. 2016) have also been documented.

The basis of drug toxicity has been the topic of several investigations and has improved our understanding of the drug's interaction with the renal tubule cells and the consequent effects on cellular function and integrity. Several xenobiotics have been shown to accumulate in the proximal convoluted tubules, inducing numerous morphologic, functional and metabolic alterations. Table 10.6 provides a comprehensive overview of the studies undertaken to assess the nephrotoxic effects as well as the mechanism of action of different toxicants.

Table 10.6 A comprehensive overview of the effects/mechanism of action of few nephrotoxicants

Nephrotoxicants	Effects/Mechanism of Action	Model and Route of Administration	References
	Drugs		
Adriamycin (6 mg/kg b.wt.), 5, 10, 15, 20, 25, 30 days	Glomerular and tubular injury as observed via heavy proteinuria, albuminuria and elevated urine excretion of N-acetyl glucosaminidase, serum ACE was increased on day 20, 25 and 30 with the excretion of ACE in urine which was parallel to the total protein excretion	Albino rats, Intravenous	(Venkatesan, Ramesh, et al. 1993)

Contd...

Nephrotoxicants	Effects/Mechanism of Action	Model and Route of Administration	References
Paracetemol (300 mg/kg b.wt.), 0.5, 1, 2, 2.5 h and 3 h	Total acid phosphatase activities increased at 0.5 h and remained elevated up to 3 h. Free as well as total cathepsin D activities increased within 2-2.5 h, elevated both free and total RNAse I1 activity at 0.5 h, Maximum activity of DNAse I1 (free and total) was seen at *2.5* h	Albino mice, Intraperitoneal	(Khandkar, Parmar, et al. 1996)
Cyclophos-phamide (150 mg/kg b.wt.), 6, 16 and 24 h	Progressive renal damage with increase in time with glomerular nephritis, cortical tubular vacuolization and interstitial edema, a reduction in the lysosomal enzymes viz acid phosphatase, β-glucuronidase and N-acetylglucosaminidase at 16 and 24 h with increase in the protein content	Wistar rats, Intraperitoneal	(Abraham, Indirani, et al. 2007)
Cyclophosph-amide (150 mg/kg b.wt.), 6, 16 h	Elevation in the nitrite levels, increased expression of nitrotyrosine and activation of PARP, decrease in oxidized NAD levels	Wistar rats, Intraperitoneal	(Abraham and Rabi 2009)
Cisplatin (0.4 mg/kg b.wt./day), 8 weeks	Rounded cisternae of smooth endoplasmic reticulum and dense chromatin in the nucleus with higher mitochondrial density, acute tubular necrosis with slogging and dilation of epithelium	Albino rats, Intraperitoneal	(Ravindra, Bhiwgade, et al. 2010)
Tenofovir disoproxil fumarate (anti-HIV drug) (600 mg/kg b.wt./day), 5 weeks	Impaired proximal tubular, mitochondrial dysfunction, reduction in the activities of the electron chain complexes I, II, IV, and V by 46%, 20%, 26%, and 21%, respectively	Wistar rats, Oral	(Rama-moorthy, Abraham, et al. 2014)
Pesticides			
Chlorpyrifos (5 and 10 mg/kg b.wt./day), 7, 14, 28, 42 and 56 days	Glomerulus shrinkage at initial stage, glomerular hypercellularity, degeneration of glomerulus and renal tubules, tubular dilation, tubular epithelium hypertrophy, deposition of eosin-positive substances in the glomerulus and renal tubules and leucocytes infiltration in a dose and time dependent manner	Wistar rats, Oral	(Tripathi and Srivastav 2010)
Methyl isocyanate (0.005 µM), 0-180 h	Stress-induced senescence, higher oxidative stress in a time dependent manner, reduction in superoxide dismutase and glutathione reductase, accumulation of 8-oxo-dG inducing abrupt expression of p21, p53, cyclin E and CDK2 proteins suggesting dysregulated cell	Human kidney epithelial HEK-293 cells	(Mishra, Raghuram, et al. 2009)

Contd...

Nephrotoxicants	Effects/Mechanism of Action	Model and Route of Administration	References
	cycle, chromosomal aberrations, centromeric amplification, aneuploidy and genomic instability		
Lambda-cyhalothrin (0.5, 1 and 2 mg/kg b.wt./day), 28 days	Increased serum urea nitrogen, creatinine, urea levels, LPO, superoxide anion generation and nitrite level and lowered the levels of reduced glutathione, reduced superoxide dismutase, catalase and glutathione-S-transferase activities	Swiss albino mice, Oral	(Pawar, Badgujar, et al. 2017)
Metals			
Cadmium (1 mg/kg b.wt.), 1, 2 and 4 weeks	Decrease in body weight and rise in blood pressure were observed as early as one week of exposure while microalbuminuria was detected in 50% of the animals after 2 weeks, Na+K+ ATPase, a renal tubular enzyme, was depressed after 1 week with maximum lowering occurring after 4 weeks	Wistar rats, Intrapeirtoneal	(Lall, Das, et al. 1997)
Flouride (5, 10, 20, and 50 mg/kg b.wt./day), 15 weeks	No clinical signs of toxicity were observed on exposure to the lowest dose, cloudy swellings in kidney, tubular epithelia degeneration, tissue necrosis, vacuolization in tubules, hypertrophy and atrophy of glomeruli, interstitial oedema, and nephritis at higher doses	Albino rabbits, Subcutaneous	(Shashi, Singh, et al. 2002)
Lead (exposure of 6 months-10 years)	Blood leads were high (24.3-62.4) µg/dL as compared to controls (19.4-30.6 µg/dL), loss of appetite, fatigue, headache, metallic taste, abdominal colic, intermittent vomiting, insomnia in workers with blood levels above 35 µg/dL, lead poisoning such aslead line, tremors, sensory and motor disturbances in the extremities were noted in 36%	Automobile workers	(Dinesh Kumar and Krishnaswamy 1995)
Lead (30 and 60 mg/kg b.wt./3 days a week), 8 weeks	Higher serum creatinine levels and lowered antioxidant enzymes (CAT, SOD & GPx) activity, severe degenerative changes, intertubular haemorrhages, atrophied and cystic glomeruli, the apoptotic bodies in the kidney elevated in the PCT epithelium	Wistar rats, Oral	(Sujatha, Srilatha, et al. 2011)
Uranyl nitrate (2 and 4 mg/kg b.wt.), 1, 3, 5, 14 and 28 days	Uranium accumulation in the kidenys, 75% tubular damage was observed after 3 days (4 mg/kg) increase in serum creatinine, urea, and blood urea nitrogen levels with	Swiss albino mice, Intraperit-oneal	(Sangeetha Vijayan, Rekha, et al. 2016)

Contd…

Nephrotoxicants	Effects/Mechanism of Action	Model and Route of Administration	References
	no progression of damage after 5 days, recovery after 14 and 28 days in a dose dependent manner		
Sodium nitrite (20, 40, 60 and 75 mg/kg b.wt.), 24 h	Increase in LPO, protein oxidation, hydrogen peroxide levels and decrease in GSH and antioxidant capacity, DNA damage ang greater crosslinking to proteins	Wistar rats, Oral	(Ansari, Ali, et al. 2018)
Miscellaneous			
Silver nanoparticles (500, 1000, 3000, and 5000 mg/kg b.wt.), 28 days	3000 and 5000 mg/kg induced irregularity in the nuclear membrane, swollen and pleomorphic mitochondria with distorted cristae, dilation of rough endoplasmic reticulum, hypertrophy and fused podocytes, thick basement membrane in the endothelial cells of the proximal tubules	Albino rats, Intraperitoneal	(Ansari, Shukla, et al. 2016)
Silver nanoparticles (50 ppm and 200 ppm) 60 days	Reduced kidney weight and loss of renal function as observed via higher serum creatinine levels and early toxicity markers such as clusterin, osteopontin, KIM- 1, damage to mitochondrial, prolonged exposure led to activation of cell proliferative, survival and proinflammatory factors (JNK/Stat, Akt/mTOR, ERK/NF-κB pathways and IL1β, MIP2, IFN-γ, TNF-α and RANTES)	Wistar rats, Oral	(Tiwari, Singh, et al. 2017)
Ochratoxin A (OTA A) (0.75 mg/kg feed), **Citrinin** (CIT) (15 mg/kg feed) and OTA+CIT (0.75 and 15 mg/kg feed), 60 days	More concentration of MDA, DNA damage and apoptosis in OTA and combination group, interstitial cells revealed nuclear fragmentation and cytoplasmic blebbing, nuclear fragmentation in proximal convoluted tubular epithelial cells	New Zealand rabbits, Oral	(Kumar, Dwivedi, et al. 2014)
Ferric nitrilo triacetate (Fe-NTA) (9mg/kg b.wt.), 3, 6, 12, 24, 48 and 72 h	Induced activity of renal ornithine decarboxylase ODC and increased renal DNA synthesis, depleted glutathione (GSH) levels, decreased glutathione S-transferase, glutathione reductase, glutathione peroxidase and glucose 6-phosphate activity contributing towards carcinogenecity	Albino rats, Intraperitoneal	(Athar and Iqbal 1998)

Malnutrition has been shown to have a profound effect on xenobiotic induced nephrotoxicity. Protein deficiency during cadmium (Cd) exposure leads to its excessive renal accumulation not bound to metallothionein (MT) proteins (Prasad and Nath 1995). Moreover, tissue-specific induction of MT in chronic Cd exposure in Rhesus monkeys undergoing nutritional stress conditions has been reported with more cadmium being directed towards the kidney than the liver (Ravi, Paliwal, et al. 1984). MT induction plays a crucial role in metabolism of metal during Cd toxicity under conditions of nutritional stress. Identification of iso-metallothioneins varying in their composition of metal, such as MTc, the main isoform in Cd-exposed, healthy and protein-calorie malnourished monkeys whereas the MTb, the main isoprotein in Cd exposed calcium deficient monkeys have shown differential capacities to reactivate apo-enzymes viz. ceruloplasmin, alkaline phosphatase, glutathione peroxidase and superoxide dismutase (Nath, Paliwal et al. 1987). Similarly, functional aspects of fetal development may be susceptible to interference by the nutritional status of the mothers. Example, iron deficiency during fetal development (15-20 days of gestation) may lead to higher xenobiotic accumulation (such as lead) in the fetus causing degeneration and pathological changes in the fetal kidney (Singh, Saxena, et al. 1991).

Excretion of urinary enzyme as an index of kidney injury has been widely studied. Infact, there has been a growing need for monitoring renal damage, particularly on therapies therapy, when nephrotoxic agents are administered together. Time-dependent alterations in serum, tissue, and urine Angiotensin I converting enzyme activity (ACE) levels as an early and sensitive indicator of adriamycin mediated renal glomerular and tubular damage has been proposed. Urinary N-acetyl-3-D-glucosaminidase activity also offers a sensitive indicator of rifampicin-induced nephrotoxicity as well as detection of blood lead and renal tubular injury (Kumar, Prasad, et al. 1992). Similarly, renal Paraoxenase 1 (PON1), acting as a defense mechanism adopted by the kidney in order to reduce or prevent cyclophosphamide (CP) induced oxidative stress activity, may be utilized as an early biochemical event in CP induced renal damage (Abraham and Sugumar 2008). Sometimes an established biomarker of renal dysfunction may not be suitable for assessing nephrotoxicity of every drug/xenobiotic. Such a case has been exemplified by the nephrotoxicity of CP which is usually overlooked as plasma creatinine, an indicator of the kidney's glomerular function, is not modified drastically in patients. However, in a study, using a rat model, the research group has provided evidence that CP causes renal injury histologically, but plasma creatinine, a reliable biomarker of kidney dysfunction, remains unchanged (Sugumar, Kanakasabapathy, et al. 2007).

The occurrence of renal failure with drug therapies has received considerable attention owing to their widespread use (Ramasubban, Majumdar, et al. 2008). Cisplatin (CIS), a frequently used broad-spectrum antineoplastic agent, is a preferred treatment option for several malignancies, such as breast cancer, despite its peripheral neuropathy, ototoxicity, and nephrotoxicity (Jamdade, Sethi et al. 2015, Mundhe, Kumar, et al. 2015). The spectrum of CIS nephrotoxicity includes tubular toxicity, DNA damage and inflammation. Inflammation plays a critical role in CIS induced nephrotoxicity via release of several cytokines (TNF-α, IL- 1β, etc.) and chemokines (MCP-1, MIP-2, etc.). TNF-α plays an important role in the induction of other inflammatory cytokines and chemokines and is a chief culprit of CIS-induced renal injury (Kumar, Prashanth, et al. 2013). Higher incidence of breast cancer in females; especially in the younger females, has demanded prompt, and intensive interventions to make the therapy more effective and less toxic (Kumar, Bolshette et al. 2013, Jamdade, Sethi, et al. 2015).

Renal carcinogenesis has been a topic of much interest in the country. Ferric-nitrilotriacetic acid (Fe-NTA), a widespread water pollutant (used as polyphosphate substitute in detergents), is a known nephrotoxic agent as well as a renal tumor promoter (Rahman, Ahmed, et al. 2003). Various mechanisms have been proposed to unravel the basis of its toxicity. Fe-NTA-induced platelet growth factor-2 through the activation of cyclooxygenase has been shown responsible for the development and maintenance of hyperplasia in the kidney (Iqbal, Giri, et al. 1997). Generation of oxidative stress and impaired antioxidant system in the kidney may play a critical role in Fe-NTA induced renal ODC activity, elevation of DNA synthesis and promotion of DEN-initiated renal tumors (Iqbal, Giri, et al. 1995, Iqbal, Sharma, et al. 1996, Athar and Iqbal 1998). Fe-NTA has also been shown to act through ROS generation, induced via Fenton's reaction and generation of oxidizing iron species such as ferryl ions (FeO_2+) which elevates LPO with a reduction in the levels of tissue GSH (Athar and Iqbal 1998, Iqbal, Sharma, et al. 1999). The involvement of LPO and oxidative stress in renal damage is also highlighted from the fact that antioxidants block Fe-NTA-induced renal damage (Iqbal, Rezazadeh, et al. 1998, Ansar, Iqbal, et al. 1999). It has also been emphasized that Fe-NTA-induced renal damage resulting in carcinogenesis may be possibly related with the generation and accumulation of 4-hydroxy-2-nonenal (HNE) altered protein adducts in the tissues. Moreover, there is also an age-dependent elevation in the vulnerability of animals to oxidant-induced kidney damage (Iqbal, Giri, et al. 1999).

Studies have hinted towards epigenetic modulation of xenobiotics in mediating nephrotoxicity. Employing human embryonic kidney cells and prenatally exposed animals, Singh, et al. 2015 have identified Interleukin-8 (IL-8) and its homologue (CINC-1) as crucial mediators in arsenic-induced kidney toxicity (Singh, Tiwari, et al. 2015). Further, embryonic kidney cells have been demonstrated to be more responsive to arsenic resulting in greater induction of IL-8 as compared with adult cells because of DNA methylation and histone acetylation (H3 acetylation) alterations in the IL-8 promoter. They have also identified arsenic altered CpG site (at 168 bases upstream of the transcription start site) associated with CREB and C/EBP binding sites in the IL-8 promoter, aberrant epigenetic modulation of which, could result in induction of IL-8 contributing to higher cell migratory and proliferative capacities, dysregulation of cell cycle and kidney toxicity. Studies have revealed for the first time how Methylmercury (MeHg) could epigenetically regulate matrix metalloproteinase 9 (MMP9) to induce nephrotoxicity. Sub-chronic exposure of MeHg interferes with the cellular and epigenetic processes, leading to aberrant alterations in MMP9 methylation, resulting in disruption of cytoskeleton and loss of kidney functions. Bisulfite sequencing has identified important CpGs in the first exon of MMP9, that were demethylated on the exposure of MeHg. ChIP studies also revealed a loss of methyl binding protein, MeCP2 and the transcription factor PEA3 at the demethylated site confirming the reduced methylation of CpG. MeHg may epigenetically alter MMP9 to induce cytoskeleton disruption and cell adhesion loss resulting in loss of kidney functions (Khan, Singh, et al. 2017).

Nephrotoxicity induced via drugs accounts for 18% to 27% of cases of acute kidney injury. Moreover, the phenotype of drug-induced kidney disease (DIKD) variates, as damage can occur in various kidney structures, such as the glomeruli, vascular endothelium, tubules, and interstitium. Moreover, DIKD may manifest as acute and/or chronic modification in the kidney functions with the onset ranging from hours to weeks. It is mostly asymptomatic, and the diagnosis is based on biomarker alteration such as elevated serum creatinine or urinary results including hematuria and proteinuria consistent with the glomerular damage. The risk factors for DIKD have been documented for individual drugs; which could be patient-specific (e.g., age, chronic kidney disease), disease-related (e.g., sepsis, volume depletion), and related process of care (e.g., drug dose and duration). In such a case, effective approaches to predict DIKD may help in reducing the risk of recurrent damage. Genetic determinants in Drug-Induced Renal Injury (DIRECT) study would be the first observational cohort study to identify the genetic factors of DIKD (Awdishu, Nievergelt, et al. 2016). The group would be employing genome-wide association and whole-genome sequencing studies; to describe the course, frequency, risk factors, resolution and the outcomes of DIKD cases; to explore the role of ethnic/racial variability in DIKD genetics; and to investigate the utilization of several tools to establish causality of DIKD.

Establishing the causality in DIKD has been challenging which requires the knowledge of the biological plausibility for the specific drug, mechanism of action, time course and accurate assessment of risk factors. Often the spectrum of injury in DIKD also goes unrecognized, as there are no standards for their identification and characterization. In recent years, the International Serious Adverse Event Consortium (iSAEC) has initiated a phenotype standardization project for drug-mediated adverse effects. In conjunction with the iSAEC, Mehta, et al 2015 have developed consensus definitions for DIKD, which takes into account the known mechanisms of renal toxicity, time course of drug setting and exposure and proposed four phenotypes based on few clinical presentations: acute kidney injury, glomerular disorder, tubular disorder, or nephrolithiasis/crystalluria; that are based on an alteration in the biomarkers and other evidences: Scr (AKI), hematuria/ proteinuria (glomerular), electrolyte alterations (tubular), ultrasound findings (nephrolithiasis). These phenotypes, standardized with expert nephrologists, adult and pediatric, and pharmacists would serve as a consistent framework for investigators, clinicians, industries and regulatory agencies to assess drug induced nephrotoxicity across different settings (Mehta, Awdishu, et al. 2015).

Diabetic nephropathy (DN), due to chronic hyperglycemia, has also been an attractive area of research among toxicologists. Clinical DN result from glomerular, tubular, interstitial and vascular lesions involving the interplay of various metabolic and biochemical pathways which contribute towards the development of diabetic renal disease and it has been suggested that renin-angiotensin-aldosterone system (RAAS), transforming growth factor (TGF)-R1 and nitric oxide pathways are significant. Research groups have utilized the streptozotocin-induced DN model to provide insights into the underlying mechanisms as well as to screen for therapeutic interventions. Numerous studies have been undertaken to identify the contributing factors towards the development of DN. Hypomagnesemia may be one of them linked with the development of DN (Prabodh, Prakash, et al. 2011). Over the years, there has been a renewed interest in understanding the role of reactive oxygen species (ROS). Chronic hyperglycemia, the main factor for the initiation and progression of DN, not only produces more reactive oxygen metabolites but also blocks the anti-oxidative mechanisms via non-enzymatic glycation of the scavenging enzymes. These results have confirmed the significance of oxidative stress in the development of DN and hint towards the possible anti-oxidative mechanisms that contribute to the nephroprotective action of antioxidants like resveratrol and quercetin (Anjaneyulu and Chopra 2004, Sharma, Anjaneyulu, et al. 2006).

Genetic susceptibility plays a pivotal role in the DN pathogenesis and several genetic tools including candidate gene association studies and genome-wide association study (GWAS) have been employed to establish the contribution of gene polymorphisms in the induction of oxidative stress in patients with DN (Ahluwalia, Ahuja, et al. 2008, Tiwari, Prasad, et al. 2009, Prasad, Tiwari, et al. 2010, Dabhi and Mistry 2015). Double deletions in GSTT1 and GSTM1 have been linked with higher oxidative stress (Datta,

Kumar, et al. 2010). Similarly, endothelial-derived nitric oxide synthase (eNOS) gene polymorphisms affecting the activity of eNOS have been related to endothelial dysfunction. Higher frequency of mutant genotypes like CC (-786T [C), TT (894G [T) and AA genotypes (27VNTR) have been found to be associated with a higher risk of nephropathy (Ahluwalia, Ahuja, et al. 2008). Studies further indicates that the allele of angiotensin-converting enzyme (ACE D) individually and in association with other renin-angiotensin system (RAS) SNPs drastically elevates the risk of nephropathy in type 2 diabetic patients (Ahluwalia, Ahuja, et al. 2009).

Among the several tested cytokine gene polymorphisms, allele 59029A of CCR5 gene is strongly linked with diabetic renal insufficiency among Asian Indians (Prasad, Tiwari, et al. 2007). The role of RAAS gene polymorphisms in DN have also been emphasized. T>C (-344) in aldosterone synthase, Met235Thr in angiotensinogen and G>A (-1903) in chymase genes have been significantly associated with diabetic chronic renal insufficiency in Indian patients (Prasad, Tiwari, et al. 2006).

In the recent years, it has been established that inflammatory mechanisms strongly contribute towards the development and progression of DN. In such a polygenic complex disease, like DN, the association of individual gene polymorphisms may be insignificant whereas particular combinations of few genotypes may have more relevance. A study examined the combined polymorphisms among five pro-inflammatory genes (TGFB1: T869C (Leu10Pro) and Tyr81His; CCL2: A-2518G and Insertion/Deletion (I/D); CCR5: Insertion/Deletion (I/D) and G59029A; IL8: T-251A; MMP9: Arg279Gln (G.A)) for their possible association with the increased susceptibility to DN. The co-occurrence of risk associated genotypes (II, -2518GG (CCL2), DD (CCR5) and 279Gln/Gln (MMP9) was observed to confer a tenfold higher risk of nephropathy among patients with type 2 diabetes, proposing them as good candidate genes for conferring vulnerability (Ahluwalia, Khullar, et al. 2009). Use of these markers for the prediction of susceptibility to diabetes-specific kidney disease in the Indian population may be promising for the purpose of risk assessment.

Chronic Kidney disease (CKD) is a global problem and the 12th major reason for death worldwide (Jha, Garcia-Garcia, et al. 2013) with few common risk-factors such as diabetes and hypertension (Vassalotti, Stevens et al. 2007). However, over the years, an increasing concern has grown for a new-form of CKD, not induced by the already known risk-factors, termed as CKD of unknown-etiology (CKDu) (Jayatilake, Mendis, et al. 2013). CKDu is prominent in few developing countries like Sri-Lanka (Wanigasuriya, Peiris-John, et al. 2011), India (Singh, Farag, et al. 2013) and some central-American countries (Correa-Rotter, Wesseling, et al. 2014) adversely affecting the kidney's tubular-interstitium belonging to type-chronic tubulointerstitial nephritis (CTN) (Mackensen and Billing 2009), induced by chronic exposure to several environmental toxins like heavy metals (arsenic, lead, cadmium), pesticides (diazinon) and mycotoxins (Weaver, Fadrowski, et al. 2015). High incidence of CKDu-cases have been documented in several parts of India in the last two decades (Rajapurkar, John, et al. 2012, Varma 2015) http://www.apiindia.org/pdf/medicine_update_2017/mu_128.pdf). With an aim to find the etiological factor for CKDu-disease, a joint-team from NIOH and ICMR (Indian Council of Medical-Research) in 2005, investigated the role of ochratoxin, arsenic and cadmium (in water and food) in mediating this disease but nothing conclusive was achieved. Recently, a study has found a strong evidence for groundwater lead (at low levels due to its bio-accumulative-potential) and silica in the causation of CKDu (Mascarenhas, Mutnuri, et al. 2017).

The phase I and II metabolizing enzymes of the kidney plays a key role in the metabolism of xenobiotic as well as endogenous compounds and proximal tubules of kidney constitute a high concentration of these metabolizing enzymes compared with the other parts. Currently, proximal tubule cell lines of human origin such as RPTEC/TERT1 and HK-2 are used to understand the pathophysiology of kidney diseases, the therapeutic efficacy of drugs, and nephrotoxicity of compounds. One of the reasons hampering efficient drug development process is the lack of translational capability, one such limitation being the differing expression of metabolizing enzymes in the kidney amongst species. A research group has been working towards developing an *in vitro* system by performing metabolic characterization of RPTEC/TERT1 cell line (human renal proximal tubular origin) and comparing it with the already established HK-2 cell line. The group found equal expression of metabolic enzymes CYP1B1, 2J2, 3A4, 3A5, UGT1A9, SULT2A1 and GSTA, higher expression of 2B6, 2D6, 4A11, 4F2, 4F8, 4F11, UGT2B7, SULT1E1 in RPTEC/TERT1 and absence of GSTT in RPTEC/TERT1 compared to HK-2 at mRNA level highlighting that such differences could affect the outcome of *in vitro* nephrotoxicity prediction as well as help in interpreting and predicting probable *in vitro* behavior of the molecule being tested (Shah, Patel et al. 2017).

Several drugs and chemicals like gentamicin, cisplatin, cyclophosphamide, Fe-NTA and potassium bromate have not just been used to understand the mechanistic basis of nephrotoxicity/neuropathy but to also screen agents for their preventive/protective effects. Different agents utilizing several mechanisms have been attempted to attenuate drug-induced nephrotoxicity. A lot of interest has been focused on the role of naturally occurring substances for the control and management of renal failures. Free radicals and oxidative stress have been found to play a crucial role in renal dysfunctions and in this context, antioxidants have got a lot of prominence due to their potential to serve as prophylactic and therapeutic agents in many diseases. In this regard, several antioxidant supplementations have been investigated for their nephroprotective effects including low doses of vitamin E and C, ascorbic acid and alpha-tocopherol, dietary compounds and free radical scavengers in different experimental models to demonstrate their effective role in the prevention of drug-induced nephrotoxicity. Several pharmacological compounds, like nordihydroguaiaretic acid, curcumin, thymoquinone, have been identified that reduce cisplatin-induced nephrotoxicity and elevates its anti-tumor activity in experimental models of breast cancer. The protective effects of Zinc-chelate of histidine (Zn-Hist) pretreatment in cisplatin toxicity, hints at the importance of Zn in the stabilization of membrane integrity via displacing the redox-active metals which may be responsible for mediating peroxidative injury at target sites (Srivastava, Farookh, et al. 1995). Several agents have been identified that abrogate the nephrotoxic and tumor-promoting effects of Fe- NTA and potassium bromate in the kidney of mice and could serve as a potential chemopreventive agent while reducing nephrotoxicity (Table 10.7).

The gradual emergence of multidrug-resistant strains of Gram-negative bacteria, have triggered worldwide interest in polymyxins. However, perceived nephrotoxicity has been a major vexation restricting their early and regular use in severe sepsis. A study undertaken to explore the efficacy and safety of polymyxin B on disease outcomes in patients with severe sepsis and septic shock has revealed nephrotoxicity with 18.7% incidence which is comparable to observed nephrotoxicity. Thus polymyxin B has been suggested to be effective and safe in patients who are not receiving any other nephrotoxic drugs, with careful administration in older patients since they are more susceptible to drug induced nephrotoxicity (Nandha, Sekhri, et al. 2013). Apart from the restoration of antioxidant systems, several agents have demonstrated to act through different mechanisms. Example, the preventive effects of vitamin B-complex on Cd induced toxicity may be attributed to interference by the various constituents of vitamin B-complex in the absorption of Cd, via formation of readily excretable complexes (Tandon, Flora, et al. 1984).

Epigenetic regulation of gene expression could be a possible mechanism underlying the protection against the pathological processes of hyperglycemia in DN. Curcumin and resveratrol treatment has shown to induce alterations of histone H3 to confer protection against the development of streptozotocin-induced DN (Tikoo, Meena, et al. 2008, Tikoo, Singh, et al. 2008). Similarly, azacytidine provides treatment against cisplatin leading to the maximum reduction in tumor size, volume and nephrotoxicity by preventing phosphorylation and acetylation of histone H3 that may be involved in inhibiting disrupted gene expression in colon tumors (Tikoo, Ali, et al. 2009). A xenobiotic may have different effects depending on the dose, duration, timing of exposure, etc., similarly protective agents may also exhibit such differential effects. Comparative studies have provided direct evidence that pre-treatment of tannic acid may reduce nephrotoxic effects of cisplatin by decreasing poly (ADP-ribose) polymerase cleavage, phosphorylation of p38 and hypoacetylation of histone H4, however, co-treatment may altogether enhance its toxicity by increasing bioavailability of cisplatin (Tikoo, Bhatt, et al. 2007).

Apart from screening natural protectants, efforts have also been directed towards synthetic protectants. Vyas, et al. 2014 have synthesized a series of ternary Mn (II) complexes using a combination of thiosemicarbazones as the main ligand and bipyridyl/aminoethanethiol as ancillary ligands which mimic the structural features of the core motif in the manganese superoxide dismutase (MnSOD) where the xenobiotic binds. Various literature reports have shown the efficacy of MnSOD and its mimetics in offering protection against oxidative stress injuries. MnSOD has a unique advantage due to its location in the mitochondrial matrix since both ROS generation via respiration and ROS removal by respiration occur in the mitochondria. The synthesized compounds have demonstrated protective effects in Xanthine-Xanthine oxidase-induced oxidative stress in HEK-293 kidney cells (Vyas, Kain, et al. 2014).

Table 10.7 Few representative studies undertaken to evaluate protective/therapeutic agents against nephrotoxicants

Nephrotoxicants	Preventive/Therapeutic interventions	Model and Route of Administration	References
Renal Carcinogens			
Potassium bromate (125 mg/kg b.wt.), 24 h	***Nigella sativa* (black cumin)** (50 and 100 mg/kg b.wt., once in 5 days): Pre-exposure resulted in reduction in renal micro somal LPO, g-glutamyl trans-peptidase, xanthine oxidase, H_2O_2, recovery of content of glutathione and antioxidant enzymes, reversed the increase in a blood urea nitrogen, serum creatinine, activity of renal ODC and DNA synthesis	Albino rats, Intraperitoneal	(Khan, Sharma, et al. 2003)
	Coumarin (10 and 20 mg/kg b.wt.,/day, oral, 5 days): Pre-exposure led to a reduction in g-glutamyl transpeptidase, LPO, generation of H_2O_2, blood urea nitrogen, xanthine oxidase, renal ODC activity, serum creatinine, and DNA synthesis, renal glutathione content and recovery of antioxidant enzymes	Wistar rats, Intraperitoneal	(Khan, Sharma, et al. 2004)

Contd...

Nephrotoxicants	Preventive/Therapeutic interventions	Model and Route of Administration	References
Potassium bromate (KBrO3) (125 mg/kg b.wt.), 24 h	***Nymphaea alba*** (100 and 200 mg/kg b.wt. oral, 1h): Pre-treatment decreases xanthine oxidase, LPO, H_2O_2 generation, γ-glutamyl transpeptidase, serum creatinine, blood urea nitrogen, renal ODC activity and synthesis of DNA	Albino rats, Intraperitoneal	(Khan and Sultana, 2005)
Potassium dichromate (15 mg/kg b.wt.), 48 h	**Vitamin C** (250 mg/kg b.wt. Intraperitoneal): Pre-exposure (6 h before the toxicant) prevented an increase in creatinine levels and serum urea nitrogen, LPO generation and decrease in total sulfhydryl groups, prevented reduction in Pi transport, activities of Cu–Zn superoxide dismutase, catalase and BBM enzymes	Wistar rats, Intraperitoneal	(Fatima and Mahmood 2007)
Ferric nitrilotriacetate (9 mg/kg b.wt.), 12 h	**Garlic oil** (50 or 100 mg/kg b.wt./day, 1 week, oral): pre-treatment resulted in reduced kidney LPO and generation of H_2O_2, recovery in glutathione depletion and inhibition of antioxidant enzymes activity, at higher dose increased serum creatinine levels and blood urea nitrogen, were decreased, prevented induction of ODC activity and increase in [³H]thymidine incorporation into DNA in a dose-dependent manner	Albino rats, Intraperitoneal	(Iqbal and Athar 1998)
Ferric nitrilotriacetate (9 mg/kg b.wt.), 12 h	**Glyceryl trinitrate** (3 and 6 mg/kg b.wt., 11 hour after exposure, Intraperitoneal): recovery of GSH metabolizing enzymes and reduction in GSH content in the tissue, prevented formation of MDA, increase in activity of ODC, increased rate of DNA synthesis in a dose-dependent manner	Wistar rats, Intraperitoneal	(Rahman, Ahmed, et al. 2003)
Ferric nitrilotriacetate (9 mg/kg b.wt.), 12 h	***Ficus racemosa*** (200 and 400 mg/kg b.wt./day Oral, 5 days): pre-treatment decreased, LPO, γ-glutamyl transpeptidase H_2O_2 generation, xanthine oxidase, serum creatinine, blood urea nitrogen, kidney ODC activity, DNA synthesis and tumor incidence, glutathione content, glutathione metabolizing enzymes and antioxidant enzymes also recovered	Albino rats, Intraperitoneal	(Khan and Sultana 2005)

Contd…

Nephrotoxicants	Preventive/Therapeutic interventions	Model and Route of Administration	References
Ferric nitrilotriacetate (Fe-NTA) (9 mg/kg b.wt.)	**Perillyl Alcohol** (0.5% per kg b.wt. and 1% per kg b.wt./daily, Oral, 7 days): pre-exposure reversed formation of MDA, activity of xanthine oxidase and ornithine decarboxylase, 3[H]thymidine incorporation in DNA with reduction in serum toxicity markers such as creatinine, blood urea nitrogen, restoration of reduced glutathione content, and its associated enzymes thereby inhibiting oxidative injury and tumor promotional events	Wistar rats, Intraperitoneal	(Jahangir and Sultana 2007)
Ferric nitrilotriacetate (Fe-NTA) (8 mg/kg b.wt.), 4 h	**Molsidomine** (10 mg/kg b.wt. perorally, 30 min): Pre-exposure decreased BUN levels and serum creatinine, lowered LPO, restored GSH levels and normal morphology, elevated total nitric oxide levels, attenuated serum levels of TNF-α, postulated due to NO donor ability	Wistar rats, Intraperitoneal	(Gupta, Sharma, et al. 2008)
Drugs			
Acetaminophen (1 g/kg b.wt.), 30 days *In vitro*: 0.5 mM, 1 mM, 2.5 mM, 5 mM and 10 mM, 24 h	**Morin** (30 mg/kg b.wt., 30 days, Oral): Pre and co-treatment prevented toxicity mediated damage by stabilization of Nrf2 nuclear retention, reduced renal damage by Akt-1/Gsk3β/Fyn kinase pathway via PHLPP2 de-activation	Wistar rats, Oral Normal rat kidney cell line NRK-52E	(Mathur, Rizvi, et al. 2016)
Cyclosporine A (15 mg/kg b.wt./day), 30 days	**Ellagic acid (EA):** EA as suspension 50 mg/kg b.wt./day, EA loaded PLGA-DMAB nanoparticles 50 mg/kg b.wt./every 3rd day: co-exposure resulted in decreased MDA levels in plasma and kidneys, prevented the increase in the BUN level, reduced glomerular collapse, nanoparticles were found to elicit more protective effect than the suspension even at one third the dose of the suspension	Sprague Dawley rats, Oral	(Sonaje, Italia, et al. 2007)
Cyclosporine (20 mg/kg b.wt./day), 21 days	**Resveratrol** (2, 5 and 10 mg/kg b.wt./day, peroral, 24 h before and co-administration for 21 days): 5 and 10 mg prominently improved kidney dysfunction; levels of total nitric oxide in tissue and urine, kidney oxidative stress and inhibited changes in morphology	Wistar rats, Subcutaneous	(Chander, Tirkey, et al. 2005)

Contd...

Nephrotoxicants	Preventive/Therapeutic interventions	Model and Route of Administration	References
Streptozotocin 45 mg/kg b.wt.), single dose	**Quercetin** (10 mg/kg b.wt./day, 4 weeks, Oral): Post exposure attenuated kidney dysfunction and oxidative stress by preventing increase in blood glucose, polyuria, proteinuria and by promoting increased creatinine and enhanced urea clearance	Sprague-Dawley rats, Intraperitoneal	(Anjaneyulu and Chopra 2004)
Streptozotocin (65 mg/kg b.wt.), single dose	**Curcumin** (15 and 30mg/kg b.wt./day, 2 weeks, Oral): Post exposure attenuated renal dysfunction and oxidative stress by preventing increase in blood glucose, polyuria, proteinuria and by promoting increased creatinine and enhanced urea clearance	Sprague-Dawley rats, Intraperitoneal	(Sharma, Kulkarni, et al. 2006)
Streptozotocin (65 mg/kg b.wt.), single dose	**Resveratrol** (5 and 10mg/kg b.wt., Oral from 4 weeks-6 weeks): Post exposure attenuated kidney dysfunction and oxidative stress by preventing increase in blood glucose, polyuria, proteinuria and by promoting increased creatinine and enhanced urea clearance	Sprague-Dawley rats, Intraperitoneal	(Sharma, Anjaneyulu, et al. 2006)
Streptozotocin (55 mg/kg b.wt.), single dose	**Tocotrienol** (25, 50 and 100 mg/kg b.wt/day.), α-tocopherol (100 mg/kg b.wt./day), 5 weeks-8 weeks, Oral): Co-exposure of tocotrienol (100 mg/kg) was demonstrated to be more effective than α-tocopherol (100 mg/kg), decreased oxidative–nitrosative stress, release of profibrotic cytokines (TNF-α, TGF-β1) and chronic inflammation parameters (active p65 subunit of NFκβ) in a dose dependent manner	Wistar rats, Intraperitoneal	(Kuhad and Chopra 2009)
Cyclophosphamide (75 mg/kg b.wt.), 24 h	**Melatonin** (0.1 mg/kg b.wt./day, 15 days, Oral): Pre-treatment prevented augmentation of the level of lipid peroxidation, blood GSSG and acid phosphatase	Swiss albino mice, Intraperitoneal	(Manda and Bhatia 2003)
Cyclophosphamide (150 mg/kg b.wt.), 16 h	**Glutamine** (1 g/kg b.wt. oral, 2 h): Pre-treatment reduced glutathione depletion and increased myeloperoxidase activity, however, it did not prevent the induced lipid peroxidation, protein carbonylation and renal damage(Abraham, Isaac et al. 2011)	Wistar rats, Intraperitoneal	(Abraham, Isaac, et al. 2011)

Contd...

Nephrotoxicants	Preventive/Therapeutic interventions	Model and Route of Administration	References
Cyclophosphamide (150 mg/kg b.wt.), 16 h	**Aminoguanidine** (200 mg/kg b.wt. 1 h, intraperitoneal): Pre-treatment attenuated induced renal damage histologically, LPO, oxidation of proteins, decrease in reduced GSH, lowered activities of the antioxidant enzymes and MPO activity	Wistar rats, Intraperitoneal	(Abraham and Rabi 2011)
Gentamicin (100 mg/kg b.wt./day), 10 days	**DLα- lipoic acid** (10 and 25 mg/kg b.wt./day, gastric intubation, 10 days): Co-administration increased the activity of glycolytic enzymes, ATPases and the TCA cycle enzymes, the protection conferred at 25 mg/kg/day of lipoic acid was greater than that at 10 mg level	Wistar rats, Intraperitoneal	(Sandhya, Mohandass, et al. 1995)
Gentamicin (80 mg/kg b.wt./day), 8 days	**Melatonin** (5 mg/kg b.wt./day, intragastric 3 days prior and 8 days co-administration): decreased blood urea and levels of serum creatinine with increased creatine clearance and decreased excretion of urinary N-acetyl-ß-D- glucosaminidase, glucose, and protein, also reduced plasma and kidney lipid peroxidation levels, reduced tubular epithelial loss in the renal cortex	Wistar rats, Intraperitoneal	(Shifow, Kumar, et al. 2000)
Gentamicin (80 mg/kg b.wt./day), 8 days	***Ginkgo biloba* extract** (300 mg/kg b.wt. oral, 2 days before and after 8 days concurrently): Alterations in blood urea, serum creatinine and creatinine clearance were inhibited, lowered kidney and plasma tissue MDA	Wistar rats, Intraperitoneal	(Naidu, Shifow, et al. 2000)
Gentamicin (80 mg/kg b.wt./day), 10 days	**Dietary fish oil** (15%, 10 days): Co-supplementationdecreased blood urea nitrogen and serum creatinine, decreased lactate and glucose-6-phosphate dehydrogenases activity, increased resistance to gentamicin's induced adverse effects and prevented reduction in ^{32}Pi uptake across brush border membrane	Wistar rats, Intraperitoneal	(Priyamvada, Priyadarshini, et al. 2008)
Gentamicin (100 mg/kg b.wt./day), 6 days	**Diallyl sulfide** (150mg/kg b.wt./day, intraperitoneal, 6 days): Co-administration prevented elevation in MPO and LPO levels, reduction in catalase, superoxide dismutase,	Albino rats, Intraperitoneal	(Kalayarasan, Prabhu, et al. 2009)

Contd...

Nephrotoxicants	Preventive/Therapeutic interventions	Model and Route of Administration	References
	glutathione peroxidase, glutathione reductase, glutathione-S-transferase and quinone reductase activities, further prevented elevation in the immunoreactivity of nitric oxide synthase, NF-κB and TNF-α		
Gentamicin (80 mg/kg b.wt./day), 10 days	**Green tea extract** ((3%), twice /day, 25 days, oral): reduced serum creatinine, cholesterol, BUN, LPO, elevated superoxide dismutase and catalase activities, restored hexokinase activity, enhanced enzymes of BBM and Pi transport	Wistar rats, Intraperitoneal	(Khan, Priyamvada, et al. 2009)
Gentamicin (85 mg/kg b.wt./day), 8 days	**Sinapic acid (10 and 20 mg/kg b.wt./day):** Co-exposurerestored renal functions, increased antioxidant levels, decreased LPO and NO levels, leading to decrease in oxidative and nitrosative stress, lowered cytokines (TNF-α and IL-6), expression of nuclear NF-κB, NF-κB-DNA binding and MPO activity, lowered apoptosis and neutrophil infiltration in renal tubules	Wistar rats, Intraperitoneal	(Ansari, Raish, et al. 2016)
Gentamicin (100 mg/kg b.wt./day), 8 days	**Hydroalcoholic leaves extracts of** *Eclipta prostrata* (250 mg/kg and 500 mg/kg,p.o. 8 days): Coexposure conferred protection via antioxidant activity	Wistar rats, Intraperitoneal	(Ahmad, Al-Subaie, et al. 2018)
Cisplatin (50 μg/ml), 30, 60, 90, and 120 min (3 mg/kg b.wt.)	**Phenolic antioxidants:** eugenol (10 mg/kg b.wt. 1 h) pre-treatment was more active (decreased MDA) in vero cells and in rat renal cortical slices than eugenol (EG) and dehydrozingerone (DZ), however none of the test compounds were able to arrest the reduction of the GSH content induced by cisplatin in either the vero cells or the renal cortical slice model	Vero (African Green Monkey Kidney) cells Wistar rats, Intraperitoneal	(Rao, Kumar, et al. 1999)
Cisplatin (6 mg/kg b.wt.)once a week for 2 weeks	**Glutathione ester** (10 mM, 10 mL/kg b.wt. /daily, 14 days, oral): Co-administration resulted in decreased nephrotoxicological parameters like urea,uric acid and creatinine, decreased the accumulation of platinum in kidney, restoration of marker enzymes, alkaline phosphalase,	Albino rats, Intraperitoneal	(Babu, Ebrahim, et al. 1999)

Contd...

Nephrotoxicants	Preventive/Therapeutic interventions	Model and Route of Administration	References
	acid phosphatase, aspartate aminotransferase and alanine aminotransferase		
Cisplatin (10 mg/kg b.wt.), 24 and 48 h	**Ascorbic acid and α-tocopherol** (250 and 500 mg/kg b.wt. perorally 1 h before and 24, 48 h post exposure):both vitamins at 500 mg/kg protected via reducing concentration of urea and creatinine, restoration of renal antioxidant enzymes only in 500 mg/kg groups, both increased the concentration of GSH and prevented the increase of LPO	Swiss albino mice, Intraperitoneal	(Ajith, Usha, et al. 2007)
Cisplatin (5 mg/kg b.wt.)	**Curcumin** (15, 30, and 60 mg/kg b.wt. 2 days before and 3 days after): restored kidney function, reduced LPO, elevated GSH levels and superoxide dismutase and catalase activities, with lowered serum TNF-α levels in a dose dependent manner	Wistar rats, Intraperitoneal	(Kuhad, Pilkhwal, et al. 2007)
Cisplatin (8 mg/kg b.wt.), on the 7th day, 3 days	**Telmisartan** (2.5, 5 and 10 mg/kg, oral, 10 days): Pretreatment normalized decreased kidney functions, changed proxidant–antioxidant balance and acute tubular necrosis, inhibited MAPK induced inflammation and apoptosis, 10mg/kg revealed maximum nephroprotective effect	Wistar rats, Intraperitoneal	(Malik, Suchal, et al. 2015)
Cisplatin (8 mg/kg b.wt.), on the 7th day	**Epicatechin gallate** (1.25, 2.5, and 5 mg/kg b.wt; intraperitoneal, 10 days):pretreatment normalized cisplatin-induced oxidative stress, renal function, and histopathological changes. ECG also prevented the activation of the MAPK pathway, and attenuated inflammation and apoptosis in rats	Albino Wistar rats, Intraperitoneal	(Malik, Suchal, et al. 2016)
Cisplatin (5 mg/kg b.wt./daily), 5 days	**Oxovanadium (IV) complex** (1 mg/kg b.wt. peroral): Co-expousre for 9 days/pre exposure for 7 days induced attenuation of kidney oxidative stress and increase of antioxidant status, lowered serum levels of creatinine and BUN, improved histopathological lesions, induced Nrf2-mediated activation of antioxidant response	Swiss albino mice, Intraperitoneal	(Basu, Bhattacharjee, et al. 2017)

Contd...

Nephrotoxicants	Preventive/Therapeutic interventions	Model and Route of Administration	References
	element (ARE) pathway and expression of ARE-driven cytoprotective proteins, heme oxygenase 1 and NAD(P)H: quinone oxidoreductase 1		
Cisplatin (8 mg/kg b.wt.), on the 8th day	**Galangin** (25, 50 and 100 mg/kg b.wt./day, oral, 10 days):100 mg/kg restored kidney function, morphology, reduced inflammation, oxidative stress and activation of apoptotis with lowered DNA fragmentation, also reduced expression of MAPK pathway proteins	Wistar rats, Intraperitoneal	(Tomar, Vasisth, et al. 2017)
Cisplatin (7.5 mg/kg b.wt.), 5 days	**Curcumin** (120 mg/kg b.wt. oral, 5 days): Pre-exposure attenuated nephrotoxicity by loweing the inflammatory markers (TNF-α, IL-6, and IL-8), increase in plasma albumin levels, inhibited disruption of renal architecture	Sprague-Dawley rats, Intraperitoneal	(Kumar, Barua, et al. 2017)
Cisplatin (5 mg/kg b.wt.)	**Disulfiram and its copper chelate (**50 mM/kg b.wt./day, 5 days, Oral: Post exposure attenuated cisplastin-induced rise in the serum/urine creatinine and BUN, reduced MDA levels and nitric oxide, reversed depletion of SOD, catalase, and GSH	Wistar rats, Intraperitoneal	(Khairnar, Mahajan, et al. 2019)

<table>
<tr><td colspan="4" align="center">Metals</td></tr>
<tr><td>Lead (8 mg/kg b.wt./day), 6 weeks</td><td>Aqueous extract of Terminalia catappa l. leaves (100mg/kg b.wt./day, 28days, Oral): Post toxicant exposure reverted the levels of transaminases, phosphatases and lysosomal marker enzymes</td><td>Wistar rats, Intraperitoneal</td><td>(Vijayaprakash, Langeswaran, et al. 2012)</td></tr>
<tr><td>Arsenic (20 mg/kg b.wt.), once in 4 days</td><td>Flax seed oil (15%, 14 days, Oral): Pre-treatment prevented increase of serum creatinine and blood urea nitrogen, reduction in particular activities of brush border membrane enzymes both in renal tissue homogenates and isolated membrane vesicles, reduction in metabolic enzymes activity and antioxidant defence system</td><td>Wistar rats, Intraperitoneal</td><td>(Rizwan, Naqshbandi, et al. 2014)</td></tr>
</table>

Contd...

Nephrotoxicants	Preventive/Therapeutic interventions	Model and Route of Administration	References
Cadmium (3 mg/kg b.wt./day), 3 days	**Selenium (2 mg/kg b.wt./day), intraperitoneal:** co-administration reduced the induced enzymuria, proteinuria and elevation of serum enzymes, also prevented inhibition in the activities of renal enzymes observed on the 4th day of Cd administration, also prevented uptake of renal copper on 4th and 8th day, did not prevent accumulation of Cd in kidney on the 8th day	Albino rats, Subcutaneous	(Flora, Behari, et al. 1982)
Cadmium (6 mg/kg. b.wt.), once	**Nickel** (6 mg/kg b.wt. Intraperitoneal, 3 days): Pre-treatment reduced enzymuria, amino aciduria, proteinuria, and elevation in serum enzymes activity	Albino rats, Intramuscular	(Tandon, Khandelwal, et al. 1984)
Cadmium (3 mg/kg. b.wt./day), 3 days	**Vitamin B complex** (10 mg/kg b.wt., Oral): Co-administration resulted in lesser cadmium accumulation in renal tissues, reduced most of the enzyme alterations (lactic dehydrogenase (LDH), glutamic oxalacetic transaminase(GOT) in urine, serum, kidney	Albino rats, Subcutaneous	(Tandon, Flora, et al. 1984)
Cadmium (20 mg/kg b.wt.), 30 days	**Calcium + Zinc** (2 mg/kg each, Oral) or **Vitamin-E** (20 mg/kg body weight, oral): Co-exposure eversed perturbations in oxidative stress marker enzymes catalase, superoxide dismutase, glutathione peroxidase, glutathione reductase, glutathione-S-transferase and lipid peroxidase in kidney mitochondrial fractions, Vit-E revealed higher inhibitory activity than Calcium + Zinc	Albino Wistar rats, Oral	(Adi, Burra, et al. 2016)
Sodium fluoride (5 mg/kg/b.wt./day) and/or arsenic trioxide (0.5 mg/kg b.wt./day), 30 days	**Calcium phosphate and vitamins C and E** (30 days): Individual andcombined supplementation post exposure restored total protein, creatinine and the activities of acid and alkaline phosphatase (ACP and ALP),	Swiss mice, Oral	(Chinoy and Shah 2004)

Contd...

Nephrotoxicants	Preventive/Therapeutic interventions	Model and Route of Administration	References
Flouride (10 mg/kg b.wt./day), 30 days	**Melatonin** (10 mg/kg b.wt./day, 30 days intraperitoneal): Co-exposure prevented decline in the activities of ACP, ALP, and SDH as well as the levels of protein and creatinine along with a restoration in kidney gravimetric data	Albino mice, Oral	(Rao, Chawla, et al. 2009)
Acetaminophen (2.5 mM) 1 mg/kg b.wt./day, 30 days	**Morin** (10 µM, 3 h, 30 mg/kg b.wt/day): Pre-exposure enhanced viability, increased glutathione levels, prevented oxidative stress, enhanced Nrf2 nuclear translocation in NRK-52E cell line Pre and co-treatment afforded protection via its intervention with Akt-1/Gsk3β/Fyn kinase pathway through PHLPP2 de-activation	NRK-52E, Wistar rats, Oral	Mathur, Rizvi, et al. 2016

10.4 Reproductive Toxicity

A crucial aspect of determining safety of chemicals is assessing their potential of reproductive toxicity, which includes deleterious effects on sexual function, adult male and female fertility, and developmental toxicity in the offspring including teratogenicity (to produce embryotoxicity and congenital disabilities). A reproductive toxicant may interfere with the sexual functions and behavior, conception, birth, growth, and development usually expressed/manifested as abnormalaties in sexual behavior, decreased fertility, adverse pregnancy outcomes, or alterations of other functions which are dependent on the integrity of the reproductive system. Teratogenesis signifies the structural abnormalties during fetal development, which is different from other types of drug-induced fetal damage such as growth retardation, dysplasia (e.g., Iodine-deficiency-related goiter), or the asymmetrical limb reduction. Human fertility is a complex phenomena, dependent on the synergy of male and female reproductive competence in which environmental, genetic, physiological and behavioral factors may interact. The need of inclusion of DART (Development and Reproductive Toxicity) screening in the safety assessment of chemicals became a significant concern worldwide in the mid-1960s post the discovery that the sedative, thalidomide, caused limb and craniofacial abnormalties in about 10,000 European babies (Brent and Holmes 1988, Ances 2002).

A number of guidelines have outlined a series of separate reproductive and developmental toxicity studies from fertilization through adulthood and in some cases to the second generation, which covers the assessment of fertility and other aspects of reproductive function in adults, prenatal developmental toxicity (including teratogenicity) and postnatal growth and development. Fertility, reproduction and multigeneration studies have been conducted in accordance with renewed OECD guidelines using the one and two-generation reproductive toxicity tests to screen metals, pesticides, pharmaceuticals, NCEs for their reproductive toxicity/teratogenic potential in compliance with the ICH guidelines. With the inclusion of new tests, India also revamped its reproductive toxicity testing activities. Complex multigeneration studies have also been undertaken to provide information on the effects of chemicals on all aspects of reproductive cycle. Improved testing paradigm using extended one generation testing have also been carried out.

Reproductive hazards from toxicant exposure in males have been one of the fastest expanding areas of concern in toxicology in India with substantial evidence piling up portending the deleterious effects of occupational/environmental toxicants on male reproduction. Since the 1970s, several authors have suggested at the appalling drop in the quality of sperm and consequently a rise in male infertility rates. Studies have shown a disturbing trend of a substantial decrease in sperm concentration (43%) and a higher abnormal sperm morphology (30%) in Indian men over a period of 10 years from the late 1980s to 1990s (Gopalkrishnan 1998). Since the 1980s, identification of various factors like exposure to various environmental toxicants like metals, pesticides, phthalates, duration of exposure (Danadevi, Rozati, et al. 2003) as well as lifestyle factors (like tobacco chewing) (Kumar and Gautam 2006) have been causally linked to reproductive anomalies, disruption of reproductive hormones, adverse effects on spermatogenesis and on the reproductive outcome of their spouse (namely stillbirths, abortion, neonatal deaths and congenital defects, as in the case of lead) (Rupa, Reddy, et al. 1991, Srinivasa, Maxim, et al. 2015). Such adversities have also been significantly correlated with the presence of toxicants in the seminal plasma and serum as well as altered sperm quality and serum levels of testicular enzymes and hormones (Kumar, Pant, et al. 2000, Pant, Mathur, et al. 2004, Pant, Shukla, et al. 2008). Kumar, et al. have been the first research group to demonstrate the detrimental effects of low-level radiation on reproductive aspects in health workers via higher incidence of hypermethylation (Kumar, Salian, et al. 2013).

Over the years the male reproductive system has been assessed for the effects of acute and chronic effects of xenobiotics using biochemical (seminal proteins), morphological (atrophy, degeneration) and behavioral (libido, sexual performance) parameters, compromised fertility associated with sperm motility, abnormal sperm concentration and semen quality (denoted in terms of number of sperm, density-viscosity, volume, sperm morphology), impaired spermatogenesis, steroidogenesis and hormonal imbalance in the exposed organisms. Various research groups have also suggested the affinity of metals and pesticides, polymers for the testis and incorporation into sperm. Table 10.8 provides a comprehensive account of the most representative studies.

Table 10.8 Few representative studies on the effects/mechanism of action of male reproductive toxicants

Reproductive toxicants	Effects on Male Reproductive System	Model	References
Pesticides			
Quinalphos (7-14 mg/kg b.wt./day), 14 days	Decreased testicular mass, increased testicular ACE acitivity, disruption of spermatogenesis with increasing doses	Sprague–Dawley rats, Oral gavage	(Sarkar, Mohanakum, ar et al. 2000)
Quinalphos (250 μg/kg b.wt./day) 13 and 26 days	Lowered activity levels of prostatic acid phosphatase and reduced fructose content of the accessory sex glands, lowered plasma levels of FSH and testosterone	Wistar rats, Intraperitoneal	(Ray, Chatterjee, et al. 1991)
Aldrin (150 μg/kg b.wt./day), 13 and 26 days	Suppression of 3β-hydroxysteroid dehydrogenase and 17β-hydroxysteroid dehydrogenase activities, along with accumulation of cholesterol in the testicular tissues, inhibits testicular testosterone production and spermatogenesis in rats by interfering with pituitary FSH and LH release	Wistar rats, Intraperitoneal	(Chatterjee, Ray, et al. 1988)
Endosulfan (2.5, 5.0, 7.5 and 10 mg/kg b.wt./day), 15 and 30 days	Disruption in pattern of steroidogenesis enzymes, inhibition of testicular androgen biosynthesis, and reduced levels of plasma gonadotrophins (FSH and LH), steroidogenic enzymes (3β and 17β hydroxysteroid dehydrogenases) were considerably lowered	Druckrey rats, Oral	(Singh and Pandey 1990)
Endosulfan (2.5, 5.0 and 10 mg/kg b.wt./day), 70 days	Reduced sperm counts in the cauda epididymis and intratesticular spermatid counts associated with increase in the activities of testicular marker enzymes (lactic dehydrogenase,sorbitol dehydrogenase, glucose-6-phosphate and gamma glutamyl transpeptidase)	Druckrey rats, Oral	(Sinha, Narayan, et al. 1995)

Contd...

Reproductive toxicants	Effects on Male Reproductive System	Model	References
Endosulfan (2.5, 5.0 and 10 mg/kg b.wt./5 day/week) from 3 weeks-90 days)	Dose dependent decrease in sperm count, spermatids number, reduction in daily sperm production, increase in the activities of LDH, GGT and G6PDH enzymes, suggestive of impaired sexual maturation	Druckrey rats, Oral	(Sinha, Narayan, et al. 1997)
Malathion (50, 150 and 250 mg/kg/b.wt./day), 60 days	Reduction in testes weight, epididymis, ventral prostate and seminal vesicle, testicular and epididymal sperm density and levels of testosterone decreased	Wistar rats, Oral	(Choudhary, Goyal, et al. 2008)
Lindane (50 mg or 100 mg/kg b.wt./day), 5 days in a week for 120 days)	Accumulation of HCH and its isomers in sperm and testes, alterations in testosterone metabolism and levels of plasma testosterone, changes in marker testicular enzymes activity viz. glucose-6-P-dehydrogenase, sorbitol dehydrogenase, β-glucuronidase and γ-glutamyl transpeptidase	Wistar rats, Dermal	(Prasad, Pant, et al. 1995)
Lindane (5 mg/kg b.wt.), (0, 3, 6, 12, 24 and 72 h)	Decreased activities of catalase and superoxide dismutase with elevation in LPO levels, significant between 6 and 24 h post-exposure, a drastic induction in the level of inducible HSP70 between 6 and 24 h of exposure, levels of secretory clusterin significantly elevated at 12 and 24 h	Wistar rats, Oral	(Saradha, Vaithinathan, et al. 2008)
Thiram (5, 10 and 25 mg/kg b.wt./day), 30, 60 and 90 days	Higher testes weight at 25 mg after exposure of 90 days, with degeneration of seminiferous tubules, dose dependent decrease in the activities of testicular enzymes such as alkaline phosphatase, lactate dehydrogenase, glucose 6-phosphate dehydrogen phoshpate, acid phosphatase and succinate dehydrogenase activities reduced significantly, serum cholesterol and testicular free sialic acid elevated at all doses	Albino rats, Oral	(Mishra, Srivastava, et al. 1993)

Contd...

Reproductive toxicants	Effects on Male Reproductive System	Model	References
Argemone oil (AO) (0.1 µl/ml, 1.5 µl/ml and 2.5 µl /ml), **argemone alkaloid(AA)** and **sanguinarine (SA)** (1 µg/ml, 15 µg/ml and 25 µg/ml, respectively) 24 h and 48 h	Dose dependent rise in germ cell detachment and reduction in viability of detached germ cells, dose and time dependent inhibition of MMP, exposure with lowest concentration of AO/AA and SA for 24 h lead to 5.2, 4.4 and 3.6-fold rise in the percentage of early apoptotic cells, respectively which further elevated to 8.3, 4.75 and 5.81-fold, respectively at 48 h in the cells undergoing early apoptosis	Rat Sertoli cell culture	(Mishra, Saxena, et al. 2009)
di(2-ethylhexyl) phthalate (DEHP) (250, 500, 1000 and 2000 mg/kg b.wt./day), 15 days	Dose dependent reduction in sperm count, γ-glutamyl transpeptidase and lactate dehydrogenase activity was elevated, a rise in β-glucuronidase activity and reduction in acid phosphatase activity at the highest dose, the sorbitol dehydrogenase activity was lowered on exposure to 1000 and 2000 mg/kg	Albino rats, Oral	(Parmar, Srivastava, et al. 1986)
Acrylonitrile (10 mg/kg b.wt./day), 60 days	Reduction in acid phosphatase and testicular sorbitol dehydrogenase activity, higher activity for β-glucuronidase and lactate dehydrogenase, seminiferous tubules degeneration, lowering of sperm counts	Albino rats, Oral	(Tandon, Saxena, et al. 1988)

Studies have not only focused on understanding the effects of xenobiotics on the adult reproductive system but also the developing system. This is significant because young, developing animals are more vulnerable to the toxicity of metals than adults (Sinha, Narayan, et al. 1995, Sinha, Narayan, et al. 1997). Xenobiotic exposure in the prepubertal stage of sexual maturity may result in permanent injuries to the gonads. These changes are suggestive of a higher risk to developing testes if they are exposed to metals like Cr^{6+} during prepubertal stages of development, which may consequently disrupt the normal testicular physiology at adult stages of life (Saxena, Murthy, et al. 1990). Similarly, exposure to endosulfan during developing phases, i.e., testicular maturation period may lead to disrupted spermatogenesis at sexual maturity (Sinha, Narayan, et al. 1995, Sinha, Narayan, et al. 1997). There are several studies of endosulfan's testicular toxicity that manifest as reduced spermatogenesis and steroidogenesis, as evidenced via a reduction in spermatid count in testes and sperm count in the cauda epididymis accompanied by alterations in marker enzymes for steroidogenesis in adult animals (Singh and Pandey 1989, Singh and Pandey 1990, Sinha, Narayan, et al. 1995, Chitra, Latchoumycandane et al. 1999). There are several situations in which outcomes of animal experiments have long before predicted reproductive effects in humans linked to environmental exposures. Chronic endosulfan exposure (of more than 20 years) in male children living near the Kasorgad district has been shown to delay the process of sexual maturation and interfere with synthesis of sex hormones (Saiyed, Dewan, et al. 2003). Detailed studies in adult rats have provided early evidence of adverse effects on spermatogenesis (reduced spermatid counts, abnormalities in the sperm, alterations in the enzymes of testicular activities, such as sorbitol dehydrogenase, lactate dehydrogenase, glucose-6-phosphate dehydrogenase and γ-glutamyl transpeptidase) (Sinha, Narayan, et al. 1995, Khan and Sinha 1996).

Extensive research over the years has resulted in the establishment of new information such as the female reproductive system is also quite vulnerable to environmentally induced reproductive abnormalities. Epidemiological studies have also established strong evidence between maternal exposure to teratogens before and during pregnancy and several birth defects (Sharma 2013). Numerous cases manifest in India with severe teratogenic effects such as congenital disorders like fetal alcoholic syndrome, velproic syndrome, congenital rubella syndrome (CRS) (Dewan and Gupta 2012). Despite a decrease in the disease burden of numerous vaccine-preventable diseases via childhood immunization, CRS (due to primary maternal rubella infection) has accounted for severe preventable morbidity such as childhood blindness, heart disease, deafness, and mental retardation (Dewan and Gupta 2012). Anticonvulsants consumed during periods of pregnancy have also been associated with a higher risk of abnormalities and delay in development. Sodium valproate, a widely employed antiepileptic drug and mood stabilizer, licensed for use in 1978, manifested its first report on adverse effect to the fetus exposed to it in 1980. Since then the potential dysmorphogenic and teratogenic effects of valproic acid have been emphasized (Sodhi, Poddar, et al. 2001, Kulkarni, Zaheeruddin, et al. 2006).

The ovaries and ova, constituting the female reproductive system, have been demonstrated to be vulnerable to direct damage by potent reproductive toxicants from an extended period of time from meiosis to ovulation. Various metals, pesticides have shown to affect various female reproductive processes such as the rate of ovulation, length of gestation, follicular development and maturation leading to atresia (Junaid, Murthy, et al. 1996, Murthy, Junaid, et al. 1996), inhibition of implantation (Bindali and Kaliwal 2002) and disruption of estrous cycle (Rao and Kaliwal 2002). Ovarian toxicity has been attributed to an alteration in the endogenous pituitary gonadotropin and/or steroidogenic secretion, progesterone values and changes in the xenobiotic metabolizing enzymes (Junaid, Chowdhuri, et al. 1997). Presence of the variant allele CYP2C19*2 has been associated with a reduced risk of ovarian toxicity in Indian patients treated with cyclophosphamide (Singh, Saxena, et al. 2007). Alterations in the onset of puberty, sexual behavior, fertility, cyclicity, gestation time, pregnancy outcomes (e.g., dystocia, sex and number of pups, live births, and runts), lactation, and premature menopause, are few of the potential manifestations of reproductive toxicity in females. Few representative studies on the effects of chemicals on the female reproductive system have been provided below (Table 10.9).

Table 10.9 Few representative studies on the effects/mechanism of action of female reproductive toxicants

Reproductive Toxicants	Effects on Female Reproductive System and/or Embryotoxic/Teratogenic Effects	Model and Route of Administration	References
Metals			
Lead (0, 2, 4 or 8 mg/kg b.wt./day) for 60 days (5 days/week)	Affects follicular development and maturation, small and medium follicles were adversely affected even at the low dose (2 mg), large follicles were adversely affected mostly at the high dose, correlated well with increased blood lead levels	Swiss Albino mice, Oral	(Junaid, Chowdhuri, et al. 1997)
Lead (266 mg/kg, 532 mg/kg and 1064 mg/kg b.wt./day), gestational exposure day 10 – day 17 and from day 10 till parturition and lactation (post natal day 21)	Reduction in the body weight and size of pups exposed *in utero*, all pups born were weak, showed delayed physical development, dose-dependent rise in the postimplantation loss (PIL)	Swiss Albino mice, Oral	(Sharma and Mogra 2013)
Chromium (250, 500, 1000 ppm, every day of gestation)	Dose-dependent embryo lethal effects, PIL at 1000 ppm, litter size reduction and reduced ossification	Albino mice, Oral	(Trivedi, Saxena, et al. 1989)
Chromium (250 ppm, 500 ppm and 750 ppm/day), 20 days and (0.05 ppm, 0.5 ppm and 5.0 ppm/day), 90 days	750 ppm revealed rise in atretic follicles and congestion in stromal tissue, decrease in the follicles' number at various stages of their maturation in a dose dependent manner, the estrus cycle duration elevated in 750 ppm group, rise in levels of blood chromium in a dose	Swiss albino mice, Oral	(Murthy, Junaid, et al. 1996)

Contd...

Reproductive Toxicants	Effects on Female Reproductive System and/or Embryotoxic/Teratogenic Effects	Model and Route of Administration	References
	dependent manner, ultrastructural results showed disintegrated cell membranes of two layered follicular cells and changed villiform mitochondria in thecal cells of 5 ppm group		
Chromium (250 ppm, 500 ppm and 750 ppm/day), gestational day 6-day 14	Dose-dependent presence of chromium in maternal blood, placenta and fetuses, abnormal fetal development, decreased fetal weight, number of fetuses (live and dead) per mother and higher incidences of dead fetuses and resorptions in 750 ppm group with increased incidences of reduced ossification	Swiss albino mice, Oral	(Junaid, Murthy, et al. 1996)
Nickel (46.125, 92.25, and 184.5) mg/kg b.w., gestational exposure day 6-13	Dose-dependent reduction in the body weight of the pregnant females and foetuses and lowered implantation sites	Swiss albino mice, Oral	(Saini, Nair, et al. 2013)
	Pesticides		
Endosulfan (1 or 2 mg/kg b.wt./day), gestational day 12 till parturition	Dose dependent alteration in spermatogenesis via changes in sorbitol dehydrogenase and testicular lactate dehydrogenase at PND 100, decrease in spermatid count in testis and sperm count in cauda epididymis, decreased weight of seminal vesicle and epididymis	Druckery rats, Oral	(Sinha, Adhikari, et al. 2001)
Methyl Parathion (5 mg/kg b.wt./day), 1,5, 10 and 15 days	10 and 15 days exposure led to drastic reduction in ovarian weight gain with -21.36% and -31.98% hypertrophy, respectively, a reduction in healthy follicles, disruption of number and duration of each phase of estrous cycle	Wistar rats, Intraperitoneal	(Asmathbanu and Kaliwal 1997)
Dimethoate (28 mg/kg b.wt.) on day 1 for 5, 10 and 15 days	Exposure for 10 or 15 days led to a reduction in ovarian weight (19.84% and 0.76% hypertrophy, respectively), lowering in healthy follicles, and higher atretic follicles, reduced number of estrous cycles, duration of proestrus, estrus, and metestrus, a rise in diestrus phase	Swiss albino mice, Oral	(Mahadevaswami and Kaliwal 2002)

Contd...

Reproductive Toxicants	Effects on Female Reproductive System and/or Embryotoxic/Teratogenic Effects	Model and Route of Administration	References
Dimethoate (4, 8, and 16 mg/kg b.wt./day), gestational day 6 to postnatal day (PND) 21	Gonadal inhibition as observed as decrease in weight and histopathological changes in epididymis and testis, lowered sperm counts, abnormalities in pituitary-testicular axis of luteinizing hormone cells, lowered size and number, decreased plasma LH and testosterone levels at 8 and 16mg/kg, adverse effects on testicular Leydig cells and steroidgenesis inhibition by lowering of testosterone levels (~70%), GD length and stillbirths were elevated with a reduction in body weight and anogenital distance of the fetus with the highest dose at PND 22, these changes persisted in young adults (PND 63)	Swiss albino mice, Oral	(Verma and Mohanty 2009)
Mancozeb (500, 600, 700, and 800 mg/kg b.wt./day), 15 days	700 and 800 mg group showed a reduction in ovarian hypertrophy with 28.2 and 22.8% hypertrophy, respectively, reduced number of estrous cycles, duration of proestrus, estrus, and metestrus with higher duration of the diestrus phase at 600, 700, and 800 mg	Wistar rats, Oral	(Mahadevaswami, Jadaramkunti, et al. 2000)
Mancozeb (18, 24, 30 and 36 mg/kg b.wt./day), 8 days	100% pre-implantation loss in 36 mg group, partial inhibition of implantation in 24 and 30 mg with 53.44 and 90.16% respectively, complete inhibition of implantation in 5 days with 100% pre-implantation loss and partial inhibition of implantation of 3 days treated mice with 75% pre-implantation loss, reduction in diestrus phase with higher estrus phase, lowered uterus weight with 24, 30 and 36 mg and for 3 and 5 days with 36 mg	Swiss albino mice, Oral	(Bindali and Kaliwal 2002)
Monocrotophos (0, 0.3, 0.6. and 1.2 mg/kg b.wt./day), 14 days	Reduced body weights of pups and resorptions, fertility and parturition indices decreased in a dose dependent manner, viability and lactation indices were greatly decrease in rats of high dose group, crown-rump length and birth weight in high-dose group were low, with no changes on average liter size	Wistar rats, Intragastric intubation	(Adilaxmamma, Janardhan, et al. 1994)

Contd...

Reproductive Toxicants	Effects on Female Reproductive System and/or Embryotoxic/Teratogenic Effects	Model and Route of Administration	References
Monocrotophos (1.6, 3.3, 6.6, 10 and 13 mg/kg b. wt./day), 30 days	Interruption in the estrous cycle, reduction in healthy follicles and higher atretic follicles	Swiss albino mice, Oral	(Rao and Kaliwal 2002)
Drugs/ Medicinal Agents			
Clomiphene (0.3 mg/kg b.wt./day), day 9,10 and 11	Marked decrease in the percentage of rats showing blastocysts and in the blastocysts number recovered from uteri in a time dependent manner	Albino rats, Oral	(Prasad and Kalra 1967)
Pippaliyadi yoga (Ayurvedic contraceptive) (525 and 1050 mg/kg b.wt./day), gestational day 6-day 16	Low birth weights and small size of fetus, mothers gained less weight during gestation, few cases of herniation of intestines into the umbilical cord in foetuses	Wistar rats, Oral	Chaudhury, Chandrasekaran, et al. 2001
Pippaliyadi yoga (140, 300 and 700 mg/kg b.wt./day), gestational exposure day 6-16	Lower body weight of pups, delayed age at which hair appeared in the pups exposed *in utero* to 700 mg (five times the therapeutic dose) and the age at which vaginal opening occurred in 300 and 700 mg groups	Holtzman strain rats, Oral	Balasinor, Bhan, et al. 2007
Ethanolic extract of *Annona squamosa* (100 µg – 1000 µg), 120 h	Only higher concentrations (900 µg and 1000 µg) showed considerable mortality and delay in hatching	Zebrafish embryos	Ponrasu, Ganeshkumar, et al 2012
Aqueous extract of *Millettia pachycarpa* (1.5, 3, 4.5, 6 or 7.5 µg/ml), 4 days post fertilization	Several developmental abnormalities such as yolk sac edema, pericardial edema, swim bladder deflation, spinal curvature, lowered heart rate, dose dependent delay in hatching, higher production of ROS and apoptosis in brain, trunk, and tail of embryos	Zebrafish embryos	Yumnamcha, Roy, et al. 2015
Food Based Toxicants			
Ochratoxin A and Aflatoxin B1 in combination (0.12+ 510.125; 0.25+ 10.50; 0.50+ 10.25 mg/kg b.wt.) gestational exposure day 6-15)	Higher resorptions and dead fetus, syndactyly and gastroschisis, increased cardiac defects in fetuses	Wistar rats, gastric intubation	Wangikar, et al 2004

Contd...

Reproductive Toxicants	Effects on Female Reproductive System and/or Embryotoxic/Teratogenic Effects	Model and Route of Administration	References
Ochratoxin A (0.004, 0.008 µg/ml) **and Aflatoxin B1** (0.5, 1.0 µg/ml) alone and in combination (0.004 + 1.0 µg/ml)	Both interfered with the development of neural tube, on combination neural tube defects reduced but heart abnormalities increased	Post implantation rat embryos from 10th day gestation period, in culture	Wangikar, Sinha, et al. 2007
Alfatoxin1 (0.025, 0.05 and 0.1 mg/kg b.wt./day), gestational day 6-day 18	Lowered crown to rump lengths at 0.05 and 0.1 mg/kg, reduced fetal weights in 0.1 mg/kg, teratogenic effects such as wrist drop and enlarged eye socket were observed, skeletal anomalies included agenesis of caudal vertebrae, incomplete ossification of skull bones and bent metacarpals, visceral anomalies of microphthalmia and cardiac problems observed at 0.1 mg/kg, distortion of normal hepatic cord pattern and lowered mega-karyocytes in liver, fusion of auriculo-ventricular valves, mild degenerative alterations in myocardial fibers, microphthalmic eyes and lenticular degeneration	New Zealand white rabbits, Oral	Wangikar, Dwivedi, et al. 2005

Early research works on female reproductive toxicity only focused on the probable effects of environmental agents on the reproductive functions rather than on the complete reproductive health. Later, it was realized that toxins, may also trigger hormonal alterations adversely affecting other aspects of reproductive health such as the menstrual cycle, fertility and ovulation. Effects of these toxins on female reproduction may result from their exposure in numerous stages starting from fetal life, during maturation and early development, and include indicators such as subfertility, infertility, intrauterine growth retardation, malformations, spontaneous abortions, birth defects, postnatal death, learning and behavior deficits, and premature aging.

Women of reproductive age have been constantly exposed to several environmental risk factors, including prenatal viral infections, smoking, drugs, hypoxia, birth complications, or stressful life events. Studies carried out on drug utilization pattern during the first trimester of pregnancy have documented consumption of alcohol consumption (2.2%), category A drugs (55.28%), category D drugs (6%) and category X drugs (5.71%) and radiation (4%) to be one of the causative agents in causing birth defects. Several substances, specifically lipophilic, to which the lactating mother has been exposed at some point in her life or is exposed, are secreted into the breast milk and may even concentrate in it (Hotham and Hotham 2015). As such, pregnancy has been recognized as a probable critical window of susceptibility to the exposure of several chemicals. Owing to the complicated nature of embryo-fetal development and maternal-fetal interactions during the gestational period, assessment of reproductive safety has historically involved *in vivo* testing employing several experimental species in the context of prenatal or lactational exposures which represent a substantial aspect of xenobiotic transmission. Innumerable studies have emphasized on the potential adverse effects of chemicals on preconception, development (embryo/fetal and newborn/pre-weaning life stages), adolescence, and adults that lead to a higher risk of fetal malformations, miscarriage, premature birth and placental insufficiency (Sengupta, Banerjee, et al. 2015). Both pregestational, as well as gestational exposure, has been shown to cause embryo lethality manifested as decreased fetal weight, number of dead fetuses and resorptions (Junaid, Murthy, et al. 1995, Junaid, Murthy, et al. 1996). Xenobiotics have been shown to cross the fetoplacental barrier and cause fetotoxic effects. A time distribution pattern of Cr^{3+} and Cr^{6+} between maternal and fetal tissue has been demonstrated as influenced by the state of gestation (Saxena, Murthy, et al. 1990). Similarly, species variation has been shown to exist in the distribution pattern of Cr^{6+} in the fetoplacental unit of rat and mouse, with mouse fetoplacental unit allowing a higher inflow of Cr+ from maternal blood to the foetuses, whereas in rats, the fetoplacental barrier restricts the transfer (Saxena, Murthy, et al. 1990).

In view of the vulnerability of the developing reproductive system, it has become all the more imperative to monitor the several developmental stages during gestation for their differential vulnerability towards toxicants. Maternal exposure of metals, pesticides and food-based toxicants during the period of organogenesis (6-14 days) has shown to retard fetal development and cause embryotoxic and teratogenic effects as observed via reduction in fetal weight, number of fetuses (live and dead) per dam, structural deformities and higher incidences of still birth (Trivedi, Saxena, et al. 1989, Wangikar, Dwivedi, et al. 2004, Saini, Nair, et al. 2013). Similarly, *in-utero* exposure to Cr^{6+} at the critical window of testis differentiation inhibits the expression of hormone receptors and Sertoli cell tight junction proteins in the adult F1 progeny rats (Kumar, Aruldhas, et al. 2017). Such early life exposure may not just cause reproductive dysfunctioning of young adult mice but may also cause perturbations that have long-lasting effects on fertility during adulthood (Verma and Mohanty 2009, Doshi, D'souza, et al. 2013). Brief maternal hypoglycemia during organogenesis has been shown to impair gestational development of offspring and induce teratogenicity (Singh, Singh, et al. 2002).

Investigations of the female in cases of poor reproductive outcome have been the primary strategy towards diagnosis. More recent advancements in the field of reproductive biology have proposed evaluation of sperm DNA integrity as a crucial assessment tool to infer the presence of DNA strand breaks, abnormalities in sperm chromosome complement, modifications in epigenetic regulation of paternal genome and oxidative stress. Correct transmission of information which is coded in the sperm genome is important for the pre and postnatal development of the offspring. Studies have highlighted the effects of low antioxidants on the integrity of sperm genome indicating it to be a more accurate prognostic tool for the evaluation of infertility as compared to simple quantitative and morphologic estimations of the spermatozoa (Venkatesh, Riyaz, et al. 2009, Shamsi, Venkatesh, et al. 2010, Shamsi, Imam, et al. 2011, Shamsi, Venkatesh, et al. 2011).

Endocrine control of reproduction has been a well-established fact and echoed by many research groups in India and over the years the focus has been diverted towards studying long term outcomes such as endocrine disruption mediated impaired fertility. The ability of endocrine-disrupting chemicals (EDCs) to modify reproductive function in females has been shown by the adverse effects of synthetic estrogen use and occupational/environmental exposure to metals leading to reduced fertility. However, a number of studies have also shown paternal factors sensitive to toxicants, such as EDCs to be involved in defective embryogenesis and affecting the pregnancy outcome (Gill-Sharma, Balasinor, et al. 2001, Balasinor, Gill-Sharma et al. 2002). Post-implantation loss (PIL) of the embryo, a common phenomenon reflecting the poor quality of the embryo or placenta has been majorly attributed to the faults in the female reproductive system, however, recent studies have been suggestive of the involvement of paternal factors as an alternative mechanism. Studies carried out by ICMR-National Institute of Research in Reproductive Health have highlighted the importance of assessing the sperm epigenome integrity for healthy embryo development. Male gametes (spermatozoa) have been shown to be vulnerable to a myriad of epigenetic insults inflicted by exposure to endocrine disruptors (such as BPA, tamoxifen, pesticides) contributing to the ensuing pathophysiology of reproductive disorders in both developing and adult animals.

Studies have supported the idea that epigenetic reprogramming in male germ line plays a vital function in the development of the embryo and any modification may attribute to male infertility. Neonatal exposure to estrogenic compounds such as Bisphenol A (BPA) induces testicular development disorders leading to impairment in HPT axis and spermatogenesis ultimately leading to subfertility during adult life (Salian, Doshi, et al. 2009). Aberrant

DNA methylation-mediated epigenetic changes in testis have been suggested as one among the probable mechanisms of BPA toxicity on spermatogenesis and impaired fertility during adulthood (Doshi, Mehta, et al. 2011). Recent developments also hint at the potential of toxic EDCs to alter epigenetic information of the gametes which could get transferred to the developing embryo and affect the immediate reproductive outcome or even persists transgenerationally (Ankolkar and Balasinor 2016). In this direction, research groups have identified various toxicant responsive imprinted genes that play an important role in embryonic development, dysregulation of which could lead to loss of chromatin integrity resulting in intrauterine and postnatal growth retardation ultimately resulting in embryo loss. Exposure of BPA could alter methylation pattern in parental-specific imprinted genes like Igf2 (Insulinlike growth factor 2) and H19 in resorbed embryo, which could have led to abnormal placental development, poor nutrient transfer and post PIL (Doshi, D'souza et al. 2013). Adult spermatogenesis also has shown to be susceptible to epigenetic modulation. A recent study has shown that exposure of adults to tamoxifen results in loss of imprinting at the ICR which were transmitted to the next generation via paternal germline thus affecting embryonic development resulting in disrupted endocrine signalling (Pathak, Kedia-Mokashi, et al. 2009).

The incidence of fetal abnormalities due to the side effects of drugs, including contraceptives is quite high. The search for antifertility agents, both natural and synthetic, has prompted research groups to evaluate them for their teratogenic effects. Chopra, et al. 1956 have reported 'Vidanga' (E. ribes) to be useful for birth control (Chopra and Nayar 1956). Munshi and Rao Shanta 1972 have shown it to be successful in preventing pregnancy without any teratogenic effects (Munshi and Rao 1972). Pippaliyadi yoga or pippaliyadi vati is an ayurvedic contraceptive derived from a powdered fruit berries using a combination of *Embelia ribes Burm.f.* (Myrsinaceae), *Piper longum L.* (Piperaceae) and borax in equal ratios. The contraceptive property of these plants has been well-known to the ayurvedic practitioners over the ages and also has been mentioned in the Sushruta Sanhita, the ancient Indian Ayurvedic treatise. Studies have been carried out to assess the effect of *in utero* exposure of pippaliyadi on postnatal development and reproductive performance of the offspring, with specific focus on the teratogenicity and embryotoxicity (Chaudhury, Chandrasekaran, et al. 2001, Balasinor, Bhan, et al. 2007). Similarly, the non-hormonal contraceptive, named RISUG (Reversible Inhibition of Sperm Under Guidance), a copolymer of styrene maleic anhydride (SMA), has aimed to provide an important addition to current options of male contraception (Guha 1996, Ananthaswamy 2002). Research groups have conducted numerous studies to ascertain the success of reproductive functionality, safety of vas occlusion by RISUG, and its reversal via dimethylsulphoxide, followed by multigenerational (F1-F3) teratogenicity studies in animals (Mishra, Manivannan, et al. 2003, Lohiya, Alam, et al. 2014). Long term studies have established its safety in contraceptive use without affecting any aspect of testicular spermatogenesis or the reproductive organs and non-toxic teratogenic potential (Sethi, Srivastava, et al. 1990, Guha 1999).

Emanating from the increasing awareness of the possibility of damage by environmental agents, the area of reproductive toxicology has drawn significant attention in recent times. Paralleling such awareness has been the pursuit of alternate *in vitro* and *in vivo* screening models for assessing the reproductive toxicity of chemicals. The conventional procedure being time and cost intensive and with the staggering number of chemicals marketed for human consumption, it would not be feasible to do complete *in vivo* teratogenicity testing on every chemical. In this regard, a lot of efforts have also been undertaken for the optimization of individual alternative *in vitro* models for identifying and characterizing the reproductive/developmental toxicity assessment. Few aspects of male reproduction have been successfully modeled *in vitro* using the rat Sertoli germ cell co-culture system. Sertoli cells closely associated with the developing germ cells are known to orchestrate spermatogenesis and testicular abnormalities may result from any disruption in the normal contact-mediated interaction between germ and Sertoli cells, that are responsible for the maintainance of the integrity of germinal epithelium, manifested by increased exfoliation. Using primary co-cultures of Sertoli and germ cells many features of the well-characterized testicular damage produced by chemicals (lead, endosulfan, argemone alkaloid) could be recapitulated *in vitro* that well correlated with their activity *in vivo* (Sinha, Adhikari, et al. 1999, Adhikari, Sinha, et al. 2000, Sinha, Adhikari, et al. 2001, Mishra, Saxena, et al. 2009, Mitra, Srivastava, et al. 2013).

Other good examples are the male germ stem cells from mouse embryonic stem cells, rodent whole embryo culture (rWEC) and zebrafish embryo assay. Research groups at CSIR-CDRI have been widely utilizing post-implantation rWEC as a model for teratogenic screening of drugs commonly used during pregnancy such as anti-inflammatory drugs, anti-cancer agents cyclophosphamide, salicylic acid, analgesics, antibiotics (mitomycin) that have shown to cause growth retardation and congenital abnormalities in experimental animals. In an attempt to establish a new *in vitro* system for teratogenicity testing by employing post-implanted rat embryos and taking apoptosis as a reference end point marker, the research group have demonstrated that these drugs on exposure during the critical periods of organogenesis may trigger apoptosis in an abnormal pattern, which may mediate teratogenicity (Singh, Sinha, et al. 2009, Singh and Sinha, 2010, Singh,

Kumar, et al. 2012, Singh, Maurya, et al. 2015). This *in vitro* model has been designed to short-list the number of chemicals tested *in vivo* and reduce the number of animals, time and money in teratological studies for assessment of toxicity.

NMR based metabolomics has offered a complementary approach for testing the teratogenicity of newly formulated drugs and chemicals/NCEs, which could bypass the inherent shortcomings of *in vitro* systems and involve less time, cost and laboratory animals. To validate this procedure, cyclophosphamide, a well-known pro-teratogen has been used as a test compound and rats as testing species that have lead to the identification of altered metabolic fingerprints, drawing a definite correlation between the teratogenic aliments and the metabolic profiles. Hence, alteration of the metabolic fingerprint of an organism may be the end point for defining teratogenicity (Sethi, Mahar, et al. 2015).

Alternate animal models have offered excellent opportunities to assess the adversities caused by xenobiotics on the reproductive systems based on the availability of certain assays/tools that are sensitive and quicker. The well-annotated genome of *Drosophila* with its well-characterized male reproductive biology and ease of experimental manipulation has facilitated the rapid preliminary screening of chemicals to assess their potential to induce reproductive toxicity. Research groups at CSIR-IITR have attempted to develop *Drosophila* based endpoints (at organismal, genetic, biochemical, and endocrine levels) that have offered new, rapid, and economical bioassay for offering evidence for reproductive adversities of chemicals (metals/pesticides) in the environment. Comprehensive analysis of sperm, as well as seminal fluid parameters and behavioral anomalies manifested in the form of reduced reproductive performance (delayed emergence and fecundity), have been used to assess biological impacts at sub-individual (tissue damages, stress gene expression) and individual levels (reproductive capacities, emergence) within the same exposure time. These have included the genetic and behavioral analysis and assessment of reproductive performance in flies that are exposed to numerous chemicals. Research groups have shown that different toxicants have a dose-dependent adverse impact on the reproductive outcome manifested in the form of decreased fecundity and delay in emergence pattern in the exposed male Drosophila (Nazir, Mukhopadhyay et al. 2001, Nazir, Mukhopadhyay, et al. 2003, Gupta, Siddique, et al. 2007).

The model has not just been validated using single chemical mixtures but instead to a combination of chemicals such as industrial effluents and leachates from municipal/industrial wastes. The impaired reproductive outcome has been shown to be either due to cellular injury or decreased expression of genes that encode seminal proteins such as Acp70A and Acp36DE which play crucial roles in induction of egg production and facilitation of sperm storage, respectively (Siddique, Mitra, et al. 2009). Interestingly, in majority of the cases, males have been found to be more vulnerable to these chemicals as compared to females which indicate that *Drosophila* males are more sensitive to environmental chemicals thus offering a valuable model to assess the candidate molecules that exhibit male reproductive adversities.

Signals at cellular and molecular levels have also been able to provide early indications of abnormal reproduction/development. Induction of stress protein hsp70, representing a universally conserved cellular defense system against environmental exposures has been found to be upregulated concurrently to the reproductive anomalies against environmental chemicals (Mukhopadhyay, Siddique, et al. 2006, Bhargav, Singh, et al. 2008). More recently, *Drosophila* has also shown to mimic organismal, biochemical, molecular and endocrine signatures similar to mammalian reproductive toxicity against the known reproductive toxicant, dibutyl phthalate (DBP). Analogous to mammals, DBP exposure lowered sperm counts, fertility, seminal proteins, elevated oxidative damage/modification in the proteins of reproductive tract and modified hormone receptor Estrogen-Related Receptor (dERR) activity, a sole *Drosophila* ortholog of the vertebrate ERR nuclear receptor subclass. In addition, as observed in the higher organism, DBP was readily metabolized to monobutyl phthalate (MBP) in the exposed male *Drosophila* and MBP was found to be more toxic than DBP. These findings are suggestive of the use of *Drosophila* as a valuable alternative to conventional animal models for pre-screening of environmental chemicals for their potential reproductive adversities and also gain reliable insights into the mechanism of chemical-induced male infertility and endocrine disruption (Misra, Singh et al. 2014). Transcriptomic analysis has further provided insights into the possible genetic perturbations underlying the harmful effects of toxicants. Microarray-based gene expression profiling has identified differential expression of 256 genes, significantly altered by endosulfan, related with cellular processes such as immune response, stress, development and metabolism (Sharma, Mishra, et al. 2011).

Mostly analysis of male reproductive effects has been limited to semen quality analysis and examination of progeny production by their mates. However, these parameters do not take into account the fate of sperms in the female environment and progeny production assay is biased towards monogamy as the assay design involves pairing of one female with a male. A study has advocated the consideration of sperm competition (which is a crucial determinant of male reproductive success) in the reproductive toxicity assessment of xenobiotics to mimic natural conditions of polyandry existing in nature. Exposure to environmental toxicants (example endosulfan) at a concentration with no toxic effects on the traditionally assayed toxicological parameters, including sperm counts and progeny production may influence the sperm competition (Misra, Kumar, et al. 2014).

QSAR modeling has aided in the development of predictive models for various endpoints of a chemicals employing the data that have been generated via experiments and information on molecular structures. Basant, et al. 2016 have developed interspecies correlated based QSAR models using decision tree forest (DTF) and decision tree boost (DTB) approaches that can accurately predict the developmental toxicity potential of chemicals which are structurally diverse in rodents (rabbits and rats) (Basant, Gupta et al. 2016). These models rigorously validated through the OECD guidelines, could reduce not only the cost and the number of animals but also streamline the risk assessment process for humans. Similarly, Kumar, et al. 2017 has utilized computational biology approaches to evaluate toxic potencies and interaction profiles of endocrine-disrupting perfluorinated chemicals with steroidogenic acute regulatory protein revealing them to be highly carcinogenic as well as a developmental toxicant (Kumar, Devi, et al. 2017).

The generation of such an extensive database on the reproductive toxicity potential of environmental agents has also simultaneously encouraged the pursuit for protective/therapeutic agents against these toxicants. CSIR-CDRI since inception has directed its research activities towards the safety evaluation of newly synthesized polymers for contraceptives for their antifertility, teratogenic activity in various experimental animals with the main objectives of drug designing, synthesis of new molecules and isolates/extracts derived from natural sources and their evaluation for development of novel leads as contraceptives, spermicides with anti-STI properties. Few of the representative studies have been provided in Table 10.10.

Table 10.10 Few representative studies for the pursuit of protective/therapeutic agents against reproductive toxicants

Reproductive Toxicants	Protective/Preventive Agents	Model and Route of Administration	Reference
Metals			
Sodium arsenite (0.4 ppm/100 g/b.wt./day, 28 days	**Vitamin C** (25 mg/100 g b.wt./day): Co-administration results in restoration of plasma gonadotrophins levels and 3β-HSD and 17β-HSD activities in the ovaries	Female albino rats, Oral	(Chattopa-dhyay, Ghosh, et al. 2001)

Contd...

Reproductive Toxicants	Protective/Preventive Agents	Model and Route of Administration	Reference
Sodium arsenite (0.4 ppm/100 g b. wt./day, 28 days)	**Sodium selenite** (0.6 mg/100 g b.w./day, 28 days): Co-administration minimized weight loss in gonads, higher activities of ovarian steroidogenic enzymes and uterine and ovarian peroxidase and restoration of plasma LH, FSH, and estradiol levels	Female Wistar rats, Oral	(Chattopadhyay, Pal, et al. 2003)
Sodium arsenite (4 ppm/day, 28 days)	**All-trans retinoic acid (ATRA)** (0.5 mg/kg b.w/day, 56 days, subcutaneous): ATRA reversed disruption of circulating levels of estradiol and gonadotropins, degenerated endometrial glands and luminal epithelial cells with an upregulation of estrogen receptor.	Female Sprague Dawley rats, Oral	(Chatterjee and Chatterji 2011)
Arsenic (3 ppm/rat/day, 30 days)	**High protein diet** (27% protein in the form of casein (20%) and pea (7%):Supplementation significantly protected steroidogenic enzyme activities and follicular growth, restoration of serum E2 levels and mitigation of oxidative stress	Female wistar rats, Oral	(Mondal, Mukherjee, et al. 2013)
Cadmium+Lead (25 ppm in combination, 120 days)	**Zinc** (50ppm, 120 days, Oral): supplementation led to restoration of sperm motility and sperm counts	Male albino rats, Oral	(Saxena, Murthy, et al. 1989)
Lead (819 mg/L), 65 days	**Zinc** (71mg/L, 65 days, Oral): Co-treatment recovered suppressed spermatogenesis, steroidogenesis (activities of 3β- HSD and 17β-HSD, elevated oxidative status, and histological damage	Male wistar rats, Oral	(Anjum, Madhu et al. 2017)
Mercuric chloride (10 mg/100 g b.wt./day, 30 days)	**Vitamin C** (40 mg/100 g b.w./day, 30 days) and **Vitamin E** (20 mg/100 g b.w./day, 30 days):Co-administration rendered significant protection by reduction in sperm abnormality and increased sperm motility and LPO, restoration of antioxidant defense enzymes SOD, GSH and CAT	Male albino rats, Oral	(Muthu and Krishnamoorthy 2012)

Contd...

Reproductive Toxicants	Protective/Preventive Agents	Model and Route of Administration	Reference
Lithium chloride (2 mg/kg b.wt./day, 21 days)	**Bovine prolactin** (0.25mg/kg b.w./day, 21 days):Co-administration rendered protection to spermatogenic (stage VII of seminiferous epithelial cycle) and steroidogenic activities of the testes, along with restoration of serum levels of FSH and testosterone	Male albino rats, Subcutaneous	(Ghosh, Biswas, et al. 1991)
Vanadium (7.5 mg/kg b.wt.), 21 days, 5days/week	**Tiron (T) alone and in combination with lipoic acid (LA), Vitamine E (Vit E) and selenium (Se)** (2days/week):The most effective combination was T+Se followed by T and Vit E+ Tand LA, cotreatment with antioxidants restored the activities of alkaline phosphatase and adenosine triphosphatase, prevented the rise in glycogen content and acid phosphatase activity in testes, seminal vesicle, ovaries and uterus, restored LPO, glutathione and glycerides level	Albino rats, Oral	(Shrivastava, Jadon, et al. 2007)
Pesticides			
Malathion (23 mg/kg b.wt./day), 24, 36 and 48 h	**Human chorionic gonadotrophin** (50IU, for 2 days at 24 h interval):Pre-treatment prevented in reduction of plasma concentration of both LH and T4 at all time points	Wistar rats, Subcutaneous	(Prakash and Venkatesh 1996)
Lindane (30 mg/kg b.wt./day), 14 and 28 days	**Curcumin** (100 mg/kg b.w) **in pretreatment** (14 days), post treatment (14 days) **and combination** (28 days): Pre, Post and co-administration of curcumin significantly ameliorated lindane induced variations in weight of testes and cauda epididymus, lipid peroxidation, sperm quality and quantity and activity of antioxidant enzymes	Male Wistar rats, Oral	(Sharma and Singh 2010)

Contd...

Reproductive toxicants	Protective/Preventive Agents	Model and Route of administration	Reference
Cypermethrin (3.38 mg/kg b.wt./day, 28 days)	**Ethanolic extract of *Tribulus terrestris*** (100mg/kg b.wt./day, 28 days): Co-administration reverted the alterations in sperm motility, FSH, LH and testosterone levels and antioxidant enzymes	Male wistar rats, Oral	(Sharma, Huq, et al. 2013)
Cypermethrin (3.83 mg/kg b.wt./day, 14 days)	**Resveratrol** (pre and post treatment, 20 mg/kg b.wt./day,14 days) : Increased sperm head counts and motility, sex hormones FSH, LH, reduced oxidative stress and LPO levels	Male Wistar rats, Oral	(Sharma, Huq, et al. 2014)
Carbendazim (25 mg/kg b.wt./48 days)	**Vitamin E** (20 mg/kg, 48days): Co-treatment prevents testicular atrophy and oxidative stress	Adult male albino rats, Oral	(Rajeswary, Mathew, et al. 2007)
Miscellaneous			
Cyclophosphamide (5 mg/kg b.wt./day, 28 days)	**Human chorionic gonadotrophin** (5 IU/kg b.wt./day for 28 days): Co-administration prevented reduction in plasma levels E2 along with activities of ovarian 3β-HSD and 17β2 HSD and degeneration of follicles	Female Wistar rats, Oral	(Ghosh, Misro, et al. 2001)
Cyclophosphamide (5 mg/kg b.wt./day, 28 days)	**a-tocopherol-succinate(Provitamin-E)** 50 mg/kg/b.wt./day for 28 days, subcutaneous: Co-administration resulted prevention of oxidative stress and restoration in activities of testicular 3β- HSD and 17β-HSD along with plasma testosterone levels and number of spermatogonia-A, preleptotene spermatocytes, midpachytene spermatocytes and step 7 spermatids at stage VII of spermatogenic cycle	Male Wistar rats, Oral	(Ghosh, Das, et al. 2002)
Bisphenol A (200 mg/kg b.wt., 30 days)	**Lycopene** (10 mg/kg b.wt./day, 30 days): Co- administration restored serum FSH, LH and testosterone levels with a decrease in ROS and LPO generation with restoration in sperm characteristics	Male Sprague Dawley rats, Oral	(Tamilselvan, Langeswaran, et al. 2014)

Contd...

Reproductive toxicants	Protective/Preventive agents	Model and Route of administration	Reference
Ethanol (4 g/kg b.wt./day, 90 days)	**Ascorbic acid** (25 mg/100 g b.wt./day, 30 days, post withdrawal of ethanol):Altered disruption of sperm morphology and motility, steroidogenesis enzymes and oxidative stress	Adult male guinea pigs, Oral	(Harikrishnan, Abhilash, et al. 2013)

10.5 Immunotoxicity

Immunotoxicity has been defined as any adverse effect on the structural and functional aspects of immune system or immune dysfunctions taking the form of an immunosuppression or alternatively, allergy, autoimmunity, or any inflammatory-based diseases. Since the immune system plays a crucial role in conferring host resistance to diseases and maintaining normal homeostasis in an organism, identification of risk of immunotoxicity is imperative for human and animal health protection and has evolved into a crucial aspect of safety evaluation of drugs/chemicals. Moreover, the inclusion of immunotoxicity endpoints as more sensitive indicators than biochemical alterations have been attributed to the fact that several environmental chemicals/drugs are capable of modulating the immune system even in low doses and short periods of exposure well before exhibiting any signs of toxicity to the other systems.

Concerns regarding increasing risks of xenobiotics to the immune system emerged shortly after the clinical introduction of potent immunosuppressive drugs to prevent kidney graft rejections in the 1960s when infections and lymphoproliferative disorders were first described in transplant patients (Muntean and Lucan 2013). These early clinical findings served as an impetus to experimental studies focused on immunosuppression not only worldwide but also in India. The immune system has been shown to be highly sensitive to environmental chemicals that may interact with its cellular and humoral components which could result in altered immune status/disruption of regulatory network leading to reduced resistance to infection, specific forms of neoplasia tumors that may escape surveillance or in some cases may exacerbate the immune response predisposing the host to allergy/hypersensitive reactions or autoimmunity. The modifications in the immune system via environmental chemicals has fascinated immunotoxicologists in India since the 1970s and increased their interest over time. Over the years India has kept itself abreast and considerable attention has been developed in assessing the vulnerability of the immune system towards several environmental chemicals.

With the steady developments in our knowledge of the immune system and its complicated regulation network, attention has been increasingly focused on the possible deleterious effects of many drugs and chemicals on the immune competence of exposed individuals. Epidemiological data from India suggests that the diseases' prevalence linked with the modifications of the immune response, such as asthma, few autoimmune disorders, and cancer have been increasing to such an extent that it cannot be solely attributed to improved diagnostics. There has been a growing concern that this could also be due to new and altered patterns of chemical exposure emphasizing the need to accurately predict/identify the immunotoxicity potential of chemicals. In several instances, effects quite same as to those observed in rodents have been reported in humans through environmental or occupational exposure to xenobiotics that may cause immunodepression leading to increased susceptibility to infections. These effects include altered immune responses in: agate industry workers, higher incidences of opportunistic infections like tuberculosis, fungal infections, and respiratory tract infections (Rastogi, Gupta, et al. 1991); impairment of macrophages with inhibited proliferation and differentiation of T cells in residents in West Bengal chronically exposed to arsenic via drinking water (Biswas, Ghosh, et al. 2008, Banerjee, Banerjee, et al. 2009), lead battery industry workers with disruption of T lymphocyte subsets and activation markers (Mishra, Singh, et al. 2003, Mishra, Rani et al. 2010) and higher risk of hepatitis and tuberculosis infections in generations of survivors exposed to Methyl isocyanate gas (Mishra, Bhargava, et al. 2011).

As immunosuppression has been the primary focus of immunotoxicologists for many years in India, there is an extensive database on the immunosuppressive potential of drugs, chemicals and xenobiotics. Several organ systems are known to be affected to different degrees following exposure in a dose and time-dependent manner. The immunotoxic effects of xenobiotics include histopathological effects in lymphoid tissues and organs (thymus, spleen, bone marrow, Peyer's patches), cellular pathology, disrupted maturation of immunocompetent cells, alterations in B and T cell populations and functional changes in immunocompetent cells. Owing to the complexity of the immune system with multiple organ involvement, a multitude of assays and models have been incorporated to predict all different kinds of adverse immune effects and to decipher the underlying mechanisms (Table 10.11). These have included an assessment of humoral immunity (i.e., antibody production), cell-mediated immunity (e.g., delayed-type hypersensitivity, lymphocyte proliferation), macrophage functions (e.g., phagocytosis or chemotaxis) and the activity of natural killer cells.

Table 10.11 Few representative studies on the immunotoxicity potential of different classes of toxicants

Immunotoxicants	Effects/Mechanism of action	Model and Route of Administration	References
Metals			
Arsenic (0.5 mg/kg b.wt.) and Lead (10 mg/kg b.wt.), daily for 15 days	Co-exposure changed cell morphology of splenic macrophages, prevented cell adhesion, release of nitric oxide, intracellular killing ability, chemotactic migration, release of myeloperoxidase release, bacterial clearance from blood and spleen and higher DNA fragmentation.	Swiss albino mice, Intraperitoneal	(Bishayi and Sengupta 2003)
Arsenic (Chronic exposure of minimum 10 years)	A dose-dependent inhibition of Concanavalin A (Con A) triggered T-cell proliferation with a reduction in secreted cytokines levels by the T cells (TNF-α, IFN-γ, IL2, IL10, IL5, and IL4)	Arsenic exposed individuals derived T-cells	(Biswas, Ghosh, et al. 2008)
Arsenic (Chronic exposure of minimum 10 years)	Loss in capacity for cell adhesion, lowered production of nitric oxide, disrupted phagocytic capacity, and lowered expression of CD 54 and F-actin via activation of the Rho A-ROCK signaling pathway	Arsenic exposed individuals derived macrophages	(Banerjee, Banerjee, et al. 2009)
Arsenic (0.038, 0.38 and 3.8 ppm), 7, 15 and 30 days	Promoted CD4 lineage commitment in a dose dependent manner supported by the expression of ThPOK in thymus, increased splenic CD^{4+} T cells and promoted their differentiation into Treg cells, induced immunosuppression characterized by low cytokine secretion from splenocytes and increased susceptibility to *Mycobacterium fortuitum* infection	Balb/c mice, Oral	(Gera, Singh, et al. 2017)
Lead (Expsoure mean duration 6.5 years)	Significant increase in serum IgA level in exposed individuals (blood lead; Pb-B > 10 µg/dL)	Lead exposed individuals	(Mishra, Chauhan, et al. 2006)
Lead (Exposure period 5 or and 10 years)	Lower percentage of CD^{4+} cells and higher of CD45RA+ cells, negative correlation among the CD^{4+} cell percentage and blood lead levels and exposure length	Lead exposed individuals	(Mishra, Rani, et al. 2010)

Contd...

Immunotoxicants	Effects/Mechanism of Action	Model and Route of Administration	References
Cadmium (1.8 mg/kg b.wt.), 18, 24, 48 and 72 h	Splenic cells were more vulnerable than thymus cells, elevation in ROS at 18 h, followed by depolarization of mitochondrial membrane, activation of caspase-3 and reduction in GSH at 24 h in spleen and later at 48 h in thymus, depletion of thymic cortical cells and higher red pulp with reduced white pulp in spleen at 48 h and beyond	BALB/c mice, Intraperitoneal	(Pathak and Khandelwal 2007)
Chromium (VI) (5.0, 10.0, and 20.0 µg/ml), 24 and 48h	Decreased gene expression of antimicrobial peptides (AMPs), reduced transcription of humoral pathway receptors (Toll and PGRP) and levels of triglyceride, decrease of activities of antioxidant enzyme, reduced resistance against bacterial infection	*Drosophila melanogaster*, Oral	(Pragya, Shukla, et al. 2015)
Mixture of eight metals (sodium arsenite, calcium chloride, lead acetate, mercuric chloride, chromium trioxide, nickel chloride, manganese chloride, ferric chloride (1X, 10X and 100X (their mode concentrations exposed daily for 90 days)	The mixture at 10X and 100X doses elevated the weight of the spleen, but that of adrenals, thymus, and popliteal lymphnodes were elevated with the 100X dose, decrease in lymphocyte count after 60 and 90 days, increase in neutrophil number after 90 days, spleen showed reduction in atrophic follicles and lymphoid cells with lowered follicular activity at 10X and 100X	Albino Wistar rats, Oral	(Jadhav, Sarkar, et al. 2007)
Pesticides			
DDT (20, 50 or 100 ppm), per day for 3-12 weeks	Depression of primary and secondary humoral immune response, a thymus dependent antigen, significant changes in spleen and liver weights in dose-time dependent pattern, 12 weeks revealed significant decrease in	Albino mice, Oral	(Banerjee, Ramachandran, et al. 1986)

Contd...

Immunotoxicants	Effects/Mechanism of action	Model and Route of Administration	References
	primary antibody titre, marked decrease of secondary antibody titre at 100 ppm, more than 6 weeks revealed a dose and time dependent reduction in primary and secondary PFC (plaque forming cells) response		
	Inhibition of primary IgM-PFC in response to a T-independent antigen (*Escherichia coli* lipopolysaccharide (LPS)), dose and time dependent supprpession of LPS-specific primary PFC response, lowered PFC response was observed after 3 weeks of exposure while reduced antibody titre was seen after six weeks only in 100 ppm group	Albino mice, Oral	(Banerjee 1987)
Endosulfan (5, 10 or 20 ppm) for 8-22 weeks	Antibody titre was significantly decreased in endosulfan-exposed rats at 10 and 20 ppm levels, significantly depressed LMI (leukpocyte migration inhibition) and MMI (macrophage migration inhibition) responses	Wistar albino rats, Oral	(Banerjee and Hussain 1986)
Endosulfan (10 mg/ml) and **Malathion** (20 mg/ml), 24 h	Suppressed LPS-triggered generation of TNF-α, malathion revealed a direct suppression on the production of nitrite and inhibition of LPS-induced generation of TNF-α	Rat peritoneal macrophages from Wistar rats	(Ayub, Verma, et al. 2003)
Lindane (5, 20 or 30 ppm of lindane), for 8-22 weeks	Decrease in globulin levels (increased A/G ratio) in the 20 ppm group exposed for 22 weeks and 30 ppm group exposed for 18-22 weeks	Wistar albino rats, Oral	(Saha and Banerjee 1993)
Deltamethrin (0.5, 1, 10, 25, 50, and 100 µM), 6 and 18 h	*In silico* studies revealed that Deltamethrin has strong binding affinity for the CD4, CD8, CD45 and CD28 receptors, Concentartion dependednt induction of apoptosis in murine splenocytes, generation of ROS and activation of caspase 3 were evident at 1 h by 25	Murine splenocytes from BALB/c mice	(Kumar, Sasmal, et al. 2014)

Contd...

Immunotoxicants	Effects/Mechanism of action	Model and Route of administration	References
	and 50 µM, depletion of glutathione observed at 3 and 6 h by 25 and 50 µM		
Cypermethrin (1.87, 3.75, 7.50, 15, or 30 μM) or **mancozeb** (0.45, 0.93, 1.87, 3.75, or 7.50 μM), 6 h	Cypermethrin caused no significant effect on proliferation or cytokine profiles Mancozeb triggered induction in lymphocyte proliferation, inhibited generation of TNFα and the TH2 cytokines IL-6 and IL-10, elevation in IFNγ (TH1 cytokine) generation, decreased IL-4 (TH2) and stimulated IL-2 (TH1) generation in a dose-dependent manner	Human Peripheral Blood Mononuclear Cells	(Mandarapu, Ajumeera, et al. 2014)
Dichlorvos (10 µM), 24 and 48 h	Increased pro-inflammatory molecules like, TNF-α, and IL-1β and CD11b, nitric oxide and microglial specific activation marker, after 24 h, activated microglial cells underwent cell death after 48 h, activation of caspase-3 and apotosis	Microglial cells from Wistar rats	(Sunkaria, Wani, et al. 2012)
Food based toxicants			
Citrinin (10 mg/kg feed) and **Endosulfan** (1 mg/kg b.wt.), gestational day 6-20	Simultaneous exposure led to increased suppression of cellular (DTH) and humoral (HA, indirect ELISA) mediated responses than individual intoxications	Pregnant Wistar rats, Oral	(Singh, Sharma, et al. 2011)
Alfatoxin B1 (70, 350 and 750µg/ml), alternate day for 4 weeks	Reduction in the weights of spleen at the 700 µg dose level and thymus at the 350 and 700 µg dose levels as well as depletion in the macrophage and phagocytic activity, inhibition of incorporation of DNA, RNA and protein precursors in peritoneal macrophages	Weanling Wistar rats, Oral	(Singh, Zaidi, et al. 1990)
Alfatoxin B1(60, 300 and 600 µg), alternate day for 4 weeks	Selectively suppressed cell mediated immunity at the 300 and 600 µg dose as measured via DTH response assay	Weanling Wistar rats, Oral	(Raisuddin, Singh, et al. 1993)

Contd...

Immunotoxicants	Effects/Mechanism of action	Model and Route of administration	References
Ochratoxin A (4ppm), 24-72 h	Induces suppression of both humoral and cell mediated immunity, leucopenia, lymphopenia and hypoproteinemia	Wistar rats, Oral	(Satheesh, Sharma, et al. 2005)
Ochratoxin A (0.75 mg/kg b.wt.), **citrinin** (15mg/kg b.wt.) and their combination, upto 60 days	More severe reduction of humoral cell mediated immunity in the OTA and combination group	New Zealand White rabbits, Oral	(Kuma Dwivedi, et al. 2010)
Red gram proteins (100 μg), once a week for 7 weeks	Allergenic response as seen by elevation in levels of IgE, IgG1, Th2 cytokine and histamine levels, anaphylactic symptoms, discernible histopathological responses and decreased IFN-c levels	BALB/c mice, Intraperitoneal	(Misra, Kumar, et al. 2010)
Green gram (100 μg), daily upto 42 days	Increased levels of total and specific IgE, Th2 cytokines in the splenocytes and histamine, β-hexosaminidase, cysteinyl leukotriene and prostaglandin D2 release from RBL-2H3 cells	BALB/c mice, Oral	(Kumar, Sharma, et al. 2014)
Rhein (from *Cassia occidentalis* seeds), 72h	Maximum dose of 10μM was non cytotoxic upto 72h, suppression of proliferation of stimulated splenocytes, significantly downregulate the expression of CD3e, CD4, CD8, CD28, CD69 molecules in T-cells and CD19, CD28, CD40 in B-cells, reduced the expression of IL2 and IL6, IL10, IFNγ and TNFα in	Splenocytes from BALB/c mice	(Panigrahi, Yadav, et al. 2016)
Piperine (1.12, 2.25 or 4.5 mg/kg b.wt.), 5 consecutive days	4.5 mg led to reduction in spleen, thymus and mesenteric lymph nodes weight, 2.25 and 4.5 mg inhibited the mitogenic response of B-lymphocytes to LPS, lower number of IgM forming cells in the spleen reduced levels of primary antibody in serum, doses of 1.12 and 2.25 inhibited mitogenic	Swiss mice, Oral	(Dogra, Khanna, et al. 2004)

Contd...

Immunotoxicants	Effects/Mechanism of action	Model and Route of administration	References
	response of T-lymphocytes to phytohaemagglutinin and nitroblue tetrazolium dye decreasing activity of peritoneal exudate cells		
Benzathrone (3.25, 7.5 mg/kg and 15 mg/kg b.wt./day), one week	Systemic inflammation as observed via heighteneda DTH response, activity of MPO, hyperplastic and dysplastic histopathological architecture of spleen and lung tissue, induction of pro-inflammatory markers (iNOS, COX-2), regulatory cytokines and DNA damage in the spleen, activation of ERK1/2, JNK MAPKs, p38, and their downstream transcription factors AP-1 (c-fos, c-jun), NF- kB and Nrf2	Balb/c mice, Intraperitoneal	(Tewari, Roy, et al. 2015)
Sunset yellow FCF (10–1000 μg/ml), 72 h	Non cytotoxic dose (250μg/ml) inhibited the mitogen triggered splenocytes proliferation and mixed lymphocyte reaction (MLR) response, altered the expression of CD3e/CD4/CD8 in T cells and CD19 in B-cells, reduced expression of IL2, IL4, IL6, IL-17, IFN-γ and TNF-α cytokines	Swiss mice isolated Splenocytes	(Yadav, Kumar, et al. 2013)
Orange II (100–1000 μg/ml), 72 h	Non-cytotoxic dose (50 μg/ml) significantly changed the distribution of T and B-cells, MLR response and the mitogen triggered proliferative response of T-cells and B-cells, reduced secretion of cytokines IL-2, IL-4, IL-6, IFN-γ, TNF-α and IL-17, higher generation of IL-10	Swiss mice isolated Splenocytes	(Yadav, Kumar, et al. 2012)
Ethanolic extract of *Boerhaavia diffusa* (plant used in Indian traditional system of medicine), 18/24 h	Inhibits human NK cell cytotoxicity *in vitro*, NO generation in mouse macrophage cells (RAW 264.7), IL-2 and TNF-a in human PBMCs	Human NK cells, mouse macrophage cells, human PBMCs	(Mehrotra, Mishra, et al. 2002)

Contd...

Immunotoxicants	Effects/Mechanism of action	Model and Route of administration	References
Tributyltin-chloride (0.1, 1, 3, 10, and 30 nM), 6 and 18 h	Dose and time dependent increase of oxidative stress and caspase dependent apoptosis	Thymocytes from BALB/c mice	(Sharma and Kumar 2014)
Styrene (50 mg/kg, 30 mg/kg or 20 mg/kg b.wt.), 5 consecutive days	Inhibition of humoral immune response in a dose dependent manner, higher blastogenic response of splenic lymphocytes, disruption in the functional activity of nonadherent and adherent peritoneal exudate cells	Swiss mice, gastric intubation	(Dogra, Khanna, et al. 1989)
Miscellaneous			
Zinc oxide nanoparticles (5, 6, and 6.6 µg/ml), 24 h	Early events involved increase in intracellular calcium level as well as ROS, 10 h caused ATP depletion with disruption of mitochondrial membrane potential and apoptosis	Mouse microglial cell line, N9	(Sharma, Singh, et al. 2017)
Methyl Isocynate (1.60 mg/l)	Protein deficient exposed rats showed diminished B-cell proliferation, significant suppression in the B-cell activation, total IgM levels were 43% less	Albino rats (protein defeicient 8% casein), Inhalation	(Saxena, Paul, et al. 1991)
Isocyanates (1.0 to 100 µg, 6 h	Induced apoptosis in the neutrophil through induction of mitochondrial-mediated pathway along with generation of ROS; reduction in status of antioxidant defense system; increased pro-inflammatory cytokine response (IL-1β, IL-6, IL-8, , IL-10, IFN-γ, TNF, and IL- 12p70)	Neutrophils isolated healthy human volunteers	(Mishra, Khan, et al. 2010)

Pesticide immunotoxicology has been one of the premier areas for research in India since the 1980s. Banerjee 1999 has been extensively involved in generating a wealth of information on the various physiological and environmental factors, which have complicated the assessment of immune toxicity of pesticides (organochlorine, organophosphate and carbamates) (Banerjee 1999). Studies have revealed immunotoxicity to be dependent on not only the dose level, duration and frequency of exposure but also on the immunological methods used (Banerjee and Hussain 1986, Banerjee, Ramachandran et al. 1986, Banerjee and Hussain 1987, Banerjee, Saha, et al.

1992, Saha and Banerjee 1993). Since the immune response is genetically regulated, modifications in responsiveness to one challenge in a particular animal model may not be reliable for a second model. For example, antibody titer to sheep red blood cell (SRBC) was decreased on sub-chronic exposure to DDT in mice, but not in the rats at the same dose level and exposure duration (Banerjee, Saha, et al. 1994). The antigen employed to monitor the immune competence, administration time of the antigen, the adjuvant utilized and the immunological parameters measured, also contribute collectively to the inference regarding the immunotoxicity potential of the pesticide. For example, immunosuppression in few of the pesticide-exposed animals, was revealed to be inconsistent with the antibody response to ovalbumin and tetanus toxoid at a shorter exposure duration (Banerjee, Saha, et al. 1994, Banerjee, Pasha, et al. 1998).

Nutritional status and pathological conditions may also influence the immunomodulation exhibited via pesticides. For example, deficiency of protein elevates the immunosuppressive effect of subchronic exposure to DDT (Banerjee, Saha, et al. 1995). Increased bacillary growth in DDT-exposed mice revealed that DDT increased the vulnerability to leprosy infection in a dose-dependent fashion (Banerjee, Koner, et al. 1997). The bio transformed products of pesticides are usually less toxic as compared to the parent compound. However, few of these products may also elicit severe toxicity or immunomodulatory capacity (Ramachandran 1984, Zaidi and Banerjee 1987, Zaidi, Bhatnagar, et al. 1989). OPs and chlorinated compounds may also adversely affect the physiological and pathological conditions and change the nutritional status and hepatic metabolism of other endogenous immunoregulatory compounds (Zaidi, Bhatnagar, et al. 1989). Moreover, the type and duration of emotional and physical stress (that may disrupt homeostasis) and probable involvement of free radicals in inducing oxidative stress are crucial in elevating pesticide-induced immune toxicity (Koner, Banerjee, et al. 1997, Banerjee, Seth, et al. 1998, Koner, Banerjee, et al. 1998).

Many environmental chemicals, instead of exerting direct toxicity, have also shown to alter the state of immunomodulation by increasing susceptibility to various infections. The use of host resistance assays (which assess susceptibility to infectious agents in whole-animal systems which is more relevant to the clinical situation) have been routinely incorporated and emphasized for better understanding and improvement of the predictive value of immunotoxicology testing of chemicals. Among industrially important chemicals, the effect of phthalate ester plasticizers (DOP), heavy metals (lead, arsenic) and pesticides on host resistance and immune surveillance to disease have been thoroughly investigated. The most popular experimental infection models incorporated for the immunotoxicity evaluation have been microbial pathogens (*Candida albicans, Staphylococcus aureus*) that have been used to delineate the possible contribution of xenobiotic-induced state of immunomodulation to infections (Rehman, Mohan, et al. 2011, Bishayi, Bandyopadhyay, et al. 2014, Nandi, Dey, et al. 2015). Some of the parasite models like *Plasmodium berghei* and *Nippostrongylus brasiliensis* and, oncogenic virus *Encephalomyocarditis* (EMCV) have also been established as suitable infection models in rodents for use as endpoints in immunotoxicity assessment of environmental chemicals reported previously to be immunotoxic such as styrene, DOP (Dogra, Chandra, et al. 1989, Dogra, Khanna, et al. 1989).

Macrophages, serving as the first line of defense, act as a link between innate and adaptive immunity and the ability of xenobiotics and natural toxins to impair macrophagic functions may increase the susceptibility to bacterial and viral infections. Research groups have generated information on the interaction of different chemicals with macrophages and their possible immunotoxicological effects (Sengupta and Bishayi 2002). Chemicals like metals and pesticides have shown to interfere with immunological responses in various experimental infection models by diminishing the functional capacities of splenic macrophages manifested as morphological alteration, adherence and chemotactic migration of cells towards infected site, nitric oxide production, significant increase in bacterial load in blood (and delayed bacterial clearance by spleen) thus highlighting an immunocompromised state (Khangarot and Rathore 1999, Bishayi and Sengupta 2003, Ghosh, Datta, et al. 2007, Barbhuiya and Sengupta 2015). All the studies described using host resistance models have demonstrated that exposure of rodents to metals, pesticides, plasticizers, etc. could markedly impair host resistance to infection challenge and supported the notion that a host resistance assay is crucial for evaluating the *in vivo* immunotoxic hazard associated with chemical exposure.

Mycobacterium tuberculosis (Mtb) is a facultative intracellular microbial pathogen and the immune abnormalties of the Mtb-infected macrophage forms the hallmark of mycobacterial pathogenesis. Bacterial pathogens are known to secrete a few virulence factors to modulate the host anti-bacterial response. Few detailed studies have been done to elucidate the putative role of Mtb secretory proteins (MTSA-10, ESAT-6) in the implication of virulence by modulating macrophage functions. Direct interaction with macrophage along with modulation of several host processes such as surface expression of co-stimulatory molecules and MHC molecules (Saha, Das et al. 1994), impaired T-cell-macrophage interaction via co-stimulatory signal (Saha, Das et al. 1995), interference with LPS signaling (Pathak, Basu et al. 2007), immune response suppression (Singh, Singh et al. 2003), miRNA induction (Kumar, Halder et al. 2012) and subversion of the macrophage immune functions by redox regulation (Basu, Kumar et al. 2009) have shown potential involvement. All these studies have suggested a novel mechanism for the immunopathogenesis of Mtb that may have implications for the prevention, diagnosis, and therapy of this disease. Considering that India accounts for one-third of the global TB burden, early and cost-effective diagnosis is a priority. A study has evaluated some of the RD1-encoded antigens of Mtb and explored their usefulness as tools for serodiagnosis by determining the immunological reactivity of these proteins with sera from healthy BCG-vaccinated and TB-infected individuals paving the way for a highly sensitive and specific diagnosis of the disease (Mukherjee, Dutta et al. 2007).

Over the years, one of the crucial revelations has been the realization that tumor regression is immunologically mediated. It has been established that many tumors are antigenic and continuously shed tumor antigens producing immunosuppressive and/or blocking factors, which may help the tumors to escape the immune attack of the host (Rabinovich, Gabrilovich, et al. 2007). Over the years studies have brought light supporting evidences in this regard. It has been shown that immunosuppression elevates metastasis facilitating tumor growth in experimental animals and immunosuppressed individuals are more vulnerable to develop cancer and infection due to compromised immune status. Many anticancer agents like cyclophosphamide when used at low doses have been found to enhance the delayed type hypersensitivity and act as an immunopotentiator, also showing immune regression (Ray, Raychaudhuri et al. 1982). Similarly, disruption of a defence mechanism by aflatoxin B1 leads to enhanced development of a transplantable tumor (Raisuddin, Zaidi, et al. 1991). The probability of immunomodulatory changes culminating in cancer has been best exemplified by arsenic exposure, wherein the profile of arsenic immunotoxicity have hinted towards arsenic-induced carcinogenesis (Acharya, Chaudhuri, et al. 2010). Moreover, studies have also established the importance to explore the nutritional status of the host while assessing the immunotoxicological effects of an environmental pollutant. While malnourishment/coexistence of xenobiotic exposure can serve as a predisposing factor for conferring the host to turn immunosuppressive, exposure of a malnourished host to toxic/carcinogenic chemicals could further elevate the risk of overall toxicity including vulnerability to infections and even carcinogenicity.

The immunosuppression triggered as a result of immunotoxicity exhibited by different chemical carcinogens has been shown to be reversed by immunopotentiation of the cancer-bearing host by employing immunomodulators, which could be either biologically derived or synthetic. Use of some immunomodulators such as Protein A, 6MFA and Poly rI.Rc have shown promising modalities against toxicities mediated by benzene and acrylamide. Amongst them, the use of Protein A (PA), a glycoprotein isolated from the cell wall of *Staphylococcus aureus Cowan* I (SAC) that binds with the Fc portion of mammalian immunoglobin G, has aroused a considerable amount of interest among the tumor immunologists. Ray, et al. 1984, 1985 documented the antitumor properties of PA for the very first time that leads to immunopotentiation and regression of different types of malignant tumors in experimental animals as well as human patients (Ray, Bandyopadhyay, et al. 1984, Ray, Dohadwala, et al. 1985, Prasad, Singh, et al. 1987). Since then, PA has been shown to abrogate the toxicity of various drugs and carcinogens. Mechanism of enhanced phagocytic response of PA at different doses and time durations against tumor regression has been attributed to its ability for immunopotentiation via increased number and macrophagic activity (Singh, Saxena, et al. 1987, Zaidi, Singh, et al. 1990), activated macrophages (Chattopadhyay, Das, et al. 2002), enhanced cytotoxic activity of peripheral blood mononuclear cells (Ray and Bandyopadhyay 1983) and natural killer cell activity (Dwivedi, Verma et al. 1992). PA-induced generation of free radicals by phagocytes is also believed to be related to its antitumor and antitoxic properties. PA activates membrane-bound electron transport system of NADPH oxidase in human neutrophils to generate O^{-2} radicals (Mishra, Dwivedi, et al. 1999). The use of other immunomodulators (non-toxic biological response modifiers) such as 6-MFA (*Aspergillus ochraceous* ATCC 28706) (Singh, George, et al. 1983), polyinosinic polycytidilic acid (an interferon inducer) (Pandya, Shanker, et al. 1986, Maheshwari, Tandon, et al. 1988, Pandya, Khan, et al. 1989, Zaidi, Raisuddin, et al. 1994) in protecting against drug/chemical mediated toxicities have also revealed very promising results.

The basic investigations such as identification of histological alterations and functional changes in the lymphoid organs have been reliable predictors of immunosuppression, but a further dissection of disrupted regulatory mechanisms has been of primary concern. Technological advancements ELISA, microarray, *in silico* approaches, have helped in understanding the mechanistic aspects of complicated immune responses and have increased our understanding to assess the immunotoxicity potential of environmental chemicals. Apart from whole animal models, efforts have also been made to use *in vitro* models as well as lower model systems. Identification of new and improvised models for better understanding of immunotoxicants have been a constant endeavor among toxicologists. To understand the complexity of the immune system, several cellular and molecular targets of immunotoxicants have to be taken into consideration. Cytokines are crucial components of the immune system which connect the several disperse elements immune system and altered regulation of cytokines gene expression has been employed as reliable markers to assess the changes in the immune system. Thakur, et al. 2013 have developed a model for prediction of the immunosuppressant nature of pesticides *in vitro* by analyzing cytokine gene expression which could be employed as an endpoint for assessing disruptions in the immune system *in vivo*. This system uses cell lines which have been transformed utilizing GFP reporter constructs which have a promoter region of Th1, Th2 cytokines and pro-inflammatory cytokines. These transformed cell lines reporter gene were made to be responsive towards the exposure to immunostimulant PMA (Phorbol Myristate Acetate)/Ionomycin and LPS and immunosuppressants like cyclosporine A (CsA) and FK506 on PMA/Ionomycin. Furthermore, three pesticides; cypermethrin, chlorpyriphos and captan have been assessed on this cytokine promoter based assay in order to establish its applicability as a fast and effective tool to assess the chemicals/pesticides mediated immunotoxicity. Using both lymphoid and myeloid cell lines of human origin and GFP as reporter gene the model offers the advantages of using cell lines derived from humans instead of murine origin making it a better model of responses that are likely to take place in humans. Moreover, using GFP as a reporter gene makes the model an economical high throughput screening tool (Thakur, Singh, et al. 2013).

Research groups have also utilized fish as an alternative model to screen out toxicants that influence lymphocyte number, viability and organosomatic indices of immunocompetent organs in fish (Fatima, Ahmad, et al. 2001). In recent years, studies have demonstrated that head kidney macrophages (HKM) from catfish (*Clarias.batrachus*) could serve as an alternative *in vitro* model to assess arsenic induced toxicity and provide insight into the underlying mechanism of arsenic toxicity (Datta, Mazumder, et al. 2009, Banerjee, Singh, et al. 2013). It has been emphasized that exposure to nonlethal concentrations of arsenic could change several hematological parameters in fish triggering tissue-specific and time-dependent alterations in fish B and T-cell functions, rendering them immune-compromised and vulnerable to pathogenic infections (Ghosh, Bhattacharya, et al. 2006, Ghosh, Datta, et al. 2007). Similarly, nonlethal concentrations of chromium could alter humoral antibody response and increase susceptibility to bacterial infections (Khangarot, Rathore, et al. 1999). B cells have also been found to be more susceptible to xenobiotics than the T cells (Ghosh, Bhattacharya, et al. 2006). Identification of novel 65 signature genes (tlr1, nitr1c, nitr1f, socs7, crfb8, abcb3/1, socs3b, ifnγ1-2, mch1uja, crlf1a and cxcl12b) as biomarkers for arsenic-induced immune changes in the adult zebrafish using global gene expression profiling has further shed insights into the involvement of major signaling pathways (JAK-STAT) in increased susceptibility to infections. Initial hyperactivation followed by immunosuppression on further stress (microbial) has been shown on chronic arsenic exposure (Ray, Bhaduri, et al. 2017). A study reveals the applicability of *D. melanogaster* in assessing the probable effects of environmental chemicals on the innate immunity which can be reliably extrapolated to higher organisms because of the evolutionary conservation of innate immune system between *Drosophila* and mammals (Pragya, Shukla, et al. 2015).

With time there has been increasing efforts in establishing an interrelationship between the immune system and the nervous system. This issue has been well taken up by CSIR-IITR that is focused to find out the molecular mechanisms of xenobiotic-induced altered immune function of microglia. Microglial cells are modified macrophages that are the key regulator of the immune response in the nervous system, acting as a double-edged sword. Resting state microglia helps to maintain healthy brain environment by phagocytosing cellular pathogen as well as cellular debris and synaptic pruning, On the other hand, activated microglia secretes cytotoxic factors like ROS and NO, leading to induction of neuroinflammation. Environmental chemicals, such as lead, trimethyltin, acrylamide and diesel exhaust have been shown to potentially hyperactivate microglia and induce neuronal anomalies (Rojo, McBean, et al. 2014). *In vitro* studies, employing cell lines or neonatal mouse primary microglia have efficiently correlated xenobiotic-mediated microglial activation and neuronal death. However, these *in vitro* studies cannot accurately portray the *in vivo* scenario. Therefore, environmental pollutant-induced *in vivo* changes in microglial function can be well assessed via *ex vivo* analysis, which has not been in use due to limitations with the isolation procedure. For the very first time, a study by Singh et al 2014 have not only optimized microglial isolation protocol (without altering their activation status) but also successfully demonstrated the applicability of the isolated microglia from adult mice for *ex vivo* analysis of xenobiotics induced immunotoxic changes for delineating the microglial response (Singh, Mitra et al. 2014).

Such a multitude of reports on xenobiotic-induced immunosuppression has also simultaneously triggered research directed towards identification of protective/preventive agents, few of which have been provided in Table 10.12.

Table 10.12 Comprehensive overview of few protective/therapeutic agents against immunotoxicants

Immunotoxicants	Preventive/protective agents and their mechanism of action	Model and Route of Administration	References
Arsenic (0.05 and 5 ppm)	**Jaggery** (250 mg/mice, daily for 180 days oral): Co-exposure prevented reduction in levels of total antioxidant, glutathione reductase and glutathione peroxidase in the serum, lowered the increased levels of serum interleukin-1β, interleukin-6 and TNF-α, reduced DNA damage, prevented necrosis and degenerative alterations in bronchiolar epithelium with emphysema and alveolar septa thickening	Swiss albino mice, Oral	(Singh, Kumar , et al. 2010)

Contd...

Immunotoxicants	Preventive/protective agents and their mechanism of action	Model and Route of Administration	References
Lead (6.3 mmol/kg b.wt.), daily for 8 weeks	**Zinc** (30 and 45mg/kg b.wt., daily for 7 days; oral) : Supplementation during chelation theraphy of lead led to recovery in changes in primary antibody forming cells to T-dependent antigen and delayed-type hypersensitivity (DTH) response	Wistar rats, Oral	(Kumar, Rai, et al. 1994)
Chromium (10 µg/ml), 18 h	*Emblica officinalis* (Amla, 100 µg/ml): Co-exposure inhibited generation of free radicals, restored the status of anti-oxidant system, relieved the immunosuppressive changes, proliferation of lymphocytes and restored the production of IL-2 and γ-IFN	Sprague- Dawley rats derived lymphocytes	(Ram, Neetu, et al. 2002)
Endosulfan (1.5, 3 and 6 mg/kg b.wt.), daily for 45 days	*Ocimum sanctum* (100mg/kg b.wt.; oral): Co-exposure restored decrease in both the HA titer and DNCB contact sensitivity score	Wistar rats, Oral	(Bharath, Anjaneyulu, et al. 2011)
Deltamethrin (25 µM), 18 h	**Piperine** (1, 10 and 50 µg/ml): Docking results revealed that piperine had good binding affinity towards CD4 and CD8 receptors Co-administration led to amerolation of Deltamethrin induced apoptosis and concentration dependent increase and decrease in the CD4+ and CD8+ cells and increase in IL-2, IFN-γ and IL-4 levels	Primary murine thymocytes from BALB/c mice	(Kumar, Sasmal, et al. 2015)
Cyclophosphamide (50 mg/kg), on the 12th day	**Alcoholic extract of green tea (*Camellia sinensis* L.)**(50, 150 and 250 mg/kg b.wt., i.p., once per day for 14 days): Elevated the thymus and spleen weight, haemagglutination titre, total leucocyte counts and decreased the DTH response	Swiss Albino mice, Intraperitoneal	(Haque and Ansari 2014)

Contd...

Immunotoxicants	Preventive/protective agents and their mechanism of action	Model and Route of Administration	References
Benzene (1.0 ml/kg b.wt.), for 3 days	**6MFA** (an interferon inducer, 100 mg/kg b.wt., i.p.): Pre-treatment normalized lipid peroxidation and iron content, increased leukocyte and lymphocyte counts, restoration of lowered organ weight (lymph nodes, thymus, and spleen)	Albino rats, intraperitoneal	(Pandya, Shanker, et al. 1986)
Benzene (1.0 ml/kg b.wt.), for 3 days	**Polyinosinic-polycytidilic acid** (Poly IC, an interferon inducer, 2500µg/kg b.wt.;i.p.): Pretreatment (24h prior) enhanced the SRBC antibody titre benzene exposed animals	Albino rats, Intraperitoneal	(Pandya, Khan, et al. 1989)
Acrylamide (50 mg/kg b.wt.), daily 10 days	**6MFA**: (100 mg/kg b.wt., single injection on the 5th day of acrylamide exposure) number of circulating lymphocyte,partially recovered the spleen and thymus weight, increase of EAC-rosettes, hemagglutination titre, IgM-PFC andDTH response against SRBC	Albino rats, intraperitoneal	(Zaidi, Raisuddin, et al. 1994)
Propoxur(10 mg/kg b.wt.), daily for 28 days	**Melatonin** (5 mg/kg b.wt.; i.p): Co-exposure reversed effects on the humoral immune response by reduction in the level of oxidative stress and normalized antibody titre and IgM Plaque forming cells	Albino Wistar rats, Oral	(Suke, Kumar, et al. 2006)
Lipopolysaccharide (1 µg/ml), 24 h	***Cymbopogon citrates*** **extract** (5 and 10 µg) pre-treatment for 1 h: decrease in the release of TNF-α and NO indicative of an anti-inflammatory effect, restored mitochondrial membrane potential	Macrophages isolated from Balb/c mice	(Tiwari, Dwivedi, et al. 2010)
Alfatoxin (300 µg/kg b.wt.), for 2 weeks on alternate days)	**Protein A** (60 µg/kg b.wt. post treatment; twice weekly for 2 weeks intravenous): Prevented depletion of peritoneal macrophage population, phagocytosis and depression of lymphocyte transformation	Wistar rats, Oral	(Raisuddin, Singh, et al. 1994)

Immunotoxicants	Preventive/protective agents and their mechanism of action	Model and Route of Administration	References
Semliki forest Virus (100 LD$_{50}$)	**Alone Panax ginseng Extract** (total of 5.4 g/kg over a period of 9 days, oral) **In combination**: extract (10 mg/mouse day for 4 consecutive days) followed by **6-MFA** (1.5 mg/mouse; i.p.) on 5th day, Gingseng could protect upto 32-40 % of lethally infected mice and the protection rate was considerably enhanced on conjunction with 6-MFA (82-100%)	Swiss mice, subcutaneous	(Singh, George, et al. 1983)

An immune response normally evokes a cascade of effector molecules that work to remove antigens by generating a subclinical localized inflammatory response. Under few circumstances, this inflammatory response may have adverse effects, resulting in tissue injury termed as hypersensitivity or allergy. In India, the burden of allergic diseases has been growing in terms of severity and prevalence. These diseases comprise of rhinitis, asthma, anaphylaxis, food, drug, and insect allergy, urticarial, eczema and angioedema. Around 20% to 30 % of the total population in India is suffering from at least one of these allergic diseases (Prasad and Kumar 2013).

In recent years, a multi-center population study, Indian Study on Epidemiology of Asthma, Respiratory Symptoms and Chronic Bronchitis (INSEARCH) has been undertaken. The study encompassed 12 centers consisting of both urban and rural urban areas spanning over several parts in India. The prevalence of combined bronchial asthma from all the 12 centers was found to be 2.05% (range, 0.4%-4.8%). Increasing age, smoking, indoor tobacco smoke (ETS) exposure, use of unclean cooking fuels have been linked with higher risks of asthma (Jindal, Aggarwal, et al. 2012). Studies have also demonstrated a relation between levels of indoor and outdoor air pollutant with several respiratory abnormalities in children (Kumar, Nagar, et al. 2007). A study to ascertain the effects of indoor air pollution (fuel employed for cooking) on respiratory allergies in children was conducted in Delhi. The study suggested that biomass fuel elevated the concentration of indoor air pollutants which may confer higher risk of rhinitis, asthma, and upper respiratory tract infections in the children (Agrawal, Anand, et al. 1983, Kumar, Nagar, et al. 2008). Sensitization to food has been strongly linked to asthma, whereas aeroallergens have been associated with rhinitis. Allergy to food has been estimated to be 4.5% in adolescents and adults having asthma, rhinitis or both. Rice, black gram, citrus fruits, and banana were identified as the main allergens for mediating allergic reactions. In addition, tobacco users had a higher incidence of rhinitis (55% of tobacco users as compared to 12.8% non-tobacco users) (Kumar and Prasad 2014).

One review has analyzed the published studies of drug-induced anaphylaxis reported from India (1998 to 2013) in relation with causative drugs and other clinical characteristics (Patel, Patel, et al. 2014). The major causative groups were antimicrobials (18.52%), NSAIDs (12.96%) neuromuscular blockers (12.96%), anesthetic agents (9.26%) and β-lactams (5.96%). The review also concisely covers the therapeutic interventions made for the management of such anaphylactic reactions using agents like adrenaline, corticosteroids, antihistaminics and many others.

Amongst the various allergies and cases of hypersensitivity, food allergy has drawn significant attention among Indian immunotoxicologists. Dietary habits of the considerable population of an area have shown to play an essential role in food allergy development. Leguminous crops are the primary source of protein in the Asian subcontinent including India and legumes such as chickpea, red gram, black gram and moong are few of the crops which consist of major food allergens for the Indian population (Singh and Kumar 2003, Misra, Kumar, et al. 2010, Mishra, Singh, et al. 2011). Instances of IgE-mediated allergic reactions in sensitized individuals have also been widely reported from India (Misra, Prasad, et al. 2008). Black gram mediates IgE mediated responses in patients with asthma and allergic rhinitis (Kumari, Kumar, et al. 2006). Similarly, chickpea mediates hypersensitivity reactions extending from rhinitis to anaphylaxis (Patil, Niphadkar, et al. 2001) as well as IgE-induced allergic reactions in patients with nasobronchial allergy and animal models (Verma, Kumar, et al. 2012).

Identification and characterization of allergens have been recognized as a crucial step for immunotherapy and clinical screening. The severity and prevalence of such legumes induced allergic reactions have prompted research groups towards the purification, characterization and assessment of allerginicity of such proteins. Stability towards digestion against gastric enzymes has been thought to be a vital aspect of the allergenic food protein. This feature of allergenic proteins has been used by assessing the effects of simulated gastric fluid (SGF) treatment on the integrity and IgE binding potential of the allergen. Various studies have screened out pepsin resistant proteins of several legumes such as black gram, chickpea, kidney bean and Bengal gram (demonstratingw stability towards gastric digestion) that have revealed IgE binding potential with respective allergic patient's sera (Niphadkar, Patil, et al. 1997, Misra, Prasad, et al. 2009). Partial characterization of red gram (*Cajanus cajan L. Millsp*) polypeptides identified by patients having bronchial asthma and rhinitis have led to identification of 5 new IgE binding proteins (Caj c1, Caj c2, Caj c3, Caj c4 and Caj c5) which bear homology to known allergens (Misra, Kumar, et al. 2010). Moreover, a number of non-digestible proteins from the black gram (10), chickpea (7), kidney bean (5) and Bengal gram (1) and IgE binding of SGF resistant soybean and chickpea proteins have been identified for the very first time (Misra, Prasad, et al. 2009). Likewise, a 26kDa protein (in Chickpea), a 47.5kDa protein phaseolin (in Red Kidney Bean) have been identified as the etiological agents for causing allergenicity (Verma, Kumar, et al. 2012, Kumar, Verma, et al. 2014). Similarly, Phytohemagglutinins (PHA), specifically PHA-L and PHA-E, the main constituents of a kidney bean, have been demonstrated to induce allergic responses via the IgE and non- IgE induced pathway as observed by the Th1/Th2 cytokines and transcription factors (Kumar, Verma, et al. 2013).

Numerous therapeutic strategies have been employed to cure food allergies, including oral immunotherapy. In oral immunotherapy, induction of oral tolerance against food allergens results in prevention of food allergy in the long term (Tang and Martino 2013). Oral tolerance induction can be mediated via initial antigen exposure (induction of inherent tolerance), and secondly, by transfer of Tregs (acquired tolerance) (Yamashita, Takahashi, et al. 2012). As an extension to their previous study, reporting allergenicity inducing capacity of green gram in the nasobronchial asthmatic patients as well as in mice in 2011, Kumar et al 2014 have explored the induction of oral tolerance (following a single acute dose) as a therapeutic approach to minimize the symptoms of green gram induced allergenicity wherein the total and specific IgE/IgG1 levels in the serum, anaphylaxis symptoms, DTH, CD^{4+} and CD^{8+} cells were observed to be lowered with higher levels of Foxp3 and IL-10 (Misra, Kumar, et al. 2011, Kumar, Sharma, et al. 2014). Moreover, computational prediction of allergenicity of transgenic proteins that are expressed in GM crops has also been carried out. Verma, et al. 2010 have tested and validated 312 allergenic, 100 non-allergenic, and 48 inserted proteins via for sequence similarity using 8-mer, 80-mer, and full FASTA search. Use of routine sequence homology has also been combined with few other bioinformatic methods like ADFS/Algpred that have helped decrease false prediction of allergenicity of novel proteins (74-78%) (Verma, Misra, et al. 2011).

As a form of hypersensitivity, modulation of the immune system may also lead to increased incidences of inflammation and allergic reactions. Environmental exposure to xenobiotics can induce oxidative stress and inflammation, which stands as one of the widely cited prominent toxicity mechanism. Macrophage, microglial disturbances have been shown to be induced by environmental exposure of xenobiotics, which in turn could initiate a multitude of inflammatory responses (Sunkaria, Wani, et al. 2012). Benzanthrone (BA), one of widely used industrial dye, manifests allergic reactions clinically as well as in animals (Trivedi and Niyogi 1968, Singh and Zaidi 1969, Singh, Das, et al. 2000, Tewari, Roy, et al. 2015). Studies have provided new mechanistic insights about the inter-relation between BA induced manifestations by identification of mediators involved in the amplification of its inflammatory responses. BA has been shown to trigger increased production of pro-inflammatory cytokines IL-17, TNF α, IFN γ and IL-1. These cytokines have been reported to play a pivotal role in the amplification of inflammatory responses and progressions of inflammatory disorders like asthma and autoimmune tissue inflammations (Tewari, Roy, et al. 2015).

Studies by Tewari, et al. 2017 using *in silico* approaches have also revealed the pivotal role of Toll-Like Receptors (TLRs) in the BA-mediated inflammatory responses in macrophages, demonstrating that activation of innate immunity receptors via agonist ligands that are prevalent as environmental pollutants may result in undesirable inflammatory changes. The apparent macrophage phenotype (with downregulated expression of MHC class I and MHC class II molecules) may lead to increase of inflammation and disrupt the homeostasis of adaptive immune responses. The study has assigned another crucial role to the new emerging functions of TLRs and emphasizes that TLRs may not just recognize pathogen-associated molecules but even xenobiotics (Tewari, Mandal, et al. 2017).

Asthma, a hypersensitivity reaction, is characterized via airway inflammation and hyper-responsiveness, higher levels of IgE, higher infiltration of inflammatory cells such as eosinophils, mast cells, neutrophils and elevated generation of cytokines and chemokines (Rogerio, Kanashiro, et al. 2007). Using an experimental murine model, the prominent role of oxidative stress with an emphasis on inflammatory responses in asthma pathophysiology has been clearly demonstrated in several studies (Cho and Moon 2010). The constant increase in the number of asthmatics and patients with allergic rhinitis has required heavy reliance on synthetic drugs and inhalers resulting in side effects which have developed a niche for exploring plant derived antioxidants for their pharmacological capacity. Studies are suggestive of anti-asthmatic effects of several plants and their constituents, which are capable of reducing the release of pro-inflammatory mediators and could better aid in the management of asthma. Results have suggested the use of cytoprotective, antioxidant and anti-inflammatory properties of *C. citratus* in the form of a potential dietary component and in formulations against lung inflammatory disorders where oxidative stress plays a crucial role (Tiwari, Dwivedi, et al. 2010). A study by Tewari et al 2014 has demonstrated potential protective efficacy of Tc extract against oxidative stress and inflammation during asthma as observed via modulation of glutathione homeostasis, elevated total antioxidant capacity of serum and lowered LPO in an animal model of asthma that could possibly prevent inflammation (Tiwari, Dwivedi, et al. 2014).

Drug hypersensitivity syndrome (DHS) is an adverse drug reaction related with various drugs, even in their therapeutic range. Identification of allele that may predispose the individual to the drug's allergic reaction may help in better management of the patients. In this context, HLA-B*58 haplotype has been recognized to be a major risk factor for DHS with imatinib therapy (Khan, Bhartia, et al. 2014). Similarly, studies have revealed a strong association between HLA-B*1502 allele and carbamazepine-mediated Stevens-Johnson syndrome among Indians (Mehta, Prajapati, et al. 2009). In this direction, an extensive database of herbal medicines showing immense potential in the management of allergic symptoms has been generated. Several medicinal plants classified as "Rasayana" in Ayurveda are suggested to be useful for immune system strengthening (Patwardhan, Kalbag, et al. 1990). Multitude of studies have been undertaken for exploration of immunopharmacological activities of several botanical drugs: *Withania somnifera* (Linn Dunal) (Solanaceae) (Ashwagandha), *Tinospora cordifolia* (Miers) (Menispermaceae) (Guduchi), and *Asparagus racemosus* (Willd.) (Liliaceae) (Shatavari) that have been screened from a large database of Rasayana (Diwanay, Chitre et al. 2004). *Withania somnifera* (conventional drug and specified in the Indian Pharmacopoeia, 1985) has been revealed to be an immunoregulator in animal modesl of immune inflammation (Agarwal, Diwanay, et al. 1999). The stems of *Tinospora cordifolia* have been reported for its several immunopharmacological activities, such as anti-oxidant properties and reduction of adverse effects of cyclophosphamide (CP) (Mathew and Kuttan 1997), anticomplementary and immunomodulatory activities (Kapil and Sharma 1997) apart from relieving symptoms of rheumatism (Agharkar 1953, Agharkar 1953) being anti-allergic, anti-arthritic and anti-inflammatory (Chopra, Chopra et al. 1958, Nadkarni and Nadkarni 1976, Kirtikar and Basu 1987). Roots of *Asparagus racemosus* have been demonstrated to induce macrophages and favorably influence long-term adaptation. It inhibits stress-mediated elevation in plasma cortisol with peritoneal macrophages activation and prevention of gastric vascular damage (Dahanukar and Thatte, 1988).

Autoimmune diseases are common, which appear in genetically vulnerable individuals, with the disease being regulated by environment. Studies have identified biomarkers of susceptibility to type 1 diabetes (TID) (a polygenic autoimmune disease, characterized by the appearance of circulating islet autoantibodies) strongly linked to the MHC. Of the 20 genomic intervals contributing to the risk of developing T1D, the MHC region on chromosome 6p21.31 (IDDM1) has been the chief contributor, which is followed by 50 regulatory region of the insulin (INS) gene on chromosome 11p15.5 (IDDM2) and many other minor loci including insulin, CTLA4 (Mehra, Kumar, et al. 2007). Antibody responses have been of importance in permitting reliable diagnosis and prediction of vulnerable individuals in developing T1D. Insulin autoantibodies (IAAs), circulating cytoplasmic islet cell autoantibodies (ICAs), and antibodies to a 65 kD antigen (glutamic acid decarboxylase or GAD) are present at diagnosis in around 70-80 per cent of patients while GAD65 and insulinoma-associated protein-2 (IA-2) antibodies are reported to be present in 20-26 per cent of cases of T1D from north India (Goswami, Kochupillai et al. 2001, Tandon, Shtauvere-Brameus et al. 2002). Research groups have also reported significant diversity in HLA class I and class II genes in the north Indian population and identified many 'novel alleles' and 'unique haplotypes'. For example, multiple DR3+ve autoimmunity that favors haplotypes have been identified, few of which are unique to the Asian North Indian T1D patients. Molecular studies have further suggested that the classical Caucasian autoimmunity favoring AH8.1 (HLA-A1 B8 DR3) is quite rare in the Indian population and has been instead replaced by a variant AH8.1v that is different from the Caucasian AH8.1 at many gene loci and there are more HLA-DR3 haplotypes HLA-A24 B8 DR3 (AH8.3), A3 B8 DR3 (AH8.4) and A31 B8 DR 3 (AH 8.5) which are prevalent in the Indian population (Mehra, Kaur et al. 2002). The two independently assorting alleles at two loci, i.e., DRB1*0301 and INS-VNTR class I, on two different chromosomes have been identified which may have the capacity to predict a prediabetic in North India (Rani, Sood et al. 2004). Similarly, HLA B27, HLA cw4 and HLA DRB1*01XX have also been linked with autoimmune hepatitis type I (Amarapurkar, Patel, et al. 2003).

10.6 Genotoxicity

Genotoxic effects are considered amongst the most serious possible side effects of xenobiotics. A genotoxin has been described as a chemical or agent that may cause DNA damage, prolonged exposure to which may also ultimately lead to impact including heritable genetic diseases (germline mutation), carcinogenesis (somatic mutation), reproductive dysfunction, and even birth defects. With an increase in the number of NCEs released into the environment, it has also become imperative to assess their potential to exert genotoxicity, mutagenicity, or carcinogenicity. Since DNA is the carrier of inheritable genetic information and any alterations in its structure may result in deleterious biological modifications that may be inherited, an understanding of the genotoxic effects of chemicals have been a significant area of research in India.

The association of habitual chewing of the "betel quid" with oral cancer has been the subject of detailed epidemiological studies in India since the 1970s (Jussawalla and Deshpande 1971, Jayant, Balakrishnan, et al. 1977, Ranadive, Ranadive, et al. 1979, Gupta, Pindborg, et al. 1982, Sen, Talukder, et al. 1986) and numerous cytogenetic studies revealed higher genomic damage among consumers of 'pan masala', cytogenetical parameters as well as identification of useful biomarkers (level of endogenous GSH and the level of p53 protein)

(Dave, Trivedi, et al. 1991, Kumpawat and Chatterjee 2003). Because of the extensive human exposure, existing information on carcinogenicity from epidemiological surveys along with well established role of the pan chewing habit in the etiology of oral, pharyngeal and oesophageal cancer in Indian populations ultimately prompted research groups to investigate the genotoxicity of the individual ingredients of betel quid (major ingredients such as betel nut, tobacco, betel leaf and slaked lime) singly and in combination using different model systems (short-term assays on mammalian cell cultures and bacterial systems) and cytogenetic endpoints such as sister chromatid exchanges (SCEs), dominant lethal mutations, chromosomal aberrations (CAs) (Jayant, Balakrishnan, et al. 1977, Abraham, Goswami, et al. 1979, Panigrahi and Rao 1982, Giri, Banerjee, et al. 1987, Adhvaryu, Dave, et al. 1989, Bagwe, Ganu, et al. 1990, Dave, Trivedi, et al. 1991, Mukherjee and Giri 1991). Lifestyle habits such as caffeine intake (Panigrahi and Rao 1983), alcohol consumption (Patel, Trivedi, et al. 1994) were found to aggravate the genetic damage further increasing the risk of oral cancer in the human population. More importantly, the carcinogenic potential of betel was found to be higher in pregnant women and oral contraceptive users owing to their elevated hormonal profile (Ghosh and Ghosh 1988). This study assumed significance owing to the ability of the alkaloid to elicit *in utero* appearance of micronuclei in the fetal cells as well as highlighting its developmental toxicity (Sinha and Rao 1985). At the same time, mutagenicity potential of alkaloids (consumed as food or drugs) from various plants was of much interest among the toxicologists. A comprehensive account of the mutagenicity and clastogenecity of food dyes used in India has been published (Giri 1991).

Over the years, studies have identified genotoxic risks associated with various occupational and environmental agents. An increase in micronuclei frequency in tobacco processing plant workers and bidi rollers (Bagwe and Bhisey 1993, Mahimkar and Bhisey 1995), higher levels of chromosomal aberrations and altered cell kinetics and mitotic index in workers exposed to pesticides (Rita, Reddy, et al. 1987, Rupa, Reddy, et al. 1989, Rupa, Reddy, et al. 1991) have been widely reported. The demonstration of chromosomal damage on exposure to arsenic-containing drinking water (Ghosh, Basu, et al. 2008, Mazumder and Dasgupta 2011) and consumption of adulterated mustard oil (Das, Ansari, et al. 2005) have also been correlated with genotoxic damage in individuals. Apart from acute exposures, the need for determining the potential genotoxic effects of long term exposure to environmental and complex workplace environment have been of particular importance in India. Arsenic-induced skin lesions, for example, have been shown to typically manifest after a latency period which ranges from a period of 6 months to 10 years of exposure, that may lead to the development of cancer, making it imperative to monitor cytogenetic damage for future preventive measures (Basu, Ghosh, et al. 2004, Mahata, Chaki, et al. 2004)

Moreover, the nature of interaction between multiple environmental pollutants in causing diseases to humans has always been debated and the same has shown to be more than true even in the case of genotoxicants where epidemiological and experimental studies have highlighted genotoxic effects due to mixture of environmental chemicals, determining the influence of various factors on the susceptibility to these genotoxicants such as increased vulnerability due to consumption of alcohol and exposure to lead in printing press workers (Rajah and Ahuja 1995), simultaneous exposure to environmental compounds like kerosene soot and cigarette smoke enhancing the sensitivity to deleterious effects of asbestos exposure (Rahman, Dopp, et al. 2000, Lohani, Dopp, et al. 2002, Arif, Khan, et al., 1992, 1994, 1997). To explore the possibilities of the effects of genotoxicants at sites other than their sites of exposure, cytogenetic analysis in peripheral blood lymphocytes of Indian population has been extensively carried out using chromosomal aberrations (CA), Micronuclei (MN) and sister chromatid exchanges (SCEs) as the endpoint for biomonitoring since they are considered to be biomarkers for early biological effects of carcinogen exposure. Since most lymphocytes belong to the redistribution pool, lymphocytes exposed to a mutagen anywhere in the body could eventually occur in peripheral blood. This system has offered an added advantage to further test the *in vivo* mutagenic/genotoxic effects of chemicals directly on human somatic cells derived from humans under long term exposure to toxicants (Rahman, et al. 2000 (Lohani, Dopp, et al. 2000, Lohani, et al. 2002).

Initially, only long-term animal bioassays, that involved lifetime studies, were conducted for classification of substances as mutagens/ carcinogens. These tests were time-consuming and exhaustive requiring a lot of facilities and labour. It was not until the 1970s that most of the current routines genetic toxicology tests were developed and short-term tests, were brought into practice, proposed by a number of regulatory authorities, that were used for identification of carcinogens and characterization for cancer risk assessment. Since the very inception, India remained in the forefront utilizing short term assays systems such as bacterial reverse test, dominant lethal and sperm shape abnormality test in *Drosophila*. Gradually other genotoxic endpoints also gained importance in routine testing and regulatory purposes and voluminous data has been generated unequivocally demonstrating the genotoxic/mutagenic potential of different categories of xenobiotics in various model systems. Several *in vitro* and *in vivo* systems for genotoxicity have been employed, using different systems and organ cell lines (bacterial systems, bone marrow cells, macrophages, lymphocytes, germ cells and somatic cells), that, with a battery of endpoints, are capable of detecting DNA damage and its consequences in prokaryotes (e.g. bacterial) or eukaryotes (e.g. mammalian, avian or yeast). These assays have been employed to assess the safety of environmental chemicals and consumer products and to explore the mechanism of action of known or suspected carcinogens. Cytogenetic endpoints such as the frequency of chromosome aberrations (CA) or sister chromatid exchanges and micronuclei (MN) have offered an excellent opportunity to quantify such genomic instability microscopically. This method has been employed in epidemiological studies to explore the impact of lifestyle factors, nutrition, exposure to genotoxin and genotype on DNA damage and cell death.

Over the years, India has made substantial progress in generating a large database on the genotoxic potential of xenobiotics viz pesticides, heavy metals, steroids, nanoparticles, food-based toxicants, drugs as well as other environmental and occupational agents using different model systems. Studies have employed various cytogenetic endpoints (CA, SCE, MN, COMET) to evaluate cytogenetic responses to chemical exposure and an excellent dose-response relationship has been established for chemicals using a panel of *in vitro* and *in vivo* short term tests. These xenobiotics have been shown to act through the multitude of mechanisms to cause chromosomal aberrations, disruption of DNA repair process, dysregulation of the cell cycle, change in the activities of tumor suppressor gene, etc., resulting in genotoxicity and carcinogenicity. Few of the studies on the effects as well as the underlying mechanisms have been outlined in Table 10.13.

Table 10.13 Few representative studies on the effects/mechanism of different categories of genotoxicants

Genotoxicants	Effects/ Mechanism of Action	Model and Route of Administration	References
Metals			
Cesium chloride (500, 250, and 125 mg/kg b.wt.), 6, 12, 18, and 24 h	Dose dependent elevation in the frequency of CA, 500 mg group was very mitostatic, 250 mg ineffective, and 125 mg slightly mitogenic	Albino mice, Oral	(Ghosh, Sharma, et al. 1991)
Zinc (1.5×10^{-4} M and 3.0×10^{-4} M), 72 h	Significant increase of micronucleated cytokinesis-blocked cells (MNCBs)	Cultured human leukocyte	(Santra, Das, et al. 2002)
Arsenic (exposed through drinking water) (368.11 µg/l)	Exposed individuals revealed a drastic rise in MN frequency in the oral mucosa, lymphocytes and urothelial cells and	Lymphocyte, oral mucosa cells, urothelial cells	(Basu, Mahata, et al. 2002)
Arsenic (exposed through drinking water) (214.7213±9.0273 µg/l)	Chronic ingestion was linked to higher incidence of MN in all cell types, slightly increased level of MN observed in lymphocytes as compared to others	Lymphocyte, oral mucosa cells, urothelial cells	(Basu, Ghosh, et al. 2004)

Contd...

Genotoxicants	Effects/ Mechanism of Action	Model and Route of Administration	References
Arsenic (exposed through drinking water 52–1055 µg/l	DNA damage as well as chromosomal aberrations were observed to be enhanced in the exposed population, within the exposed, only CA was enhanced in exposed individuals with hyperkeratosis as compared to those exposed individuals without hyperkeratosis, DNA repair capacity in the exposed individuals with premalignant hyperkeratosis was reduced than those without skin lesion	Lymphocytes	(Banerjee, Sarma, et al. 2008)
Pesticides			
Rogor (dimethoate)(1.5 x 10^{-5} % (w/w) for both first and second stage larvae and 2x10^{-5} % for third stage), entire larvae life	Triggered sex linked recessive lethals in immature germ cells and was mutagenic/and or recombinogenic in both somatic cells and the germ line cells	Drosophila Melanogaster larvae, Oral	(Tripathy, Majhi, et al. 1988)
Lindane (50, 75 and 100 mg/kg b.wt.), 24 and 48 h	Highest dose (100 mg/kg) caused significant enhancement of chromosome aberrations after 24 and 48 h and with the second highest dose (75 mg/kg) after 24 h, higher frequency of MN in bone marrow cells was induced by all three doses (100, 75 and 50 mg/kg) given either intraperitoneally or orally orally while in peripheral erythrocytes only	Chicks (*Gallus domesticus*), Intraperitoneal/Oral	(Bhunya and Jena 1992)
Cypermethrin (30, 40, and 50 mg/kg b.wt.), For the micronucleus assay, each of the three doses given twice with an interval of 24 h, and the animals were	Dose dependent induction in the micronucleated PCEs than NCEs Various abnormal head shapes and sizes, including giant sperm and branched sperm were induced by cypermethrin that were not dose dependent	Swiss mice, intraperitoneal	(Bhunya and Pati 1988)

Contd...

Genotoxicants	Effects/ Mechanism of Action	Model and Route of Administration	References
sacrificed 6 h after the second injection. For the sperm abnormality assay, each dose was fractionated into five equal parts and each part was injected at 24 h intervals			
Cypermethrin (12.5, 25, 50, 100, 200 mg/kg b.wt., 5 days)	Induces dose dependent systemic genotoxicity, brain revealed maximum DNA damage followed by spleen > kidney > bone marrow> liver > lymphocytes	Swiss albino mice, intraperitoneal	(Patel, Pandey, et al. 2006)
Deltamethrin (5.6, 8.4, or 11.2 mg/kg b.wt.) 5 consecutive days	The mitotic index decreased in a dose-dependent manner, an induction in the incidence of CA in the bone marrow at 24 h post exposure, most prevalent abnormality was endomitotic reduplication of chromosomes along with mitotic inhibition and micronucleus induction. Parenteral administration more effective in elicitin genotoxicity than oral administration	Albino rats, Oral, Intraperitoneal and subcutaneous	(Agarwal, Chauhan, et al. 1994)
Carbosulfan (1.25, 2.5 and 5 mg/kg b.wt.) 5 times	Significant increases in the frequency of sister chromatid exchanges in bone marrow cells, induced a delay in the cell cycle, as observed by elevation in average generation time along with accumulation of cells in the first division cycle	Swiss albino mice, intraperitoneal	(Giri, Giri, et al. 2002)
Carbofuran (1.9, 3.8 or 5.7 mg/kg b.wt.), 24 h for CA 5.7 mg/kg b.wt., 24 and 48 h for MN	All the test doses induced mitotic inhibition, CAs, micronucleus MN. formation and sperm abnormalities in a dose dependent manner	Swiss albino mice, oral	(Chauhan, Pant, et al. 2000)

Contd...

Genotoxicants	Effects/ Mechanism of Action	Model and Route of Administration	References
Dichlorvos and pendimethalin (1 µM, 10 µM, 100 µM, 1000 µM, and 10,000 µM, 3 h)	Pendimethalin produced significant concentration dependent (0.1–100 µM) induction in DNA damage, while dichlorvos induced significantly high extent of DNA damage in CHO cells at comparatively lower concentrations (0.01–10 µM)	Chinese Hamster Ovary cells	(Patel, Bajpayee, et al. 2007)
Chlorpyrifos (50 mg and 100 mg/kg b.wt. daily for 1, 2, and 3 days and 1.12 mg and 2.24 mg/kg b. wt. for 90 days)	Both acute and chronic exposure caused a dose-dependent induction in DNA damage in the brain and liver of rats	Albino rats, intramuscular	(Mehta, Verma, et al. 2008)
Chlorphyifos (CPF)(77.5 mg/kg b.wt.), **Methyl Parathion** (MPT) (6.5 mg/kg b.wt.) and Malathion (MLT)(687.5 mg/kg b.wt), 24, 48 and 72 hrs	Acute and chronic exposure resulted in marked DNA damage in the brain, liver, spleen, and kidney, time dependent DNA repair was observed, MPT triggered highest amount of DNA damage and brain was affected maximum by these OP compounds	Wistar albino rats, Oral	(Ojha, Yaduvanshi, et al. 2011)
Chlorpyrifos (CPF, LC50 0.2 mg/L), **methyl parathion** (MPT, LC50 0.135 mg/L) and **malathion** (MLT, LC50 5.2 mg/L), individually and mixture to give 1/20, 1/10, 1/8, 1/6 and 1/4 LC50, 2 and 4 h	Increase in ROS namely, superoxide anion and hydrogenperoxide and oxidative stress, on exposure with CPF, MPT and MLT individually and in combination of different period of time, MPT exposure caused maximum DNA damage (single and double strand breaks) followed by CPF and MLT	Cultured lymphocytes from albino Wistar rats, Oral	(Ojha and Srivastava 2014)
Monocrotophos (0.046, 0.093, 0.186, 0.373 and 0.746 mg/kg b.wt.), 24, 48 and 72h	Dose related induction and time dependent decrease in the comet tail length indicating DNA damage	Swiss albino mice, Oral	(Mahboob, Rahman, et al. 2002)

Contd...

Genotoxicants	Effects/ Mechanism of Action	Model and Route of Administration	References
Endosulfan (9.8, 12.7 and 16.6 mg/kg b.wt./day), 5 days	At higher doses, triggered dominant lethal mutations in one mating interval (36-42 days) after exposure, dose-dependent induction in sperm abnormalities	Swiss albino mice, Intraperitoneal	(Pandey, Gundevia, et al. 1990)
Endosulfan (0.5, 0.25 and 0.2 µg/l) day 1, 7, 15, 22, 29, 36, and 43	Tissues (kidney gill and blood erythrocytes) at all concentrations resulted in the highest DNA damage on day 1, after which nonlinear reduction in tail DNA percentage	Teleost fish Mystus vittatus	(Sharma, Nagpure, et al. 2007)
Quinalphos (0.1, 0.2, 0.4 and 0.8 µg/ml) **Methyl parathion** (0.02, 0.04, 0.08 and 0.16 µg/ml), 24, 48 and 72 h	Quinalphos induced CA and SCE in a time and dose dependent manner Methyl-parathion did not induce chromosomal aberrations but it did induce SCEs significantly over all time periods	Human peripheral lymphocytes	(Rupa, Reddy, et al. 1990)
Chlorpyrifos (0.28 to 8.96 mg/kg b.wt.), **Acephate** (12.25 to 392.00 mg/kg b.wt.) 24,48,72 and 96 h	Dose dependent increase in DNA damage, DNA damage repair by 96 h	Swiss albino mice, Oral	(Rahman, Mahboob, et al. 2002)
Nanoparticles			
Stable aqueous suspensions of colloidal C60 fullerenes prepared by ethanol to water solvent exchange (EthOH/nC60suspensions) and extended mixing in water (aqu/nC60 suspensions)	Comet assay revealed genotoxicity for both suspensions with a strong association between the genotoxic response and nC60 concentration, genotoxicity seen at concentrations as low as 2.2 µg/L for aqu/nC60 and 4.2 µg/L for EtOH/nC60	Human lymphocytes	(Dhawan, Taurozzi, et al. 2006)
Nanosilver (10, 20, 40 and 50 ppm) 0.5, 1, 2 and 4h 24, 48 and 72 h	Dose dependent induction in the incidence of CA and decrease in mitotic index, alterations such as fragments, stickiness, C-metaphase, laggard, anaphasic bridge and disrupted anaphase	Allium cepa root meristem	(Babu, Deepa, et al. 2008)

Contd...

Genotoxicants	Effects/ Mechanism of Action	Model and Route of Administration	References
Zinc oxide nanoparticles (300 and 2000 mg/kg b.wt.) 24, 48, and 72 h	Reactive oxygen species (ROS), 8-oxo-20-deoxyguanosine and CAs were increased at the highest dosage (2000 mg/kg) of ZnONPs, abnormal sperm morphology observed at day 34.5	Swiss mice, Oral	(Srivastav, Kumar, et al. 2017)
Nano-titanium dioxide (10 and 50 mg/ml) 6–24 h	Induction of oxidative stress, induced the generation of apoptotic bodies and MN	A549 cell line	(Srivastava, Rahman, et al. 2013)
Amphibole asbestos fibers (amosite, crocidolite and tremolite) (2–40 mg/mL) of each asbestos fiber) 24, 48, and 72 h.	Concentration dependent induction in the incidence of MN in binucleated (BN) cells, crocidolite was most genotoxic, followed by tremolite, and amosite, parallel ROS formation by crocidolite, tremolite and amosite	A549 cell line	(Srivastava, Lohani, et al. 2010)
Mobile phone radiations 2The average daily duration of exposure to mobile phone radiations is 61.26 min with an overall average duration of exposure in term of years is 2.35 years)	Slight elevation in frequency of karyorrhexis, broken egg and bi nucleated cells positive correlation between years of exposure and the frequency of MNC and TMN	Exfoliated cells from buccal mucosa	(Yadav and Sharma 2008)
Miscellaneous			
Erythromycin (clinically equivalent dose (CED; EMC 14.2 mg/kg b.wt.) and a lower dose (EMC 10 mg/ kg b.wt.), gestation (14, 15, 16, 17, 18 and 19) and lactation (PND 1, 2, 3, 4, 5 and 6)	Transplacental exposure of 14.2 mg/kg showed a significant increase in micronucleated reticulocytes (MnRETs) and micronucleated normochromatocytes (MnNCEs) in peripheral blood erythrocytes as well as bone marrow of pups in comparison 10 mg/kg group and a parallel a significant reduction in percentage of RETs	Mice, Intraperitoneal	(Singh, Singh, et al. 2014)

Contd...

Genotoxicants	Effects/ Mechanism of Action	Model and Route of Administration	References
Norethynodrel (20,40 and 60 µg/ml), 72 h	Under metabolic activation affected cell growth kinetics, caused chromatids and chromosome breaks at 60 µg/ml	Human lymphocytes	(Siddique and Afzal 2005)
Norgestrel (10, 25 and 50 µg/ml), 24, 48 and 72 h	Time and dose dependent induction in CA, SCE and inhibition of lymphocyte proliferation at 25 and 50 µg/ml only	Human lymphocytes	(Ahmad, Shadab, et al. 2001)
Norethindrone (20, 40 and 75 µg/ml), 24, 48 and 72 h	The drug norethindrone was found to be non-genotoxic at any concentration		
Benzene and its major metabolites p-benzoquinone (BQ), hydroquinone (HQ), catechol (CT), 1,2,4-benzenetriol (BT) and trans–trans muconic acid (MA)] at concentrations 0.5–50µM, 3 h	Concentration-dependent adverse effects in all end points (Comet assay, cytokinesis blocked micronucleus (CBMN) assay, MN and CA, HQ was found to be the most potent DNA damaging metabolite followed by BQ> BT > CT > BZ >MA *In silico* studies employing several genotoxicity endpoints and molecular docking studies with human topoisomerase-II alpha, a major DNA repair enzyme were undertaken, corroborated with the *in vitro* results, observed genotoxicity associated with the structural features and several interactions of metabolites with the enzyme	Chinese Hamster Ovary cells	(Pandey, Gurbani, et al. 2009)
Argemone oil (0.5, 1, 2 and 4 ml/kg b. wt. chromosome aberrations (24h) and micronucleus test (30 min), while 0.25, 0.5, 1.0 and 2.0 ml/kg b. wt. for alkaline comet assay (24h)	Frequencies of CA and MN formation in erythrocytes in the mouse bone marrow cells elevated in a dose-dependent manner (0.5mg), comet assay demonstrated DNA damage in blood, bone marrow and liver cells (1 ml/kg)	Swiss albino mice, Intraperitoneal	(Ansari, Chauhan, et al. 2004)

Contd...

Genotoxicants	Effects/ Mechanism of Action	Model and Route of Administration	References
Sanguinarine alkaloid (1.35, 2.70, 5.40, 10.80 and 21.60 mg/kg b.wt.), 24 h	Dose dependent induction in DNA damage in blood and bone marrow cells by Comet assay, all the parameters including Olive tail moment, tail length and tail DNA revealed induction (33–51%) at a dose of 10.80 mg sanguinarine alkaloid/kg bwt.	Swiss albino mice, Intraperitoneal	(Ansari, Dhawan, et al. 2005)
Argemone oil (0.15–0.3 ml) or isolated sanguinarine (4.5–18 mmol), 25 weeks	The increased p53 and p21/WAF1 expression in the skin, DNA damage in terms of olive tail moment (89–129%), tail length (54%) and tail DNA (153– 205%)	Swiss albino mice, Topical application	(Das, Ansari, et al. 2005)
Arecoline, betel-nut alkaloid (0.25, 0.5, 1 and 2 mg/kg b.wt./daily), 10, 20 and 30 days	Dose dependent rise in the numbers of aberrations were observed in the form of chromatid breaks, ring structure chromosome breaks, multiple breaks and ceils with pulverized chromosomal complements	Swiss albino mice, Intraperitoneal	(Panigrahi and Rao 1982)
Arecoline (20, 40 and 80 mg/kg b.wt./daily), 5 days	Dose-related rise in the number of abnormal sperm heads, as well as the unscheduled [3H] thymidine incorporation into the DNA of early spermatids	Swiss albino mice, Intraperitoneal	(Sinha and Rao 1985)
Nicotine (150, 250, 375, 500, 625 µg/ml and 1000 µg/ml) 2, 4, 24 and 48 h	Induction of CA and SCE frequency in a dose and duration dependent manner	CHO cells	(Trivedi, Dave, et al. 1990)
Pan masala (betel quid) (5, 12.5, 25, 50, 100 or 200 mg /kg b.wt.), 24 h	Dose-related increase in sister chromatid exchanges, with the minimum effective dose being 25 mg/kg, two highest doses resulted in a prominent cell cycle delay	Swiss albino mice, Intraperitoneal	(Mukherjee and Giri 1991)
Metanil yellow and nitrite (2.5, 5,10, 20, 40, 100 and 200 mg/kg b.wt.) individually and in combination, 24 h	The SCEs incidence was high in both groups, a combination of half the concentrations of both resulted in a higher frequency of SCE than individual exposures, suggesting the stronger clastogenicity of the formed nitrosamine	Swiss albino mice, Intraperitoneal	(Giri, Talukder, et al. 1986)

Contd...

Genotoxicants	Effects/ Mechanism of Action	Model and Route of Administration	References
Contraceptive pills (combination containing 50 or 30 µg ethenyl estradiol and 150 µg d-norgestrel/day), 10 to 25 months	Showed significantly higher mean sister chromatid exchanges	Isolated blood lymphocytes	(Murthy and Prema 1979)
Fast green FCF, indigo carmine, orange G and tartrazine, and metanil yellow (200, 500 and 1000 ppm), 6,12 and 24 h	Induction in polyploid cells, higher doses triggered chromosome breaks and formation of MN, all dyes caused mitotic aberrations, metanil yellow and fast green FCF revealed stronger clastogenic activity	Allium cepa root	(Roychoudhury and Giri 1989)
Aziridinyl steroid (50-500 µM), 30 min	Induced a high degree of strand separation and sensitivity/susceptibility to S1 nuclease hydrolysis, increased number of strand breaks per molecule of DNA in calf thymus DNA, caused cell death in human promyelocytic leukemia cell line HL-60 and induced DNA degradation, characteristic of apoptosis, the test steroid has the ability to produce reactive oxygen intermediates	Calf thymus DNA and human promyelocytic leukemia cell line HL-60	(Quadri, Qadri, et al. 1997)

The induction and accumulation of genetic damage can cause genomic instability and the measurement of DNA damage using genotoxicity assays has been known as a critical approach for understanding the carcinogenesis and assessing the risk of cancer incidence against few environmental toxicants. Genotoxic end-points have been employed successfully as biomarkers, as they are believed to be markers of early biological effects of carcinogen exposure. Several authors have reported elevated levels of spontaneous and mutagen-induced CAs and/or SCEs in peripheral blood lymphocytes or skin fibroblasts of individuals suffering from genetic instability syndromes such as uterine cancer (Mitra, Murty, et al. 1982, Murty, Mitra, et al. 1987, Adhvaryu, Rawal, et al. 1988) with an association between lifestyle habits such as smoking and chewing (Desai, Ghaisas, et al. 1996). Apart from peripheral lymphocytes, the assessment of micronuclei in exfoliated cells such as buccal epithelial cells have also been extensively validated as a cytogenetic marker for the differential prevalence of DNA damage among oral cancers, pre-cancers and non-malignant oral pathologies (Chatterjee, Dhar, et al. 2009, Devi, Thimmarasa, et al. 2011, Joshi, Verma, et al. 2011). Genetic variation or polymorphisms in the miRNA pathway have shown potential involvement, concomitant to the prognosis and progression of oral cancer. A relation between miR-499 A/G and miR-149 C/T polymorphisms with vulnerability towards the development of different grades of various stages of oral squamous cell carcinoma has been established in the Indian population (Sushma, Jamil et al. 2015, Tandon, Dewangan, et al. 2018)

Arsenic-induced genotoxicity and carcinogenesis have been a topic of much interest in the country. Cytogenetic assessment of individuals exposed to arsenic has demonstrated DNA damage, corresponding to an increased vulnerability to arsenic-induced toxicity (Basu, Ghosh, et al. 2004, Mahata, Chaki, et al. 2004). Arsenic-induced keratosis has been regarded as a precancerous state of *in situ* skin carcinoma. The exact mechanism of its carcinogenicity has been challenging to understand since it does not directly trigger cancer in animal models. CSIR-IGIB has been involved in deciphering the contributing factors that may result in a higher risk to arsenic vulnerability. Several possible mechanisms have been suggested in causing DNA damage due to chronic arsenic toxicity and have been well associated with disease manifestations. In these endemic areas, although a large proportion was exposed to arsenic via drinking water, only 15–20% revealed arsenic-induced skin lesions hinting that genetic variations may perform a crucial role in arsenic-induced toxicity and genotoxicity via a complex interplay of multiple gene products.

Over the years, multiple candidate genes have been identified in arsenic-induced cytogenetic damage and carcinogenicity that have shed light on the underlying mechanisms. Association of particular p53 polymorphisms with keratosis have been observed in individuals exposed to arsenic via drinking water (De Chaudhuri, Mahata, et al. 2006). Moreover, the role of few genes such as GSTM1 null (Ghosh, Basu, et al. 2006), polymorphism in XRCC3 T241M (Kundu, Ghosh, et al. 2011) have also been shown to confer protection against arsenic exposure. Further, individual variations in the metabolism of arsenic (purine nucleoside phosphorylase) may also underlie vulnerability towards arsenic carcinogenesis (De Chaudhuri, Ghosh, et al. 2008). Deficiency in DNA repair capacity due to ERCC2 codon 751 Lys/Lys genotype/polymorphism (Banerjee, Sarkar et al. 2007, Banerjee, Sarma, et al. 2008), has been majorly postulated to be involved in arsenic-induced carcinogenesis. DNA methylation has also been proposed as one of the epigenetic mechanisms which perpetuates cancer and perturbations of methylation status in tumor suppressor genes (p53 and p16) as well as DNA repair genes have been identified on chronic arsenic exposure (Chanda, Dasgupta, et al. 2005, Banerjee, Paul, et al. 2013, Paul, Banerjee, et al. 2014). Abnormalties in the DNA repair mechanism has also been linked with arsenic-triggered genetic damage and several cancers.

Initial studies relied mostly on genotoxic endpoints such as CA, MN and SCEs that were extensively employed to derive a quantitative association between DNA damage and genotoxic exposure. Over the years, the single cell gel electrophoresis (SCGE or Comet assay) has become one of the most promising genotoxicity assays. It is less resource intensive as compared with traditional genotoxic assays and allows qualitative as well as quantitative estimation of DNA damage in any eukaryotic cell with the added advantage of detecting cells in G0 phase against CA or SCE that require proliferating cells. During the last 2 decades, comet assay protocols (*in vitro* models such as lymphocytes, CHO cells, and *in vivo* testicular and bone marrow cells) have been adopted and optimized by many laboratories in India. The sensitivity and simplicity of the Comet assay has led to fast and widespread progression/full acceptance of this assay in several arenas, e.g. environmental monitoring (Rajaguru, Suba, et al. 2003), basic research studies of DNA damage and repair (Siddique, Sharma, et al. 2008), for comparison of the sensitivities of different organs *in vivo* (Anderson, Dhawan, et al. 1996), epidemiological and biomonitoring studies in human populations exposed occupationally (Kumaravel and Jha 2006, Singh, Kumar, et al. 2011), environmentally or clinically (Basu, Som, et al. 2005, Pandey, Bajpayee, et al. 2005) (Dhawan, Bajpayee, et al. 2009). It has also given sufficient insight into the DNA damage, resulting from gender differences (Bajpayee, Dhawan, et al. 2002), and lifestyle (such as smoking and eating habits) (Dhawan, Mathur, et al. 2001, Mohankumar, Janani, et al. 2002). Research groups at CSIR-IITR have further modified the protocols for the conventional comet assay by incorporating changes in composition of lysis solution, optimized the experimental conditions and decreased the times of unwinding and electrophoresis to 10 and 15 min, respectively, leading to improved performance of the assay in detecting DNA damage (Mukhopadhyay, Chowdhuri, et al. 2004).

Various possible mechanisms have been put forward such as inhibition of DNA repair enzymes, metabolic activation, disruption of the cell cycle, ROS generation and oxidative stress, etc. to elucidate the effect of genotoxicants. One of the most common mechanism involves the formation of strong chemical bonds between the genotoxins and the molecules such as in the case of steroidal hormones and their synthetic derivatives that perform their functions by forming steroid receptor complexes with DNA to influence gene expression (Siddique and Afzal 2008). Metabolic activation and possible conversion to reactive species have also been attributed in the genotoxicity of steroids (Ahmad, Shadab, et al. 2000). This is also observed in arsenic metabolism, that generates hydroxyl radicals, which are known to elicit genotoxic effects. Using QSTR models, attempts have also been made to comprehensively explore the differential genotoxicity of benzene in association with its metabolites employing sensitive and particular genotoxicity end points. Data points to a direct association of the observed genotoxicity with the structural features and several interactions of benzene metabolites thus leading to inhibition of the DNA repair enzyme, human topoisomerase-II alpha (Pandey, Gurbani, et al. 2009). Similarly, ROS has been implicated in genotoxicity induced by particles and fibers (Srivastava, Lohani, et al. 2010). The probable involvement of different mechanisms for induction of SCEs and structural CA have been documented in other studies (Giri, Sharma, et al. 2002, Giri, Giri, et al. 2003).

DNA damage in an organism is inhibited by activation of the repair process, which is one of the important steps used by a cell for maintaining the DNA integrity. When mammalian cells encounter damage to the DNA, several defensive mechanisms are triggered (checkpoint pathways), to stop the DNA replication and repair the damage and any deficiency in checkpoint regulation may result in chromosomal abnormalities. A systematic analysis established the stability of 23 replication factors extending from replication initiator to processive DNA polymerase epsilon post exposure to several forms of DNA damage (bleomycin, cisplatin, doxorubicin and cyclophosphamide), highlighting various types of stress development of a model for inhibiting replication machinery in which the mammalian cells target particular important replication factors based on experienced stress (Sharma, Kar, et al. 2010). DNA/chromosomal instability and DNA repair deficiencies have also been suggested in contributing to cancer risks. The equilibrium from replication fidelity (in normal or damaged DNA) and DNA repair processes may result in triggering of mutations (Sarasin 2003).

Most of the toxicity testing models have relied on small mammals such as rats or mice and hence are expensive, time-consuming, and have attracted ethical criticism (Tsuda, Murakami, et al. 2001, Fatima and Ahmad 2006). The complexity of environmental pollutants has demanded more genotoxicity testing tools with increased sensitivity, economic viability and simplicity. Genotoxicity testing of industrial effluents and surface waters employing a battery of bioassays have demonstrated that these mixtures may contain several unidentified and unregulated toxins that may pose genotoxic risks of unknown levels. Several reports are suggestive of direct evidence between mutagenicity and pollutant levels such as heavy metals and pesticides (Malik and Ahmad 1995, Rehana, Malik, et al. 1995, Alam, Ahmad, et al. 2010). Studies have explored the application of various systems for the genotoxicity testing of complex water samples and several *in vitro* methods have been developed that employ bacterial or plant cells.

Various bioassays (*E. coli* survival assay, Ames testing, comet assay, *Allium cepa* genotoxicity assay, and plasmid nicking assays) have been performed for mutagenicity testing data on different Indian surface waters and major rivers for pollutants heavy metals and nitrates, pesticides, phenolics that has been concisely summarized (Tabrez, Shakil, et al. 2011). Among the tests that are routinely recommended, the Ames plate incorporation test, the Ames fluctuation test and the *Allium cepa* test for anaphase aberrations, have occupied a prominent position (Siddiqui, Tabrez, et al. 2011). The efficacy of the tester strains TA98 and TA102 and others, to accurately detect the genotoxicity of industrial wastewater has been shown in numerous studies (Fatima and Ahmad 2006, Tabrez and Ahmad 2011). It has been suggested that it is important to employ several strains of *S. typhimurium* because particular mutations at hot spots within the tester strains renders them more vulnerable to different mutagens (Siddiqui and Ahmad 2003, Tabrez and Ahmad 2011). Employing several strains instead of a single one for testing of complex samples has been well justified since a single strain would neither reflect the accurate potency nor the multiplicity of mutagens in the samples that contain a range of hazardous substances.

Similarly, another study affirms the feasibility using one *in vitro* assay i.e. plasmid nicking assay and two *in vivo* assays i.e. survival pattern of *Escherichia coli* K-12 repair defective mutants and the λ-prophage induction test for assessing the genotoxic potential of several water bodies in India and environmental biomonitoring of toxicants (Siddiqui, Tabrez, et al. 2011). The efficacy of the *E. coli* K-12 repair defective mutants in estimating the genotoxicity of industrial waste and surface waters has been established (Malik and Ahmad 1995). Rehana, et al. 1996 in their studies have also documented the sensitivity of recA and polA mutants for assessing the genotoxicity of the Ganges water samples validating the system for determination of genotoxicity in complex environmental mixtures (Rehana, Malik, et al. 1996). Moreover, the results are consistent with the hypothesis that test water samples trigger the SOS responses which could induce mutations in bacterial DNA under *in vivo* conditions. These systems are suggestive of preliminary carcinogenicity testing model for the test samples/compounds as well as the possible role of SOS repair in *E.coli* (Siddiqui, Tabrez, et al. 2011). Steroids have been shown to initiate the SOS response and thus induce mutation in bacterial DNA (recA and lexA of *E.coli*) by oxygen radical formation that may not just increase the risk of chemical carcinogenesis but also provide a favorable microenvironment for the generation of toxin radicals (Islam and Ahmad 1991, Qadri, Islam, et al. 1992). Similarly, Chaudhuri, et al. 1999 analysed differential sensitivity of different bacterial systems against genotoxicity of endosulfan and the role of the recA gene in the repair of endosulfan-induced DNA damage (Chaudhuri, Selvaraj, et al. 1999).

Plant-based bioassays for genotoxicity testing in aquatic systems have gradually gained immense popularity among the toxicity testing procedures owing to their sensitivity, simplicity, cost-effectiveness and strong correlation with other toxicity systems (Fatima and Ahmad 2006). Use of two plant bioassays, *Allium cepa* test and seed germination test toxicity/genotoxicity determination of industrial wastewater and river water and standardization with the common pollutants in Indian waters such as pesticides, heavy metals, and phenolics have been undertaken (Siddiqui, Tabrez, et al. 2011). Biomarkers have been incorporated in routine monitoring of aquatic systems for screening for toxicity. *Allium cepa* derived EROD as a potential biomarker for the detection of few pesticides in water, and metallothioneins as a marker of heavy metal exposure have been widely employed. While the Ames plate incorporation test and the Ames fluctuation test have been employed to assess the ROS induced mutagenic and carcinogenic potential of the samples, the *Allium cepa* test has been particularly helpful in establishing the injury caused by ROS producing substances at the chromosomal level since it targets the chromosomal aberrations (Fatima and Ahmad 2006). Indian contributions on the development of plant systems to assess the genotoxic effects of metals has been concisely reviewed (Patra, Bhowmik, et al. 2004). Similarly, safety evaluation of genotoxicity of plant-based drug systems has also been carried out (Sharma, Singh, et al. 2009).

Bioassays have been undertaken on environmental toxicants employing fresh-water fishes (Ali, Nagpure, et al. 2008, Ali, Nagpure et al. 2009, Malik, Kumar, et al. 2009, Malik, Parmesh, et al. 2009, Nagpure, Srivastava, et al. 2015), reporting a battery of toxicological effects in economically important fishes. To this end, the fish *C. catla* has been regarded as a suitable aquatic biomonitoring species of contaminated waters. Several cytogenetic techniques like CA assay, MN assay, SCEs and comet assay have been routinely employed to evaluate the effects of pollutants and radiations in the aquatic ecosystem. Among the cytogenetic endpoints, the erythrocyte MN assay has gained popularity over other assays owing to its simplicity, sensitivity, and reliability for accurately detecting DNA damage (Anbumani and Mohankumar 2012, Anbumani and Mohankumar 2015).

Emphasis has also been given to the utilization of alternative animal models. Encouraging re-suits have been obtained using embryonic and neonatal chicks for screening for chemically induced cellular and genetic damage (Bhunya and Jena 1992, Bhunya and Jena 1993, Jena and Bhunya 1994). *Drosophila* has been well established as an insect model for toxicological research in India for detection of DNA damage due to its well-elucidated genetics and developmental biology. *D.melanogaster* as a suitable and sensitive test system for the *in vivo* evaluation of genotoxicity employing modified alkaline and neutral Comet assay has been successfully validated by CSIR-IITR (Siddique, Dhawan, et al. 2003, Siddique, Chowdhuri, et al. 2005, Siddique, Gupta et al. 2005). Majority of the genotoxicity studies in this organism have been restricted to its germ cells whereas several chromosomal alterations (deletion, breaks, and duplication) have been observed in its brain cells. Most of the chemicals enter the organism via gut through food in take, however, gut cells have been ignored for monitoring somatic cell genotoxicity. In this context, the research group has shown that similar to brain cells, the gut cells could also be a potential candidate for estimating the genotoxicity of chemicals (cypermethrin, industrial leachates) employing alkaline version of Comet assay (Mukhopadhyay, Chowdhuri, et al. 2004).

Genomic instability because of double-strand breaks (DSBs) generation has been one of the crucial parameters causally linked to carcinogenesis. However, its detection in different experimental systems employing neutral Comet assay have been available from *in vitro* systems with little information from *in vivo*. In this direction, efforts have also led to validation of the efficacy of neutral Comet assay for assessment of genotoxicity in the model organism against well known DSBs inducers, i.e. cyclophosphamide, cisplatin, bleomycin, alkylating agents i.e. methyl methanesulfonate, ethyl methanesulfonate and N-ethyl-N-nitrosourea which are identified carcinogens by the International Agency for Research on Cancer (Sharma, Shukla, et al. 2011). Interestingly, the modified comet assay under *in vivo* conditions exhibits more sensitivity than the traditional methods with drastic elevation in comet parameters in the gut cells as early as 24 h as compared with 2-5 days in the other methods (Graf, Frei, et al. 1989, Vogel and Nivard 1993).

For understanding the DNA damage and repair mechanims, chemical-triggered mutagenesis and subsequent generation of *Drosophila* based mutants have been very helpful. Microarray approaches using *Drosophila* have further led to the identification of misregulated DNA repair responsive genes (ku80 and DNA ligase IV) of the non-homologous end joining repair pathway (involved in the repair of DSBs) on Cr(VI) exposure offering fresh insights into the toxicant-induced probable mechanism of carcinogenesis (Mishra, Sharma et al. 2013). Similarly, oxidative damage to DNA, caused by free radicals, may affect disease progression (e.g., carcinogenesis and inflammation) making it imperative to accurately detect oxidative damage induced DNA damage. Alterations to the alkaline Comet assay by employing lesion-specific endonucleases, such as formamidopyrimidine-DNA glycosylase and endonuclease III, have been established for detecting DNA bases with oxidative injury against three well known environmental chemicals: cadmium chloride, hydrogen peroxide, and copper sulfate (Shukla, Pragya, et al. 2011).

A loss or defect in the DNA repair pathway may result in accumulation of mutations and CA contributing to genotoxicity. Efforts to characterize the role of DNA repair pathways against the effects of genotoxicants have shown potential involvement (misregulation) of both pre (mei-9, mus201, and mus207) and post-replication (mei-41 and mus209) DNA repair pathways against dichlorvos-induced DNA damage in *Drosophila* (Mishra, Sharma et al. 2014). Leachates induced high levels of DNA damage in mutant strains mei41 (deficient in cell cycle check-point protein), mus201 (deficient in excision repair protein), mus308 (deficient in postreplication repair protein), and rad54 (deficient in double-strand break repair protein) than in the OregonR1 wild-type strain. Suggesting that DNA damage repair in organisms that are exposed to leachates is dependent upon many DNA repair proteins, these results have been indicative of the contribution of several overlapping repair pathways. The study also suggested the potential of Comet assay in assessing the DNA repair mechanisms in *Drosophila* (Siddique, Sharma, et al. 2008).

Genotoxicity testing has been crucial for ensuring drug safety and is mandatory before Phase I/II clinical trials of new drugs. The exiting battery of tests suggested by regulatory authorities (Ames test, CA; *in vitro* gene mutation in eukaryotic cells and *in vivo* test) are quite time-consuming, laborious, and require large amount of test compounds (Committee 2011). In addition, they are restricted by variations in other factors such as uptake, metabolism, structure of chromosome and process of DNA repair between prokaryotic and mammalian cells, identification of chemicals which do not interact with DNA but disrupt cellular response to DNA damage and so on. In such a scenario, a high-throughput screen which is mammalian cell-based and can help in detecting the potential genotoxins at an early stage of drug discovery have been the need of the hour. A new, versatile, human-based reporter screen (Anthem's Genotoxicity screen) has been developed and rigorously validated employing 62 ECVAM recommended compounds (aneugens, clastogens, alkylating agents, nucleoside analogues, topoisomerase inhibitor and others which were tested with and without metabolic activation) in p53-proficient human colon carcinoma HCT116 cell line (Kirkland, Kasper et al. 2008). The screening is conducted on genetically transformed human single cell clone which expresses three reporter genes which are under the transcriptional control of promoters of DNA damage-inducible genes (p21, GADD153 and p53) that get triggered via genotoxic stress (Fornace, Alamo et al. 1988, Amundson, Myers et al. 1998, Zhou and Elledge 2000). This assay could enable fast screening and early detection of potential genotoxins from several sources such as pesticides, food additives, cosmetics, and environmental pollutants and also provide information on the possible mechanisms thus helping in rational drug design. The concordance of the screen with *in vivo* method was found to be 95.5% with a sensitivity of 95.2% and specificity of 95.7% (Rajakrishna, Unni et al. 2014).

The pursuit of alternative testing systems for genotoxicity have also led to the validation of Umbilical Cord derived-Mesenchymal Stem Cells (UC-MSCs) as a better replacement of peripheral lymphocytes and cancer cell lines for more efficient screening of compounds for micronuclei detection. Validated against two known mutagens (hydrogen peroxide and mitomycin-C), two solvents (ethanol and dimethyl sulfoxide), and two drugs (rapamycin and metformin), the culture demonstrated higher sensitivity and efficacy in comparison with lymphocytes and A549 cell line (Sharma, Venkatesan, et al. 2014).

Apart from generating a large database on the genotoxic/mutagenic potential of toxicants, studies have also been directed towards the identification of protective/preventive agents. Example, genotoxic damage caused by the steroids has been demonstrated to be decreased by the use of antioxidants (Siddique, Beg, et al. 2006, Siddique, Beg, et al. 2007), antimutagenic profile of antioxidants and natural plant products (Karekar, Joshi et al. 2000, Gupta, Vikram et al. 2010, Kumar, Sushama et al. 2011). Micronutrients and other vitamins have been shown to significantly decrease MN levels in healthy tobacco users, as well as in individuals with precancerous lesions (Prasad, Mukundan, et al. 1995). Dietary supplements against the clastogenic effects of heavy metals have also been documented (Azuine, Kayal, et al. 1992, Das, Roychoudhury, et al. 1993, Singh, Kumar, et al. 2008). Few of the representative studies can be found in Table 10.14.

Table 10.14 Few representative studies on the protective/therapeutic agents against different genotoxicants

Genotoxicants	Preventive/Protective Agents	Model and Route of Administration	References
Metals			
Lead (10, 20 and 40 mg/kg b.wt.)and **aluminium** (250, 500 and 1000 mg/kg b.wt.) 24 h	***Phyllanthus emblica* fruit extract** (685 mg/kg b.wt./day, 7 days, Oral): Pre-exposure increased the cell division frequency and decreased the frequency of chromosmal breaks in all the doses of the metals	Swiss albino mice, Intraperitoneal	(Dhir, Roy, et al. 1990)
Arsenic (0.1 mg/kg b.wt.), on day 7, 14, 21 and 30	**Dietary garlic extract** (100 mg/kg and mustard oil (0.643 mg/kg b.wt./day, 30 days, Oral): Co exposure reduced the degree of clastogenic effects of sodium arsenite	Swiss albino mice, Subcutaneous	(Choudhury, Das, et al. 1997)

Contd...

Phototoxicant	Effects/Mechanism of Action	Model and Route of Administration	References
Arsenic (2.5 mg/kg b.wt.), 24 h	**Iron** (152 mg/kg b.wt, oral): Pre exposure for 2 h and co-exposure bothreduced the clastogenic effects of arsenic induced chromosomal aberrations	Swiss albino mice, Oral	(Poddar, Mukherjee, et al. 2000)
Mercuric chloride (1.052, 5.262 and 10.524 µM), 70 h	**Ascorbic acid** (9.734 µM): Prevented mercuric chloride induced C-anaphases (abnormal mitosis)	Human peripheral blood lymphocytes	(Rao, Chinoy, et al. 2001)
Drugs			
Cyclophoshamide (25 mg/kg b.wt.), 24 h	**β-carotene** (2.7 and 27 mg/kg b.wt. 7 days): Oral pre exposure resulted in dose dependent reduction of clastogenicity in bone marrow cells	Swiss albino mice, Intraperitoneal	(Mukherjee, Agarwal, et al. 1991)
Hydrocortisone (25 and 50 µg/mL, 24, 48, and 72 h)	**Ascorbic acid** (20 µg/mL and 30 µg/mL) **and Vitamin E** (15 µg/mL and 20 µg/mL): Co-administration rendered an additive effect against hydrocortisone induced levels of chromosomal aberrations and sister chromatid exchanges	Human lymphocytes	(Ahmad, Hoda, et al. 2002)
Chlormadinone acetate (40 µM, 24 h)	**Allicin** (5 and 10 µM) and L-ascorbic acid (40-80 µM, 48h: Post treatment led to a reduction in abnormal cells assessed by CAs analysis, dose dependent decrease in SCEs	Human lymphocytes	(Siddique and Afzal 2005)
Norethynodrel (60 mg/ml), 48 h	**Ascorbic acid** (20, 40 and 80 mM): Decrease in genotoxic damage, employing CA and SCEs as parameters	Human Peripheral blod lymphocytes	(Siddique, Beg, et al. 2007)
Diethylstilbestrol (1.3 x 10^{-5} M), 24,48 and 72h	**Vitamin C** (5×10^{-6} M, 10^{-5} M 5×10^{-5} M):Co-administration of 1st and 2nd concentration for 72 h led to a reduction in the incidence of anomalies in metaphase chromosomes, decreased the mean frequency of SCE	Human lymphocytes	(Shadab, Ahmad, et al. 2006)
Cyproterone acetate (20 and 30 µM), 24 h	***Centella asiaticaL*. Extract** (1.075×10^{-4}, 2.125×10^{-4}, 3.15×10^{-4} and 4.17×0^{-4} g/ml): A dose dependent reduction in the number of abnormal metaphase chromosomes and SCEs	Human lymphocytes	(Siddique, Ara, et al. 2008)

Contd...

Genotoxicants	Preventive/Protective Agents	Model and Route of Administration	References
Miscellaneous			
Argemone oil (2 ml/kg, 24 h, i.p.)	**Combination of riboflavin** (50 mg/kg, i.p.) **and α-tocopherol** (150 mg/kg, i.p.) 4 h prior to or immediately after AO exposure:Reduction in tail length (37–44%), tail moment (70–72%), and tail DNA (49–53%) in bone marrow cells	Swiss albino mice	(Ansari, Dhawan, et al. 2006)
Aflatoxin B1(15 nM), 24 h	**Piperine** (100 μM, 24 h):Co-exposure restored the growth rate of cells and decreased MN formation in a concentration dependent manner	H4IIEC3 rat hepatoma cells	(Singh, Reen, et al. 1994)
Aflatoxin B1 (4 mg/kg b.wt.), 26 h	**Ouercetin pentaacetate** (300 mg/kg b.wt. intraperitoneal preexposure and second dose (co-exposure with alfatoxin B1): demonstrated time-dependent inhibition of liver microsome catalysed AFB1 epoxidation resulting in inhibition of toxicity	Albino rats, Intraperitoneal	(Kohli, Raj, et al. 2002)
X-radiation (2, 3 and 4 Gy)	**Cysteine** (30 μg, 1 mg or 2 mg/ml): 30 min pre and post treatmentprotected only against chromosomal deletions in 4 Gy-treated cells while 1 mg protected against deletions by all three doses of X-rays whereas cysteine at 2mg also protected against aberrations with a prominent reduction in the frequency of aberrant metaphases, reduced X-ray-induced cell cycle delay	Indian muntjac, Muntiacus muntjak vaginalis and human lymphocytes	(Chatterjee and Mercy 1993)
Asbestos (crocidolite and chrysotile 1 mg/cm^2)	**Diallylsulfide** (5 and 10 μM) 48 and 66 h:Simultaneous exposure resulted in reduction in micronuclei induction after treatment of cells with 5 μM but not with 10 μM	Human mesothelial cells	(Lohani, Yadav, et al. 2003)
Benzene, toluene and zylene (1, 10, 50 and 100 mM, 12, 24 and 48 h), individually	**Quercetin and Curcumin** (100 μM, 24 and 48 h): Co-exposure decreased activity of cytochrome P450, levels of GST, parameters of oxidative stress, genotoxic and apoptotic endpoints	*Drosophila melanogaster*, Oral	(Singh, Mishra, et al. 2011)

10.7 Phototoxicity

Skin, constituting approximately 15% of body weight and may be regarded as the largest organ of the body (Parrish 1982), is the most sensitive organ to the effects of toxicants exposure ubiquitously persistent in the environment. Phototoxicity has been defined as an abnormal cutaneous response generated after skin exposure to xenobiotics and subsequent exposure to light/UV or which is similarly caused via skin irradiation after topical or systemic administration of a chemical. Any compound or cosmetic which absorbs UVA, UVB or visible light in the range of 290-700 nm and can reach the skin or eyes is required to be tested for its potential phototoxicity as mandated by regulatory authorities (FDA Guidance for Industry on Photosafety Testing 2003 and EMEA Note for Guidance on Photosafety Testing 2002).

Perception of phototoxic hazards to the biological system has been growing because of the expanding use of chemicals in industry, agriculture, and medicine and the concomitant exposure to UV radiation (UVR), making it all the more imperative to estimate the photodynamic potential of chemicals. Shortwave and longwave UV light have been classified as class I carcinogen by the WHO International Agency for Research on Cancer Monograph Working Group (El Ghissassi, Baan, et al. 2009). Moreover, India being a tropical country amounts to most of the human activities taking place in bright sunlight, which has triggered much interest in this arena. Phototoxicity evaluation has also gained immense significance in general owing to the increasing concern over health effects due to gradual stratospheric ozone depletion resulting in a rising penetration of UVR which could further contribute to activation of chemical and biological molecules to potential phototoxic agents affecting not only human life but also other forms of life (Soni and Joshi 1997, Farooq, Babu, et al. 2000, Misra, Lal, et al. 2005)

Since inception CSIR-IITR has been at the forefront in addressing issues related to phototoxicity. Effects of UVR and sunlight on xenobiotics /biomolecules with specific focus on the carcinogenic impacts due to DNA damage and oxidative damage due to ROS generation have been the prime area of concern. The earliest studies focused on the synergistic action of a widely employed industrial dye benzanthrone (BZ) and sunlight that was shown to induce hyperpigmentation of the epidermis, hyperplasia and histological alterations such as fibrosis and vascularity in the skin of mice (Singh, Sharma, et al. 1967). Many follow up studies brought to limelight the generation of two ROS, singlet oxygen ($^1O_2$) and superoxide radicals (O^-), from illuminated BZ (Srivastava, Misra, et al. 1986). Similarly, in a skin photosensitization study on guinea pigs, BA was reported to induce erythema, edema and photodynamic oxidation potential in a dose-dependent manner (Srivastava, Misra, et al. 1990). Studies also brought to the limelight the DNA-damaging property of sensitized riboflavin (Vitamin B2), a common nutrient distributed in human tissues, blood, skin, and milk in free and conjugated forms. With riboflavin being an important element of our dietary system, the concern over its photosensitization properties resulting in cellular damage triggered a lot of studies to understand its mechanism of photosensitization (Joshi 1985, Ali, Upreti, et al. 1991).

Since then, a wealth of information on the experimental evidence revealing strong correlation between the production of ROS and skin photosensitization and phototoxicity manifested by several exogenous and endogenous molecules such as nutritional factors like riboflavin (Misra, Bajpai, et al. 2001), psoralens (Pathak and Joshi 1984), drugs used for photochemotherapy in skin diseases (Saha, Das, et al. 2012), antibiotics (Pandey, Mehrotra, et al. 2002), cosmetics (Kyadarkunte, Patole, et al. 2014), dyestuffs (Tobit, Verma, et al. 2012, Goyal, Srivastav, et al. 2018) and environmental pollutants (Srivastava, Singh, et al. 1999, Tobit, Verma, et al. 2011) have been generated by using the radiation intensity which reaches the earth surface. The drugs, antibiotics, cosmetics, PAHs are nontoxic or less toxic in perse but photoactivation (upon absorption) may sensitize them to produce ROS and trigger phototoxicity. Such generation of ROS has been responsible for causing alteration in the normal functioning of cellular constituents resulting in erythema or edema, erythrocyte photohaemolysis, damage to cell membranes, lipid-peroxidation reactions, protein fragmentation, the formation of photoadducts, photodynamic oxidation potential, DNA damage and induction of carcinogenic effects. The *in-situ* ROS generated due to photosensitization may also play an important role in a tumor-promoting response (Giri, Iqbal, et al. 1996) (Table 10.15).

Table 10.15 Few representative studies on the effects/mechanism of different categories of phototoxicants

Phototoxicant	Effects/Mechanism of Action	Model and Route of Administration	References
Polyaromatic Hydrocarbons			
Benzathrone (5 to 25 µM), 24-36 h	UVA (1.8 ±0.1 mW/cm^2) and UVB (0.5± 0.05 mW/cm^2) caused generation of singlet oxygen by benzanthrone that was dependent on the concentration of the test chemical and the dose of solar radiation, photohaemolysis and lipid peroxidation	Albino rat erythrocytes	(Srivastava, Misra, et al. 1990)
Benzathrone (25 and 50 mg/kg b.wt.), 24 h	Co-exposure with UV B (50 mJ/cm^2) causes enhanced ROS generation, increased epidermal thickness, mast cell number, MPO activity via activation of MAPKs-NF-kB/AP-1 signaling, increased expression of inflammatory markers (COX-2 and iNOS)	SKH-1 hairless mice, Topical	(Abbas, Alam, et al. 2016)

Contd...

Phototoxicant	Effects/Mechanism of Action	Model and Route of Administration	References
Chrysene (1.0 µg/ml), 0, 1, 3, 6, 12, 24, 48 and 72 h	Co-exposure with UVB 0.6mW/cm^2 induced ROS that was elevated in a concentration dependent manner, triggered apoptosis via caspases-3 activation and translocation of phosphatidylserine, reduced glutathione and activity of catalse, DNA damage	Human skin epidermal cell line HaCaT	(Ali, Verma, et al. 2011)
Benzathrone (5-50 ppm) and **Anthracene** (20-50 ppm), 60 min	Co-exposure with UV-A (5.76 J/cm^2)/UV-B (2.16 J/cm^2)/sunlight generated singlet oxygen ($^1O_2$), benzanthrone produced higher amount of singlet oxygen and superoxide as compared to anthracene	Mouse fibroblast cell lines NIH-3T3 and L-929	(Tobit, Verma, et al. 2012)
Benzo(a)pyrene and **pyrene** (5-50 ppm), 60 min	Co-exposure with UV-A (5.76 J/cm^2)/UV-B (2.16 J/cm^2)/sunlight generated singlet oxygen ($^1O_2$), pyrene prosduced higher level of singlet oxygen as compared to benzo(a)pyrene while benzo(a)pyrene produced more superoxide	Mouse fibroblast cell lines NIH-3T3 and L-929	(Tobit, Verma, et al. 2011)
Benz(e) acephenanthryle ne (0.5–8.0 µg/ml), 24 h	Exposure with UVA (1.40 mW/cm^2) generates singlet oxygen, superoxide anion radical and hydroxyl radical (•OH) in a concentration-dependent manner, glutathione reduced and activity of catalase was lowered while DNA damage and cell death were triggered	Human skin cell line A375	(Ali, Ray, et al. 2010)
Anthrone (0.1–1 µg/ml)	Co-exposure with UV-A (2.16 J/cm^2)/UV-B (0.72 J/cm^2) and sunlight (30 min) caused type-II photodynamic reaction by producing $^1O_2$, induced cell cycle arrest (G2/M-phase) and DNA damage in a concentration dependent manner up-regulation of p21 and bax and caspase concomitantly down regulation of bcl2 genes expression, phosphotidylserine translocation	Human skin epidermal cell line HaCaT	(Mujtaba, Dwivedi, et al. 2013)
Anthracene (5 µg mL^{-1}), 60 min-4h	Degraded within 4 h, co-exposure with sunlight/UVR caused photodegradation of 2-deoxyguanosine and linoleic acid peroxidation, causes cell cycle arrest in G0/G1 phases, induced expression of CYP 1A1 and 1B1 genes, generation of $^1O_2$, $O_2^{•1}$ and •OH through photosensitized mechanisms	Human skin epidermal cell line (HaCaT)	(Mujtaba, Dwivedi, et al. 2011)

Contd...

Phototoxicant	Effects/Mechanism of Action	Model and Route of Administration	References
Cosmetics and Dyes			
Benzophenone (5–50 µg/mL), 30-60 min	Co-exposure with UVA (2.7 J/cm^2)/ UVB/ (1.08 J/cm^2) and sunlight generates ROS, singlet oxygen, superoxide anion and hydroxyl radicals through type-I and type-II photodynamic mechanisms, cyclo-butane pyrimidine dimer (CPD) formation (DNA damage), lipid peroxidation, cell cycle arrest in G1 phase	Human skin epidermal cell line HaCaT	(Amar, Goyal, et al. 2015)
Paraphenylenedi amine (5–100 µg/mL), 30 min-4 h	Co-exposure with UV A (2.88 J/cm^2)/ UV B (1.08 J/cm^2)/ sunlight (30 min) caused Type I photodynamic reaction mediated oxidative DNA damage via single stranded DNA breaks, micronuclei and CPD formation, lysosomal destabilization, release of lysosomal cathepsin B and activation of Bid, mitochondrial depolarization, cell cycle arrest at G1 phase	Human skin epidermal cell line HaCaT	(Goyal, Amar, et al. 2015)
Rose Bengal	Time dependent photodegradation, generates $^1O_2$ via Type-II photodynamic pathway, 2'dGuO degradation, micronuclei formation, single and double strand breakage, p53 mediated apoptosis with increased of caspase-3 activity, decreased mitochondrial membrane potential as well as PS translocation	Human melanoma cell line A375	(Srivastav, Mujtaba, et al. 2016)
Antibiotics and drugs			
Ciprofloxacin (5–400 µg mL^{-1}), 60 min	Co- exposure with UV-A (1.14, 1.6 and 2.2 mW cm^2), UV-B (0.6, 0.9 and 1.2 mW cm^2) and sunlight resulted in time and concentration dependent ROS generation and degradation of nucleotide, linoleic acid peroxidation by Type I and II photodynamic reactions, the order of $O_2^{\cdot-}$ generating potential of ciprofloxacin at various concentrations was sunlight>UV-A>UV-B. The NIH-3T3 cell line showed a higher photosensitizing potential than L-929	Mouse fibroblast cell lines L-929 and NIH-3T3	(Agrawal, Ray, et al. 2007)
Antibiotics cephaloridine, cephalexin, cephradine, nystatin and nafcillin (0–100 µg/ml)	UV B radiation (0.0–10.8 J/cm^2) caused production of $^1O_2$ by various antibiotics was both concentration and UV-B dose dependent. The $^1O_2$ generation was in the order: cephaloridine> cephalexin> nystatin> cephradine> nafcillin, the rate of photodegradation of dGuo was found to be dose and concentration dependent in following order: cephaloridine> nystatin> cephalexin> cephradine.	Photochemical method	(Ray, Misra, et al. 2002)

Contd...

Phototoxicant	Effects/Mechanism of Action	Model and Route of Administration	References
Tetracycline (0–1.0 mM), 2h	Co-exposure to white light triggered time and concentration dependent generation of hydroxyl radicals (•OH) induced protein (serum albumin) fragmentation	Human blood	(Khan and Musarrat 2002)
Fluoroquinolones (Enoxacin, lomefloxacin, ofloxacin, norfloxacin) (0-50 µg/ml)	UVA, B, sunlight triggered oxygen dependent Type I and Type II photosensitizing reactions producing ^1O and $O_2^{\bullet1}$ radicals, significant photodegradation of 2-deoxyguanosine, TBARS formation	Human blood	(Ray, Agrawal, et al. 2006)
Ketoprofen (1-50 µg/ml)	Co-exposure to UV-B (0.72 J/cm^2) and UV-A (2.16 J/cm^2) and sunlight (30 min) generated $_1O^2$ through Type-II photodynamic reaction, 2'dGuO photodegradation, single and double strand breakage, cell cycle arrest in G2/M phase, caspase-3 activation, cytochrome-c release from mitochondria, upregulation of Bax protein and phosphatidylserine translocation	Human skin epidermal cell line HaCaT	(Ray, Mujtaba, et al. 2013)
Quinine (5, 10 and 25 µg/ml), 30-120 min	Degradation of 2-deoxyguanosine, significant reduction in cell viability at 25µg/ml increase in ROS in a concentration dependent manner, cell cycle arrest in G2 phase, upregulation of p21 and p53 genes expression	Human melanocyte cell line A375	(Yadav, Dwivedi, et al. 2013)
Mefloquine, (5–100 µg/ml)	UVB (0.6 mW/cm^2) and sunlight for 60 min Generated superoxide radical, hydroxyl radical, and singlet oxygen through type I and type II photodynamic reactions, single-stranded DNA damage and formation of CPDs, mitochondrial membrane depolarization and lysosomal destabilization, upregulation of bax and p21 and downregulation of Bcl-2 genes, G2/M phase cell cycle arrest	Human skin epidermal cell line HaCaT	(Yadav, Dwivedi, et al. 2014)
Ophthalmic formulations (Sulphacetamide (10, 20, and 30 % w/v), ketoconazole (1, 2, and 3 % w/v), voriconazole (0.5, 1, and 1.5 % w/v), diclofenac (0.05, 0.1, and 0.15 % w/v) and ketorolac (0.2, 0.4, and 0.5 % w/v)), 30 min-4h	Sulphacetamide is moderately toxic in the presence of light/UV-A, Ketoconazole and voriconazole were found slightly irritant in presence of light/UV-A, Diclofenac and ketorolac demonstrated slight irritancy in the light	HET-CAM Test; ICE Test; NSAIDs; RBC Test	(Sahu, Singh, et al. 2014)

Phototoxicant induced *in vivo* photoirritation with a reversible inflammatory reaction of the skin after chemical contact and UV irradiation exposure has increasingly been observed as a side effect associated with the use of some cosmetics and systemic drugs. Over the years increasing evidence of phototoxicity cases such as polymorphic light eruptions, chronic actinic dermatitis, solar urticaria, photoallergic reactions and pellagra (Srinivas, Sekar, et al. 2012, Gayathri, Kanaki, et al. 2013) which constitute different types of photodermatoses in India has prompted the assessment of phototoxicity and photocarcinogenicity of various drugs, cosmetics and food supplements/additives for the safety of human beings. In a study, photoallergic dermatitis has been observed in 35% of the population, only to hair dyes and lipsticks (Dogra, Minocha, et al. 2003).

The earliest approaches for phototoxicity evaluation were based on physicochemical assessment under ambient environmental intensities using animal-based skin-sensitization tests (erythema, edema and melanogenesis), erythrocyte photohaemolysis and photochemical methods for biodegradation of 2'–Deoxyguanosine (2 ϕ -dGuO) and estimation of free radical formation. ROS generation and photodegradation of 2 ϕ -dGuO have been important factors incorporated in phototoxicity assessment (Ray, Mehrotra, et al. 1996, Ray, Mehrotra, et al. 2001, Ray, Misra, et al. 2002, Ray, Agrawal, et al. 2006). The photo-excited form of various drugs is known to produce phototoxic responses to cellular biomolecules. Due to the relatively high sensitivity of the guanine base of DNA and RNA to photo-oxidation via ROS formation, dGuo has been used as a model compound for nuclear damaging studies.

Skin sensitization has been the most conspicuous response of the exposure of UVR on the skin and a variety of chemical agents, dyes, drugs, agricultural and health care products are capable of acting as a photosensitizer at environmentally relevant levels of UV radiation. These photosensitizers have shown to either react directly with the biological substrate to produce damage to the cellular ingredients or undergo photoexcitation to transfer energy to molecular oxygen, which in turn, causes oxidative stress. In the photosensitization reaction, it is now recognized that $^1O_2$, superoxide anion radicals (O_{-2}), hydroxyl radicals (OH) and hydrogen peroxide (H_2O_2) serve as the major ROS producers. The chemicals have shown to undergo Type I and/or Type II photodynamic reactions. In Type-I reaction, the photosensitized molecule transfers an electron to molecular oxygen leading to the formation of O_2.-, .OH and H_2O_2. In a Type-II reaction, the Photoexcited molecule transfers energy to O_2 molecules and $^1O_2$ is formed. Both the O_2 dependent and independent reactions have shown to contribute to the oxidation of target molecules of the cellular system (Ray, Agrawal, et al. 2006).

The formation of ROS has been of special interest because this reactive moiety is largely responsible for the damage to DNA and cytoplasmic constituents (lysosomes, mitochondria, etc.). ROS generation potential has also been proposed as a suitable marker for *in vitro* testing and the majority of the studies have evaluated the possible role of ROS in the manifestation of phototoxicity. Although the cell is well equipped to minimize harmful effects induced by oxidative stress through its endogenous defense mechanism, however, some photosensitive chemicals and drugs have potential to generate excess ROS, which suppresses the defense mechanism and damage the cell organelles (Dwivedi, Mujtaba, et al. 2014). Studies have unambiguously demonstrated that a large number of antibiotics (at concentrations used in treatments) are a potential source of $O_{2.-}$ under UV light and natural sunlight. The drugs are used generally for a period of 3 to 15 days during treatment which warrants due precaution to minimize their photosensitizing potential that may cause additional phototoxicity over more extended usage (Ray, Mehrotra, et al. 2001). Hans, et al. 2008 have assessed the phototoxic potential of cosmetic products and found some of the lipsticks and facial creams generated ROS, produced hemolysis, and caused LPO in human erythrocytes (*in vitro*) when exposed to sunlight (Hans, Agrawal, et al. 2008). Many ophthalmic solutions and commonly used antibiotics have been reported to get sensitized and photodegraded in the presence of light which might cause irritation leading to toxicity upon continuous usage (Sahu, Singh, et al. 2014). The selection of different intensities of UVA irradiation has further proved the viewpoint that higher intensities of UVA during peak hours in sunlight would be more deleterious (Yadav, Dwivedi, et al. 2013).

Studies have also highlighted the crucial factors that may augment xenobiotic-induced phototoxic responses. In the presence of divalent cations, tetracycline binds non-covalently to serum albumin, which alters the protein's helicity (Khan, Muzammil, et al. 1998). Increased fragmentation of albumin and generation of •OH radicals with the addition of Cu(II) ions also support the role of metal ions in augmenting tetracycline-induced toxicity. Although $O_{2.-}$ is considered to be a less reactive species, the presence of transition metal ions are likely to transform it into a highly cytotoxic species, hydroxyl radical (Khan and Musarrat 2002). Similarly, the phototoxic characteristic of riboflavin to cause damage to RBC membrane takes place only in the presence of serum/plasma (Misra, Bajpai, et al. 2001).

Photooxidation is a potentially important pathway for biomodification in the environment. Upon absorbing sunlight, chemicals can be rapidly transformed/biodegraded to a variety of compounds, most of which are oxidation products. The earliest study recording the photodegradation along with identification of photoproducts was the UV radiation-induced photodegradation of riboflavin into limichrome and lumiflavin (Joshi 1989). CSIR-IITR has remained at the forefront in shedding insights into the mechanisms of phototoxicity/photogenotoxicity and photodegradation of different compounds that have a widespread use, demonstrating for the very first time the photosensitized nature and photodegradation of antibiotics, sunscreen ingredients (Ray, Mujtaba, et al. 2013, Amar, Goyal, et al. 2015), hair dyes (Goyal, Amar, et al. 2015) and synthesized antimalarial drugs (Dwivedi, Mujtaba, et al. 2012, Dwivedi, and Mujtaba, et al. 2014). Many of them have been hypothesized to be hazardous to human skin due to its photodegradation and photoproducts accumulation, as well as ROS, mediated DNA and membrane damage and apoptosis, which could possibly lead to a variety of skin diseases and ultimately skin cancer. Most of them have shown to be photounstable, leading to the generation of photoproducts within 4 h, indicating the need to identify and assess the biological responses evoked by the photoproducts itself to understand the total environmental impact. Advancement of techniques such as LC-MS has allowed the identification of different photoproducts generated upon photooxidation.

For example, sunscreens have been an effective tool in protecting against the known carcinogenic effects of UV radiation. However, several controversies are surrounding the safety and efficacy of sunscreens as a form of photoprotection. Benzophenone (BP) and its derivatives are commonly used in sunscreens as a UV blocker. Amar, et al. 2015 have been the first to elucidate the mechanism of BP phototoxicity and its photomodification under sunlight exposure into photoproducts P1 and P2 that also form ROS via type I and type II photodynamic mechanism (Amar, Goyal et al. 2015). Similarly, Levofloxacin (LVFX), is a broad spectrum third-generation fluoroquinolone antibiotic, used in the treatment of severe or life-threatening bacterial infections. Results identified for the time three photoproducts of LVFX at ambient levels of UV-R by LC-MS / MS. The generation of ROS was investigated photochemically as well as intracellularly in HaCaT cell line (Dwivedi, Mujtaba, et al. 2012). Paraphenylenediamine (PPD), a derivative of paranitroaniline has been most commonly used as an ingredient of oxidative hair dye and permanent tattoos. PPD is photodegraded and forms a novel photoproduct under UV A exposure (Goyal, Amar, et al. 2015). Photosensitized quinine (antimalarial drug) also produced a photoproduct 6-methoxy-quinoline-4-ylm- ethyl-oxonium identified through LC-MS/MS (Yadav, Dwivedi, et al. 2013). Similarly, anthracene photomodifies into anthrone and anthraquinone under ambient environmental intensities of sunlight/UV exposure (Mujtaba, Dwivedi, et al. 2011).

Moreover, the photo-instability of few fluoroquinolones (FQ) has also been associated with attenuated antimicrobial activity. Ofloxacin (OFLX) is a member of the FQs drug family and active against both Gram-positive and Gram-negative bacteria by inhibiting DNA gyrase (Joshi 1985). Such changes by antibiotics have also been accompanied with induced expression of p21 and p53 genes (photosensitive genes), that play a pivotal role in cell cycle regulation, DNA repair and apoptosis mechanisms which may lead to aberrant cell kinetics (Yadav, Dwivedi, et al. 2013, Dwivedi, Mujtaba, et al. 2014, Yadav, Dwivedi, et al. 2014). All these studies have warranted the cautious use of such compounds as they may undergo photomodification and become more deleterious.

In light of certain commonly used antibiotics undergoing photosensitization reactions, it has been imperative to assess the phototoxic response and the establishment of their mechanism of action in different alternate test systems. Paralleling to *in vivo* approaches and photochemical methods, the utilization of human erythrocytes (RBCs) has been utilized as an alternate biological tool to study the phototoxic potential of chemicals on the basis of their ability to haemolyze RBC membrane and/or to oxidize haemoglobin under sunlight exposure (Srivastava, Misra, et al. 1990, Ali, Upreti, et al. 1991, Misra, Ray, et al. 2005). In view of the clinical importance, the speed, easy and low cost of RBC, has made this model the most time-honored for the study of phototoxicity *in vitro* and in postulation of the anomalies to human beings because the equivalent of the entire blood volume of an adult passes through the skin and is potentially irradiated in about 20 min under sunlight exposure (Kornhauser, Wamer, et al. 1996).

Due to the complexity of the biological system, it has also been challenging to demonstrate the specific role of ROS in the manifestation of phototoxicity in *in vivo* studies. In this regard, development of new test models for phototoxicity by using human/mouse skin and ocular cell lines/human skin dermal models and primary skin cell culture have received much attention since 2007, that have provided insights into the phototoxicity mechanisms. The reliability and suitability of the L-929, a mouse fibroblast cell line, as an *in vitro* test system for the phototoxicity has been evaluated that provides information regarding the lethality of higher intensities of UVR and its importance in view of increasing UV intensities on the earth's surface due to ozone depletion (Ray, Agrawal, et al. 2008). NIH-3T3, HaCaT, A375 have been suitably employed for the phototoxicity assessment of wide range of chemicals using different cytotoxic endpoints. Furthermore, these cell lines have been provided sufficient insights into the process of photodegradation, identification of its photoproducts and role of ROS in the manifestation of phototoxicity. Similarly the suitable models viz Hen's Egg Test Chorioallantoic Membrane (HET-CAM) test, Isolated Chicken Eye (ICE) test as recommended by ECVAM, ICCVAM, and OECD guidelines has been utilized as an *ex-vivo* systems to predict the potential ocular irritancy of the test substance (Velpandian, Bankoti, et al. 2006, Sahu, Singh, et al. 2014).

Apart from using well-established cell lines and primary cultures, the development of alternative models have also been generously pursued. In view of the speed, easiness, sensitivity and low cost, *E.coli* and *Paramecium*, as an alternate test system for phototoxic assessment has been examined for possible inclusion in the battery of tests to investigate UVA-radiation assisted phototoxicity of various chemical ingredients or formulations used in cosmetics and drugs (Joshi and Misra 1986, Misra, Sundararaman, et al. 1987, Verma, Agrawal, et al. 2008). Similarly, Tubifex has shown to be a convenient model for evaluation of wide range of phototoxic alterations in biochemical parameters in aquatic biomass owing to its sensitivity to determine even low doses of UV radiation and less than ppm level of test chemical is sufficient to produce noticeable phototoxic response (Soni and Joshi 1997, Misra and Joshi 1999, Misra, Babu, et al. 2002). The usefulness of the test has also extended towards the assessment of the effect of UV radiation on aquatic organisms (Zooplankton and phytoplankton) in relation to the stratospheric ozone depletion which is threatening to affect even the marine food life chain. Protozoa and ciliate *Tetrahymena* have also offered themselves as a promising alternative means to study phototoxicity both in presence and absence of photoreactive chemical agents. These models have provided scope for studying the biological effects of UV radiation, DNA damage, and defense against oxidative stress (Misra and Joshi 1999).

The limited studies have been conducted on the identification of protective compounds against phototoxicity. Relying on its proven anti-oxidant and anti-inflammatory capabilities in restoring the various neurodegenerative disorders, wound healing, antimicrobial activities, etc, curcumin has been supplemented as an active ingredient in a variety of cosmetic and personal health care products. However, the phototoxic/photosensitizing responses of curcumin are the issue of concern in terms of its applicability as an active ingredient in sunscreen topical creams/lotions (Dahll, Bilski, et al. 1994). To overcome its limitation, Chopra, et al 2016 have synthesized biodegradable and non- toxic polymer-poly (lactic-co-glycolic) acid (PLGA) encapsulated formulation of curcumin (PLGA-Cur-NPs, 150 nm) and have demonstrated that low level sustained release of curcumin from PLGA-Cur-NPs could be a promising way to protect the adverse biological interactions of photo-degradation products of curcumin upon the exposure of UVA and UVB (Chopra, Ray, et al. 2016).

CHAPTER 11

Mapping the Publication Output of Toxicology Research in India

In India, bibliometric studies have been carried out for several areas viz. medical research, neuroscience, engineering, fisheries, and agricultural research; however, toxicology research remains to be analyzed (Arunachalam 1997, Kumar, et al. 2009, Raghavan and Rao 2015, Bala and Gupta 2010). Despite the fact that research publications are not complete indicators of R&D output, they have been widely used in scientometric studies as they are generally available and measurable. An attempt has therefore been made here to analyze India's research output in terms of publications available on ISI's Web of Science. The Web of Science database is available from 1900 and covers IF journals only.

This study is an appraisal of toxicological research in India and is indicative of the research trends during the last 69 years (1950-April 2019). The years have been broken down into slots of 10 years. Search was done for the different fields using the following keywords: 'Occupational Toxicology and India', 'Environmental Toxicology and India', 'Medical toxicology and India', 'Nanomaterial toxicity and India', 'Toxicogenomics and India', 'Regulatory Toxicology and India', 'Neurotoxicity and India', 'Hepatotoxicity and India', 'Nephrotoxicity and India', 'Reproductive toxicity and India', 'Immunotoxicity and India', 'Genotoxicity and India' and 'Phototoxicity and India'. This study analyzes the research output in toxicology over a period of every 10 years and the analysis includes global publications' share, research growth and trends, most productive institutions and profile journals. We would like to bring this to the kind consideration of the readers, that these analysis and trends are based on the records available on the database, which could be subject to discrepancies. The only reason for carrying out this analysis is to get a reflection of the changing trends in the different areas of toxicology in India.

Global publication share and rank

The total global publication output on Toxicology from 1950-2019 is 1781172 papers. India is among the top 10 most productive countries. United States of America topped the list, with a global publication share of 656499 articles (36.86%) (Figure 11.1) United Kingdom ranked second, followed by Japan,

Canada, France, Germany, China, Italy (their global publications share ranging from (3-11%), India and Spain. India ranks at the 9th position with its global publications' share of 2.86%. India has witnessed a growth in the global output share from 0.61% (1950-1960s) to 2.45% (1980-1990) and a current value of 4.15%.

(a)

Country	Total Publication Output	% Global Contribution
USA	656499	36.86
UK	195938	11.00
Japan	99950	5.61
Canada	80522	4.52
France	70500	3.95
Germany	70373	3.95
China	69550	3.94
Italy	62398	3.50
India	**51003**	**2.86**
Spain	42413	2.38

(b)

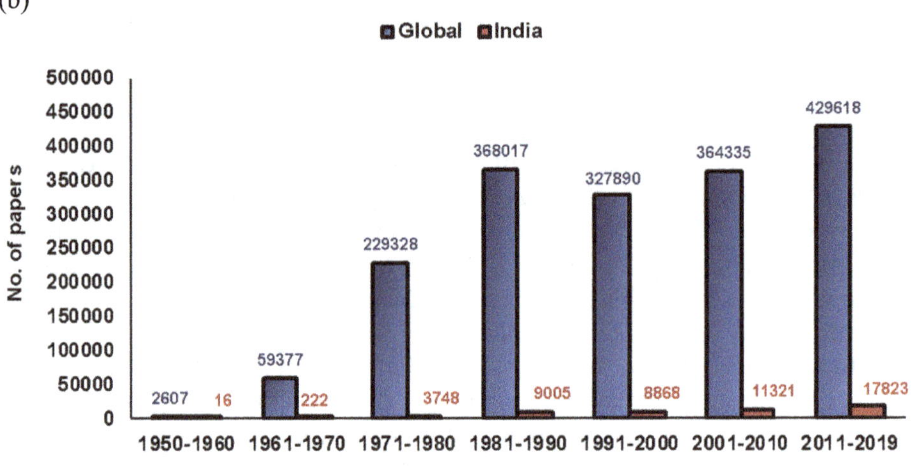

Figure 11.1 (a) List of top 10 countries with their global output in Toxicology (b) Global publication output vs India

We next looked at the trends of Toxicology growth in India. India's cumulative publications' output during 1950-2019 consists of 51003 papers. As evident from the Figure 11.2, there has been an increasing trend of publication output over the years. India has witnessed a growth from 0.03% (1951-1960), to 18.63% (1981-1990) and to a current high value of 34.95%. The authors would like to point out that the year slot from 2011-2019 (end of April) holds the highest number of publications (17823 papers) even though it just includes almost 9 years, indicating this number to further increase if we consider a time period of complete 10 years.

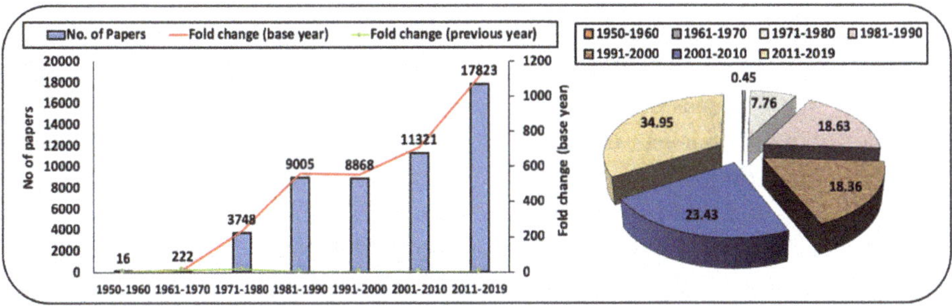

Figure 11.2 Increasing trend of publication output in India from 1950 to 2019

The top 10 research institutions and journals from which maximum publications have emerged are shown in the Table 11.1. These 10 Indian institutions together have contributed 26.85% share (with 13699 papers) of the publications' output of India.

Table 11.1 The top 10 research institutions and journals with maximum research publications

Journal name	Publications
Indian Journal of Experimental Biology	1768
The Indian Journal of Medical Research	1123
Bulletin of Environmental Contamination and Toxicology	1121
Indian Journal of Medical Research	1048
Indian Veterinary Journal	978
Indian Journal of Animal Sciences	962
Journal of Environmental Biology	925
Current Science	881
Indian Journal of Pharmacology	880
Current Science Bangalore	836
Institute	**Publications**
CSIR-Indian Institute of Toxicology Research	2541
Banaras Hindu University	1813
Indian Institute of Technology	1678
All India Institute of Medical Sciences	1467
Bhabha Atomic Research Center	1388
University of Calcutta	1292
PGIMER	999
University of Madras	866
Defense Research Development Organization	816
Punjab University	809

Similarly, we next mapped the publication trends in the different arenas viz, occupational toxicology, environmental toxicology, medical toxicology, nano-toxicology, toxicogenomics, regulatory toxicology as well as organ specific toxicity.

For **occupational toxicology,** a total of 1359 papers have been recorded. The increasing concerns of workplace exposures have prompted interest in epidemiological assessment and intervention strategies. However, as per the quantum of work that has been conducted in this field, the number of papers recorded do not do justice to it. One of the reasons for this small number maybe the absence of the word 'occupational' in the abstracts. India has witnessed a growth from 0.15% (1961-1970s), to a significant percentage 20.08% (1981-1990) and to a current high value of 32.74%. From just 2 papers in the year 1961-1970, there has been almost a fold change of 63 in the next 10 year slot (with 126 papers) (Figure 11.3).

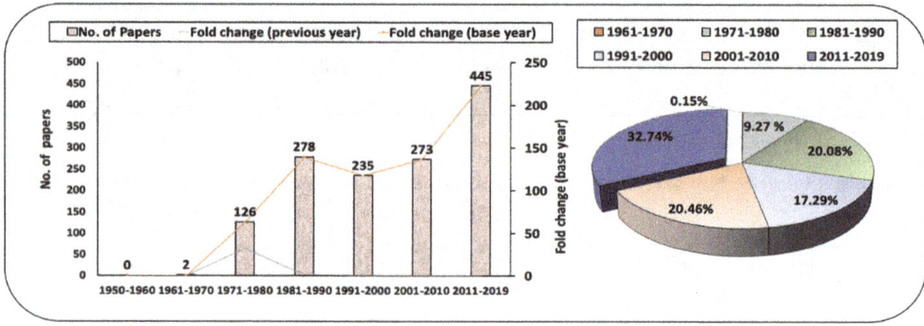

Figure 11.3 Trend of publications in Occupational Toxicology

The top 10 research institutions and journals from which maximum publications have emerged are shown in the Table 11.2. These 10 Indian institutions together have contributed to 42.68% share (with 629 papers) of the publications' output of India.

Table 11.2 The top 10 research institutions and journals with maximum publications in occupational toxicology

Institutions	Publications	% Contribution
CSIR-Indian Institute of Toxicology Research	261	19.21%
ICMR-National Institute of Occupational Health	76	5.60%
Bhabha Atomic Research Center	59	4.34%
Osmania University	48	3.53%
Indian Institrute of Technology	47	3.46%
University of Calcutta	34	2.50%
All India Institute of Medical Sciences	29	2.13%
CSIR-Indian Institute of Chemical Technology	26	1.92%
Defence Research Development Organisation	25	1.84%
PGIMER	24	1.77%

Contd...

Journal name	Publications
The Indian Journal of Medical Research	96
Indian Journal of Occupational and Environmental Medicine	47
Bulletin of Environmental Contamination and Toxicology	41
Industrial Health	33
Mutation Research	31
Environmental Research	30
Toxicology Letters Shannon	26
Toxicology Letters	26
Toxicology and Industrial Health	25
Human Experimental Toxicology	25

For **environmental toxicology,** a total of 10,672 papers have been recorded. As evident from the Figure 11.4, there has been an increasing trend of publication output over the years. From merely 3 papers in 1961-1971 (0.03%), India has witnessed a growth from 591 papers (1971-1980s, contributing to 6% total), to a drastic increase to 1842 and 4172 papers from 1991-2000 and 2011-2019 respectively. The year 2011-2019 slot has contributed maximum number of papers (39%).

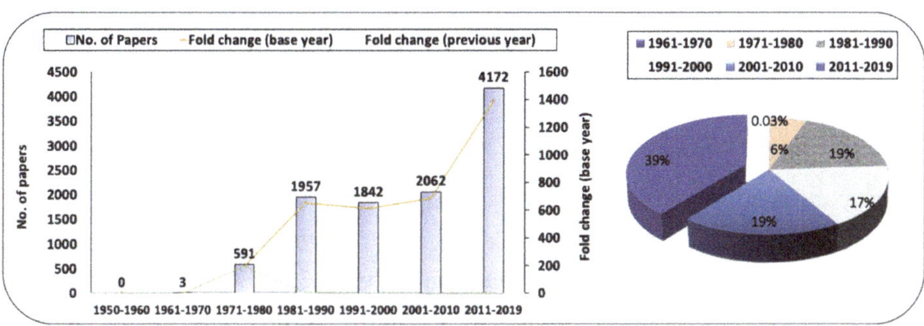

Figure 11.4 Trend of publications in Environmental Toxicology

Table 11.3 The top 10 research institutions and journals with maximum publications in Environmental Toxicology

Institutions	Publications	% Contribution
CSIR-Indian Institute of Toxicology Research	666	6.24%
Indian Institute of Technology	596	5.58%
Banaras Hindu University	527	4.94%
Bhabha Atomic Research Center	439	4.11%
University of Calcutta	339	3.18%

Contd...

Institutions	Publications	% Contribution
Aligarh Muslim University	287	2.69%
University of Delhi	243	2.28%
National Botanical Research Institute	177	1.66%
Sri Venkateswara University	153	1.43%
National Institute of Oceanography	150	1.41%

Journal name	Publications
Bulletin of Environmental Contamination And Toxicology	678
Journal of Environmental Biology	406
Environmental Monitoring and Assessment	330
Ecotoxicology and Environmental Safety	247
Current Science	236
Current Science Bangalore	234
Chemosphere	196
Indian Journal of Experimental Biology	191
Journal of Hazardous Materials	181
Science of the Total Environment	163

The top 10 research institutions and journals from which maximum publications have emerged are shown in the Table 11.3. These 10 Indian institutions together have contributed almost 33.5% share (with 3577 papers) of the publications' output of India.

For **medical toxicology,** a total of 9691 papers have been recorded. As evident from the Figure 11.5, there has been an increasing trend of publication output over the years. From merely 13 papers in 1961-1971 (0.13%), India has witnessed a growth from 763 papers (1971-1980s, contributing to 7.87% total), to a drastic increase to 1385 and 3846 papers from 1991-2000 and 2011-2019 respectively. The year 2011-2019 slot has contributed to maximum number of papers (39.69%).

The top 10 research institutions and journals from which maximum publications have emerged are shown in the Table 11.4. These 10 Indian institutions together have contributed almost 30.32% share (with 2939 papers) of the publications' output of India.

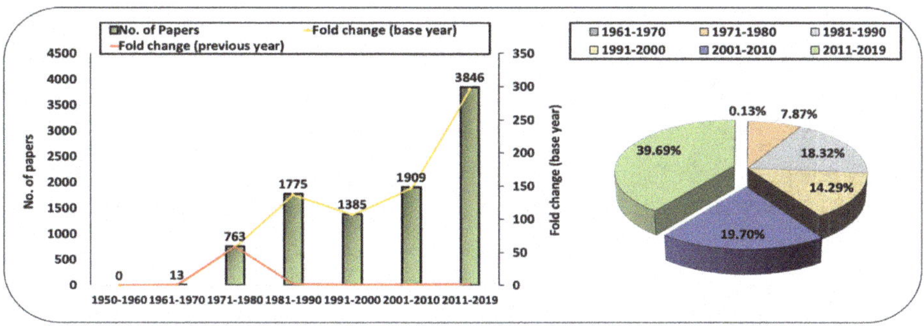

Figure 11.5 Trend of publications in Medical Toxicology

Table 11.4 The top 10 research institutions and journals with maximum publications in Medical Toxicology

Institutions	Publications	% Contribution
All India Institute of Medical Sciences	747	7.71%
PGIMER	629	6.50%
Christian Medical College	246	2.54%
Tata Memorial Hospital	238	2.46%
CSIR-Indian Institute of Toxicology Research	222	2.30%
Banaras Hindu University	182	1.88%
Indian Veterinary Research Institute	177	1.83%
University of Delhi	176	1.82%
Manipal University	169	1.74%
National Institute Of Cholera Enteric Diseases	153	1.58%
National Institute of Oceanography	150	1.55%

Journal name	Publications
The Indian Journal of Medical Research	1061
Indian Journal of Pharmacology	465
Indian Veterinary Journal	323
Indian Journal of Animal Sciences	315
Indian Journal of Experimental Biology	174
Indian Journal of Pediatrics	136
Indian Journal of Cancer	123
Current Science	109
Indian Pediatrics	81
PLOS One	79

Nanomaterial toxicology has been a nascent field in India, finding its earliest mention after 2005. As such comparatively lesser number of papers have been recorded as compared to the rest of the fields. A total of 2034 papers have been recorded. As evident from the Figure 11.6, India has witnessed a growth from 171 papers (2001-2010, contributing to 8.41% of total), to a current drastic increase of 1863 papers, which is almost a 133 fold change within a short span of time).

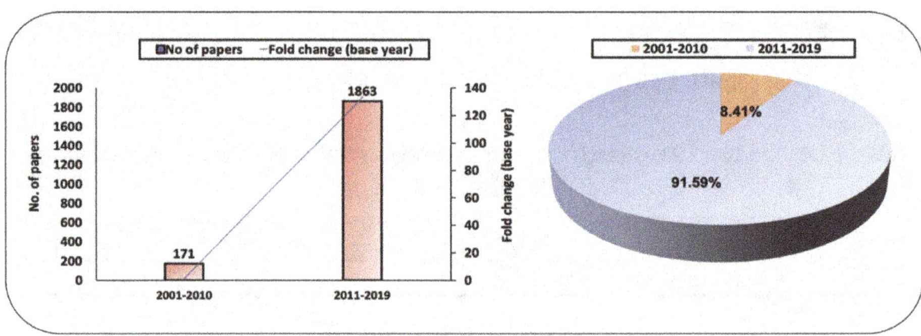

Figure 11.6 Trend of publications in Nanomaterial Toxicology

The top 10 research institutions and journals from which maximum publications have emerged are shown in the Table 11.5. These 10 Indian institutions together have contributed almost 10.57 % share (with 215 papers) of the publications' output of India.

Table 11.5 The top 10 research institutions and journals with maximum publications in Nanomaterial Toxicology

Institutions	Publications	% Contribution
Indian Institute of Technology	50	2.46%
Vellore Institute of Technology	48	2.36%
CSIR-Indian Institute of Toxicology Research	26	1.28%
University of Calcutta	18	0.89%
Ahmedabad University	16	0.79%
Bharathiar University	14	0.69%
Sree Chitra Tirunal Institute for Medical Sciences Technology	12	0.59%
National Institute of Chemical Physics Biophysics	11	0.54%
Bhabha Atomic Research Centre	10	0.49%
Alagappa University	10	0.49%

Journal name	Publications
Aquatic Toxicology	12
Environmental Science And Pollution Research International	8
Nanotoxicology	7
Ecotoxicology and Environmental Safety	7
Mutation Research	6
Chemosphere	6
Journal of Hazardous Materials	5
Journal of Applied Toxicology	5
International Journal of Biological Macromolecules	5
Chemical Engineering Journal	5

The rapid evolution of genome-based technologies has greatly accelerated the application of **toxicogenomics** in toxicology studies in India. However, a quick search at the database yielded a total of only 70 papers that have been recorded. As per the quantum of work undertaken in this field, the number of papers recorded are clearly quite low. One of the reasons for this small number maybe the absence of the word '**toxicogenomics**' in the abstracts. Using the available values, the same analysis was carried out. The number of papers have increased from 10 (14.29%) in the year 2001-2010 to 60 in 2011-2019 (85.71%) (Figure 11.7).

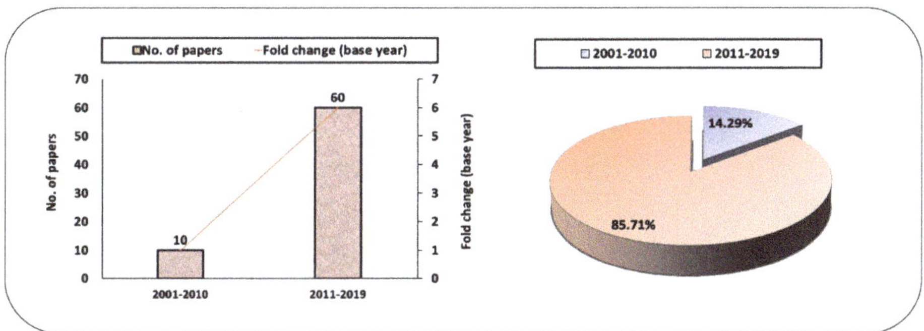

Figure 11.7 Trend of publications in Toxicogenomics

Even the list of research institutions and related journals have displayed only a few results as shown in Table 11.6. Even the names of the institutes (like CSIR-IITR, CSIR-IGIB, NEERI, etc.) known to undertake appreciable work in this field do not find a mention here.

Table 11.6 Few research institutions and journals with maximum publications in Toxicogenomics

Institutions	Publications	% Contribution
Council of Scientific and Industrial Research	11	15.71%
Dr DY Patil University	5	7.14%
Vellore Institute of Technology	2	2.90%
Piramal Life Sciences Ltd	2	2.90%
Central Drug Research Institute	2	2.90%

Journal name	Publications
Environmental Toxicology and Pharmacology	5
Current Drug Metabolism	3
Biochemical and Biophysical Research Communications	3
Toxicology	2

As expected, the total number of papers recorded for the field **regulatory toxicology** were also low (755). The reason for this small number maybe the absence of the word '**regulatory**' in the abstracts. Using the available values, the same analysis was carried out. As observed in other fields, a time dependent increase in the number of papers have been observed. From 9 papers reported from 1971 to 1980s there has been an increase from 46 and 530 publications from 1991-2000 to 2011-2019 respectively. The current year slot has contributed 70.2% of the total publication share (Figure 11.8).

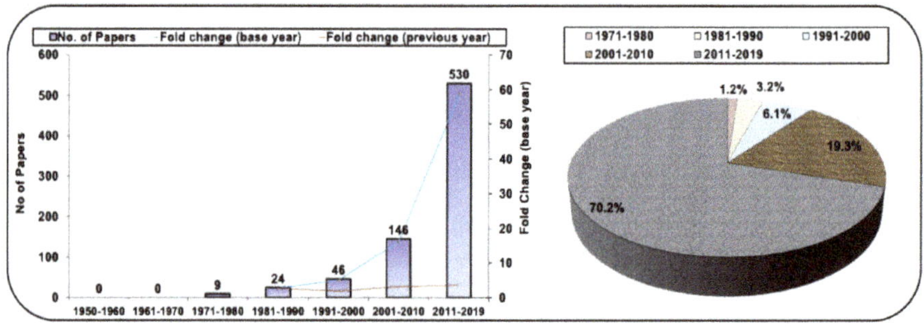

Figure 11.8 Trend of publications in Regulatory Toxicology

The top 10 research institutions and journals from which maximum publications have emerged are shown in the Table 11.7. These 10 Indian institutions together have contributed to almost 36.42% of share (with 275 papers) of the publications' output of India.

Table 11.7 Top 10 research institutions and journals with maximum publications in Regulatory Toxicology

Institutions	Publications	% Contribution
CSIR-Indian Institute of Toxicology Research	75	9.93%
Banaras Hindu University	35	4.63%
Indian Institute of Technology	25	3.31%
Jawaharlal Nehru University	25	3.31%
Central Food Technological Research Institute India	24	3.18%
University of Madras	20	2.65%
Punjab Agricultural University	18	2.38%
PGIMER	15	1.99%
All India Institute of Medical Sciences	14	1.85%
Indian Agricultural Research Institute	12	1.59%

Journal name	Publications
Bulletin of Environmental Contamination and Toxicology	48
Indian Journal of Medical Research	18
Toxicology and Applied Pharmacology	14
Journal of Food Science and Technology	14
Toxicology	9
Journal of Hazardous Materials	9
Current Science	8
Food and Chemical Toxicology	7
Chemosphere	7
Molecular and Cellular Biochemistry	6

For **neurotoxicity,** a total of 2265 papers have been recorded. As evident from the Figure 11.9, there has been an increasing trend of publication output over the years. From merely 6 papers in 1971-1980 (0.26%), India has witnessed a growth from 116 papers (1981-1990s, contributing to 5.12% total), almost a 19 fold change to a drastic increase of 544 and 1368 papers from 2001-2010 and 2011-2019 respectively. The year 2011-2019 slot has contributed to maximum number of papers (60.40%).

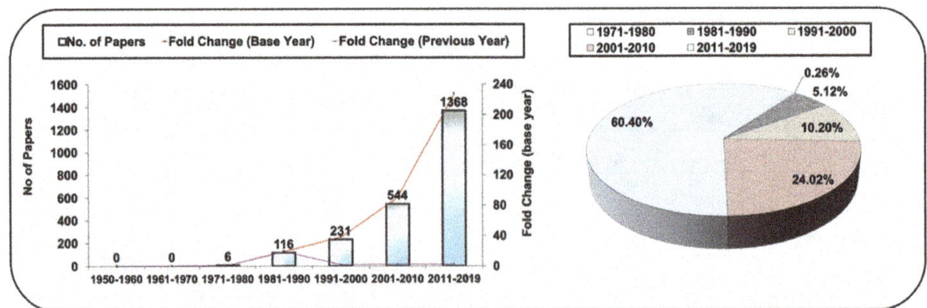

Figure 11.9 Trend of publications in Neurotoxicity

Table 11.8 Top 10 research institutions and journals with maximum publications in Neurotoxicity

Institutions	Publications	% Contribution
CSIR-Indian Institute of Toxicology Research	75	9.93%
Banaras Hindu University	35	4.63%
Indian Institute of Technology	25	3.31%
Jawaharlal Nehru University	25	3.31%
Central Food Technological Research Institute India	24	3.18%
University of Madras	20	2.65%
Punjab Agricultural University	18	2.38%
PGIMER	15	1.99%
All India Institute of Medical Sciences	14	1.85%
Indian Agricultural Research Institute	12	1.59%

Journal name	Publications
Bulletin of Environmental Contamination and Toxicology	48
Indian Journal of Medical Research	18
Toxicology and Applied Pharmacology	14
Journal of Food Science and Technology	14
Toxicology	9
Journal of Hazardous Materials	9
Current Science	8
Food and Chemical Toxicology	7
Chemosphere	7
Molecular and Cellular Biochemistry	6

The top 10 research institutions and journals from which maximum publications have emerged are shown in the Table 11.8. These 10 Indian institutions together have contributed almost 31.74% share (with 719 papers) of the publications' output of India.

For **hepatotoxicity,** a total of 2280 papers have been recorded. As evident from the Figure 11.10, there has been an increasing trend of publication output over the years. From merely 7 papers in 1971-1980 (0.31%), India has witnessed a growth from 77 papers (1981-1990s, contributing to 3.37% total), almost a 11 fold change to a drastic increase of 715 and 1260 papers from 2001-2010 and 2011-2019 respectively. The year 2011-2019 slot has contributed to maximum number of papers (55.26%).

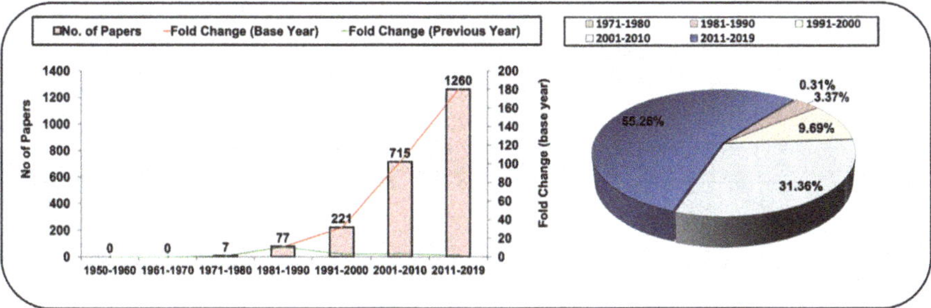

Figure 11.10 Trend of publications in Hepatotoxicity

Table 11.9 Top 10 research institutions and journals with maximum publications in Hepatotoxicity

Institutions	Publications	% Contribution
Annamalai University	156	6.84%
Jamia Hamdard	147	6.45%
University of Madras	114	5.00%
Bose Institute	79	3.46%
Panjab University	75	3.29%
All India Institute of Medical Sciences	75	3.29%
CSIR-Indian Institute of Technology Research	67	2.94%
Jadavpur University	52	2.28%
PGIMER	48	2.11%
Indian Veterinary Research Institute	38	1.67%

Journal name	Publications
Indian Journal of Pharmacology	73
Indian Journal of Experimental Biology	64
Phytotherapy Research	62
Journal of Ethnopharmacology	59
Food and Chemical Toxicology	45
Pharmaceutical Biology	28
Chemico-Biological Interactions	25
The Indian Journal of Medical Research	24
Toxicology Mechanisms And Methods	23
Human Experimental Toxicology	23

The top 10 research institutions and journals from which maximum publications have emerged are shown in the following Table 11.9. These 10 Indian institutions together have contributed to almost 37.32% share (with 851 papers) of the publications' output of India.

For **nephrotoxicity,** a total of 1155 papers have been recorded. As evident from the Figure 11.11, there has been an increasing trend of publication output over the years. From merely 4 papers in 1971-1980 (0.30%), India has witnessed a growth from 25 papers (1981-1990s, contributing to 2.2% total), to a drastic increase 333 and 696 papers from 2001-2010 and 2011-2019 respectively. The year 2011-2019 slot has contributed to maximum number of papers (60.3%).

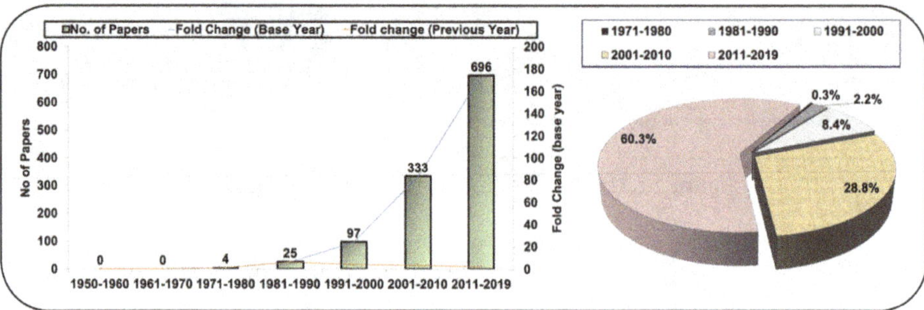

Figure 11.11 Trend of publications in Nephrotoxicity

The top 10 research institutions and journals from which maximum publications have emerged are shown in the Table 11.10. These 10 Indian institutions together have contributed almost 51.95% share (with 600 papers) of the publications' output of India.

Table 11.10 Top 10 research institutions and journals with maximum publications in Nephrotoxicity

Institutions	Publications	% Contribution
Jamia Hamdard	99	8.57%
Aligarh Muslim University	91	7.88%
University of Madras	90	7.80%
All India Institute of Medical Sciences	64	5.54%
Panjab University	62	5.37%
Annamalai University	46	4.00%
Christian medical College	45	3.90%
National Institute of Pharmaceutical and Education Research	44	3.81%
PGIMER	34	2.94%
Indian Veterinary Research Institute	25	2.16%

Contd...

Journal name	Publications
Food and Chemical Toxicology	35
Renal Failure	29
Indian Journal of Pharmacology	29
Indian Journal of Animal Sciences	22
Human Experimental Toxicology	22
The Indian Journal of Medical Research	21
Molecular and Cellular Biochemistry	16
Indian Journal of Experimental Biology	15
Toxicology	14
Experimental and Toxicological Pathology	23

For **reproductive toxicity,** a total of 3274 papers have been recorded. This has been one of the few fields that gained momentum right from the 1960s, as evident from few papers during this period. As evident from the Figure 11.12, there has been an increasing trend of publication output over the years. From merely 2 papers in 1961-1971 (0.06%), India has witnessed a growth from 127 papers (1971-1980s, contributing to 3.88% total), to a drastic increase of 486, 905 and 1404 papers in 1991-2000, 2001-2010 and 2011-2019 respectively. The year 2011-2019 slot has contributed to maximum number of papers (42.88%).

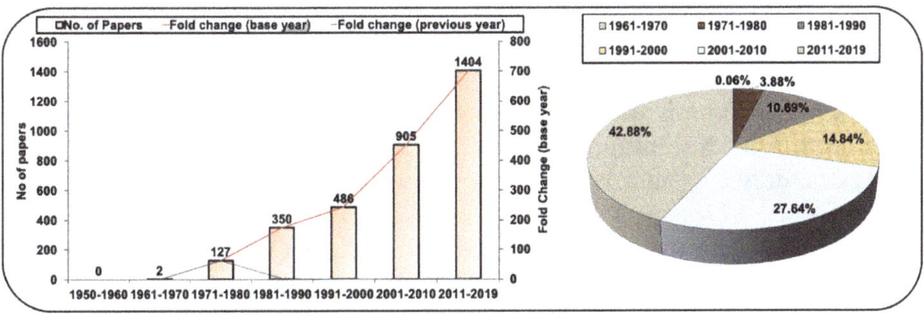

Figure 11.12 Trend of publications in Reproductive Toxicity

The top 10 research institutions and journals from which maximum publications have emerged are shown in the Table 11.11. These 10 Indian institutions together have contributed almost 32.59% share (with 1067 papers) of the publications' output of India.

Table 11.11 Top 10 research institutions and journals with maximum publications in Reproductive Toxicity

Institutions	Publications	% Contribution
CSIR-Indian Institute of Toxicology Research	238	7.27%
University of Madras	200	6.11%
Banaras Hindu University	109	3.33%
All India Institute of Medical Sciences	106	3.23%
Tata Memorial Hospital	97	2.96%
Panjab university	76	2.32%
University of Rajasthan	71	2.17%
Gujarat University	63	1.92%
University of Calcutta	61	1.86 %
Indian Veterinary Research Institute	46	1.41%

Journal name	Publications
Indian Journal of Experimental Biology	140
Journal of Environmental Biology	91
Bulletin of Environmental Contamination and Toxicology	78
Reproductive Toxicology	75
Mutation Research	55
Indian Journal of Medical Research	50
Toxicology Letters	46
Food and Chemical Toxicology	46
Ecotoxicology and Environmental Safety	45
Toxicology	43

As evident from the previous section, substantial amount of work has been undertaken on the **immunotoxicity** potential of different environmental pollutants, drugs, chemicals etc. However, according to the database record, a total of only 177 papers seem to exist (beginning from 1981), a number unbelievable as this has been one of the few fields that gained momentum right from the 1960s. However, like others, an increasing trend has also been observed here. From 8 papers in 1981-1971 (4.52%), India has witnessed a growth from 55 papers (2001-2010, contributing to 31.07% total), to an increase of 96 papers in 2011-2019 (54.24%) (Figure 11.13).

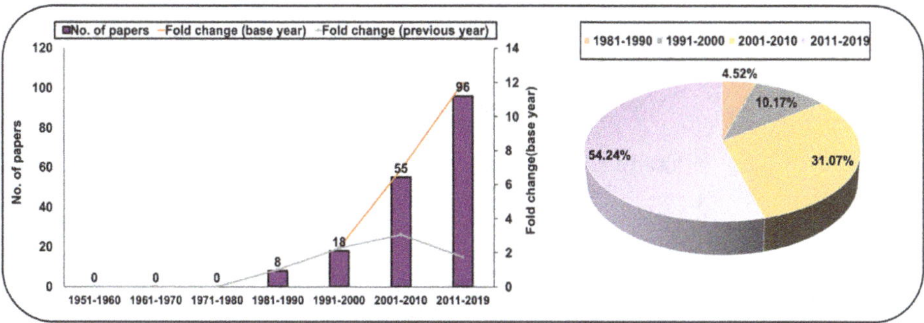

Figure 11.13 Trend of publications in Immunotoxicity

The top 10 research institutions and journals from which maximum publications have emerged are shown in the Table 11.12.

Table 11.12 Top 10 research institutions and journals with maximum immunotoxicity

Institutions	Publications	% Contribution
CSIR-Indian Institute of Toxicology Research	48	27.12%
University of Delhi	28	15.82%
Indian Veterinary Research Institute	19	10.73%
University of Calcutta	18	10.17%
Jamia Hamdard	11	6.21%
Banaras Hindu University	8	4.52%
Indian institute of Science	8	4.52%
Univ Coll Med Sci	7	3.95%
Defence Research Development Organization	6	3.39%
Defence Research Development Establishment	4	2.26%

Journal name	Publications
Toxicology	11
Indian Journal of Experimental Biology	11
Toxicology Letters	9
Journal of Immunotoxicology	7
Environmental Toxicology and Pharmacology	6
Immunopharmacology and Immunotoxicology	5
Ecotoxicology and Environmental Safety	5
Drug and Chemical Toxicology	5
Toxicology *in Vitro*	3
Indian Journal of Animal Sciences	3

For **genotoxicity,** a total of 2267 papers have been recorded. As evident from the Figure 11.14, there has been an increasing trend of publication output over the years. From 79 papers in 1981-1990 (3.48%), India has witnessed a growth from 256 papers (1991-2000), contributing to 11.29% total), to a further increase of 595 and 1337 papers in 2001-2010 and 2011-2019 respectively.

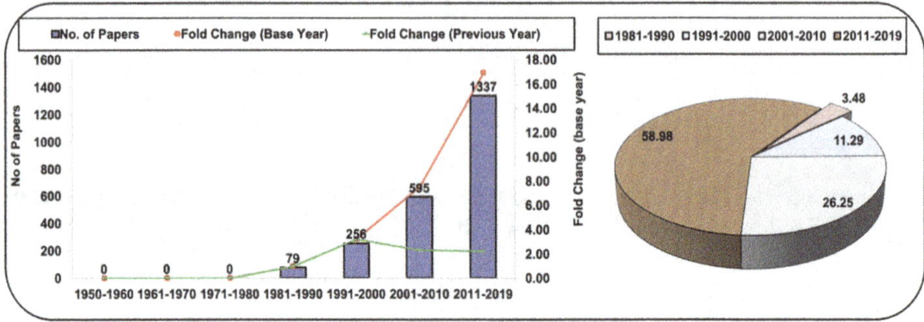

Figure 11.14 Trend of publications in Genotoxicity

The top 10 research institutions and journals from which maximum publications have emerged are shown in Table 11.13. These 10 Indian institutions together have contributed almost 49.54 % share (with 1123 papers) of the publications' output of India.

Table 11.13 Top 10 research institutions and journals with maximum publications in Genotoxicity

Institutions	Publications	% Contribution
Aligarh Muslim University	237	10.45%
Indian Institute of Toxicology Research	212	9.35%
University of Calcutta	143	6.31%
Jawaharlal Nehru University	132	5.82%
Indian Institute of Chemical Technology	70	3.09%
Manipal University	69	3.04%
University of Madras	67	2.96%
Lucknow University	66	2.91%
Guru Nanak Dev University	64	2.82%
Bhabha Atomic Research Center	63	2.78%

Contd...

Journal name	Publications
Mutation Research	339
Food and Chemical Toxicology	74
Ecotoxicology and Environmental Safety	47
Drug and Chemical Toxicology	45
Environmental Science and Pollution Research International	41
Journal of Environmental Biology	34
Indian Journal of Experimental Biology	33
Mutagenesis	32
Chemosphere	32
Toxicology Mechanisms and Methods	26

As evident from the previous section, substantial amount of work has been undertaken on the **phototoxicity** potential of different environmental pollutants, drugs, chemicals etc. However, according to the database record, a total of only 137 papers seem to exist (beginning from 1981). However, like others, an increasing trend has also been observed here. From 1 paper in 1981-1990 (0.73%), India has witnessed a growth from 18 papers (1991-2000, contributing to 13.14% total), to an increase of 40 (29.20%) and 78 papers (56.93%) in 2001-2010 and 2011-2019 respectively (Figure 11.15).

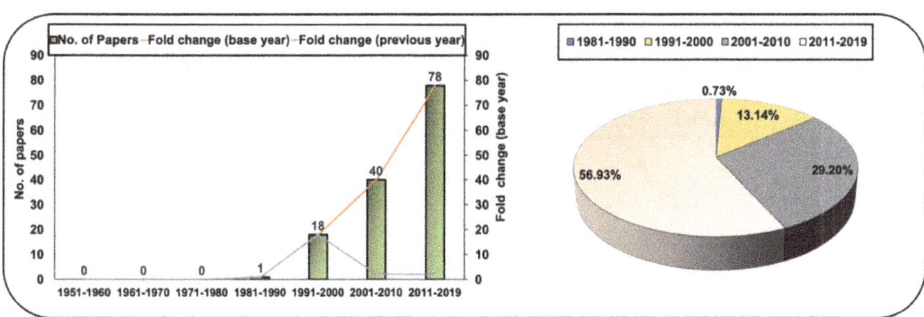

Figure 11.15 Trend of publications in Phototoxicity

The top 10 research institutions and journals from which maximum publications have emerged are shown in the Table 11.14.

Table 11.14 Top 10 research institutions and journals with maximum publications in Phototoxicity

Institutions	Publications	% Contribution
Indian Institute of Toxicology Research	55	40.15%
Indian Institute of Technology	14	10.22%
Aligarh Muslim University	10	7.30%
Raja Ramanna Centre for Advance Technologies	7	5.11%
Panjab University	6	4.38%
All India Institute of Medical Sciences	5	3.65%
Kurukshetra University	5	3.65%
Devi Ahilyabai University, Indore	5	3.65%
PGIMER	4	2.92%
Indian Oil Corporation Ltd	3	2.19%

Journal name	Publications
Photochemistry and Photobiology	6
Toxicology In-vitro	5
Indian Journal of Experimental Biology	5
Toxicology Letters	4
Indian Journal of Chemistry	4
Food and Chemical Toxicology	4
RSC Advances	3
Ecotoxicology and Environmental Safety	3
Bioorganic Medicinal Chemistry Letters	3
Alternatives to Laboratory Animals	3

CHAPTER 12

Future Prospects and Recommendations

Traditionally toxicology was considered no more than a scion of forensic medicine, and a poor cousin of clinical medicine. However, with the subject gaining national importance, undergoing constant improvements and refinements in methodology and implementation of novel approaches, it is one of the important disciplines practiced in India. From the 'science of poisons' to the 'science of protection', toxicology research in India, today, stands as a highly evolved, multidisciplinary endeavor that develops its own conceptual frameworks while also drawing upon advances in the chemical, medical and biological sciences.

There has been an exponential growth in the discipline, not in terms of just publications, but also in terms of professional societies, journals, research scientists, specialized departments with state-of-the-art infrastructure, and institutes with research facilities, which is a vivid reflection of the increasing interest in the discipline. A number of educational institutions and universities have been teaching and researching toxicology, at undergraduate, graduate and postgraduate levels for several years. Over the years from essentially being a data generating process on the toxicogenic potential of chemicals such as pesticides, heavy metals, drugs, dyes and food colors mainly for regulatory purposes, the scope of toxicology has been further extended towards understanding the mechanistic basis of toxicants. The development in the post-genomics era has also provided immense opportunities for pragmatic assessment of environmental and occupational exposure to noxious substances. Identification and validation of various biomarkers, toxicogenomic effects, and genes susceptibilities have revolutionized our understanding of human occupational and environmental diseases. The concept of biomarkers, alternatives to animal models, mathematical modeling, predictive toxicology, detection and development of methods for toxins/adulterants/environmental chemicals in different matrices are to name a few that have paved the way for a paradigm shift in the way toxicology is being practiced today.

Today's technologies have provided great opportunities, although many challenges remain regarding their development, implementation, and validation to adequately assess human health effects. To bring the envisioned toxicology closer to concrete implementation, it is important to identify the current knowledge gaps in the vision and develop solutions to strengthen the discipline. Through the 'Make in India' initiative, India is striving hard to be at the forefront of innovation and self-sustainable methods. Research into the development of indigenous alternative approaches for toxicity models have so far resulted in the incorporation of a panel of new cell and tissue culture systems and *in-silico* models, but their maximum utilization have been hampered as regulatory acceptance requires time, prior validation and robust financial and scientific investment. This draws attention to the need of having a national body to monitor, regulate and validate these newly developed models to facilitate their efficient utilization. Such reproducible, rapid, economical and high-throughput models will not only generate accurate results but will also be entirely instrumental in reducing the clinical trial failure rates and getting rid of the ethical burden of animal euthanasia.

Publications in high impact factor journals are limited in the area of toxicology, however, with an expansion in the activities of the institutes in this multidisciplinary field of toxicology, the number of publications in high IF journals would hopefully increase. There should be an increase in international collaboration to increase the output and also to improve the quality of research. In addition, there should be more collaboration among Indian institutions. There is an urgent need for a substantial increase in research and development investments, both at the institutional level as well as in terms of extramural funding from different scientific agencies. Academic institutes should take steps to create interest in research in toxicology among graduate and postgraduate students and also among young clinicians and scientists. This is one of the reasons that prompted us to write this book in the very first place. This book, providing insights into the rich history of toxicology in India as well as its transition into a fully-fledged discipline, could be a rich reservoir of information for students, budding young toxicologists and an asset to the entire scientific fraternity, leaving them marvelled over the outstanding efforts made by the Indian scientific fraternity to contribute to the understanding of the complexities the subject offers.

We believe that India has the necessary academic and industrial strengths to develop and employ new technologies, which could position it as a global powerhouse in this area. Through this book, we not just appraise the unstinted strides India has made in carving a niche, but also emphasize the need for India to catch up with the developed and the rest of the developing nations in practicing the available technologies and contributing globally. We hope that the delivery of the recommendations in this book will be able to drive innovation in development, validation and utilization of various toxicological approaches in the country.

Conclusion

Understanding the toxicity of compounds could never be a 'closed book' situation. The arena of toxicology has been continuously expanding and diversifying, driven by the need to investigate and understand the human and ecological risks of exposure to newer chemicals and other toxicants. India has made great strides to keep itself abreast of this evolving discipline, which has placed the country on the pedestal of toxicology research. However, many gaps remain to be bridged when it comes to the transition from conventional into technologically assisted methods, and a great deal still needs to be done in this arena.

Any substance introduced into the body or environment has the potential to cause toxicity.

The Real Danger exists in knowing and not acknowledging the danger and doing nothing about it.

From the inability to let alone; from too much zeal for the new and contempt for what is old;

From putting knowledge before wisdom, and Science before art and cleverness before common sense;

From treating patients as cases; and from making a cure of the disease more grievous than the endurance of the same, Good Lord, deliver us.

-Sir Robert Hutchison

References

Abbas, S., S. Alam, A. Pal, M. Kumar, D. Singh and K. M. Ansari (2016). "UVB exposure enhanced benzanthrone-induced inflammatory responses in SKH-1 mouse skin by activating the expression of COX-2 and iNOS through MAP kinases/NF-κB/AP-1 signalling pathways." Food and Chemical Toxicology 96: 183-190.

Abhilash, P. and N. Singh (2009). "Pesticide use and application: an Indian scenario." Journal of Hazardous Materials 165(1-3): 1-12.

Abraham, P., K. Indirani and E. Sugumar (2007). "Effect of cyclophosphamide treatment on selected lysosomal enzymes in the kidney of rats." Experimental and Toxicologic Pathology 59(2): 143-149.

Abraham, P., B. Isaac, H. Ramamoorthy and K. Natarajan (2011). "Oral glutamine attenuates cyclophosphamide-induced oxidative stress in the bladder but does not prevent hemorrhagic cystitis in rats." Journal of Medical Toxicology 7(2): 118-124.

Abraham, P. and S. Rabi (2009). "Nitrosative stress, protein tyrosine nitration, PARP activation and NAD depletion in the kidneys of rats after single dose of cyclophosphamide." Clinical and Experimental Nephrology 13(4): 281-287.

Abraham, P. and S. Rabi (2011). "Protective effect of aminoguanidine against cyclophosphamide-induced oxidative stress and renal damage in rats." Redox Report 16(1): 8-14.

Abraham, P. and E. Sugumar (2008). "Enhanced PON1 activity in the kidneys of cyclophosphamide treated rats may play a protective role as an antioxidant against cyclophosphamide induced oxidative stress." Archives of Toxicology 82(4): 237-238.

Abraham, S. K., V. Goswami and P. Kesavan (1979). "A preliminary assessment of possible mutagenicity of betel nut and ingredients of the betel quid when administered alone or in combinations to larvae of Drosophila melanogaster." Mutation Research/Genetic Toxicology 66(3): 261-266.

Acharya, S., S. Chaudhuri, S. Chatterjee, P. Kumar, Z. Begum, S. Dasgupta, S. Flora and S. Chaudhuri (2010). "Immunological profile of arsenic toxicity: a hint towards arsenic-induced carcinogenesis." Asian Pacific Journal of Cancer Prevention 11(2): 479-490.

Adhikari, N., N. Sinha and D. Saxena (2000). "Effect of lead on Sertoli–germ cell coculture of rat." Toxicology Letters 116(1-2): 45-49.

Adhvaryu, S., B. Dave and A. Trivedi (1989). "An *in vitro* assessment of the genotoxic potential of pan masalas." The Indian Journal of Medical Research 90: 131-134.

Adhvaryu, S. G., U. M. Rawal, J. V. Patel, D. D. Patel and D. B. Balar (1988). "Increased frequency of sister chromatid exchanges in lymphocytes of breast cancer patients." International Journal of Cancer 41(3): 394-398.

Adi, P. J., S. P. Burra, A. R. Vataparti and B. Matcha (2016). "Calcium, zinc and vitamin E ameliorate cadmium-induced renal oxidative damage in albino Wistar rats." Toxicology Reports 3: 591-597.

Adilaxmamma, K., A. Janardhan and K. Reddy (1994). "Monocrotophos: reproductive toxicity in rats." Indian Journal of Pharmacology 26(2): 126.

Afaq, F., P. Abidi and Q. Rahman (2000). "N-acetyl L-cysteine attenuates oxidant-mediated toxicity induced by chrysotile fibers." Toxicology Letters 117(1-2): 53-60.

Agarwal, D., L. Chauhan, S. Gupta and V. Sundararaman (1994). "Cytogenetic effects of deltamethrin on rat bone marrow." Mutation Research/Fundamental and Molecular Mechanisms of Mutagenesis 311(1): 133-138.

Agarwal, R., S. Diwanay, P. Patki and B. Patwardhan (1999). "Studies on immunomodulatory activity of Withania somnifera (Ashwagandha) extracts in experimental immune inflammation." Journal of Ethnopharmacology 67(1): 27-35.

Aggrawal, A. (2005). "History of toxicology."

Agharkar, S. (1953). "Gazetteer of Bombay State." General-Ar Botany.

Agharkar, S. (1953). Gazetteer of Bombay State, Part I—Medicinal Plants, Bombay.

Agrahari, A., A. Singh, A. Srivastava, R. R. Jha, D. K. Patel, S. Yadav, V. Srivastava and D. Parmar (2019). "Overexpression of cerebral cytochrome P450s in prenatally exposed offspring modify the toxicity of lindane in rechallenged offspring." Toxicology and Applied Pharmacology.

Agrawal, A. K., M. Anand, N. F. Zaidi and P. K. Seth (1983). "Involvement of serotonergic receptors in endosulfan neurotoxicity." Biochemical Pharmacology 32(23): 3591-3593.

Agrawal, M., V. Kumar, M. P. Kashyap, V. K. Khanna, G. S. Randhawa and A. B. Pant (2011). "Ischemic insult induced apoptotic changes in PC12 cells: protection by trans resveratrol." European Journal of Pharmacology 666(1-3): 5-11.

Agrawal, M., V. Kumar, A. K. Singh, M. P. Kashyap, V. K. Khanna, M. A. Siddiqui and A. B. Pant (2012). "*Trans-Resveratrol* protects ischemic PC12 Cells by inhibiting the hypoxia associated transcription factors and increasing the levels of antioxidant defense enzymes." ACS Chemical Neuroscience 4(2): 285-294.

Agrawal, N., R. S. Ray, M. Farooq, A. B. Pant and R. K. Hans (2007). "Photosensitizing potential of ciprofloxacin at ambient level of UV radiation." Photochemistry and Photobiology 83(5): 1226-1236.

Agrawal, S., A. Singh, P. Tripathi, M. Mishra, P. K. Singh and M. P. Singh (2015). "Cypermethrin-induced nigrostriatal dopaminergic neurodegeneration alters the mitochondrial function: a proteomics study." Molecular Neurobiology 51(2): 448-465.

Ahamed, M., M. Fareed, A. Kumar, W. Siddiqui and M. Siddiqui (2008). "Oxidative stress and neurological disorders in relation to blood lead levels in children." Redox Report 13(3): 117-122.

Ahamed, M., M. A. Siddiqui, M. J. Akhtar, I. Ahmad, A. B. Pant and H. A. Alhadlaq (2010). "Genotoxic potential of copper oxide nanoparticles in human lung epithelial cells." Biochemical and Biophysical Research Communications 396(2): 578-583.

Ahamed, M., S. Verma, A. Kumar and M. Siddiqui (2005). "Environmental exposure to lead and its correlation with biochemical indices in children." Science of the Total Environment 346(1-3): 48-55.

Ahamed, M., S. Verma, A. Kumar and M. K. Siddiqui (2010). "Blood lead levels in children of Lucknow, India." Environmental Toxicology: An International Journal 25(1): 48-54.

Ahluwalia, T. S., M. Ahuja, T. S. Rai, H. S. Kohli, A. Bhansali, K. Sud and M. Khullar (2009). "ACE variants interact with the RAS pathway to confer risk and protection against type 2 diabetic nephropathy." DNA and Cell Biology 28(3): 141-150.

Ahluwalia, T. S., M. Ahuja, T. S. Rai, H. S. Kohli, K. Sud, A. Bhansali and M. Khullar (2008). "Endothelial nitric oxide synthase gene haplotypes and diabetic nephropathy among Asian Indians." Molecular and Cellular Biochemistry 314(1-2): 9-17.

Ahluwalia, T. S., M. Khullar, M. Ahuja, H. S. Kohli, A. Bhansali, V. Mohan, R. Venkatesan, T. S. Rai, K. Sud and P. K. Singal (2009). "Common variants of inflammatory cytokine genes are associated with risk of nephropathy in type 2 diabetes among Asian Indians." PLoS One 4(4): e5168.

Ahmad, A. S., M. A. Ansari, M. Ahmad, S. Saleem, S. Yousuf, M. N. Hoda and F. Islam (2005). "Neuroprotection by crocetin in a hemi-parkinsonian rat model." Pharmacology Biochemistry and Behavior 81(4): 805-813.

Ahmad, F., A. M. Al-Subaie, A. I. Al-Ohali and A. S. Mohammed (2018). "Phytochemical and Nephroprotective Activity of Eclipta prostrata against Gentamicin Induced Nephrotoxicity in Wistar Rats." International Journal of Pharma Research and Health Sciences 6(2): 2559-2564.

Ahmad, I., M. I. Khan and G. Patil (2011). Nanotoxicity of occupational dust generated in granite stone saw mill. 2011 International Conference on Nanoscience, Technology and Societal Implications, IEEE.

Ahmad, I., M. I. Khan, G. Patil and L. Chauhan (2012). "Evaluation of cytotoxic, genotoxic and inflammatory responses of micro-and nano-particles of granite on human lung fibroblast cell IMR-90." Toxicology Letters 208(3): 300-307.

Ahmad, I., S. Shukla, A. Kumar, B. K. Singh, V. Kumar, A. K. Chauhan, D. Singh, H. P. Pandey and C. Singh (2013). "Biochemical and molecular mechanisms of N-acetyl cysteine and silymarin-mediated protection against maneb and paraquat-induced hepatotoxicity in rats." Chemico-Biological Interactions 201(1-3): 9-18.

Ahmad, I., S. Shukla, A. Kumar, B. K. Singh, D. K. Patel, H. P. Pandey and C. Singh (2010). "Maneb and paraquat-induced modulation of toxicant responsive genes in the rat liver: comparison with polymorphonuclear leukocytes." Chemico-Biological Interactions 188(3): 566-579.

Ahmad, M., S. Saleem, A. S. Ahmad, M. A. Ansari, S. Yousuf, M. N. Hoda and F. Islam (2005). "Neuroprotective effects of Withania somnifera on 6-hydroxydopamine induced Parkinsonism in rats." Human and Experimental Toxicology 24(3): 137-147.

Ahmad, M., D. Sharma, S. Ansari and B. Ansari (2012). "Effect of lambda-cyhalothrin and Neemgold on some biochemical parameters in the gill, liver, and ovary of zebrafish, Danio rerio (Cyprinidae)." Archiwum Rybactwa Polskiego 20(1): 19-25.

Ahmad, M. E., G. Shadab, M. A. Azfer and M. Afzal (2001). "Evaluation of genotoxic potential of synthetic progestins-norethindrone and norgestrel in human lymphocytes *in vitro*." Mutation Research/Genetic Toxicology and Environmental Mutagenesis 494(1-2): 13-20.

Ahmad, M. E., G. Shadab, A. Hoda and M. Afzal (2000). "Genotoxic effects of estradiol-17β on human lymphocyte chromosomes." Mutation Research/Genetic Toxicology and Environmental Mutagenesis 466(1): 109-115.

Ahmad, S., A. Hoda and M. Afzal (2002). "Additive action of vitamins C and E against hydrocortisone-induced genotoxicity in human lymphocyte chromosomes." International Journal for Vitamin and Nutrition Research 72(4): 204-209.

Ahmad, S., M. B. Khan, M. N. Hoda, K. Bhatia, R. Haque, I. S. Fazili, A. Jamal, J. S. Khan and D. P. Katare (2012). "Neuroprotective effect of sesame seed oil in 6-hydroxydopamine induced neurotoxicity in mice model: cellular, biochemical and neurochemical evidence." Neurochemical Research 37(3): 516-526.

Ahmed, B., S. Dwivedi, M. Z. Abdin, A. Azam, M. Al-Shaeri, M. S. Khan, Q. Saquib, A. A. Al-Khedhairy and J. Musarrat (2017). "Mitochondrial and chromosomal damage induced by oxidative stress in Zn 2+ ions, ZnO-bulk and ZnO-NPs treated Allium cepa roots." Scientific Reports 7: 40685.

Ahmed, G., M. A. Khandkar and S. S. Katyare (1995). "Mitochondrial ATPase: a target for paracetamol-induced hepatotoxicity." European Journal of Pharmacology: Environmental Toxicology and Pharmacology 293(3): 225-229.

Aithal, A. P., L. K. Bairy, R. N. Seetharam and M. K. Rao (2019). "Human bone marrow-derived mesenchymal stromal cells in combination with silymarin regulate hepatocyte growth factor expression and genotoxicity in carbon tetrachloride induced hepatotoxicity in Wistar rats." Journal of Cellular Biochemistry.

Ajith, T., S. Usha and V. Nivitha (2007). "Ascorbic acid and α-tocopherol protect anticancer drug cisplatin induced nephrotoxicity in mice: a comparative study." Clinica Chimica Acta 375(1-2): 82-86.

Ajmal, M., R. A. K. Rao, S. Anwar, J. Ahmad and R. Ahmad (2003). "Adsorption studies on rice husk: removal and recovery of Cd (II) from wastewater." Bioresource Technology 86(2): 147-149.

Alam, M. Z., S. Ahmad, A. Malik and M. Ahmad (2010). "Mutagenicity and genotoxicity of tannery effluents used for irrigation at Kanpur, India." Ecotoxicology and Environmental Safety 73(7): 1620-1628.

Aleem, A. and A. Malik (2003). "Genotoxicity of water extracts from the River Yamuna at Mathura, India." Environmental Toxicology: An International Journal 18(2): 69-77.

Aleem, A. and A. Malik (2005). "Genotoxicity of the Yamuna river water at Okhla (Delhi), India." Ecotoxicology and Environmental Safety 61(3): 404-412.

Ali, D., N. Nagpure, S. Kumar, R. Kumar, B. Kushwaha and W. Lakra (2009). "Assessment of genotoxic and mutagenic effects of chlorpyrifos in freshwater fish Channa punctatus (Bloch) using micronucleus assay and alkaline single-cell gel electrophoresis." Food and Chemical Toxicology 47(3): 650-656.

Ali, D., N. S. Nagpure, S. Kumar, R. Kumar and B. Kushwaha (2008). "Genotoxicity assessment of acute exposure of chlorpyrifos to freshwater fish Channa punctatus (Bloch) using micronucleus assay and alkaline single-cell gel electrophoresis." Chemosphere 71(10): 1823-1831.

Ali, D., R. Ray and R. Hans (2010). "UVA-induced cyototoxicity and DNA damaging potential of benz (e) acephenanthrylene." Toxicology Letters 199(2): 193-200.

Ali, D., A. Verma, F. Mujtaba, A. Dwivedi, R. Hans and R. Ray (2011). "UVB-induced apoptosis and DNA damaging potential of chrysene via reactive oxygen species in human keratinocytes." Toxicology Letters 204(2-3): 199-207.

Ali, M., N. Mathur and S. Chandra (1990). "Effect of chronic cadmium exposure on locomotor behaviour of rats." Indian Journal of Experimental Biology 28(7): 653-656.

Ali, M., R. Murthy, D. Saxena and S. Chandra (1983). "Effect of low protein diet on manganese neurotoxicity: II. Brain GABA and seizure susceptibility." Neurobehavioral Toxicology and Teratology 5(3): 385-389.

Ali, M. M., B. Lal, N. Mathur and S. Chandra (1991). "Behavioral toxicity of cadmium in rats in relation to the level of protein nutrition." Nutrition Research 11(4): 325-335.

Ali, N., R. Upreti, L. Srivastava, R. Misra, P. Joshi and A. Kidwai (1991). "Membrane damaging potential of photosensitized riboflavin." Indian Journal of Experimental Biology 29(9): 818-822.

Ali, S. J. and P. S. Rajini (2016). "Effect of monocrotophos, an organophosphorus insecticide, on the striatal dopaminergic system in a mouse model of Parkinson's disease." Toxicology and Industrial Health 32(7): 1153-1165.

Amar, S. K., S. Goyal, D. Dubey, A. K. Srivastav, D. Chopra, J. Singh, J. Shankar, R. K. Chaturvedi and R. S. Ray (2015). "Benzophenone 1 induced photogenotoxicity and apoptosis via release of cytochrome c and Smac/DIABLO at environmental UV radiation." Toxicology Letters 239(3): 182-193.

Amar, S. K., S. Goyal, S. F. Mujtaba, A. Dwivedi, H. N. Kushwaha, A. Verma, D. Chopra, R. K. Chaturvedi and R. S. Ray (2015). "Role of type I & type II reactions in DNA damage and activation of caspase 3 via mitochondrial pathway induced by photosensitized benzophenone." Toxicology Letters 235(2): 84-95.

Amarapurkar, D., N. Patel, A. D. Amarapurkar and S. Kankonkar (2003). "HLA genotyping in type-I autoimmune hepatitis in Western India." Association of Physicians of India 51: 967-979.

Amba, A., K. Seth, M. Ali, M. Das, A. Agarwal, S. K. Khanna and P. Seth (2002). "Comparative effect of dietary administration of Lathyrus sativus pulse on behaviour, neurotransmitter receptors and membrane permeability in rats and guinea pigs." Journal of Applied Toxicology: An International Journal 22(6): 415-421.

Ameen, M., M. S. Musthapa, P. Abidi, I. Ahmad and Q. Rahman (2003). "Garlic attenuates chrysotile-mediated pulmonary toxicity in rats by altering the phase I and phase II drug metabolizing enzyme system." Journal of Biochemical and Molecular Toxicology 17(6): 366-371.

Amundson, S. A., T. G. Myers and A. J. Fornace Jr (1998). "Roles for p53 in growth arrest and apoptosis: putting on the brakes after genotoxic stress." Oncogene 17(25): 3287.

Anand, A. S., U. Gahlot, D. N. Prasad, Amitabh and E. Kohli (2019). "Aluminum oxide nanoparticles mediated toxicity, loss of appendages in progeny of Drosophila melanogaster on chronic exposure." Nanotoxicology: 1-13.

Anand, M., A. Agrawal, B. Rehmani, G. Gupta, M. Rana and P. Seth (1998). "Role of GABA receptor complex in low dose lindane (HCH) induced neurotoxicity: neurobehavioural, neurochemical and electrophysiological studies." Drug and Chemical Toxicology 21(1): 35-46.

Anandatheerthavarada, H. K., S. K. Shankar and V. Ravindranath (1990). "Rat brain cytochromes P-450: catalytic, immunochemical properties and inducibility of multiple forms." Brain Research 536(1-2): 339-343.

Ananthaswamy, A. (2002). "Now It's Men's Turn: A Contraceptive Injection Makes Its Debut in India." New Scientist 174(2346): 5.

Anbumani, S. and M. N. Mohankumar (2012). "Gamma radiation induced micronuclei and erythrocyte cellular abnormalities in the fish Catla catla." Aquatic Toxicology 122: 125-132.

Anbumani, S. and M. N. Mohankumar (2015). "Cytogenotoxicity assessment of monocrotophos and butachlor at single and combined chronic exposures in the fish Catla catla (Hamilton)." Environmental Science and Pollution Research 22(7): 4964-4976.

Anbumani, S. and M. N. Mohankumar (2015). "Gamma radiation induced cell cycle perturbations and DNA damage in Catla Catla as measured by flow cytometry." Ecotoxicology and Environmental Safety 113: 18-22.

Ances, B. M. (2002). "New concerns about thalidomide." Obstetrics and Gynecology 99(1): 125-128.

Anderson, D., A. Dhawan, T.-W. Yu and M. J. Plewa (1996). "An investigation of bone marrow and testicular cells *in vivo* using the comet assay." Mutation Research/Genetic Toxicology 370(3-4): 159-174.

Angeline, T., N. Jeyaraj, S. Granito and G. J. Tsongalis (2004). "Prevalence of MTHFR gene polymorphisms (C677T and A1298C) among Tamilians." Experimental and Molecular Pathology 77(2): 85-88.

Anjaneyulu, M. and K. Chopra (2004). "Quercetin, an anti-oxidant bioflavonoid, attenuates diabetic nephropathy in rats." Clinical and Experimental Pharmacology and Physiology 31(4): 244-248.

Anjum, M. R., P. Madhu, K. P. Reddy and P. S. Reddy (2017). "The protective effects of zinc in lead-induced testicular and epididymal toxicity in Wistar rats." Toxicology and Industrial Health 33(3): 265-276.

Ankolkar, M. and N. Balasinor (2016). "Endocrine control of epigenetic mechanisms in male reproduction." Hormone Molecular Biology and Clinical Investigation 25(1): 65-70.

Ansar, S., M. Iqbal and M. Athar (1999). "Nordihydroguairetic acid is a potent inhibitor of ferric-nitrilotriacetate-mediated hepatic and renal toxicity, and renal tumour promotion, in mice." Carcinogenesis 20(4): 599-606.

Ansari, B. and K. Kumar (1986). "Malathion toxicity: Embryotoxicity and survival of hatchlings of zebrafish (Brachydanio rerio)." Acta Hydrochimica et Hydrobiologica 14(5): 567-570.

Ansari, F. A., S. N. Ali, A. A. Khan and R. Mahmood (2018). "Acute oral dose of sodium nitrite causes redox imbalance and DNA damage in rat kidney." Journal of Cellular Biochemistry 119(4): 3744-3754.

Ansari, K. M., L. K. Chauhan, A. Dhawan, S. K. Khanna and M. Das (2004). "Unequivocal evidence of genotoxic potential of argemone oil in mice." International Journal of Cancer 112(5): 890-895.

Ansari, K. M., A. Dhawan, S. K. Khanna and M. Das (2005). "*In vivo* DNA damaging potential of sanguinarine alkaloid, isolated from argemone oil, using alkaline Comet assay in mice." Food and Chemical Toxicology 43(1): 147-153.

Ansari, K. M., A. Dhawan, S. K. Khanna and M. Das (2006). "Protective effect of bioantioxidants on argemone oil/sanguinarine alkaloid induced genotoxicity in mice." Cancer Letters 244(1): 109-118.

Ansari, M. A., M. Raish, A. Ahmad, S. F. Ahmad, S. Mudassar, K. Mohsin, F. Shakeel, H. M. Korashy and S. A. Bakheet (2016). "Sinapic acid mitigates gentamicin-induced nephrotoxicity and associated oxidative/nitrosative stress, apoptosis, and inflammation in rats." Life Sciences 165: 1-8.

Ansari, M. A., A. K. Shukla, M. Oves and H. M. Khan (2016). "Electron microscopic ultrastructural study on the toxicological effects of AgNPs on the liver, kidney and spleen tissues of albino mice." Environmental Toxicology and Pharmacology 44: 30-43.

Ansari, R. W., R. K. Shukla, R. S. Yadav, K. Seth, A. B. Pant, D. Singh, A. K. Agrawal, F. Islam and V. K. Khanna (2012). "Cholinergic dysfunctions and enhanced oxidative stress in the neurobehavioral toxicity of lambda-cyhalothrin in developing rats." Neurotoxicity Research 22(4): 292-309.

Ansari, R. W., R. K. Shukla, R. S. Yadav, K. Seth, A. B. Pant, D. Singh, A. K. Agrawal, F. Islam and V. K. Khanna (2012). "Involvement of dopaminergic and serotonergic systems in the neurobehavioral toxicity of lambda-cyhalothrin in developing rats." Toxicology Letters 211(1): 1-9.

Anu Prathap, M., A. K. Chaurasia, S. N. Sawant and S. Apte (2012). "Polyaniline-based highly sensitive microbial biosensor for selective detection of lindane." Analytical Chemistry 84(15): 6672-6678.

Arif, E., A. Ahsan, A. Vibhuti, C. Rajput, D. Deepak, M. Athar, B. Singh and M. Q. Pasha (2007). "Endothelial nitric oxide synthase gene variants contribute to oxidative stress in COPD." Biochemical and Biophysical Research Communications 361(1): 182-188.

Arif, E., A. Vibhuti, D. Deepak, B. Singh, M. S. Siddiqui and M. Q. Pasha (2008). "COX2 and p53 risk-alleles coexist in COPD." Clinica Chimica Acta 397(1-2): 48-50.

Arif, J., S. Khan, N. Mahmood, M. Aslam and Q. Rahman (1994). "Effect of coexposure to asbestos and kerosene soot on pulmonary drug-metabolizing enzyme system." Environmental Health Perspectives 102(suppl 5): 181-183.

Arif, J. M., S. G. Khan, I. Ahmad, L. Joshi and Q. Rahman (1997). "Effect of kerosene and its soot on the chrysotile-mediated toxicity to the rat alveolar macrophages." Environmental Research 72(2): 151-161.

Arif, J. M., S. G. Khan, M. Aslam, N. Mahmood and Q. Rahman (1992). "Diminution in Kerosene-Mediated Induction of Drug Metabolizing Enzymes by Asbestos in Rat Lungs." Pharmacology and Toxicology 71(1): 37-40.

Arif, M., S. K. Tripathi, K. C. Gupta and P. Kumar (2013). "Self-assembled amphiphilic phosphopyridoxyl-polyethylenimine polymers exhibit high cell viability and gene transfection efficiency *in vitro* and *in vivo*." Journal of Materials Chemistry B 1(32): 4020-4031.

Arora, D., M. H. Siddiqui, P. K. Sharma and Y. Shukla (2016). "Deltamethrin induced RIPK3-mediated caspase-independent non-apoptotic cell death in rat primary hepatocytes." Biochemical and Biophysical Research Communications 479(2).

Arora, D., M. H. Siddiqui, P. K. Sharma, S. P. Singh, A. Tripathi, P. Mandal, U. S. Singh, P. K. Singh and Y. Shukla (2016). "Evaluation and physiological correlation of plasma proteomic fingerprints for deltamethrin-induced hepatotoxicity in Wistar rats." Life Sciences 160: 72-83.

Arunachalam, K. D., S. K. Annamalai and J. K. Kuruva (2013). *"In-vivo* evaluation of hexavalent chromium induced DNA damage by alkaline comet assay and oxidative stress in catla catla." American Journal of Environmental Science 9(6): 470-482.

Arya, B. D., S. Mittal, P. Joshi, A. K. Pandey, J. E. Ramirez-Vick and S. P. Singh (2018). "Graphene oxide–chloroquine nanoconjugate induce necroptotic death in A549 cancer cells through autophagy modulation." Nanomedicine 13(18): 2261-2282.

Ashok, A., N. K. Rai, S. Tripathi and S. Bandyopadhyay (2014). "Exposure to As-, Cd-, and Pb-mixture induces Aβ, amyloidogenic APP processing and cognitive impairments via oxidative stress-dependent neuroinflammation in young rats." Toxicological Sciences 143(1): 64-80.

Asmathbanu, I. and B. Kaliwal (1997). "Temporal effect of methyl parathion on ovarian compensatory hypertrophy, follicular dynamics and estrous cycle in hemicastrated albino rats." Journal of Basic and Clinical Physiology and Pharmacology 8(4): 237-254.

Athar, M. and M. Iqbal (1998). "Ferric nitrilotriacetate promotes N-diethylnitrosamine-induced renal tumorigenesis in the rat: implications for the involvement of oxidative stress." Carcinogenesis 19(6): 1133-1139.

Attri, S., S. Rana, K. Vaiphei, C. Sodhi, R. Katyal, R. Goel, C. Nain and K. Singh (2000). "Isoniazid–and rifampicin–induced oxidative hepatic injury–protection by N–acetylcysteine." Human and Experimental Toxicology 19(9): 517-522.

Awasthi, A., N. Singh, S. Mittal, P. K. Gupta and R. Agarwal (2010). "Effects of agriculture crop residue burning on children and young on PFTs in North West India." Science of the Total Environment 408(20): 4440-4445.

Awasthi, N., A. Kumar, R. Makkar and S. S. Cameotra (1999). "Biodegradation of soil-applied endosulfan in the presence of a biosurfactant." Journal of Environmental Science and Health Part B 34(5): 793-803.

Awasthi, Y., A. Ratn, R. Prasad, M. Kumar and S. P. Trivedi (2018). "An *in vivo* analysis of Cr6+ induced biochemical, genotoxicological and transcriptional profiling of genes related to oxidative stress, DNA damage and apoptosis in liver of fish, Channa punctatus (Bloch, 1793)." Aquatic Toxicology 200: 158-167.

Awdishu, L., C. M. Nievergelt, A. Davenport, P. T. Murray, E. Macedo, J. Cerda, R. Chakaravarthi, S. P. R. Rao, A. Holden and S. L. Goldstein (2016). "Rationale and design of the genetic contribution to Drug Induced Renal Injury (DIRECT) study." Kidney International Reports 1(4): 288-298.

Ayub, S., J. Verma and N. Das (2003). "Effect of endosulfan and malathion on lipid peroxidation, nitrite and TNF-α release by rat peritoneal macrophages." International Immunopharmacology 3(13-14): 1819-1828.

Azuine, M., J. Kayal and S. Bhide (1992). "Protective role of aqueous turmeric extract against mutagenicity of direct-acting carcinogens as well as benzo [a] pyrene-induced genotoxicity and carcinogenicity." Journal of Cancer Research and Clinical Oncology 118(6): 447-452.

Babu, C. K., K. M. Ansari, S. Mehrotra, R. Khanna, S. K. Khanna and M. Das (2008). "Alterations in redox potential of glutathione/glutathione disulfide and cysteine/cysteine disulfide couples in plasma of dropsy patients with argemone oil poisoning." Food and Chemical Toxicology 46(7): 2409-2414.

Babu, E., A. S. Ebrahim, N. Chandramohan and D. Sakthisekaran (1999). "Case Report: Rehabilitating Role of Glutathione Ester on Cisplatin Induced Nephrotoxicity." Renal Failure 21(2): 209-217.

Babu, K., M. Deepa, S. G. Shankar and S. Rai (2008). "Effect of nano-silver on cell division and mitotic chromosomes: a prefatory siren." International Journal of Nanotechnology 2: 2-5.

Babu, S. and I. Shenolikar (1995). "Health & nutritional implications of food colours." The Indian Journal of Medical Research 102: 245-249.

Baccarelli, A. and V. Bollati (2009). "Epigenetics and environmental chemicals." Current Opinion in Pediatrics 21(2): 243.

Baghel, A., B. Singh, P. Pandey and K. Sekhar (2007). "A rapid field detection method for arsenic in drinking water." Analytical Sciences 23(2): 135-137.

Bagwe, A. N. and R. A. Bhisey (1993). "Occupational exposure to tobacco and resultant genotoxicity in bidi industry workers." Mutation Research/Genetic Toxicology 299(2): 103-109.

Bagwe, A. N., U. K. Ganu, S. V. Gokhale and R. A. Bhisey (1990). "Evaluation of the mutagenicity of 'pan masala', a chewing substitute widely used in India." Mutation Research/Genetic Toxicology 241(4): 349-354.

Bahekar, S., R. Kale and S. Nagpure (2012). "A review on medicinal plants used in scorpion bite treatment in India." Mintage Journal of Pharmaceutical and Medical Sciences1(1): 1-6.

Baig, M. S. and N. Manickam (2010). "Homology modeling and docking studies of Comamonas testosteroni B-356 biphenyl-2, 3-dioxygenase involved in degradation of polychlorinated biphenyls." International Journal of Biological Macromolecules 46(1): 47-53.

Bajaj, A., S. Mayilraj, M. K. R. Mudiam, D. K. Patel and N. Manickam (2014). "Isolation and functional analysis of a glycolipid producing Rhodococcus sp. strain IITR03 with potential for degradation of 1, 1, 1-trichloro-2, 2-bis (4-chlorophenyl) ethane (DDT)." Bioresource Technology 167: 398-406.

Bajaj, A., A. Pathak, M. Mudiam, S. Mayilraj and N. Manickam (2010). "Isolation and characterization of a Pseudomonas sp. strain IITR01 capable of degrading α-endosulfan and endosulfan sulfate." Journal of Applied Microbiology 109(6): 2135-2143.

Bajaj, R. and H. S. Wasir (1990). "Epidemiology of aluminium phosphide poisoning. Need for a survey." Journal of the Association of Physicians of India 38(3): 197-198.

Bajpayee, M., A. Dhawan, D. Parmar, A. K. Pandey, N. Mathur and P. K. Seth (2002). "Gender-related differences in basal DNA damage in lymphocytes of a healthy Indian population using the alkaline Comet assay." Mutation Research/Genetic Toxicology and Environmental Mutagenesis 520(1-2): 83-91.

Bala, R., M. Kumar, K. Bansal, R. K. Sharma and N. Wangoo (2016). "Ultrasensitive aptamer biosensor for malathion detection based on cationic polymer and gold nanoparticles." Biosensors and Bioelectronics 85: 445-449.

Balachandran, S., B. R. Meena and P. Khillare (2000). "Particle size distribution and its elemental composition in the ambient air of Delhi." Environment International 26(1-2): 49-54.

Balakrishna, K., A. Rath, Y. Praveenkumarreddy, K. S. Guruge and B. Subedi (2017). "A review of the occurrence of pharmaceuticals and personal care products in Indian water bodies." Ecotoxicology and Environmental Safety 137: 113-120.

Balakrishnan, K., S. Ghosh, B. Ganguli, S. Sambandam, N. Bruce, D. F. Barnes and K. R. Smith (2013). "State and national household concentrations of PM 2.5 from solid cookfuel use: results from measurements and modeling in India for estimation of the global burden of disease." Environmental Health 12(1): 77.

Balakrishnan, K., P. Ramaswamy, S. Sambandam, G. Thangavel, S. Ghosh, P. Johnson, K. Mukhopadhyay, V. Venugopal and V. Thanasekaraan (2011). "Air pollution from household solid fuel combustion in India: an overview of exposure and health related information to inform health research priorities." Global Health Action 4(1): 5638.

Balakrishnan, K., S. Sambandam, P. Ramaswamy, S. Mehta and K. R. Smith (2004). "Exposure assessment for respirable particulates associated with household fuel use in rural districts of Andhra Pradesh, India." Journal of Exposure Science and Environmental Epidemiology 14(S1): S14.

Balani, S., G. Umarji, R. Bellare and H. Merchant (1967). "Chronic manganese poisoning." Journal of Postgraduate Medicine 13: 116-122.

Balasinor, N., A. Bhan, N. Paradkar, A. Shaikh and T. Nandedkar (2007). "Postnatal development and reproductive performance of F1 progeny exposed in utero to ayurvedic contraceptive: Pippaliyadi yoga." Journal of Ethnopharmacology 109(3): 406-411.

Balasinor, N., M. K. Gill-Sharma, P. Parte, S. D'Souza, N. Kedia and H. Juneja (2002). "Effect of paternal administration of an antiestrogen, tamoxifen on embryo development in rats." Molecular and Cellular Endocrinology 190(1-2): 159-166.

Banerjee, A., S. Ghatak and S. K. Sikdar (2016). "l-Lactate mediates neuroprotection against ischaemia by increasing TREK 1 channel expression in rat hippocampal astrocytes *in vitro*." Journal of Neurochemistry 138(2): 265-281.

Banerjee, A., N. K. Mondal, D. Das and M. R. Ray (2012). "Neutrophilic inflammatory response and oxidative stress in premenopausal women chronically exposed to indoor air pollution from biomass burning." Inflammation 35(2): 671-683.

Banerjee, B. (1987). "Sub-chronic effect of DDT on humoral immune response to a thymus-independent antigen (bacterial lipopolysaccharide) in mice." Bulletin of Environmental Contamination and Toxicology 39(5): 822-826.

Banerjee, B. (1999). "The influence of various factors on immune toxicity assessment of pesticide chemicals." Toxicology Letters 107(1-3): 21-31.

Banerjee, B. and Q. Hussain (1986). "Effect of sub-chronic endosulfan exposure on humoral and cell-mediated immune responses in albino rats." Archives of Toxicology 59(4): 279-284.

Banerjee, B. and Q. Hussain (1987). "Effects of endosulfan on humoral and cell-mediated immune responses in rats." Bulletin of Environmental Contamination and Toxicology 38(3): 435-441.

Banerjee, B., S. Pasha, Q. Hussain, B. Koner and A. Ray (1998). "A comparative evaluation of immunotoxicity of malathion after subchronic exposure in experimental animals." Indian Journal of Experimental Biology 36(3): 273-282.

Banerjee, B., M. Ramachandran and Q. Hussain (1986). "Sub-chronic effect of DDT on humoral immune response in mice." Bulletin of Environmental Contamination and Toxicology 37(1): 433-440.

Banerjee, B., S. Saha, K. Ghosh and P. Nandy (1992). "Effect of tricresyl phosphate on humoral and cell-mediated immune responses in albino rats." Bulletin of Environmental Contamination and Toxicology 49(2): 312-317.

Banerjee, B., S. Saha, T. Mohapatra and A. Ray (1995). "Influence of dietary protein on DDT-induced immune responsiveness in rats." Indian Journal of Experimental Biology 33(10): 739-744.

Banerjee, B., S. Saha, S. Pasha and Q. Hussain (1994). "Comparative assessment of immunotoxicity of pesticides using different antigens: Quantitative studies of immunosuppression by DDT, lindane, endosulfan and malathion." Journal of Basic and Applied Biomedicine 2: 15-25.

Banerjee, B., V. Seth, A. Bhattacharya, A. Chakraborty and S. Pasha (1998). "Oxidatives stress in human poisoning cases following malathion and propoxur ingestion." Toxicology Letters 95(1001): 58-58.

Banerjee, B., V. Seth, B. Koner, R. S. Ahmed, M. Sharma, S. Grover, R. Rautala, R. Avasthi and S. Pasha (2000). "Evaluation of oxidative stress in some cases of argimone oil poisoning during a recent outbreak of epidemic dropsy in India." International Journal of Environmental Health Research 10(4): 341-346.

Banerjee, B. D., B. C. Koner and S. T. Pasha (1997). "Influence of DDT exposure on susceptibility to human leprosy bacilli in mice." International Journal of Leprosy and Other Mycobacterial Diseases 65(1): 97.

Banerjee, C., A. Singh, R. Raman and S. Mazumder (2013). "Calmodulin–CaMKII mediated alteration of oxidative stress: interplay of the cAMP/PKA–ERK 1/2-NF-κB–NO axis on arsenic-induced head kidney macrophage apoptosis." Toxicology Research 2(6): 413-426.

Banerjee, G., S. Pandey, A. K. Ray and R. Kumar (2015). "Bioremediation of heavy metals by a novel bacterial strain Enterobacter cloacae and its antioxidant enzyme activity, flocculant production, and protein expression in presence of lead, cadmium, and nickel." Water, Air, and Soil Pollution 226(4): 91.

Banerjee, M., J. Sarkar, J. K. Das, A. Mukherjee, A. K. Sarkar, L. Mondal and A. K. Giri (2007). "Polymorphism in the ERCC2 codon 751 is associated with arsenic-induced premalignant hyperkeratosis and significant chromosome aberrations." Carcinogenesis 28(3): 672-676.

Banerjee, M., N. Sarma, R. Biswas, J. Roy, A. Mukherjee and A. K. Giri (2008). "DNA repair deficiency leads to susceptibility to develop arsenic-induced premalignant skin lesions." International Journal of Cancer 123(2): 283-287.

Banerjee, M., S. Siddique, S. Mukherjee, S. Roychoudhury, P. Das, M. Ray and T. Lahiri (2012). "Hematological, immunological, and cardiovascular changes in individuals residing in a polluted city of India: a study in Delhi." International Journal of Hygiene and Environmental Health 215(3): 306-311.

Banerjee, N., A. K. Bandyopadhyay, S. Dutta, J. K. Das, T. R. Chowdhury, A. Bandyopadhyay and A. K. Giri (2017). "Increased microRNA 21 expression contributes to arsenic induced skin lesions, skin cancers and respiratory distress in chronically exposed individuals." Toxicology 378: 10-16.

Banerjee, N., S. Banerjee, R. Sen, A. Bandyopadhyay, N. Sarma, P. Majumder, J. K. Das, M. Chatterjee, S. N. Kabir and A. K. Giri (2009). "Chronic arsenic exposure impairs macrophage functions in the exposed individuals." Journal of Clinical Immunology 29(5): 582-594.

Banerjee, N., S. Paul, T. J. Sau, J. K. Das, A. Bandyopadhyay, S. Banerjee and A. K. Giri (2013). "Epigenetic modifications of DAPK and p16 genes contribute to arsenic-induced skin lesions and nondermatological health effects." Toxicological Sciences 135(2): 300-308.

Banerjee, R., S. Sreetama, K. S. Saravanan, S. N. Dey and K. P. Mohanakumar (2007). "Apoptotic mode of cell death in substantia nigra following intranigral infusion of the parkinsonian neurotoxin, MPP+ in sprague-dawley rats: Cellular, molecular and ultrastructural evidences." Neurochemical Research 32(7): 1238-1247.

Banerjee, T., V. Murari, M. Kumar and M. Raju (2015). "Source apportionment of airborne particulates through receptor modeling: Indian scenario." Atmospheric Research 164: 167-187.

Banik, R., R. Prakash and S. Upadhyay (2008). "Microbial biosensor based on whole cell of Pseudomonas sp. for online measurement of p-Nitrophenol." Sensors and Actuators B: Chemical 131(1): 295-300.

Bansal, R., S. Tripathi, K. Gupta and P. Kumar (2012). "Lipophilic and cationic triphenylphosphonium grafted linear polyethylenimine polymers for efficient gene delivery to mammalian cells." Journal of Materials Chemistry 22(48): 25427-25436.

Banu, G. S., G. Kumar and A. Murugesan (2009). "Effect of ethanolic leaf extract of Trianthema portulacastrum L. on aflatoxin induced hepatic damage in rats." Indian Journal of Clinical Biochemistry 24(4): 414.

Barbhuiya, S. A. S. and M. Sengupta (2015). "The toxic effects of lead on testicular macrophage immunomodualation and sperm cell parameters in mice." British Journal of Medicine and Medical Research 9(5): 1-10.

Barman, A., R. Goel, M. Sharma and P. Mahanta (2016). "Acute kidney injury associated with ingestion of star fruit: Acute oxalate nephropathy." Indian Journal of Nephrology 26(6): 446.

Barthwal, M., N. Srivastava and M. Dikshit (2001). "Role of nitric oxide in a progressive neurodegeneration model of Parkinson's disease in the rat." Redox Report 6(5): 297-302.

Basant, N., S. Gupta and K. P. Singh (2015). "Predicting toxicities of diverse chemical pesticides in multiple avian species using tree-based QSAR approaches for regulatory purposes." Journal of Chemical Information and Modeling 55(7): 1337-1348.

Basant, N., S. Gupta and K. P. Singh (2016). "*In silico* prediction of the developmental toxicity of diverse organic chemicals in rodents for regulatory purposes." Toxicology Research 5(3): 773-787.

Basant, N., S. Gupta and K. P. Singh (2016). "A three-tier QSAR modeling strategy for estimating eye irritation potential of diverse chemicals in rabbit for regulatory purposes." Regulatory Toxicology and Pharmacology 77: 282-291.

Bashyam, M. D., G. Purushotham, A. K. Chaudhary, K. M. Rao, V. Acharya, T. A. Mohammad, H. A. Nagarajaram, V. Hariram and C. Narasimhan (2012). "A low prevalence of MYH7/MYBPC3 mutations among familial hypertrophic cardiomyopathy patients in India." Molecular and Cellular Biochemistry 360(1-2): 373-382.

Basu, A., A. Bhattacharjee, S. Hajra, A. Samanta and S. Bhattacharya (2017). "Ameliorative effect of an oxovanadium (IV) complex against oxidative stress and nephrotoxicity induced by cisplatin." Redox Report 22(6): 377-387.

Basu, A., P. Ghosh, J. K. Das, A. Banerjee, K. Ray and A. K. Giri (2004). "Micronuclei as biomarkers of carcinogen exposure in populations exposed to arsenic through drinking water in West Bengal, India: a comparative study in three cell types." Cancer Epidemiology and Prevention Biomarkers 13(5): 820-827.

Basu, A., J. Mahata, A. Roy, J. Sarkar, G. Poddar, A. Nandy, P. Sarkar, P. Dutta, A. Banerjee and M. Das (2002). "Enhanced frequency of micronuclei in individuals exposed to arsenic through drinking water in West Bengal, India." Mutation Research/Genetic Toxicology and Environmental Mutagenesis 516(1-2): 29-40.

Basu, A., A. Som, S. Ghoshal, L. Mondal, R. C. Chaubey, H. N. Bhilwade, M. M. Rahman and A. K. Giri (2005). "Assessment of DNA damage in peripheral blood lymphocytes of individuals susceptible to arsenic induced toxicity in West Bengal, India." Toxicology Letters 159(1): 100-112.

Basu, D., M. Aggarwal, P. P. Das, S. K. Mattoo, P. Kulhara and V. K. Varma (2012). "Changing pattern of substance abuse in patients attending a de-addiction centre in north India (1978-2008)." The Indian Journal of Medical Research 135(6): 830.

Basu, S. K., D. Kumar, N. Ganguly, K. V. S. Rao and P. Sharma (2009). "Mycobacterium tuberculosis secreted antigen (MTSA-10) inhibits macrophage response to lipopolysaccharide by redox regulation of phosphatases." Indian Journal of Experimental Biology 47: 509-519.

Bawaskar, H. and P. Bawaskar (2000). "Prazosin therapy and scorpion envenomation." The Journal of the Association of Physicians of India 48(12): 1175-1180.

Bedi, J., J. Gill, P. Kaur and R. Aulakh (2018). "Pesticide residues in milk and their relationship with pesticide contamination of feedstuffs supplied to dairy cattle in Punjab (India)." Journal of Animal and Feed Sciences 27(1): 18-25.

Bedi, O., K. R. V. Bijjem, P. Kumar and V. Gauttam (2016). "Herbal induced hepatoprotection and hepatotoxicity: A critical review." Indian Journal of Physiology and Pharmacology 60(1): 6-21.

Beg, K. and S. Ali (2008). "Chemical contaminants and toxicity of Ganga river sediment from up and down stream area at Kanpur." American Journal of Environmental Sciences 4(4): 362.

Beg, M., Q. Rahman, P. Viswanathan and S. Zaidi (1973). "The effect of asbestos dust on mitochondrial enzymes of rat lung." Environmental Physiology and Biochemistry 3: 185-191.

Bhadauria, S., R. Mishra, R. Kanchan, C. Tripathi, A. Srivastava, A. Tiwari and S. Sharma (2010). "Isoniazid-induced apoptosis in HepG2 cells: generation of oxidative stress and Bcl-2 down-regulation." Toxicology Mechanisms and Methods 20(5): 242-251.

Bhagia, L., S. Dave, S. Shah, J. Vyas, P. Kulkarni and D. Parikh (1994). "Size distribution of airborne asbestos fibers in milling process." Indian Aerosol Science and Technology Association Bulletin 7(3): 1-4.

Bhagia, L. J. and H. Sadhu (2008). "Cost–benefit analysis of installing dust control devices in the agate industry, Khambhat (Gujarat)." Indian Journal of Occupational and Environmental Medicine 12(3): 128.

Bhagwat, V. R., A. J. Patil, J. A. Patil and A. V. Sontakke (2008). "Occupational lead exposure and liver functions in battery manufacture workers around Kolhapur (Maharashtra)." Al Ameen Journal of Medical Sciences 1(1): 2-9.

Bhanti, M. and A. Taneja (2007). "Contamination of vegetables of different seasons with organophosphorous pesticides and related health risk assessment in northern India." Chemosphere 69(1): 63-68.

Bharath, B., Y. Anjaneyulu and C. Srilatha (2011). "Imunno-modulatory effect of Ocimum sanctum against endosulfan induced immunotoxicity in Wistar Rat." Veterinary World 4(1): 25.

Bhardwaj, J. R., R. Chawla and R. K. Sharma (2007). "Chemical disaster management: Current status and perspectives." Journal of Scientific and Industrial Research 66: 110-119.

Bhardwaj, T. and J. Sharma "Impact of Pesticides Application in Agricultural Industry: An Indian Scenario." International Journal of Agriculture and Food Science Technology 4(8): 817-822.

Bhargav, D., M. P. Singh, R. C. Murthy, N. Mathur, D. Misra, D. K. Saxena and D. K. Chowdhuri (2008). "Toxic potential of municipal solid waste leachates in transgenic Drosophila melanogaster (hsp70-lacZ): hsp70 as a marker of cellular damage." Ecotoxicology and Environmental Safety 69(2): 233-245.

Bhargava, A., R. Khanna, S. Bhargava and S. Kumar (2004). "Exposure risk to carcinogenic PAHs in indoor-air during biomass combustion whilst cooking in rural India." Atmospheric Environment 38(28): 4761-4767.

Bhargava, A., R. P. Punde, N. Pathak, S. Dabadghao, P. Desikan, A. Jain, K. K. Maudar and P. K. Mishra (2010). "Status of inflammatory biomarkers in the population that survived the Bhopal gas tragedy: a study after two decades." Industrial Health 48(2): 204-208.

Bhat, R. V. and P. Mathur (1998). "Changing scenario of food colours in India." Current Science 74(3): 198-202.

Bhatia, A., A. Sharma, S. Patni and A. L. Sharma (2007). "Prophylactic effect of flaxseed oil against radiation-induced hepatotoxicity in mice." Phytotherapy Research: An International Journal Devoted to Pharmacological and Toxicological Evaluation of Natural Product Derivatives 21(9): 852-859.

Bhatia, T., M. K. Gupta, P. Singh, A. Chauhan, P. N. Saxena and M. K. R. Mudiam (2016). "Sol-gel approach for extracting highly versatile aspirin and its metabolites using MISPE followed by GC–MS/MS analysis." Bioanalysis 8(8): 795-805.

Bhatnagar, A. and A. Minocha (2006). "Conventional and non-conventional adsorbents for removal of pollutants from water–A review." Indian Journal of Chemical Technology 13:213-217.

Bhatnagar, M., P. Rao, S. Jain and R. Bhatnagar (2002). "Neurotoxicity of fluoride: neurodegeneration in hippocampus of female mice." Indian Journal of Experimental Biology 40(5):546-54.

Bhatnagar, S. and R. Kumari (2013). "Bioremediation: a sustainable tool for environmental management–a review." Annual Research and Review in Biology: 974-993.

Bhatnagar, V., A. Karnik, A. Suthar, S. Zaidi, R. Kashyap, M. Shah, P. Kulkarni and H. Saiyed (2002). "Biological indices in formulators exposed to a combination of pesticides." Bulletin of Environmental Contamination and Toxicology 68(1): 22-28.

Bhatnagar, V., R. Kashyap, S. Zaidi, P. Kulkarni and H. Saiyed (2004). "Levels of DDT, HCH, and HCB residues in human blood in Ahmedabad, India." Bulletin of Environmental Contamination and Toxicology 72(2): 261-265.

Bhatnagar, V., S. Saigal, S. Singh, L. Khemani and A. Malviya (1982). "Survey amongst workers in pesticide factories." Toxicology Letters 10(2-3): 129-132.

Bhatt, M. H., M. A. Elias and A. K. Mankodi (1999). "Acute and reversible parkinsonism due to organophosphate pesticide intoxication: five cases." Neurology 52(7): 1467-1467.

Bhattacharjee, N. and A. Borah (2016). "Oxidative stress and mitochondrial dysfunction are the underlying events of dopaminergic neurodegeneration in homocysteine rat model of Parkinson's disease." Neurochemistry International 101: 48-55.

Bhattacharjee, N., M. K. Mazumder, R. Paul, A. Choudhury, S. Choudhury and A. Borah (2016). "L-DOPA treatment in MPTP-mouse model of Parkinson's disease potentiates homocysteine accumulation in substantia nigra." Neuroscience Letters 628: 225-229.

Bhattacharjee, P., T. Sanyal and S. Bhattacharjee (2018). "Epigenetic alteration of mismatch repair genes in the population chronically exposed to arsenic in West Bengal, India." Environmental Research 163: 289-296.

Bhattacharya, A. and S. Khare (2016). "Sustainable options for mitigation of major toxicants originating from electronic waste." Current Science 111(12): 1946.

Bhattacharya, A. and S. Khare (2017). "Biodegradation of 4-chlorobiphenyl by using induced cells and cell extract of Burkholderia xenovorans." Bioremediation Journal 21(3-4): 109-118.

Bhattacharya, A., S. Naik and S. Khare (2018). "Harnessing the bio-mineralization ability of urease producing Serratia marcescens and Enterobacter cloacae EMB19 for remediation of heavy metal cadmium (II)." Journal of Environmental Management 215: 143-152.

Bhattacharya, A., S. Naik and S. Khare (2019). "Efficacy of ureolytic Enterobacter cloacae EMB19 mediated calcite precipitation in remediation of Zn (II)." Journal of Environmental Science and Health, Part A: 1-7.

Bhattacharya, R., P. Lakshmana Rao, A. Bhaskar, S. Pant and S. Dube (1996). "Liver slice culture for assessing hepatotoxicity of freshwater cyanobacteria." Human and Experimental Toxicology 15(2): 105-110.

Bhattacharya, S., A. Jayanthi and S. Shilpa (2012). "Nanotechnology Development in India: Investigating Ten years of India's efforts in Capacity Building." CSIR-NISTADS Policy Brief I. Delhi: NISTADS. 'Moving Forward Responsibly': From Agribiotechnology to Agrinanotechnology.

Bhattacharyya, N. and D. Chakrabarti (2012). "Ergonomic basket design to reduce cumulative trauma disorders in tea leaf plucking operation." Work 41 (Supplement 1): 1234-1238.

Bhunya, S. and G. Jena (1992). "Genotoxic potential of the organochlorine insecticide lindane (γ-BHC): an *in vivo* study in chicks." Mutation Research/Environmental Mutagenesis and Related Subjects 272(2): 175-181.

Bhunya, S. and G. Jena (1993). "Studies on the genotoxicity of monocrotophos, an organophosphate insecticide, in the chick *in vivo* test system." Mutation Research/Environmental Mutagenesis and Related Subjects 292(3): 231-239.

Bhunya, S. and P. Pati (1988). "Genotoxic effects of a synthetic pyrethroid insecticide, cypermethrin, in mice *in vivo*." Toxicology Letters 41(3): 223-230.

Bhuvaneshwari, M., V. Iswarya, S. Archanaa, G. Madhu, G. S. Kumar, R. Nagarajan, N. Chandrasekaran and A. Mukherjee (2015). "Cytotoxicity of ZnO NPs towards fresh water algae Scenedesmus obliquus at low exposure concentrations in UV-C, visible and dark conditions." Aquatic Toxicology 162: 29-38.

Bihari, V., C. Kesavachandran, B. Pangtey, A. Srivastava and N. Mathur (2011). "Musculoskeletal pain and its associated risk factors in residents of National Capital Region." Indian Journal of Occupational and Environmental Medicine 15(2): 59.

Bijetri, B. and D. Sen (2014). "Occupational stress among women moulders: A study in manual brick manufacturing industry of West Bengal." International Journal of Scientific and Research Publications 4(6).

Bindali, B. B. and B. B. Kaliwal (2002). "Anti-implantation effect of a carbamate fungicide mancozeb in albino mice." Industrial Health 40(2): 191-197.

Binukumar, B., A. Bal, R. J. Kandimalla and K. D. Gill (2010). "Nigrostriatal neuronal death following chronic dichlorvos exposure: crosstalk between mitochondrial impairments, α synuclein aggregation, oxidative damage and behavioral changes." Molecular Brain 3(1): 35.

Bishayi, B., D. Bandyopadhyay, A. Majhi and R. Adhikary (2014). "Possible Role of Toll-like Receptor-2 in the Intracellular Survival of S taphylococcus aureus in Murine Peritoneal Macrophages: Involvement of Cytokines and Anti-Oxidant Enzymes." Scandinavian Journal of Immunology 80(2): 127-143.

Bishayi, B. and M. Sengupta (2003). "Intracellular survival of Staphylococcus aureus due to alteration of cellular activity in arsenic and lead intoxicated mature Swiss albino mice." Toxicology 184(1): 31-39.

Bishi, D. K., S. Mathapati, J. R. Venugopal, S. Guhathakurta, K. M. Cherian, S. Ramakrishna and R. S. Verma (2013). "Trans-differentiation of human mesenchymal stem cells generates functional hepatospheres on poly (L-lactic acid)-co-poly (ε-caprolactone)/collagen nanofibrous scaffolds." Journal of Materials Chemistry B 1(32): 3972-3984.

Bishnoi, N. R., M. Bajaj, N. Sharma and A. Gupta (2004). "Adsorption of Cr (VI) on activated rice husk carbon and activated alumina." Bioresource Technology 91(3): 305-307.

Bisset, N. G. and G. Mazars (1984). "Arrow poisons in South Asia Part 1. Arrow poisons in Ancient India." Journal of Ethnopharmacology 12(1): 1-24.

Biswas, G., S. Sarkar and T. Chatterjee (1994). "Surveillance on Artificial Colors in Food-Products Marketed in Calcutta and Adjoining Areas." Journal of Food Science and Technology-Mysore 31(1): 66-67.

Biswas, R., P. Ghosh, N. Banerjee, J. Das, T. Sau, A. Banerjee, S. Roy, S. Ganguly, M. Chatterjee and A. Mukherjee (2008). "Analysis of T-cell proliferation and cytokine secretion in the individuals exposed to arsenic." Human and Experimental Toxicology 27(5): 381-386.

Bondarenko, O. M., M. Heinlaan, M. Sihtmäe, A. Ivask, I. Kurvet, E. Joonas, A. Jemec, M. Mannerström, T. Heinonen and R. Rekulapelly (2016). "Multilaboratory evaluation of 15 bioassays for (eco) toxicity screening and hazard ranking of engineered nanomaterials: FP7 project NANOVALID." Nanotoxicology 10(9): 1229-1242.

Borah, A., R. Paul, M. K. Mazumder and N. Bhattacharjee (2013). "Contribution of β-phenethylamine, a component of chocolate and wine, to dopaminergic neurodegeneration: implications for the pathogenesis of Parkinson's disease." Neuroscience Bulletin 29(5): 655-660.

Boro, R. C., J. Kaushal, Y. Nangia, N. Wangoo, A. Bhasin and C. R. Suri (2011). "Gold nanoparticles catalyzed chemiluminescence immunoassay for detection of herbicide 2, 4-dichlorophenoxyacetic acid." Analyst 136(10): 2125-2130.

Bose, P. D., M. P. Sarma, S. Medhi, B. C. Das, S. A. Husain and P. Kar (2011). "Role of polymorphic N-acetyl transferase2 and cytochrome P4502E1 gene in antituberculosis treatment-induced hepatitis." Journal of Gastroenterology and Hepatology 26(2): 312-318.

Bové, J., D. Prou, C. Perier and S. Przedborski (2005). "Toxin-induced models of Parkinson's disease." NeuroRx 2(3): 484-494.

Brent, R. L. and L. B. Holmes (1988). "Clinical and basic science lessons from the thalidomide tragedy: what have we learned about the causes of limb defects?" Teratology 38(3): 241-251.

Burman, U., M. Saini and P.- Kumar (2013). "Effect of zinc oxide nanoparticles on growth and antioxidant system of chickpea seedlings." Toxicological and Environmental Chemistry 95(4): 605-612.

Caussy, E. and W. H. Organization (2005). A field guide for detection, management and surveillance of arsenicosis cases, World Health Organization.

Ch, R., A. K. Singh, M. K. Pathak, S. Amarnath, C. N. Kesavachandran, V. Bihari and M. K. R. Mudiam (2019). "Saliva and urine metabolic profiling reveals altered amino acid and energy metabolism in male farmers exposed to pesticides in Madhya Pradesh State, India." Chemosphere.

Chakraborti, D., M. M. Rahman, K. Paul, U. K. Chowdhury, M. K. Sengupta, D. Lodh, C. R. Chanda, K. C. Saha and S. C. Mukherjee (2002). "Arsenic calamity in the Indian subcontinent: what lessons have been learned?" Talanta 58(1): 3-22.

Chakraborty, P., S. Sampath, M. Mukhopadhyay, S. Selvaraj, G. K. Bharat and L. Nizzetto (2019). "Baseline investigation on plasticizers, bisphenol A, polycyclic aromatic hydrocarbons and heavy metals in the surface soil of the informal electronic waste recycling workshops and nearby open dumpsites in Indian metropolitan cities." Environmental Pollution 248: 1036-1045.

Chakraborty, T., S. K. Das, V. Pathak and S. Mukhopadhyay (2018). "Occupational stress, musculoskeletal disorders and other factors affecting the quality of life in Indian construction workers." International Journal of Construction Management 18(2): 144-150.

Chanda, S., U. B. Dasgupta, D. GuhaMazumder, M. Gupta, U. Chaudhuri, S. Lahiri, S. Das, N. Ghosh and D. Chatterjee (2005). "DNA hypermethylation of promoter of gene p53 and p16 in arsenic-exposed people with and without malignancy." Toxicological Sciences 89(2): 431-437.

Chander, V., N. Tirkey and K. Chopra (2005). "Resveratrol, a polyphenolic phytoalexin protects against cyclosporine-induced nephrotoxicity through nitric oxide dependent mechanism." Toxicology 210(1): 55-64.

Chandra, A., N. Rao, K. Malhotra, M. Rastogi and R. Khurana (2017). "Everolimus-associated acute kidney injury in patients with metastatic breast cancer." Indian Journal of Nephrology 27(5): 406.

Chandra, G., P. K. Gangopadhyay, K. S. S. Kumar and K. P. Mohanakumar (2006). "Acute intranigral homocysteine administration produces stereotypic behavioral changes and striatal dopamine depletion in Sprague–Dawley rats." Brain Research 1075(1): 81-92.

Chandra, S., A. Pandey and D. K. Chowdhuri (2015). "MiRNA profiling provides insights on adverse effects of Cr (VI) in the midgut tissues of Drosophila melanogaster." Journal of Hazardous Materials 283: 558-567.

Chandra, S., T. Saxena, S. Nehra and M. K. Mohan (2016). "Quality assessment of supplied drinking water in Jaipur city, India, using PCR-based approach." Environmental Earth Sciences 75(2): 153.

Chandra, S. V. (1972). "Histological and histochemical changes in experimental manganese encephalopathy in rabbits." Archives of Toxicology 29(1): 29-38.

Chandra, S. V., M. M. Ali, D. Saxena and R. Murthy (1981). "Behavioral and neurochemical changes in rats simultaneously exposed to manganese and lead." Archives of Toxicology 49(1): 49-56.

Chandra, S. V., Z. Imam and N. Nagar (1973). "Significance of serum calcium, inorganic phosphates and alkaline phosphatase in experimental manganese toxicity." Industrial Health 11(1-2): 43-47.

Chandra, S. V., P. Seth and J. Mankeshwar (1974). "Manganese poisoning: clinical and biochemical observations." Environmental Research 7(3): 374-380.

Chandra, S. V. and G. S. Shukla (1976). "Role of iron deficiency in inducing susceptibility to manganese toxicity." Archives of Toxicology 35(4): 319-323.

Chandra, S. V. and G. S. Shukla (1978). "Manganese encephalopathy in growing rats." Environmental Research 15(1): 28-37.

Chandra, S. V., G. S. Shukla and D. Saxena (1979). "Manganese-induced behavioral dysfunction and its neurochemical mechanism in growing mice." Journal of Neurochemistry 33(6): 1217-1221.

Chandra, S. V. and S. Srivastava (1970). "Experimental production of early brain lesions in rats by parenteral administration of manganese chloride." Acta Pharmacologica et Toxicologica 28(3): 177-183.

Chandrasekaran, K., K. Swaminathan, S. Chatterjee and A. Dey (2010). "Apoptosis in HepG2 cells exposed to high glucose." Toxicology *In Vitro* 24(2): 387-396.

Chandravanshi, L. P., R. S. Yadav, R. K. Shukla, A. Singh, S. Sultana, A. B. Pant, D. Parmar and V. K. Khanna (2014). "Reversibility of changes in brain cholinergic receptors and acetylcholinesterase activity in rats following early life arsenic exposure." International Journal of Developmental Neuroscience 34: 60-75.

Chatterjee, A. and U. Chatterji (2011). "All-trans retinoic acid protects against arsenic-induced uterine toxicity in female Sprague–Dawley rats." Toxicology and Applied Pharmacology 257(2): 250-263.

Chatterjee, A., D. Das, B. K. Mandal, T. R. Chowdhury, G. Samanta and D. Chakraborti (1995). "Arsenic in ground water in six districts of West Bengal, India: the biggest arsenic calamity in the world. Part I. Arsenic species in drinking water and urine of the affected people." Analyst 3.

Chatterjee, A. and J. Mercy (1993). "Protective effect of cysteine against X-ray-and bleomycin-induced chromosomal aberrations and cell cycle delay." Mutation Research/Fundamental and Molecular Mechanisms of Mutagenesis 290(2): 231-238.

Chatterjee, S., S. Dhar, B. Sengupta, A. Ghosh, M. De, S. Roy, R. Raychowdhury and S. Chakrabarti (2009). "Cytogenetic monitoring in human oral cancers and other oral pathology: the micronucleus test in exfoliated buccal cells." Toxicology Mechanisms and Methods 19(6-7): 427-433.

Chatterjee, S., A. Ray, S. Ghosh, K. Bhattacharya, A. Pakrashi and C. Deb (1988). "Effect of aldrin on spermatogenesis, plasma gonadotrophins and testosterone, and testicular testosterone in the rat." Journal of Endocrinology 119(1): 75-81.

Chattopadhyay, B., P. Gangopadhyay, A. Das, S. J. Alam, M. Hossain, A. Chowdhury and A. Kundu (2014). "Respiratory response to tobacco dust exposure among biddi binders: A follow up and bronchodilator study." Indian Journal of Occupational and Environmental Medicine 18(2): 57.

Chattopadhyay, B., P. Gangopadhyay and H. Saiyed (1995). "Effect of jute dust exposure on ventilatory function and the pertinence of cough and smoking to the response." Journal of University of Occupational and Environmental Health 17(2): 91-104.

Chattopadhyay, B., H. Saiyed, S. J. Alam, S. Roy, S. Thakur and T. Dasgupta (1999). "Inquiry into occurrence of byssinosis in jute mill workers." Journal of Occupational Health 41(4): 225-231.

Chattopadhyay, P., A. Karnik, K. Thakore, B. Lakkad, S. Nigam and S. Kashyap (1988). "Health effects among workers involved in the manufacture of hexachlorocyclohexane." Occupational Medicine 38(3): 77-81.

Chattopadhyay, S., S. Bhaumik, M. Purkayastha, S. Basu, A. N. Chaudhuri and S. D. Gupta (2002). "Apoptosis and necrosis in developing brain cells due to arsenic toxicity and protection with antioxidants." Toxicology Letters 136(1): 65-76.

Chattopadhyay, S., T. Das, G. Sa and P. Ray (2002). "Protein A-activated macrophages induce apoptosis in Ehrlich's ascites carcinoma through a nitric oxide-dependent pathway." Apoptosis 7(1): 49-57.

Chattopadhyay, S., S. Ghosh, J. Debnath and D. Ghosh (2001). "Protection of sodium arsenite-induced ovarian toxicity by coadministration of L-ascorbate (vitamin C) in mature wistar strain rat." Archives of Environmental Contamination and Toxicology 41(1): 83-89.

Chattopadhyay, S., S. Pal, D. Ghosh and J. Debnath (2003). "Effect of dietary co-administration of sodium selenite on sodium arsenite-induced ovarian and uterine disorders in mature albino rats." Toxicological Sciences 75(2): 412-422.

Chaturvedi, V., A. Kumar and J. Singh (2012). "Power tiller: vibration magnitudes and intervention development for vibration reduction." Applied Ergonomics 43(5): 891-901.

Chaudhari, P. R., R. Gupta, D. G. Gajghate and S. R. Wate (2012). "Heavy metal pollution of ambient air in Nagpur City." Environmental Monitoring and Assessment 184(4): 2487-2496.

Chaudhary, S., M. Behari, M. Dihana, P. V. Swaminath, S. T. Govindappa, S. Jayaram, S. Singh, U. B. Muthane, R. C. Juyal and B. Thelma (2005). "Association of N-acetyl transferase 2 gene polymorphism and slow acetylator phenotype with young onset and late onset Parkinson's disease among Indians." Pharmacogenetics and Genomics 15(10): 731-735.

Chaudhary, S. and S. Parvez (2012). "An *in vitro* approach to assess the neurotoxicity of valproic acid-induced oxidative stress in cerebellum and cerebral cortex of young rats." Neuroscience 225: 258-268.

Chaudhuri, K., S. Selvaraj and A. Pal (1999). "Studies on the genotoxicity of endosulfan in bacterial systems." Mutation Research/Genetic Toxicology and Environmental Mutagenesis 439(1): 63-67.

Chaudhury, M., R. Chandrasekaran and S. Mishra (2001). "Embryotoxicity and teratogenicity studies of an ayurvedic contraceptive--pippaliyadi vati." Journal of Ethnopharmacology 74(2): 189.

Chaudhury, N., A. Phatak, R. Paliwal and C. Raichaudhari (2010). "Silicosis among agate workers at Shakarpur: An analysis of clinic-based data." Lung India: Official Organ of Indian Chest Society 27(4): 221.

Chauduri, R. (1959). "Clinical and experimental research." Bulletin of the Calcutta School of Tropical Medicine 7: 157-161.

Chauhan, A. K., N. Mittra, B. K. Singh and C. Singh (2019). "Inhibition of glutathione S-transferase-pi triggers c-jun N-terminal kinase-dependent neuronal death in Zn-induced Parkinsonism." Molecular and Cellular Biochemistry 452(1-2): 95-104.

Chauhan, L., N. Pant, S. Gupta and S. Srivastava (2000). "Induction of chromosome aberrations, micronucleus formation and sperm abnormalities in mouse following carbofuran exposure." Mutation Research/Genetic Toxicology and Environmental Mutagenesis 465(1-2): 123-129.

Chhillar, N., N. K. Singh, B. Banerjee, K. Bala, M. Mustafa, D. Sharma and M. Chhillar (2013). "Organochlorine pesticide levels and risk of Parkinson's disease in north Indian population." ISRN Neurology.

Chinoy, N. and S. Shah (2004). "Beneficial Effects of Some Antidotes in Fluoride and Arsenic induced Toxicity in Kidney of Mice." Fluoride 37(3): 151-161.

Chitra, K., C. Latchoumycandane and P. Mathur (1999). "Chronic Effect of Endosulfan on the Testicular Functions of Rat." DNA 1(11.131): 35.

Chitrangi, S., P. Nair and A. Khanna (2017). "3D engineered *In vitro* hepatospheroids for studying drug toxicity and metabolism." Toxicology *in Vitro* 38: 8-18.

Cho, Y. S. and H.-B. Moon (2010). "The role of oxidative stress in the pathogenesis of asthma." Allergy, Asthma and Immunology Research 2(3): 183-187.

Chopra, D., L. Ray, A. Dwivedi, S. K. Tiwari, J. Singh, K. P. Singh, H. N. Kushwaha, S. Jahan, A. Pandey and S. K. Gupta (2016). "Photoprotective efficiency of PLGA-curcumin nanoparticles versus curcumin through the involvement of ERK/AKT pathway under ambient UV-R exposure in HaCaT cell line." Biomaterials 84: 25-41.

Chopra, R., I. Chopra, K. Handa and L. Kapur (1958). "Indigenous drugs of India." N. Dhur and Sons: Calcutta, India: 308.

Chopra, R. N. and S. L. Nayar (1956). Glossary of Indian medicinal plants, Council of Scientific and Industrial Research; New Delhi.

Choudhary, N., R. Goyal and S. Joshi (2008). "Effect of malathion on reproductive system of male rats." Journal of Environmental Biology 29(2): 259.

Choudhary, S., K. Joshi and K. D. Gill (2001). "Possible role of enhanced microtubule phosphorylation in dichlorvos induced delayed neurotoxicity in rat." Brain Research 897(1-2): 60-70.

Choudhury, A. R., T. Das and A. Sharma (1997). "Mustard oil and garlic extract as inhibitors of sodium arsenite-induced chromosomal breaks *in vivo*." Cancer Letters 121(1): 45-52.

Chowdhuri, D. K., D. Saxena and P. Viswanathan (1999). "Effect of Hexachlorocyclohexane (HCH), Its Isomers, and Metabolites on Hsp70 Expression in Transgenic Drosophila melanogaster." Pesticide Biochemistry and Physiology 63(1): 15-25.

Chowdhury, A., A. Santra, K. Bhattacharjee, S. Ghatak, D. R. Saha and G. K. Dhali (2006). "Mitochondrial oxidative stress and permeability transition in isoniazid and rifampicin induced liver injury in mice." Journal of Hepatology 45(1): 117-126.

Chowgule, R., V. Shetye and J. Parmar (1995). "Lung function tests in normal Indian children." Indian Pediatrics 32: 185-185.

Chugh, K. (1989). "Snake-bite-induced acute renal failure in India." Kidney International 35(3): 891-907.

Chugh, K., P. Singhal and S. Banejee (1977). "Acute tubular necrosis following intravesical instillation of formalin." Urologia Internationalis 32(6): 454-459.

Chugh, K. S., Y. Pal, R. Chakravarty, B. Datta, R. Mehta, V. Sakhuja, A. K. Mandal and S. C. Sommers (1984). "Acute renal failure following poisonous snakebite." American Journal of Kidney Diseases 4(1): 30-38.

Chugh, S. (1992). "Aluminium phosphide poisoning: present status and management." Journal of the Association of Physicians of India 40(6): 401-405.

Chugh, S. (1995). "Aluminium phosphide poisoning with special reference on its diagnosis and management. Review article." Journal of Indian Association of Clinical Medicine 1: 20-22.

Chugh, S., P. Kamar, A. Sharma, K. Chugh, A. Mittal and B. Arora (1994). "Magnesium status and parenteral magnesium sulphate therapy in acute aluminum phosphide intoxication." Magnesium Research 7(3-4): 289.

Chugh, S., S. Ram, B. Arora and K. Malhotra (1991). "Incidence and outcome of aluminium phosphide poisoning in a hospital study." The Indian Journal of Medical Research 94: 232-235.

Chugh, S., S. Ram, K. Chugh and K. Malhotra (1989). "Spot diagnosis of aluminium phosphide ingestion: an application of a simple test." The Journal of the Association of Physicians of India 37(3): 219.

Clerk, S., B. Gupta, S. Rastogi and H. Chandra (1983). "Respiratory morbidity in agate workers: A case study in Khambhat, Gujarat, India." Industrial Toxicology Research Centre Report, Lucknow, India.

Clifford, D. B. and B. M. Ances (2013). "HIV-associated neurocognitive disorder." The Lancet Infectious Diseases 13(11): 976-986.

Committee, E. S. (2011). "Scientific opinion on genotoxicity testing strategies applicable to food and feed safety assessment." EFSA Journal 9(9): 2379.

Correa-Rotter, R., C. Wesseling and R. J. Johnson (2014). "CKD of unknown origin in Central America: the case for a Mesoamerican nephropathy." American Journal of Kidney Diseases 63(3): 506-520.

CPCB, F. (2010). "Air quality monitoring, emission inventory and source apportionment study for Indian cities." Central Pollution Control Board.

D'Silva, T. D., A. Lopes, R. L. Jones, S. Singhawangcha and J. K. Chan (1986). "Studies of methyl isocyanate chemistry in the Bhopal incident." The Journal of Organic Chemistry 51(20): 3781-3788.

Dabhi, B. and K. N. Mistry (2015). "Oxidative stress and its association with TNF-α-308 G/C and IL-1α-889 C/T gene polymorphisms in patients with diabetes and diabetic nephropathy." Gene 562(2): 197-202.

Dahal, S., S. V. Chitti, M. P. Nair and S. K. Saxena (2015). "Interactive effects of cocaine on HIV infection: implication in HIV-associated neurocognitive disorder and neuroAIDS." Frontiers in Microbiology 6: 931.

Dahanukar S. A. and U. M. Thatte (1988). "Comparative study of immunomodulating activity of Indian medicinal plants, lithium carbonate and glucan". Methods and Findings in Experimental and Clinical Pharmacology, 10(10), 639-644.

Dahll, T. A., P. Bilski, K. J. Reszka and C. F. Chignell (1994). "Photocytotoxicity of curcumin." Photochemistry and Photobiology 59(3): 290-294.

Dale, W. E., M. F. Copeland and W. J. Hayes Jr (1965). "Chlorinated insecticides in the body fat of people in India." Bulletin of the World Health Organization 33(4): 471.

Danadevi, K., R. Rozati, B. S. Banu and P. Grover (2004). "Genotoxic evaluation of welders occupationally exposed to chromium and nickel using the Comet and micronucleus assays." Mutagenesis 19(1): 35-41.

Danadevi, K., R. Rozati, B. S. Banu, P. H. Rao and P. Grover (2003). "DNA damage in workers exposed to lead using comet assay." Toxicology 187(2-3): 183-193.

Danadevi, K., R. Rozati, P. Reddy and P. Grover (2003). "Semen quality of Indian welders occupationally exposed to nickel and chromium." Reproductive Toxicology 17(4): 451-456.

Dangi, B. M. and A. R. Bhise (2017). "Cotton dust exposure: Analysis of pulmonary function and respiratory symptoms." Lung India: Official Organ of Indian Chest Society 34(2): 144.

Das, B., T. Ghosh and S. Gangopadhyay (2013). "Child work in agriculture in West Bengal, India: assessment of musculoskeletal disorders and occupational health problems." Journal of Occupational Health: 12-0185-OA.

Das, J., A. Sarkar and P. C. Sil (2015). "Hexavalent chromium induces apoptosis in human liver (HepG2) cells via redox imbalance." Toxicology Reports 2: 600-608.

Das, J., P. Sarkar, J. Panda and P. Pal (2014). "Low-cost field test kits for arsenic detection in water." Journal of Environmental Science and Health, Part A 49(1): 108-115.

Das, K., M. Ghosh, C. Nag, S. P. Nandy, M. Banerjee, M. Datta, G. Devi and G. Chaterjee (2011). "Role of familial, environmental and occupational factors in the development of Parkinson's disease." Neurodegenerative Diseases 8(5): 345-351.

Das, M., K. M. Ansari, A. Dhawan, Y. Shukla and S. K. Khanna (2005). "Correlation of DNA damage in epidemic dropsy patients to carcinogenic potential of argemone oil and isolated sanguinarine alkaloid in mice." International Journal of Cancer 117(5): 709-717.

Das, M., K. Babu, N. P. Reddy and L. M. Srivastava (2005). "Oxidative damage of plasma proteins and lipids in epidemic dropsy patients: alterations in antioxidant status." Biochimica et Biophysica Acta (BBA)-General Subjects 1722(2): 209-217.

Das, M., K. Garg, A. Joshi, G. B. Singh and S. K. Khanna (1991). "Interaction of benzanthrone with cytochrome p450: Altered patterns of hepatic xenobiotic metabolism in rats." Journal of Biochemical Toxicology 6(1): 37-44.

Das, M., K. Garg, G. B. Singh and S. K. Khanna (1994). "Attenuation of benzanthrone toxicity by ascorbic acid in guinea pigs." Fundamental and Applied Toxicology 22(3): 447-456.

Das, M. and S. K. Khanna (1997). "Clinicoepidemiological, toxicological, and safety evaluation studies on argemone oil." Critical Reviews in Toxicology 27(3): 273-297.

Das, M., H. Mukhtar and P. K. Seth (1982). "Effect of acrylamide on brain and hepatic mixed-function oxidases and glutathione-S-transferase in rats." Toxicology and Applied Pharmacology 66(3): 420-426.

Das, M., P. K. Seth and H. Mukhtar (1981). "Characterization of microsomal aryl hydrocarbon hydroxylase of rat brain." Journal of Pharmacology and Experimental Therapeutics 216(1):156-61.

Das, M., K. K. Upreti and S. K. Khanna (1991). "Biochemical toxicology of argemone oil. Role of reactive oxygen species in iron catalyzed lipid peroxidation." Bulletin of Environmental Contamination and Toxicology 46(3): 422-430.

Das, R. N. and K. Roy (2014). "Predictive modeling studies for the ecotoxicity of ionic liquids towards the green algae *Scenedesmus vacuolatus*." Chemosphere 104: 170-176.

Das, S., P. Roy, R. G. Auddy and A. Mukherjee (2011). "Silymarin nanoparticle prevents paracetamol-induced hepatotoxicity." International Journal of Nano-medicine 6: 1291.

Das, S., A. Santra, S. Lahiri and D. G. Mazumder (2005). "Implications of oxidative stress and hepatic cytokine (TNF-α and IL-6) response in the pathogenesis of hepatic collagenesis in chronic arsenic toxicity." Toxicology and Applied Pharmacology 204(1): 18-26.

Das, T., A. Roychoudhury, A. Sharma and G. Talukder (1993). "Modification of clastogenicity of three known clastogens by garlic extract in mice *in vivo*." Environmental and Molecular Mutagenesis 21(4): 383-388.

Datta, D., S. Mitra, P. Chhuttani and R. Chakravarti (1979). "Chronic oral arsenic intoxication as a possible aetiological factor in idiopathic portal hypertension (non-cirrhotic portal fibrosis) in India." Gut 20(5): 378-384.

Datta, P. (1970). "*In vivo* detoxication of p, p'-DDT via p, p'-DDE to p, p'-DDA in rats." IMS, Industrial Medicine and Surgery 39(4): 190-194.

Datta, S., S. Mazumder, D. Ghosh, S. Dey and S. Bhattacharya (2009). "Low concentration of arsenic could induce caspase-3 mediated head kidney macrophage apoptosis with JNK–p38 activation in Clarias batrachus." Toxicology and Applied Pharmacology 241(3): 329-338.

Datta, S. K., V. Kumar, R. S. Ahmed, A. K. Tripathi, O. P. Kalra and B. D. Banerjee (2010). "Effect of GSTM1 and GSTT1 double deletions in the development of oxidative stress in diabetic nephropathy patients." Indian Journal of Biochemistry and Biophysics 47(2):100-3.

Dave, B. J., A. H. Trivedi and S. G. Adhvaryu (1991). "Cytogenetic studies reveal increased genomic damage among 'pan masala'consumers." Mutagenesis 6(2): 159-163.

Dave, S., N. Ghodasara, N. Mohanrao, G. Patel and B. Patel (1997). "The relation of exposure to asbestos and smoking habit with pulmonary function tests and chest radiograph." Indian Journal of Public Health 41(1): 16-24.

Dave, S.K., N. Mohanrao and N.B. Ghodasara (1995). "The effect of asbestos exposure and smoking habit on pulmonary function tests of asbestos cement factory workers". Indian Journal of Occupational Health 38:27–35.

Dave, S. K. and W. S. Beckett (2005). "Occupational asbestos exposure and predictable asbestos-related diseases in India." American Journal of Industrial Medicine 48(2): 137-143.

Dayal, M., D. Parmar, M. Ali, A. Dhawan, U. N. Dwivedi and P. K. Seth (2001). "Induction of rat brain cytochrome P450s (P450s) by deltamethrin: regional specificity and correlation with neurobehavioral toxicity." Neurotoxicity Research 3(4): 351-357.

Dayal, M., D. Parmar, A. Dhawan, M. Ali, U. Dwivedi and P. Seth (2003). "Effect of pretreatment of cytochrome P450 (P450) modifiers on neurobehavioral toxicity induced by deltamethrin." Food and Chemical Toxicology 41(3): 431-437.

Dayal, M., D. Parmar, A. Dhawan, U. N. Dwivedi, J. Doehmer and P. K. Seth (1999). "Induction of rat brain and liver cytochrome P450 1A1/1A2 and 2B1/2B2 isoenzymes by deltamethrin." Environmental Toxicology and Pharmacology 7(3): 169-178.

De, B. K., S. Gangopadhyay, D. Dutta, S. D. Baksi, A. Pani and P. Ghosh (2009). "Pentoxifylline versus prednisolone for severe alcoholic hepatitis: a randomized controlled trial." World Journal of Gastroenterology: WJG 15(13): 1613.

De Chaudhuri, S., P. Ghosh, N. Sarma, P. Majumdar, T. J. Sau, S. Basu, S. Roychoudhury, K. Ray and A. K. Giri (2008). "Genetic variants associated with arsenic susceptibility: study of purine nucleoside phosphorylase, arsenic (+ 3) methyltransferase, and glutathione S-transferase omega genes." Environmental Health Perspectives 116(4): 501-505.

De Chaudhuri, S., J. Mahata, J. K. Das, A. Mukherjee, P. Ghosh, T. J. Sau, L. Mondal, S. Basu, A. K. Giri and S. Roychoudhury (2006). "Association of specific p53 polymorphisms with keratosis in individuals exposed to arsenic through drinking water in West Bengal, India." Mutation Research/Fundamental and Molecular Mechanisms of Mutagenesis 601(1-2): 102-112.

DeBethizy, J. and J. R. Hayes (1994). "Metabolism: a determinant of toxicity." Principles and Methods of Toxicology: 59-100.

Debnath, S., S. Ghosh and B. Hazra (2013). "Inhibitory effect of Nymphaea pubescens Willd. flower extract on carrageenan-induced inflammation and CCl4-induced hepatotoxicity in rats." Food and Chemical Toxicology 59: 485-491.

Desai, S., S. Ghaisas, S. Jakhi and S. Bhide (1996). "Cytogenetic damage in exfoliated oral mucosal cells and circulating lymphocytes of patients suffering from precancerous oral lesions." Cancer Letters 109(1-2): 9-14.

Deshmukh, D. K., M. K. Deb and S. L. Mkoma (2013). "Size distribution and seasonal variation of size-segregated particulate matter in the ambient air of Raipur city, India." Air Quality, Atmosphere and Health 6(1): 259-276.

Devarbhavi, H. (2011). "Antituberculous drug-induced liver injury: current perspective." Tropical Gastroenterology 32(3): 167-174.

Devarbhavi, H. (2012). "An update on drug-induced liver injury." Journal of Clinical and Experimental Hepatology 2(3): 247-259.

Devi, I. (2007). "Facing Hazards at Work: Agricultural Workers and Pesticide Exposure in Kuttanad, Kerala." SANDEE Policy Brief(19-07): 4.

Devi, P., V. Thimmarasa, V. Mehrotra and P. Arora (2011). "Micronucleus assay for evaluation of genotoxicity in potentially malignant and malignant disorders." Journal of Indian Academy of Oral Medicine and Radiology 23(2): 97.

Dewan, A., V. K. Bhatnagar, M. L. Mathur, T. Chakma, R. Kashyap, H. G. Sadhu, S. N. Sinha and H. N. Saiyed (2004). "Repeated episodes of endosulfan poisoning." Journal of Toxicology: Clinical Toxicology 42(4): 363-369.

Dewan, A. and M. Shoukat (2014). "Evaluation of risk of nephrotoxicity with high dose, extended-interval colistin administration." Indian Journal of Critical Care Medicine: Peer-reviewed, Official Publication of Indian Society of Critical Care Medicine 18(7): 427.

Dewan, P. and P. Gupta (2012). "Burden of congenital rubella syndrome (CRS) in India: a systematic review." Indian Pediatrics 49(5): 377-399.

Dey, S., L. Di Girolamo, A. van Donkelaar, S. Tripathi, T. Gupta and M. Mohan (2012). "Variability of outdoor fine particulate (PM2. 5) concentration in the Indian Subcontinent: A remote sensing approach." Remote Sensing of Environment 127: 153-161.

Dhar, P., M. Jaitley, M. Kalaivani and R. D. Mehra (2005). "Preliminary morphological and histochemical changes in rat spinal cord neurons following arsenic ingestion." Neurotoxicology 26(3): 309-320.

Dhar, S., S. Chatterjee, B. Sengupta, S. Chakrabarti, S. Ray and A. Dutta (2010). "Polymorphisms of methylenetetrahydrofolate reductase gene as the genetic predispositions of coronary artery diseases in eastern India." Journal of Cardiovascular Disease Research 1(3): 152-157.

Dhara, R. (1994). "Health effects of the Bhopal gas leak: A review." New Solutions: A Journal of Environmental and Occupational Health Policy 4(3): 35-48.

Dhara, V. R. and R. Dhara (2002). "The Union Carbide disaster in Bhopal: a review of health effects." Archives of Environmental Health: An International Journal 57(5): 391-404.

Dhatrak, S. V. and S. S. Nandi (2009). "Risk assessment of chronic poisoning among Indian metallic miners." Indian Journal of Occupational and Environmental Medicine 13(2): 60.

Dhawan, A., M. Bajpayee and D. Parmar (2009). "Comet assay: a reliable tool for the assessment of DNA damage in different models." Cell Biology and Toxicology 25(1): 5-32.

Dhawan, A., N. Mathur and P. K. Seth (2001). "The effect of smoking and eating habits on DNA damage in Indian population as measured in the Comet assay." Mutation Research/Fundamental and Molecular Mechanisms of Mutagenesis 474(1-2): 121-128.

Dhawan, A., D. Parmar, M. Das and P. K. Seth (1989). "Characterization of cerebral 7-ethoxycoumarin-O-deethylase: Evidence for multiplicity of cytochrome P450 in brain." Biochemical Medicine and Metabolic Biology 41(3): 184-192.

Dhawan, A., D. Parmar, M. Das and P. K. Seth (1990). "Cytochrome P-450 dependent monooxygenases in neuronal and glial cells: Inducibility and specificity." Biochemical and Biophysical Research Communications 170(2): 441-447.

Dhawan, A., D. Parmar, M. Dayal and P. K. Seth (1999). "Cytochrome P450 (P450) isoenzyme specific dealkylation of alkoxyresorufins in rat brain microsomes." Molecular and Cellular Biochemistry 200(1-2): 169-176.

Dhawan, A., R. Shanker, M. Das and K. C. Gupta (2011). "Guidance for safe handling of nanomaterials." Journal of Biomedical Nanotechnology 7(1): 218-224.

Dhawan, A., R. Shanker, B. Laffon, J. F. Tajes, D. Fuchs, H. Becker, H. Moriske, J. Teixeira, M. Carriere and N. Herlin-Boime (2011). "NanoLINEN: nanotoxicology link between India and European Nations." Journal of Biomedical Nanotechnology 7(1): 203-204.

Dhawan, A. and V. Sharma (2010). "Toxicity assessment of nanomaterials: methods and challenges." Analytical and Bioanalytical Chemistry 398(2): 589-605.

Dhawan, A., V. Sharma and D. Parmar (2009). "Nanomaterials: a challenge for toxicologists." Nanotoxicology 3(1): 1-9.

Dhawan, A., J. S. Taurozzi, A. K. Pandey, W. Shan, S. M. Miller, S. A. Hashsham and V. V. Tarabara (2006). "Stable colloidal dispersions of C60 fullerenes in water: evidence for genotoxicity." Environmental Science and Technology 40(23): 7394-7401.

Dhawan, M., S. Flora and S. Tandon (1992). "Biochemical changes and essential metals concentration in lead-intoxicated rats pre-exposed to ethanol." Alcohol 9(3): 241-245.

Dheenan, P. S., D. K. Jha, A. K. Das, N. V. Vinithkumar, M. P. Devi and R. Kirubagaran (2016). "Geographic information systems and multivariate analysis to evaluate fecal bacterial pollution in coastal waters of Andaman, India." Environmental Pollution 214: 45-53.

Dherani, M. (2003). "Indoor air pollution due to biomass fuels in north India." Transactions of the Royal Society of Tropical Medicine and Hygiene 97(6): 626.

Dhikav, V., S. Singh and K. Anand (2004). "Adverse drug reaction monitoring in India." Journal, Indian Academy of Clinical Medicine 5: 27-33.

Dhir, H., A. K. Roy, A. Sharma and G. Talukder (1990). "Modification of clastogenicity of lead and aluminium in mouse bone marrow cells by dietary ingestion of Phyllanthus emblica fruit extract." Mutation Research/Genetic Toxicology 241(3): 305-312.

Dhobale, M. and S. Joshi (2012). "Altered maternal micronutrients (folic acid, vitamin B12) and omega 3 fatty acids through oxidative stress may reduce neurotrophic factors in preterm pregnancy." The Journal of Maternal-Fetal and Neonatal Medicine 25(4): 317-323.

Dhuriya, Y. K., P. Srivastava, R. K. Shukla, R. Gupta, D. Singh, D. Parmar, A. B. Pant and V. K. Khanna (2017). "Prenatal exposure to lambda-cyhalothrin alters brain dopaminergic signaling in developing rats." Toxicology 386: 49-59.

Dhuriya, Y. K., P. Srivastava, R. K. Shukla, R. Gupta, D. Singh, D. Parmar, A. B. Pant and V. K. Khanna (2017). "Prenatal exposure to lambda-cyhalothrin impairs memory in developing rats: Role of NMDA receptor induced post-synaptic signalling in hippocampus." Neurotoxicology 62: 80-91.

Dikshith, T., K. Datta and P. Chandra (1976). "90 day dermal toxicity of DDVP in male rats." Bulletin of Environmental Contamination and Toxicology 15(5): 574-580.

Dikshith, T., P. Gupta, J. Gaur, K. Datta and A. K. Mathur (1976). "Ninety day toxicity of carbaryl in male rats." Environmental Research 12(2): 161-170.

Dikshith, T., S. Kumar, G. Tandon, R. Raizada and P. Ray (1989). "Pesticide residues in edible oils and oil seeds." Bulletin of Environmental Contamination and Toxicology 42(1): 50-56.

Dikshith, T., R. Raizada and K. Datta (1980). "Response of female guinea pigs to repeated oral administration of quinalphos." Bulletin of Environmental Contamination and Toxicology 24(1): 739-745.

Dinesh Kumar, B. and K. Krishnaswamy (1995). "Detection of occupational lead nephropathy using early renal markers." Journal of Toxicology: Clinical Toxicology 33(4): 331-335.

Diwanay, S., D. Chitre and B. Patwardhan (2004). "Immunoprotection by botanical drugs in cancer chemotherapy." Journal of Ethnopharmacology 90(1): 49-55.

Dixit, R., M. Das, M. Mushtaq, S. Srivastava and P. K. Seth (1982). "Depletion of glutathione content and inhibition of glutathione-S-transferase and aryl hydrocarbon hydroxylase activity of rat brain following exposure to styrene." Neurotoxicology 3(1): 142-145.

Dixit, R., R. Husain, H. Mukhtar and P. Seth (1981). "Acrylamide induced inhibition of hepatic glutathione-S-transferase activity in rats." Toxicology Letters 7(3): 207-210.

Dixit, R., R. Husain, H. Mukhtar and P. K. Seth (1981). "Effect of acrylamide on biogenic amine levels, monoamine oxidase, and cathepsin D activity of rat brain." Environmental Research 26(1): 168-173.

Dixit, R., H. Mukhtar, P. K. Seth and C. R. K. Murti (1981). "Conjugation of acrylamide with glutathione catalysed by glutathione-S-transferases of rat liver and brain." Biochemical Pharmacology 30(13): 1739-1744.

Dixit, R., S. Verma, V. Nitnaware and N. Thacker (2003). "Heavy metals contamination in surface and groundwater supply of an urban city." Indian Journal of Environmental Health 45(2): 107-112.

Dixit, S., S. K. Khanna and M. Das (2013). "All India survey for analyses of colors in sweets and savories: exposure risk in Indian population." Journal of Food Science 78(4): T642-T647.

Dixit, S., R. Pandey and M. Das (1995). "Food quality surveillance on colours in eatables." Journal of Food Science and Technology 32: 373-376.

Dixit, S., S. Purshottam, S. Khanna and M. Das (2011). "Usage pattern of synthetic food colours in different states of India and exposure assessment through commodities preferentially consumed by children." Food Additives and Contaminants: Part A 28(8): 996-1005.

Dixit, S., S. K. Purshottam, S. K. Khanna and M. Das (2009). "Surveillance of the quality of turmeric powders from city markets of India on the basis of curcumin content and the presence of extraneous colours." Food Additives and Contaminants 26(9): 1227-1231.

Dogra, A., Y. Minocha and S. Kaur (2003). "Adverse reactions to cosmetics." Indian Journal of Dermatology, Venereology, and Leprology 69(2): 165.

Dogra, R., K. Chandra, S. Chandra, S. Gupta, S. Khanna, S. Srivastava, L. Shukla, J. Katiyar and R. Shanker (1992). "Host resistance assays as predictive models in styrene immunomodulation." International Journal of Immunopharmacology 14(6): 1003-1009.

Dogra, R., K. Chandra, S. Chandra, S. Khanna, S. Srivastava, L. Shukla, J. Katiyar and R. Shanker (1989). "Di-octyl phthalate induced altered host resistance: viral and protozoal models in mice." Industrial Health 27(2): 83-87.

Dogra, R., S. Khanna, S. Srivastava, L. Shukla and R. Shanker (1989). "Styrene-induced immunomodulation in mice." International Journal of Immuno-pharmacology 11(5): 577-586.

Dogra, R. K., S. Khanna and R. Shanker (2004). "Immunotoxicological effects of piperine in mice." Toxicology 196(3): 229-236.

Dogra, S. and K. Donaldson (1995). "Effect of long and short fibre amosite asbestos on *in vitro* TNF production by rat alveolar macrophages: the modifying effect of lipopolysaccharide." Industrial Health 33(3): 131-141.

Dohadwala, M. and P. K. Ray (1985). "*In vivo* protection by protein A of hepatic microsomal mixed function oxygenase system of cyclophosphamide-treated rats." Cancer Chemotherapy and Pharmacology 14(2): 135-138.

Doshi, T., C. D'souza and G. Vanage (2013). "Aberrant DNA methylation at Igf2–H19 imprinting control region in spermatozoa upon neonatal exposure to bisphenol A and its association with post implantation loss." Molecular Biology Reports 40(8): 4747-4757.

Doshi, T., S. S. Mehta, V. Dighe, N. Balasinor and G. Vanage (2011). "Hypermethylation of estrogen receptor promoter region in adult testis of rats exposed neonatally to bisphenol A." Toxicology 289(2-3): 74-82.

Dubey, J., K. M. Kumari and A. Lakhani (2015). "Chemical characteristics and mutagenic activity of PM2.5 at a site in the Indo-Gangetic plain, India." Ecotoxicology and Environmental Safety 114: 75-83.

Dureja, G. and R. Saxena (1987). "The methyl isocyanate (MIC) gas tragedy in Bhopal (India)." Indian Journal of Anaesthesia 35: 264-268.

Dureja, P., A. Nair and M. Pillai (1991). "Aldrin and dieldrin in maternal serum, cord serum and breast milk in human samples from Delhi, India." International Journal of Environmental Analytical Chemistry 44(4): 253-256.

Dutta, A., B. Mukherjee, D. Das, A. Banerjee and M. Ray (2011). "Hypertension with elevated levels of oxidized low-density lipoprotein and anticardiolipin antibody in the circulation of premenopausal Indian women chronically exposed to biomass smoke during cooking." Indoor Air 21(2): 165-176.

Dwivedi, A., S. F. Mujtaba, H. N. Kushwaha, D. Ali, N. Yadav, S. Singh and R. S. Ray (2012). "Photosensitizing mechanism and identification of levofloxacin photoproducts at ambient UV radiation." Photochemistry and Photobiology 88(2): 344-355.

Dwivedi, A., S. F. Mujtaba, N. Yadav, H. N. Kushwaha, S. K. Amar, S. K. Singh, M. C. Pant and R. Ray (2014). "Cellular and molecular mechanism of ofloxacin induced apoptotic cell death under ambient UV-A and sunlight exposure." Free Radical Research 48(3): 333-346.

Dwivedi, H. P., R. D. Smiley and L.-A. Jaykus (2010). "Selection and characterization of DNA aptamers with binding selectivity to Campylobacter jejuni using whole-cell SELEX." Applied Microbiology and Biotechnology 87(6): 2323-2334.

Dwivedi, M. and B. Prasad (1964). "An epidemiological study of lathyrism in the district of Rewa, Madhya Pradesh." Indian Journal of Medical Research 52: 81-116.

Dwivedi, N., Y. D. Bhutia, V. Kumar, P. Yadav, P. Kushwaha, H. Swarnkar and S. Flora (2010). "Effects of combined exposure to dichlorvos and monocrotophos on blood and brain biochemical variables in rats." Human and Experimental Toxicology 29(2): 121-129.

Dwivedi, P., A. Verma, A. Mishra, K. Singh, A. Prasad, A. Saxena, K. Dutta, N. Mathur and P. Ray (1989). "Protein A protects mice from depletion of biotransformation enzymes and mortality induced by Salmonella typhimurium endotoxin." Toxicology Letters 49(1): 1-13.

Dwivedi, P., A. Verma and P. Ray (1992). "Induction of immune rejection of tumors by protein A in mice bearing transplantable solid tissue Dalton's lymphoma tumors." Immunopharmacology and Immunotoxicology 14(1-2): 105-128.

Dwivedi, P. C., J. K. Raizada, V. K. Saini and P. C. Mittal (1985). "Ocular lesions following methyl isocyanate contamination: the Bhopal experience." Archives of Ophthalmology 103(11): 1627-1627.

Dwivedi, S., S. Mishra and R. D. Tripathi (2018). "Ganga water pollution: a potential health threat to inhabitants of Ganga basin." Environment International 117: 327-338.

Dwivedi, S. K. and S. Dey (2002). "Medicinal herbs: a potential source of toxic metal exposure for man and animals in India." Archives of Environmental Health: An International Journal 57(3): 229-231.

El Ghissassi, F., R. Baan, K. Straif, Y. Grosse, B. Secretan, V. Bouvard, L. Benbrahim-Tallaa, N. Guha, C. Freeman and L. Galichet (2009). "A review of human carcinogens—part D: radiation." The Lancet Oncology 10(8): 751-752.

Embrandiri, A., R. P. Singh, H. M. Ibrahim and A. B. Khan (2012). "An epidemiological study on the health effects of endosulfan spraying on cashew plantations in Kasaragod District, Kerala, India." Asian Journal of Epidemiology 5(1): 22-31.

Eruvaram, N. R. and M. Das (2009). "Phenotype of hepatic xenobiotic metabolizing enzymes and CYP450 isoforms of sanguinarine treated rats: effect of P450 inducers on its toxicity." Toxicology Mechanisms and Methods 19(8): 510-517.

Fareed, M., C. N. Kesavachandran, M. K. Pathak, V. Bihari, M. Kuddus and A. K. Srivastava (2012). "Visual disturbances with cholinesterase depletion due to exposure of agricultural pesticides among farm workers." Toxicological and Environmental Chemistry 94(8): 1601-1609.

Fareed, M., M. K. Pathak, V. Bihari, R. Kamal, A. K. Srivastava and C. N. Kesavachandran (2013). "Adverse respiratory health and hematological alterations among agricultural workers occupationally exposed to organophosphate pesticides: a cross-sectional study in North India." PLoS One 8(7): e69755.

Farooq, M., G. S. Babu, R. Ray, R. Misra, U. Shankar and R. Hans (2000). "Sensitivity of duckweed (Lemna major) to ultraviolet-B radiation." Biochemical and Biophysical Research Communications 276(3): 970-973.

Fatima, M., I. Ahmad, R. Siddiqui and S. Raisuddin (2001). "Paper and pulp mill effluent-induced immunotoxicity in freshwater fish Channa punctatus (Bloch)." Archives of Environmental Contamination and Toxicology 40(2): 271-276.

Fatima, R. A. and M. Ahmad (2005). "Certain antioxidant enzymes of Allium cepa as biomarkers for the detection of toxic heavy metals in wastewater." Science of the Total Environment 346(1-3): 256-273.

Fatima, R. A. and M. Ahmad (2006). "Genotoxicity of industrial wastewaters obtained from two different pollution sources in northern India: a comparison of three bioassays." Mutation Research/Genetic Toxicology and Environmental Mutagenesis 609(1): 81-91.

Fatima, S. and R. Mahmood (2007). "Vitamin C attenuates potassium dichromate-induced nephrotoxicity and alterations in renal brush border membrane enzymes and phosphate transport in rats." Clinica Chimica Acta 386(1-2): 94-99.

Flora, G. J., V. K. Khanna and P. K. Seth (1999). "Changes in neurotransmitter receptors and neurobehavioral variables in rats co-exposed to lead and ethanol." Toxicology Letters 109(1-2): 43-49.

Flora, S., J. R. Behari, M. Ashquin and S. Tandon (1982). "Time-dependent protective effect of selenium against cadmium-induced nephrotoxicity and hepatotoxicity." Chemico-Biological Interactions 42(3): 345-351.

Flora, S., M. Dhawan and S. Tandon (1999). "Lead-ethanol interaction in rats during protein deficiency." Trace Elements and Electrolytes 16(2): 93-98.

Flora, S., D. Kumar, S. Sachan and S. D. Gupta (1991). "Combined exposure to lead and ethanol on tissue concentration of essential metals and some biochemical indices in rat." Biological Trace Element Research 28(2): 157-164.

Flora, S., S. Pant, P. Malhotra and G. Kannan (1997). "Biochemical and histopathological changes in arsenic-intoxicated rats coexposed to ethanol." Alcohol 14(6): 563-568.

Flora, S. J. (2008). Status of toxicological research in India, ACS Publications. Chemical Research in Toxicology 21(7):1317-1319

Flora, S. J., G. Saxena and A. Mehta (2007). "Reversal of lead-induced neuronal apoptosis by chelation treatment in rats: role of reactive oxygen species and intracellular Ca2+." Journal of Pharmacology and Experimental Therapeutics 322(1): 108-116.

Flora, S. J. and S. K. Tandon (1987). "Effect of combined exposure to lead and ethanol on some biochemical indices in the rat." Biochemical Pharmacology 36(4): 537-541.

Fornace, A. J., I. Alamo and M. C. Hollander (1988). "DNA damage-inducible transcripts in mammalian cells." Proceedings of the National Academy of Sciences 85(23): 8800-8804.

Gaikwad, A. S., P. Karunamoorthy, S. J. Kondhalkar, M. Ambikapathy and R. Beerappa (2015). "Assessment of hematological, biochemical effects and genotoxicity among pesticide sprayers in grape garden." Journal of Occupational Medicine and Toxicology 10(1): 11.

Ganapathy, K. and M. Dwivedi (1961). "Studies on clinical epidemiology of lathyrism." Lathyrism Enquiry Field Unit, Indian Council of Medical Research, Ghandi Memorial Hospital, Rewa, Madhya Pradesh, India.

Gandhi, N., Z. M. Saiyed, J. Napuri, T. Samikkannu, P. V. Reddy, M. Agudelo, P. Khatavkar, S. K. Saxena and M. P. Nair (2010). "Interactive role of human immunodeficiency virus type 1 (HIV-1) clade-specific Tat protein and cocaine in blood-brain barrier dysfunction: Implications for HIV-1–associated neurocognitive disorder." Journal of Neurovirology 16(4): 294-305.

Gangadhar, B., B. Subrahmanya, H. Venkatesh and S. Channabasavanna (1982). "Clonidine in opiate detoxification." Indian Journal of Psychiatry 24(4): 387.

Gangopadhyay, S., T. Das, G. Ghoshal and T. Ghosh (2006). "Work organization in sand core manufacturing for health and productivity." International Journal of Industrial Ergonomics 36(10): 915-920.

Gangopadhyay, S. and S. Dev (2014). "Design and evaluation of ergonomic interventions for the prevention of musculoskeletal disorders in India." Annals of Occupational and Environmental Medicine 26(1): 18.

Gargava, P. and V. Rajagopalan (2016). "Source apportionment studies in six Indian cities—drawing broad inferences for urban PM 10 reductions." Air Quality, Atmosphere and Health 9(5): 471-481.

Gayathri, A., A. R. Kanaki, B. Patil, A. Binjawadgi and B. V. Anandi (2013). "A case of sulfonylurea induced phototoxicity in an elderly subject-a rare case report." Journal of Evolution of Medical and Dental Sciences 2(39): 7472-7475.

Gera, R., V. Singh, S. Mitra, A. K. Sharma, A. Singh, A. Dasgupta, D. Singh, M. Kumar, P. Jagdale and S. Patnaik (2017). "Arsenic exposure impels CD4 commitment in thymus and suppress T cell cytokine secretion by increasing regulatory T cells." Scientific Reports 7(1): 7140.

Ghafur, A., S. Gohel, V. Devarajan, T. Raja, J. Easow, M. Raja, S. Sreenivas, B. Ramakrishnan, T. Ramakrishnan and S. Raman (2017). "Colistin nephrotoxicity in adults: single centre large series from India." Indian Journal of Critical Care Medicine: Peer-reviewed, Official Publication of Indian Society of Critical Care Medicine 21(6): 350.

Ghosh, A., A. Sharma, G. Talukder and F. Oleson (1991). "Cytogenetic damage induced *in vivo* to mice by single exposure to cesium chloride." Environmental and Molecular Mutagenesis 18(2): 87-91.

Ghosh, A. and P. C. Sil (2007). "Anti-oxidative effect of a protein from Cajanus indicus L against acetaminophen-induced hepato-nephro toxicity." Journal of Biochemistry and Molecular Biology 40(6): 1039.

Ghosh, B. B., S. Sengupta, A. Roy, S. Maity, S. Ghosh, G. Talukder and A. Sharma (1990). "Cytogenetic studies in human populations exposed to gas leak at Bhopal, India." Environmental Health Perspectives 86: 323-326.

Ghosh, D., S. Bhattacharya and S. Mazumder (2006). "Perturbations in the catfish immune responses by arsenic: organ and cell specific effects." Comparative Biochemistry and Physiology Part C: Toxicology and Pharmacology 143(4): 455-463.

Ghosh, D., N. Biswas and P. Ghosh (1991). "Studies on the effect of prolactin treatment on testicular steroidogenesis and gametogenesis in lithium-treated rats." European Journal of Endocrinology 125(3): 313-318.

Ghosh, D., U. B. Das and M. Misro (2002). "Protective role of α-tocopherol-succinate (provitamin-E) in cyclophosphamide induced testicular gametogenic and steroidogenic disorders: a correlative approach to oxidative stress." Free Radical Research 36(11): 1209-1218.

Ghosh, D., S. Datta, S. Bhattacharya and S. Mazumder (2007). "Long-term exposure to arsenic affects head kidney and impairs humoral immune responses of Clarias batrachus." Aquatic Toxicology 81(1): 79-89.

Ghosh, D., S. Ghosh, S. Sarkar, A. Ghosh, N. Das, K. D. Saha and A. K. Mandal (2010). "Quercetin in vesicular delivery systems: evaluation in combating arsenic-induced acute liver toxicity associated gene expression in rat model." Chemico-Biological Interactions 186(1): 61-71.

Ghosh, P. (1964). "Industrial Pulmonary Disease in India." Industrial Medicine and Surgery 33(10): 732-737.

Ghosh, P., A. Basu, J. Mahata, S. Basu, M. Sengupta, J. K. Das, A. Mukherjee, A. K. Sarkar, L. Mondal and K. Ray (2006). "Cytogenetic damage and genetic variants in the individuals susceptible to arsenic-induced cancer through drinking water." International Journal of Cancer 118(10): 2470-2478.

Ghosh, P., A. Basu, K. K. Singh and A. K. Giri (2008). "Evaluation of cell types for assessment of cytogenetic damage in arsenic exposed population." Molecular Cancer 7(1): 45.

Ghosh, P. and R. Ghosh (1988). "Effect of betel chewing on the frequency of sister chromatid exchanges in pregnant women and women using oral contraceptives." Cancer Genetics and Cytogenetics 32(2): 211-215.

Ghosh, S., I. Maisnam, B. K. Murmu, P. K. Mitra, A. Roy and I. D. Simpson (2008). "A Locally Developed Snakebite Management Protocol Significantly Reduces Overall Anti Snake Venom Utilization in West Bengal, India." Wilderness and Environmental Medicine 19(4): 267-275.

Ghosh, S., M. Misro, U. B. Das, R. Maiti, J. M. Debnath and D. Ghosh (2001). "Effect of human chorionic gonadotrophin coadministration on ovarian steroidogenic and folliculogenic activities in cyclophosphamide treated albino rats." Reproductive Toxicology 15(2): 221-225.

Ghosh, S., J. Parikh, V. Gokani, S. Kashyap and S. Chatterjee (1979). "Studies on occupational health problems during agricultural operation of Indian tobacco workers: a preliminary survey report." Journal of Occupational Medicine.: Official Publication of the Industrial Medical Association 21(1): 45-47.

Ghosh, S., J. Parikh, V. Gokani, M. Rao, S. Kashyap and S. Chatterjee (1980). "Studies on occupational health problems in agricultural tobacco workers." Occupational Medicine 30(3): 113-117.

Ghosh, T. and S. Gangopadhyay (2012). "Effect of an ergonomic intervention on muscle fatigue and respiratory stress of goldsmiths during blowing pipe activity in India." Work 43(4): 427-435.

Gill-Sharma, M., N. Balasinor and P. Parte (2001). "Effect of intermittent treatment with tamoxifen on reproduction in male rats." Asian Journal of Andrology 3(2): 115-120.

Gill, K., V. Gupta and R. Sandhir (2003). "Ca2+/calmodulin-mediated neurotransmitter release and neurobehavioural deficits following lead exposure." Cell Biochemistry and Function: Cellular Biochemistry and its Modulation by Active Agents or Disease 21(4): 345-353.

Giri, A. K. (1991). "Food dyes of India: mutagenic and clastogenic potentials - a review." Proceedings of the Indian National Science Academy 57(3/4): 183-198.

Giri, A. K., T. S. Banerjee, G. Talukder and A. Sharma (1987). "Induction of sister chromatid exchange and dominant lethal mutation by 'katha'(catechu) in male mice." Cancer Letters 36(2): 189-196.

Giri, A. K., G. Talukder and A. Sharma (1986). "Sister chromatid exchange induced by metanil yellow and nitrite singly and in combination *in vivo* on mice." Cancer Letters 31(3): 299-303.

Giri, S., A. Giri, G. D. Sharma and S. B. Prasad (2002). "Mutagenic effects of carbosulfan, a carbamate pesticide." Mutation Research/Genetic Toxicology and Environmental Mutagenesis 519(1-2): 75-82.

Giri, S., A. Giri, G. D. Sharma and S. B. Prasad (2003). "Induction of sister chromatid exchanges by cypermethrin and carbosulfan in bone marrow cells of mice *in vivo*." Mutagenesis 18(1): 53-58.

Giri, S., G. Sharma, A. Giri and S. Prasad (2002). "Fenvalerate-induced chromosome aberrations and sister chromatid exchanges in the bone marrow cells of mice *in vivo*." Mutation Research/Genetic Toxicology and Environmental Mutagenesis 520(1-2): 125-132.

Giri, S. and A. K. Singh (2019). "Assessment of metal pollution in groundwater using a novel multivariate metal pollution index in the mining areas of the Singhbhum copper belt." Environmental Earth Sciences 78(6): 192.

Giri, U., M. Iqbal and M. Athar (1996). "Porphyrin-mediated photosensitization has a weak tumor promoting activity in mouse skin: possible role of *in situ-generated* reactive oxygen species." Carcinogenesis 17(9): 2023-2028.

Goel, S., G. Rao and K. Pandya (1988). "Hepatotoxic effects elicited by n-hexane or n-heptane." Journal of Applied Toxicology 8(2): 81-84.

Goel, S., O. Rao and K. Pandya (1982). "Toxicity of n-hexane and n-heptane: some biochemical changes in liver and serum." Toxicology Letters 14(3-4): 169-174.

Gopalkrishnan, K. (1998). "Characteristics of semen parameters in a selected population of Indian men over a period of 10 years." Current Science: 939-942.

Goswami, R., N. Kochupillai, N. Gupta, A. Kukreja, M. Lan and N. Maclaren (2001). "Islet cell autoimmunity in youth onset diabetes mellitus in Northern India." Diabetes Research and Clinical Practice 53(1): 47-54.

Gourie-Devi, M. (2014). "Epidemiology of neurological disorders in India: Review of background, prevalence and incidence of epilepsy, stroke, Parkinson's disease and tremors." Neurology India 62(6): 588.

Govil, N., S. Chaudhary, M. Waseem and S. Parvez (2012). "Postnuclear supernatant: an *in vitro* model for assessing cadmium-induced neurotoxicity." Biological Trace Element Research 146(3): 402-409.

Govil, P. K. and A. K. Krishna (2018). Soil and water contamination by potentially hazardous elements: a case history from India. Environmental Geochemistry, Elsevier: 567-597.

Goyal, S., S. K. Amar, D. Dubey, M. K. Pal, J. Singh, A. Verma, H. N. Kushwaha and R. S. Ray (2015). "Involvement of cathepsin B in mitochondrial apoptosis by p-phenylenediamine under ambient UV radiation." Journal of Hazardous Materials 300: 415-425.

Goyal, S., A. K. Srivastav, S. K. Amar, S. Agnihotry and R. S. Ray (2018). Phototoxicity of Hair Dyes: Challenge for Tropical Countries. Photocarcinogenesis and Photoprotection, Springer: 101-108.

Graf, U., H. Frei, A. Kägi, A. Katz and F. Würgler (1989). "Thirty compounds tested in the Drosophila wing spot test." Mutation Research/Genetic Toxicology 222(4): 359-373.

Grover, P. S. and K. Thakur (2001). "Shimla drinking water: A bacteriological analysis." Journal of Communicable Diseases 33(1): 44-52.

Guha Mazumder, D. (2003). "Chronic arsenic toxicity: clinical features, epidemiology, and treatment: experience in West Bengal." Journal of Environmental Science and Health, Part A 38(1): 141-163.

Guha Mazumder, D. N., B. K. De, A. Santra, N. Ghosh, S. Das, S. Lahiri and T. Das (2001). "Randomized placebo-controlled trial of 2, 3-dimercapto-1-propanesulfonate (DMPS) in therapy of chronic arsenicosis due to drinking arsenic-contaminated water." Journal of Toxicology: Clinical Toxicology 39(7): 665-674.

Guha, S. (1996). "Contraceptive for use by a male." US patent 54880705.

Guha, S. K. (1999). "Non-invasive reversal of intraluminal vas deferens polymer injection-induced azoospermia-technology." Asian Journal of Andrology 1: 131-134.

Gummeneni, S., Y. B. Yusup, M. Chavali and S. Samadi (2011). "Source apportionment of particulate matter in the ambient air of Hyderabad city, India." Atmospheric Research 101(3): 752-764.

Gunturu, K. S., P. Nagarajan, P. McPhedran, T. R. Goodman, M. E. Hodsdon and M. P. Strout (2011). "Ayurvedic herbal medicine and lead poisoning." Journal of Hematology and Oncology 4(1): 51.

Gupta, A., R. Agarwal and G. S. Shukla (1999). "Functional impairment of blood-brain barrier following pesticide exposure during early development in rats." Human and Experimental Toxicology 18(3): 174-179.

Gupta, A., A. Gupta and G. S. Shukla (1998). Effects of neonatal quinalphos exposure and subsequent withdrawal on free radical generation and antioxidative defenses in developing rat brain. Journal of Applied Toxicology: 18(1):71–77.

Gupta, A., R. S. Patil and S. Gupta (2004). "Influence of meteorological factors on air pollution concentration for a coastal region in India." International Journal of Environment and Pollution 21(3): 253-262.

Gupta, A., S. Sharma and K. Chopra (2008). "Reversal of iron-induced nephrotoxicity in rats by molsidomine, a nitric oxide donor." Food and Chemical Toxicology 46(2): 537-543.

Gupta, A. and G. Shukla (1997). "Enzymatic antioxidants in erythrocytes following heavy metal exposure: Possible role in early diagnosis of poisoning." Bulletin of Environmental Contamination and Toxicology 58(2): 198-205.

Gupta, C., A. Vikram, D. Tripathi, P. Ramarao and G. Jena (2010). "Antioxidant and antimutagenic effect of quercetin against DEN induced hepatotoxicity in rat." Phytotherapy Research: 24(1): 119-128.

Gupta, G. and Tarique (2013). Prevalence of Musculoskeletal Disorders in Farmers of Kanpur-Rural." Journal of Community Medicine and Health Education 3(249).

Gupta, G. S., A. Kumar, V. A. Senapati, A. K. Pandey, R. Shanker and A. Dhawan (2017). "Laboratory scale microbial food chain to study bioaccumulation, biomagnification, and ecotoxicity of cadmium telluride quantum dots." Environmental Science and Technology 51(3): 1695-1706.

Gupta, J. D., P. Satishchandra, K. Gopukumar, F. Wilkie, D. Waldrop-Valverde, R. Ellis, R. Ownby, D. Subbakrishna, A. Desai and A. Kamat (2007). "Neuropsychological deficits in human immunodeficiency virus type 1 clade C-seropositive adults from South India." Journal of Neurovirology 13(3): 195-202.

Gupta, K., B. Radotra, V. Sakhuja, A. Banerjee and K. Chugh (1989). "Mucormycosis in patients with renal failure." Renal Failure 11(4): 195-199.

Gupta, P. (2004). "Pesticide exposure-Indian scene." Toxicology 198(1-3): 83-90.

Gupta, P., R. Singh, M. Murali, S. Bhargava and P. Sharma (1992). "Kerosene oil poisoning--a childhood menace." Indian Pediatrics 29(8): 979-984.

Gupta, P. C., J. J. Pindborg and F. S. Mehta (1982). "Comparison of carcinogenicity of betel quid with and without tobacco: an epidemiological review." Ecology of Disease 1(4): 213-219.

Gupta, R., R. Shukla, A. Pant and V. Khanna (2018). "A dopamine-dependent activity in controlling the motor functions in cadmium induced neurotoxicity: Neuroprotective potential of quercetin." Parkinsonism and Related Disorders 46: e39.

Gupta, R., R. K. Shukla, L. P. Chandravanshi, P. Srivastava, Y. K. Dhuriya, J. Shanker, M. P. Singh, A. B. Pant and V. K. Khanna (2017). "Protective role of quercetin in cadmium-induced cholinergic dysfunctions in rat brain by modulating mitochondrial integrity and MAP kinase signaling." Molecular Neurobiology 54(6): 4560-4583.

Gupta, S., A. Bajaj and S. Bhagwan (1976). "Simple lung function studies in silicosis amongst stone-cutters." The Indian Journal of Chest Diseases and Allied Sciences 18(2): 73.

Gupta, S., A. Bajaj, A. Jain and Y. Vasudeva (1972). "Clinical and radiological studies in silicosis: based on a study of the disease amongst stonecutters." Indian Journal of Medical Research 60(9): 1309-1315.

Gupta, S., A. Garg and O. Gupta (1969). "Silicosis amongst stone-cutters. (A clinical and radiological study.)." Journal of the Association of Physicians of India 17(3): 163-172.

Gupta, S., P. Kapoor, K. Chaudhary, A. Gautam, R. Kumar, G. P. Raghava and O. S. D. D. Consortium (2013). "*In silico* approach for predicting toxicity of peptides and proteins." PLoS One 8(9): e73957.

Gupta, S., T. Kushwah, A. Vishwakarma and S. Yadav (2015). "Optimization of ZnO-NPs to investigate their safe application by assessing their effect on soil nematode Caenorhabditis elegans." Nanoscale Research Letters 10(1): 303.

Gupta, S. C., H. R. Siddique, N. Mathur, R. K. Mishra, D. K. Saxena and D. K. Chowdhuri (2007). "Adverse effect of organophosphate compounds, dichlorvos and chlorpyrifos in the reproductive tissues of transgenic Drosophila melanogaster: 70 kDa heat shock protein as a marker of cellular damage." Toxicology 238(1): 1-14.

Gupta, V. and K. D. Gill (2000). "Lead and ethanol coexposure: implications on the dopaminergic system and associated behavioral functions." Pharmacology Biochemistry and Behavior 66(3): 465-474.

Gupta, V., A. Shrivastava and N. Jain (2001). "Biosorption of chromium (VI) from aqueous solutions by green algae Spirogyra species." Water Research 35(17): 4079-4085.

Gupta, V. H., M. Singh, D. N. Amarapurkar, P. Sasi, J. M. Joshi, R. Baijal, P. K. HR, A. D. Amarapurkar, K. Joshi and P. P. Wangikar (2013). "Association of GST null genotypes with anti-tuberculosis drug induced hepatotoxicity in Western Indian population." Annals of Hepatology 12(6): 959-965.

Gupta, Y., M. Sharma and G. Chaudhary (2002). "Pyrogallol-induced hepatotoxicity in rats: a model to evaluate antioxidant hepatoprotective agents." Methods and Findings in Experimental and Clinical Pharmacology 24(8): 497-500.

Gupta, Y., M. Sharma, G. Chaudhary and C. Katiyar (2004). "Hepatoprotective effect of New Livfit®, a polyherbal formulation, is mediated through its free radical scavenging activity." Phytotherapy Research: 18(5): 362-364.

Gupta, Y. K. and S. S. Peshin (2014). "Snake bite in India: current scenario of an old problem." Journal of Clinical Toxicology 4(1): 182.

Guttikunda, S. K., R. Goel and P. Pant (2014). "Nature of air pollution, emission sources, and management in the Indian cities." Atmospheric Environment 95: 501-510.

Hans, R. K., N. Agrawal, K. Verma, R. B. Misra, R. S. Ray and M. Farooq (2008). "Assessment of the phototoxic potential of cosmetic products." Food and Chemical Toxicology 46(5): 1653-1658.

Haque, M. R. and S. H. Ansari (2014). "Immunostimulatory effect of standardised alcoholic extract of green tea (Camellia sinensis L.) against cyclophosphamide-induced immunosuppression in murine model." International Journal of Green Pharmacy (IJGP) 8(1).

Haque, N., S. Rizvi and M. Khan (1987). "Malathion induced alterations in the lipid profile and the rate of lipid peroxidation in rat brain and spinal cord." Pharmacology and Toxicology 61(1): 12-15.

Harikrishnan, R., P. Abhilash, S. S. Das, P. Prathibha, S. Rejitha, F. John, S. Kavitha and M. Indira (2013). "Protective effect of ascorbic acid against ethanol-induced reproductive toxicity in male guinea pigs." British Journal of Nutrition 110(4): 689-698.

Harish, D., B. Sharma, V. Sharma and K. Vij (2002). "The present day poisoning scenario and the role of chemical analysis;"Role of Forensic Science in the New Millennium"." Department of Anthropology, University of Delhi, Delhi, India: 19-25.

Hasan, M., S. F. Ali and M. Tariq (1978). "Levels of Dopamine, Norepinephrine and 5-Hydroxytryptamine in Different Regions of the Rat Brain in Thallium Toxicosis." Acta Pharmacologica et Toxicologica 43(3): 169-173.

Hasan, M., S. Maitra and S. F. Ali (1979). "Organophosphate pesticide DDVP-induced alterations in the rat cerebellum and spinal cord — an electron microscopic study." Experimental Pathology 17(2): 88-94.

Hotham, N. and E. Hotham (2015). "Drugs in breastfeeding." Australian Prescriber 38(5): 156.

Husain, R., R. Dixit, M. Das and P. Seth (1987). "Neurotoxicity of acrylamide in developing rat brain: changes in the levels of brain biogenic amines and activities of monoamine oxidase and acetylcholine esterase." Industrial Health 25(1): 19-28.

Husain, R., R. Husain, V. M. Adhami and P. Seth (1996). "Behavioral, neurochemical, and neuromorphological effects of deltamethrin in adult rats." Journal of Toxicology and Environmental Health Part A 48(5): 515-516.

Husain, R., M. Malaviya, P. K. Seth and R. Husain (1992). "Differential responses of regional brain polyamines following in utero exposure to synthetic pyrethroid insecticides: A preliminary report." Bulletin of Environmental Contamination and Toxicology 49(3): 402-409.

Husain, R., S. P. Srivastava, M. Mushtaq and P. K. Seth (1980). "Effect of styrene on levels of serotonin, noradrenaline, dopamine and activity of acetyl cholinesterase and monoamine oxidase in rat brain." Toxicology Letters 7(1): 47-50.

Husain, R., S. P. Srivastava and P. K. Seth (1985). "Methyl methacrylate induced behavioural and neurochemical changes in rats." Archives of Toxicology 58(1): 33-36.

Husain, R., S. P. Srivastava and P. K. Seth (1985). "Some behavioral effects of early styrene intoxication in experimental animals." Archives of Toxicology 57(1): 53-55.

Hussain, S. and S. F. Ali (2002). "Zinc potentiates 1-methyl-4-phenyl-1, 2, 3, 6-tetrahydropyridine induced dopamine depletion in caudate nucleus of mice brain." Neuroscience Letters 335(1): 25-28.

Ikhar, D., V. Deshpande and S. Untawale (2013). "Work Related Musculoskeletal Disorders in Cotton Spinning Occupation: An Ergonomic Intervention." Engineering 38(8.96): 18-60.

Imran, M., A. K. Najmi, M. F. Rashid, S. Tabrez and M. A. Shah (2013). "Clinical research regulation in India - history, development, initiatives, challenges and controversies: Still long way to go." Journal of Pharmacy and Bioallied Sciences 5(1): 2.

Iqbal, M. and M. Athar (1998). "Attenuation of iron-nitrilotriacetate (Fe-NTA)-mediated renal oxidative stress, toxicity and hyperproliferative response by the prophylactic treatment of rats with garlic oil." Food and Chemical Toxicology 36(6): 485-495.

Iqbal, M., U. Giri and M. Athar (1995). "Ferric nitrilotriacetate (Fe-NTA) is a potent hepatic tumor promoter and acts through the generation of oxidative stress." Biochemical and Biophysical Research Communications 212(2): 557-563.

Iqbal, M., U. Giri, D. K. Giri and M. Athar (1997). "Evidence that Fe-NTA-induced renal prostaglandin F2α is responsible for hyperplastic response in kidney: Implications for the role of cyclooxygenase-dependent arachidonic acid metabolism in renal tumor promotion." IUBMB Life 42(6): 1115-1124.

Iqbal, M., H. Rezazadeh, S. Ansar and M. Athar (1998). "α-Tocopherol (vitamin-E) ameliorates ferric nitrilotriacetate (Fe-NTA)-dependent renal proliferative response and toxicity: diminution of oxidative stress." Human and Experimental Toxicology 17(3): 163-171.

Iqbal, M., S. Sharma, H. Rezazadeh, N. Hasan, M. Abdulla and M. Athar (1996). "Glutathione metabolizing enzymes and oxidative stress in ferric nitrilotriacetate mediated hepatic injury." Redox Report 2(6): 385-391.

Iqbal, M., S. D. Sharma, A. Rahman, P. Trikha and M. Athar (1999). "Evidence that ferric nitrilotriacetate mediates oxidative stress by down-regulating DT-diaphorase activity: implications for carcinogenesis." Cancer Letters 141(1-2): 151-157.

Islam, S. and M. Ahmad (1991). "Mutagenic activity of aziridinyl steroids and their mechanism of action in biological systems." Mutagenesis 6(4): 271-278.

Islam, S. and M. Ahmad (1991). "Mutagenic activity of certain synthetic steroids: structural requirement for the mutagenic activity in Salmonella and E. coli." Mutation Research/Genetic Toxicology 259(2): 177-187.

Jadhav, K. B. and P. Rajini (2009). "Neurophysiological alterations in Caenorhabditis elegans exposed to dichlorvos, an organophosphorus insecticide." Pesticide Biochemistry and Physiology 94(2-3): 79-85.

Jadhav, K. B. and P. S. Rajini (2009). "Evaluation of sublethal effects of dichlorvos upon Caenorhabditis elegans based on a set of end points of toxicity." Journal of Biochemical and Molecular Toxicology 23(1): 9-17.

Jadhav, S., S. Sarkar, R. Patil and H. Tripathi (2007). "Effects of subchronic exposure via drinking water to a mixture of eight water-contaminating metals: a biochemical and histopathological study in male rats." Archives of Environmental Contamination and Toxicology 53(4): 667-677.

Jadhav, S., S. Sarkar, G. Ram and H. Tripathi (2007). "Immunosuppressive effect of subchronic exposure to a mixture of eight heavy metals, found as groundwater contaminants in different areas of India, through drinking water in male rats." Archives of Environmental Contamination and Toxicology 53(3): 450-458.

Jadiya, P. and A. Nazir (2012). "Environmental toxicants as extrinsic epigenetic factors for parkinsonism: studies employing transgenic C. elegans model." CNS and

Neurological Disorders-Drug Targets (Formerly Current Drug Targets-CNS and Neurological Disorders) 11(8): 976-983.

Jafri Ali, S. and P. Sharda Rajini (2012). "Elicitation of dopaminergic features of Parkinson's disease in C. elegans by monocrotophos, an organophosphorous insecticide." CNS and Neurological Disorders-Drug Targets (Formerly Current Drug Targets-CNS and Neurological Disorders) 11(8): 993-1000.

Jaga, K. and C. Dharmani (2003). "Global surveillance of DDT and DDE levels in human tissues." International Journal of Occupational Medicine and Environmental Health 16(1): 7-20.

Jagota, S. and J. Rajadas (2012). "Effect of phenolic compounds against Aβ aggregation and Aβ-induced toxicity in transgenic C. elegans." Neurochemical Research 37(1): 40-48.

Jagota, S. and J. Rajadas (2013). "Synthesis of d-amino acid peptides and their effect on beta-amyloid aggregation and toxicity in transgenic caenorhabditis elegans." Medicinal Chemistry Research 22(8): 3991-4000.

Jagwani, D. and J. Bhawsar (2015). "decision-making frameworks to predict ecological effects and environmental fate of chemical substances." Journal of Chemical and Pharmaceutical Research 7(8): 137-145.

Jahan, S., D. Kumar, A. Kumar, C. S. Rajpurohit, S. Singh, A. Srivastava, A. Pandey and A. Pant (2017). "Neurotrophic factor mediated neuronal differentiation of human cord blood mesenchymal stem cells and their applicability to assess the developmental neurotoxicity." Biochemical and Biophysical Research Communications 482(4): 961-967.

Jahan, S., D. Kumar, S. Singh, V. Kumar, A. Srivastava, A. Pandey, C. Rajpurohit, V. Khanna and A. Pant (2018). "Resveratrol Prevents the Cellular Damages Induced by Monocrotophos via PI3K Signaling Pathway in Human Cord Blood Mesenchymal Stem Cells." Molecular Neurobiology 55(11): 8278-8292.

Jahan, S., S. Singh, A. Srivastava, V. Kumar, D. Kumar, A. Pandey, C. Rajpurohit, A. Purohit, V. Khanna and A. Pant (2018). "PKA-GSK3β and β-catenin signaling play a critical role in trans-resveratrol mediated neuronal differentiation in human cord blood stem cells." Molecular Neurobiology 55(4): 2828-2839.

Jahangir, T. and S. Sultana (2007). "Perillyl alcohol protects against Fe-NTA-induced nephrotoxicity and early tumor promotional events in rat experimental model." Evidence-based Complementary and Alternative Medicine 4(4): 439-445.

Jain, A. K., D. Singh, K. Dubey, R. Maurya and A. K. Pandey (2019). "Zinc oxide nanoparticles induced gene mutation at the HGPRT locus and cell cycle arrest associated with apoptosis in V-79 cells." Journal of Applied Toxicology. 39(5):735-750.

Jain, A. K., N. K. Swarnakar, C. Godugu, R. P. Singh and S. Jain (2011). "The effect of the oral administration of polymeric nanoparticles on the efficacy and toxicity of tamoxifen." Biomaterials 32(2): 503-515.

Jain, A. K., K. Thanki and S. Jain (2013). "Co-encapsulation of tamoxifen and quercetin in polymeric nanoparticles: implications on oral bioavailability, antitumor efficacy, and drug-induced toxicity." Molecular Pharmaceutics 10(9): 3459-3474.

Jain, K., N. Kumar Mehra and N. K Jain (2015). "Nanotechnology in drug delivery: safety and toxicity issues." Current Pharmaceutical Design 21(29): 4252-4261.

Jain, R., M. K. Gupta, A. Chauhan, V. Pandey and M. K. Reddy Mudiam (2015). "Ultrasound-assisted dispersive liquid–liquid microextraction followed by GC–MS/MS analysis for the determination of valproic acid in urine samples." Bioanalysis 7(19): 2451-2459.

Jain, S. and S. Dave (1986). "Working Manual-1 on 'The Health Problems of Bhopal Gas Victims: Assessment and Management'." Indian Council of Medical Research, New Delhi.

Jain, S., G. Sepaha, K. Khare and V. Dubey (1980). "Ventilatory functions and sputum cytology in slate pencil workers silicosis." The Indian Journal of Chest Diseases and Allied Sciences 22(2): 103-109.

Jain, S., G. Sepaho, K. Khare and V. Dubey (1977). "Silicosis in Slate Pencil Workers: A Clinicoradiologic Study." Chest 71(3): 423-426.

Jain, S., G. Spandana, A. K. Agrawal, V. Kushwah and K. Thanki (2015). "Enhanced antitumor efficacy and reduced toxicity of docetaxel loaded estradiol functionalized stealth polymeric nanoparticles." Molecular Pharmaceutics 12(11): 3871-3884.

Jain, S., V. S. Thakare, M. Das, C. Godugu, A. K. Jain, R. Mathur, K. Chuttani and A. K. Mishra (2011). "Toxicity of multiwalled carbon nanotubes with end defects critically depends on their functionalization density." Chemical Research in Toxicology 24(11): 2028-2039.

Jamal, F., Q. Haque and S. Singh (2016). "The influence of pesticides on hepatic and renal functions in occupational sprayers of rural Malihabad, Lucknow (India)." Toxicology 1: 2-7.

Jamdade, V. S., N. Sethi, N. A. Mundhe, P. Kumar, M. Lahkar and N. Sinha (2015). "Therapeutic targets of triple-negative breast cancer: a review." British Journal of Pharmacology 172(17): 4228-4237.

Jameel, A. A. (2002). "Evaluation of drinking water quality in Tiruchirapalli, Tamil Nadu." Indian Journal of Environmental Health 44(2): 108-112.

Jamil, K., G. P. Das, A. P. Shaik, S. S. Dharmi and S. Murthy (2007). "Epidemiological studies of pesticide-exposed individuals and their clinical implications." Current Science: 340-345.

Jayant, K., V. Balakrishnan, L. Sanghvi and D. Jussawalla (1977). "Quantification of the role of smoking and chewing tobacco in oral, pharyngeal, and oesophageal cancers." British Journal of Cancer 35(2): 232.

Jayaprabha, K. and K. Suresh (2016). "Endosulfan contamination in water: a review on to an efficient method for its removal." Journal of Chemical Sciences 6: 182-191.

Jayatilake, N., S. Mendis, P. Maheepala and F. R. Mehta (2013). "Chronic kidney disease of uncertain aetiology: prevalence and causative factors in a developing country." BMC Nephrology 14(1): 180.

Jena, G. and S. Bhunya (1994). "Mutagenicity of an organophosphate insecticide acephate—an *in vivo* study in chicks." Mutagenesis 9(4): 319-324.

Jha, V., G. Garcia-Garcia, K. Iseki, Z. Li, S. Naicker, B. Plattner, R. Saran, A. Y.-M. Wang and C.-W. Yang (2013). "Chronic kidney disease: global dimension and perspectives." The Lancet 382(9888): 260-272.

Jindal, S. K. (2013). "Silicosis in India: past and present." Current Opinion in Pulmonary Medicine 19(2): 163-168.

Jindal, S. K., A. Aggarwal, D. Gupta, R. Agarwal, R. Kumar, T. Kaur, K. Chaudhry and B. Shah (2012). "Indian study on epidemiology of asthma, respiratory symptoms and chronic bronchitis in adults (INSEARCH)." The International Journal of Tuberculosis and Lung Disease 16(9): 1270-1277.

Jindal, S. K., A. N. Aggarwal and D. Gupta (2001). "Dust-induced interstitial lung disease in the tropics." Current Opinion in Pulmonary Medicine 7(5): 272-277.

Johri, A., A. Dhawan, R. L. Singh and D. Parmar (2006). "Effect of prenatal exposure of deltamethrin on the ontogeny of xenobiotic metabolizing cytochrome P450s in the brain and liver of offsprings." Toxicology and Applied Pharmacology 214(3): 279-289.

Johri, A., A. Dhawan, R. L. Singh and D. Parmar (2007). "Persistence in alterations in the ontogeny of cerebral and hepatic cytochrome P450s following prenatal exposure to low doses of lindane." Toxicological Sciences 101(2): 331-340.

Johri, A., S. Yadav, A. Dhawan and D. Parmar (2007). "Overexpression of cerebral and hepatic cytochrome P450s alters behavioral activity of rat offspring following prenatal exposure to lindane." Toxicology and Applied Pharmacology 225(3): 278-292.

Johri, A., S. Yadav, R. L. Singh, A. Dhawan, M. Ali and D. Parmar (2006). "Long lasting effects of prenatal exposure to deltamethrin on cerebral and hepatic cytochrome P450s and behavioral activity in rat offspring." European Journal of Pharmacology 544(1-3): 58-68.

Jones, W. R. (1933). "Silicotic lungs: the minerals they contain." Epidemiology and Infection 33(3): 307-329.

Joshi, M., Y. Verma, A. Gautam, G. Parmar, B. Lakkad and S. Kumar (2011). "Cytogenetic alterations in buccal mucosa cells of chewers of areca nut and tobacco." Archives of Oral Biology 56(1): 63-67.

Joshi, P. (1989). "Ultraviolet radiation-induced photodegradation and $1O_2$, O2-. production by riboflavin, lumichrome and lumiflavin." Indian Journal of Biochemistry and Biophysics 26(3): 186-189.

Joshi, P. C. (1985). "Comparison of the DNA-damaging property of photosensitised riboflavin via singlet oxygen (1O2) and superoxide radical (O2−) mechanisms." Toxicology Letters 26 (2-3): 211-217.

Joshi, P. C. and R. Misra (1986). "Evaluation of chemically-induced phototoxicity to aquatic organism using Paramecium as a model." Biochemical and Biophysical Research Communications 139(1): 79-84.

Joshi, R., H. Janagama, H. P. Dwivedi, T. S. Kumar, L.-A. Jaykus, J. Schefers and S. Sreevatsan (2009). "Selection, characterization, and application of DNA aptamers for the capture and detection of Salmonella enterica serovars." Molecular and Cellular Probes 23(1): 20-28.

Junaid, M., D. Chowdhuri and R. N. R. S. D. Saxena (1997). "Lead-induced changes in ovarian follicular development and maturation in mice." Journal of Toxicology and Environmental Health Part A 50(1): 31-40.

Junaid, M., R. Murthy and D. Saxena (1995). "Chromium fetotoxicity in mice during late pregnancy." Veterinary and Human Toxicology 37(4): 320-323.

Junaid, M., R. Murthy and D. Saxena (1996). "Embryo - and fetotoxicity of chromium in pregestationally exposed mice." Bulletin of Environmental Contamination and Toxicology 57(2): 327-334.

Junaid, M., R. C. Murthy and D. K. Saxena (1996). "Embryotoxicity of orally administered chromium in mice: exposure during the period of organogenesis." Toxicology Letters 84(3): 143-148.

Jussawalla, D. and V. Deshpande (1971). "Evaluation of cancer risk in tobacco chewers and smokers: an epidemiologic assessment." Cancer 28(1): 244-252.

Jyothi, P., M. P. Rudra and S. Rao (1998). "*In vivo* metabolism of β-N-oxalyl-L-α, β-diaminopropionic acid: the Lathyrus sativus neurotoxin in experimental animals." Natural Toxins 6(5): 189-195.

Jyoti, A., S. Ram, P. Vajpayee, G. Singh, P. D. Dwivedi, S. K. Jain and R. Shanker (2010). "Contamination of surface and potable water in South Asia by Salmonellae: Culture-independent quantification with molecular beacon real-time PCR." Science of the Total Environment 408(6): 1256-1263.

Jyoti, A., S. P. Singh, M. Yashpal, P. D. Dwivedi and R. Shanker (2011). "Rapid detection of enterotoxigenic Escherichia coli gene using bio-conjugated gold nano-particles." Journal of Biomedical Nanotechnology 7(1): 170-171.

Kala, S. V. and A. L. Jadhav (1995). "Low level lead exposure decreases *in vivo* release of dopamine in the rat nucleus accumbens: a microdialysis study." Journal of Neurochemistry 65(4): 1631-1635.

Kalahasthi, R., R. Hirehal Raghavendra Rao, R. Bagalur Krishna Murthy and M. Karuna Kumar (2006). "Effect of Cadmium Exposure on Serum Amylase Activity in Cadmium Electroplating Workers." Environmental Bioindicators 1(4): 260-267.

Kalahasthi, R., R. Tapu Barman, B. S. Bagepally and R. Beerappa (2016). "Effectiveness of interventions on biological monitoring among workers exposed to Pb from lead-acid storage battery plant." International Journal of Medical Science and Public Health 5(09): 1770.

Kalaiselvan, V., P. Thota and G. N. Singh (2016). "Pharmacovigilance Programme of India: Recent developments and future perspectives." Indian Journal of Pharmacology 48(6): 624.

Kalaria, D., G. Sharma, V. Beniwal and M. R. Kumar (2009). "Design of biodegradable nanoparticles for oral delivery of doxorubicin: *in vivo* pharmacokinetics and toxicity studies in rats." Pharmaceutical Research 26(3): 492-501.

Kalayarasan, S., P. N. Prabhu, N. Sriram, R. Manikandan, M. Arumugam and G. Sudhandiran (2009). "Diallyl sulfide enhances antioxidants and inhibits inflammation through the activation of Nrf2 against gentamicin-induced nephrotoxicity in Wistar rats." European Journal of Pharmacology 606(1-3): 162-171.

Kale, A., S. Kulkarni, G. Joglekar and J. Balwani (1966). "Effect of Liv. 52 on growth and alcohol induced hepatic dysfunction in rats." Current Medical Practice 10: 240.

Kale, S., N. Murthy, K. Raghu, P. Sherkhane and F. Carvalho (1999). "Studies on degradation of 14C-DDT in the marine environment." Chemosphere 39(6): 959-968.

Kamat, S., A. Mahashur, A. K. Tiwari, P. Potdar, M. Gaur, V. Kolhatkar, P. Vaidya, D. Parmar, R. Rupwate and T. Chatterjee (1985). "Early observations on pulmonary changes and clinical morbidity due to the isocyanate gas leak at Bhopal." Journal of Postgraduate Medicine 31(2): 63-72.

Kamboj, A., R. Kiran and R. Sandhir (2006). "Carbofuran-induced neurochemical and neurobehavioral alterations in rats: attenuation by N-acetylcysteine." Experimental Brain Research 170(4): 567.

Kamboj, S. S., V. Kumar, A. Kamboj and R. Sandhir (2008). "Mitochondrial oxidative stress and dysfunction in rat brain induced by carbofuran exposure." Cellular and Molecular Neurobiology 28(7): 961-969.

Kandinov, B., N. Giladi and A. D. Korczyn (2009). "Smoking and tea consumption delay onset of Parkinson's disease." Parkinsonism and Related Disorders 15(1): 41-46.

Kanthasamy, A., H. Jin, V. Anantharam, G. Sondarva, V. Rangasamy, A. Rana and A. Kanthasamy (2012). "Emerging neurotoxic mechanisms in environmental factors-induced neurodegeneration." Neurotoxicology 33(4): 833-837.

Kapil, A. and S. Sharma (1997). "Immunopotentiating compounds from Tinospora cordifolia." Journal of Ethnopharmacology 58(2): 89-95.

Kapley, A., H. J. Purohit, S. Chhatre, R. Shanker, T. Chakrabarti and P. Khanna (1999). "Osmotolerance and hydrocarbon degradation by a genetically engineered microbial consortium." Bioresource Technology 3(67): 241-245.

Kapoor, N., A. B. Pant, A. Dhawan, U. N. Dwievedi, Y. K. Gupta, P. K. Seth and D. Parmar (2006). "Differences in sensitivity of cultured rat brain neuronal and glial cytochrome P450 2E1 to ethanol." Life Sciences 79(16): 1514-1522.

Kapoor, N., A. B. Pant, A. Dhawan, U. N. Dwievedi, P. K. Seth and D. Parmar (2006). "Cytochrome P450 1A isoenzymes in brain cells: Expression and inducibility in cultured rat brain neuronal and glial cells." Life Sciences 79(25): 2387-2394.

Kapoor, R. and P. Kakkar (2012). "Protective role of morin, a flavonoid, against high glucose induced oxidative stress mediated apoptosis in primary rat hepatocytes." PLoS One 7(8): e41663.

Kar, S. and P. Dhara (2007). "An evaluation of musculoskeletal disorder and socioeconomic status of farmers in West Bangal, India." Nepal Medical College Journal 9(4): 245-249.

Kar, S. and K. Roy (2010). "QSAR modeling of toxicity of diverse organic chemicals to Daphnia magna using 2D and 3D descriptors." Journal of Hazardous Materials 177(1-3): 344-351.

Karar, K. and A. Gupta (2006). "Seasonal variations and chemical characterization of ambient PM10 at residential and industrial sites of an urban region of Kolkata (Calcutta), India." Atmospheric Research 81(1): 36-53.

Karar, K. and A. Gupta (2007). "Source apportionment of PM10 at residential and industrial sites of an urban region of Kolkata, India." Atmospheric Research 84(1): 30-41.

Karekar, V., S. Joshi and S. Shinde (2000). "Antimutagenic profile of three antioxidants in the Ames assay and the Drosophila wing spot test." Mutation Research/Genetic Toxicology and Environmental Mutagenesis 468(2): 183-194.

Karmakar, R., R. Bhattacharya and M. Chatterjee (2000). "Biochemical, haematological and histopathological study in relation to time-related cadmium-induced hepatotoxicity in mice." Biometals 13(3): 231-239.

Karthikeyan, S. (2005). "Isoniazid and rifampicin treatment on phospholipids and their subfractions in liver tissue of rabbits." Drug and Chemical Toxicology 28(3): 273-280.

Karunakaran, C. (1958). "The Kerala food poisoning." Journal of the Indian Medical Association 31(5): 204-207.

Karunasagar, D., M. B. Krishna, Y. Anjaneyulu and J. Arunachalam (2006). "Studies of mercury pollution in a lake due to a thermometer factory situated in a tourist resort: Kodaikkanal, India." Environmental Pollution 143(1): 153-158.

Kashyap, M., A. Singh, M. Siddiqui, V. Kumar, V. Tripathi, V. Khanna, S. Yadav, S. Jain and A. Pant (2010). "Caspase cascade regulated mitochondria mediated apoptosis in monocrotophos exposed PC12 cells." Chemical Research in Toxicology 23(11): 1663-1672.

Kashyap, M. P., V. Kumar, A. K. Singh, V. K. Tripathi, S. Jahan, A. Pandey, R. K. Srivastava, V. K. Khanna and A. B. Pant (2015). "Differentiating neurons derived from human umbilical cord blood stem cells work as a test system for developmental neurotoxicity." Molecular Neurobiology 51(2): 791-807.

Kashyap, M. P., A. K. Singh, V. Kumar, V. K. Tripathi, R. K. Srivastava, M. Agrawal, V. K. Khanna, S. Yadav, S. K. Jain and A. B. Pant (2011). "Monocrotophos induced apoptosis in PC12 cells: role of xenobiotic metabolizing cytochrome P450s." PLoS One 6(3): e17757.

Kashyap, M. P., A. K. Singh, V. Kumar, D. K. Yadav, F. Khan, S. Jahan, V. K. Khanna, S. Yadav and A. B. Pant (2012). "Pkb/Akt1 mediates Wnt/GSK3β/β-catenin signaling-induced apoptosis in human cord blood stem cells exposed to organophosphate pesticide monocrotophos." Stem Cells and Development 22(2): 224-238.

Kashyap, M. P., A. K. Singh, D. K. Yadav, M. A. Siddiqui, R. K. Srivastava, V. Chaturvedi and N. Rai (2015). "4-Hydroxy-trans-2-nonenal (4-HNE) induces neuronal SH-SY5Y cell death via hampering ATP binding at kinase domain of Akt1." Archives of Toxicology 89(2): 243-258.

Kasturiratne, A., A. R. Wickremasinghe, N. de Silva, N. K. Gunawardena, A. Pathmeswaran, R. Premaratna, L. Savioli, D. G. Lalloo and H. J. de Silva (2008). "The global burden of snakebite: a literature analysis and modelling based on regional estimates of envenoming and deaths." PLoS Medicine 5(11): e218.

Katyare, S. S. and J. G. Satav (1989). "Impaired mitochondrial oxidative energy metabolism following paracetamol-induced hepatotoxicity in the rat." British Journal of Pharmacology 96(1): 51-58.

Kaur, S., K. Senthilkumar, V. Verma, B. Kumar, S. Kumar, J. K. Katnoria and C. Sharma (2013). "Preliminary analysis of polycyclic aromatic hydrocarbons in air particles (PM10) in Amritsar, India: sources, apportionment, and possible risk implications to humans." Archives of Environmental Contamination and Toxicology 65(3): 382-395.

Kaushik, A., A. Kansal, S. Kumari and C. Kaushik (2009). "Heavy metal contamination of river Yamuna, Haryana, India: assessment by metal enrichment factor of the sediments." Journal of Hazardous Materials 164(1): 265-270.

Kaushik, G., A. Chel, S. Patil and S. Chaturvedi (2018). "Status of Particulate Matter Pollution in India: A Review." Handbook of Environmental Materials Management: 1-28.

Kaw, J., A. Khanna and M. Waseem (1990). "Modification of pulmonary silicotic reaction in rats exposed to coal fly ash." Experimental Pathology 39(1): 49-57.

Kaw, J. and S. Zaidi (1970). "Pathogenesis of pulmonary silicosis in rats fed stock and multi-deficient diet since weaning." Environmental Research 3(3): 199-211.

Kazi, A. I. and A. Oommen (2012). "The effect of acute severe monocrotophos poisoning on inhibition, expression and activity of acetylcholinesterase in different rat brain regions." Neurotoxicology 33(5): 1284-1290.

Kazi, A. I. and A. Oommen (2014). "Chronic noise stress-induced alterations of glutamate and gamma-aminobutyric acid and their metabolism in the rat brain." Noise and Health 16(73): 343.

Kesavachandran, C. and M. Mudiam (2010). "Adverse sub-clinical health effects in pesticide-exposed population: challenges and need for developing non-invasive clinical biomarkers." Current Science 99(12).

Kesavachandran, C., B. Pangtey, V. Bihari, M. Fareed, M. Pathak, A. Srivastava and N. Mathur (2013). "Particulate matter concentration in ambient air and its effects on lung functions among residents in the National Capital Region, India." Environmental Monitoring and Assessment 185(2): 1265-1272.

Kesavachandran, C., M. Pathak, M. Fareed, V. Bihari, N. Mathur and A. Srivastava (2009). "Health risks of employees working in pesticide retail shops: an exploratory study." Indian Journal of Occupational and Environmental Medicine 13(3): 121.

Kesavachandran, C., V. K. Singh, N. Mathur, S. Rastogi, M. Siddiqui, M. Reddy, R. Bharti and A. M. Khan (2006). "Possible mechanism of pesticide toxicity-related oxidative stress leading to airway narrowing." Redox Report 11(4): 159-162.

Kesavachandran, C. N., M. Fareed, M. K. Pathak, V. Bihari, N. Mathur and A. K. Srivastava (2009). Adverse health effects of pesticides in agrarian populations of developing countries. Reviews of Environmental Contamination and Toxicology 200, 33-52.

Kesavachandran, C. N., S. K. Rastogi, N. Mathur, M. K. J. Siddiqui, V. K. Singh, V. Bihari and R. S. Bharti (2008). "Health status among pesticide applicators at a mango plantation in India." Journal of Pesticide Safety Education 8: 1-9.

Khairnar, S. I., U. B. Mahajan, K. R. Patil, H. M. Patel, S. D. Shinde, S. N. Goyal, S. Belemkar, S. Ojha and C. R. Patil (2019). "Disulfiram and its Copper Chelate Attenuate Cisplatin-Induced Acute Nephrotoxicity in Rats Via Reduction of Oxidative Stress and Inflammation." Biological Trace Element Research: 1-11.

Khan, A. J., G. Choudhuri, Q. Husain and D. Parmar (2009). "Polymorphism in glutathione-S-transferases: a risk factor in alcoholic liver cirrhosis." Drug and Alcohol Dependence 101(3): 183-190.

Khan, A. J., Q. Husain, G. Choudhuri and D. Parmar (2010). "Association of polymorphism in alcohol dehydrogenase and interaction with other genetic risk factors with alcoholic liver cirrhosis." Drug and Alcohol Dependence 109(1-3): 190-197.

Khan, A. J., M. Ruwali, G. Choudhuri, N. Mathur, Q. Husain and D. Parmar (2009). "Polymorphism in cytochrome P450 2E1 and interaction with other genetic risk factors and susceptibility to alcoholic liver cirrhosis." Mutation Research/ Fundamental and Molecular Mechanisms of Mutagenesis 664(1-2): 55-63.

Khan, A. J., A. Sharma, G. Choudhuri and D. Parmar (2011). "Induction of blood lymphocyte cytochrome P450 2E1 in early stage alcoholic liver cirrhosis." Alcohol 45(1): 81-87.

Khan, F. H., K. Ambreen, G. Fatima and S. Kumar (2012). "Assessment of health risks with reference to oxidative stress and DNA damage in chromium exposed population." Science of the Total Environment 430: 68-74.

Khan, H., R. D. Singh, R. Tiwari, S. Gangopadhyay, S. K. Roy, D. Singh and V. Srivastava (2017). "Mercury exposure induces cytoskeleton disruption and loss of renal function through epigenetic modulation of MMP9 expression." Toxicology 386: 28-39.

Khan, J. A., B. Pillai, T. K. Das, Y. Singh and S. Maiti (2007). "Molecular effects of uptake of gold nanoparticles in HeLa cells." ChemBio Chem 8(11): 1237-1240.

Khan, M. A. and J. Musarrat (2002). "Tetracycline–Cu (II) photo-induced fragmentation of serum albumin." Comparative Biochemistry and Physiology Part C: Toxicology and Pharmacology 131(4): 439-446.

Khan, M. A., S. Muzammil and J. Musarrat (1998). "Interactions of photosensitized tetracycline with serum albumin." IUBMB Life 46(5): 943-950.

Khan, M. B., M. N. Hoda, S. Yousuf, T. Ishrat, M. Ahmad, A. S. Ahmad, S. H. Alavi, N. Haque and F. Islam (2006). "Prevention of cognitive impairments and neurodegeneration by Khamira Abresham Hakim Arshad Wala." Journal of Ethnopharmacology 108(1): 68-73.

Khan, M. M., A. Ahmad, T. Ishrat, M. B. Khan, M. N. Hoda, G. Khuwaja, S. S. Raza, A. Khan, H. Javed and K. Vaibhav (2010). "Resveratrol attenuates 6-hydroxydopamine-induced oxidative damage and dopamine depletion in rat model of Parkinson's disease." Brain Research 1328: 139-151.

Khan, M. M., M. N. Hoda, T. Ishrat, A. Ahmad, M. B. Khan, G. Khuwaja, S. S. Raza, M. M. Safhi and F. Islam (2010). "Amelioration of 1-methyl-4-phenyl-1, 2, 3, 6-tetrahydropyridine-induced behavioural dysfunction and oxidative stress by Pycnogenol in mouse model of Parkinson's disease." Behavioural Pharmacology 21(5-6): 563-571.

Khan, M. W. A. and M. Ahmad (2006). "Detoxification and bioremediation potential of a Pseudomonas fluorescens isolate against the major Indian water pollutants." Journal of Environmental Science and Health, Part A 41(4): 659-674.

Khan, N., S. Sharma and S. Sultana (2003). "Nigella sativa (black cumin) ameliorates potassium bromate-induced early events of carcinogenesis: diminution of oxidative stress." Human and Experimental Toxicology 22(4): 193-203.

Khan, N., S. Sharma and S. Sultana (2004). "Attenuation of potassium bromate-induced nephrotoxicity by coumarin (1, 2-benzopyrone) in Wistar rats: chemoprevention against free radical-mediated renal oxidative stress and tumor promotion response." Redox Report 9(1): 19-28.

Khan, N. and S. Sultana (2005). "Chemomodulatory effect of Ficus racemosa extract against chemically induced renal carcinogenesis and oxidative damage response in Wistar rats." Life Sciences 77(11): 1194-1210.

Khan, N. and S. Sultana (2005). "Inhibition of potassium bromate-induced renal oxidative stress and hyperproliferative response by Nymphaea alba in Wistar rats." Journal of Enzyme Inhibition and Medicinal Chemistry 20(3): 275-283.

Khan, P. and S. Sinha (1996). "Ameliorating effect of vitamin C on murine sperm toxicity induced by three pesticides (endosulfan, phosphamidon and mancozeb)." Mutagenesis 11(1): 33-36.

Khan, S., S. Bhartia and S. Roy (2014). "Multiple Drug Induced Hypersensitivity Syndrome Reactions in a Patient with Drugs that Have Known HLA Associations for Reactions." General Medicine 2(133): 2.

Khan, S., T. Bhatia, P. Trivedi, G. Satyanarayana, K. Mandrah, P. N. Saxena, M. K. R. Mudiam and S. K. Roy (2016). "Selective solid-phase extraction using molecularly imprinted polymer as a sorbent for the analysis of fenarimol in food samples." Food Chemistry 199: 870-875.

Khan, S. and K. Pandya (1980). "Biochemical studies on the toxicity of n-octane and n-nonane." Environmental Research 22(2): 271-276.

Khan, S. A. and S. A. Ali (1993). "Assessment of certain hematological responses of factory workers exposed to pesticides." Bulletin of Environmental Contamination and Toxicology 51(5): 740-747.

Khan, S. A., S. Priyamvada, N. Farooq, S. Khan, M. W. Khan and A. N. Yusufi (2009). "Protective effect of green tea extract on gentamicin-induced nephrotoxicity and oxidative damage in rat kidney." Pharmacological Research 59(4): 254-262.

Khandelwal, S., M. Ashquin and S. Tandon (1984). "Influence of essential elements on manganese intoxication." Bulletin of Environmental Contamination and Toxicology 32(1): 10-19.

Khandelwal, S., D. Kachru and S. Tandon (1980). "Chelation in metal intoxication IX. Influence of amino and thiol chelators on excretion of manganese in poisoned rabbits." Toxicology Letters 6(3): 131-135.

Khandkar, M. A., D. V. Parmar, M. Das and S. S. Katyare (1996). "Is Activation of Lysosomal Enzymes Responsible for Paracetamol-induced Hepatotoxicity and Nephrotoxicity?" Journal of Pharmacy and Pharmacology 48(4): 437-440.

Khangarot, B. and R. Rathore (1999). "Copper exposure reduced the resistance of the catfish Saccobranchus fossilis to Aeromonas hydrophila infection." Bulletin of Environmental Contamination and Toxicology 62(4): 490-495.

Khangarot, B., R. Rathore and D. Tripathi (1999). "Effects of chromium on humoral and cell-mediated immune responses and host resistance to disease in a freshwater catfish, Saccobranchus fossilis (Bloch)." Ecotoxicology and Environmental Safety 43(1): 11-20.

Khanna, S. (1991). "Toxicity, carcinogenic potencial and clinicoepidemiological studies on dyes and dye intermedites." Journal of Scientific and Industrial Research 50: 965-974.

Khanna, S., P. Tewari, A. Joshi and G. Singh (1987). "Studies on the skin uptake and efflux kinetics of N-phenyl-p-phenylenediamine: an aromatic amine intermediate." International Journal of Cosmetic Science 9(3): 137.

Khanna, V. K., R. Husain, J. P. Hanig and P. K. Seth (1991). "Increased neurobehavioral toxicity of styrene in protein-malnourished rats." Neurotoxicology and Teratology 13(2): 153-159.

Khanna, V. K., R. Husain and P. Seth (1988). "Low protein diet modifies acrylamide neurotoxicity." Toxicology 49(2-3): 395-401.

Khanna, V. K., R. Husain and P. K. Seth (1994). "Effect of protein malnutrition on the neurobehavioural toxicity of styrene in young rats." Journal of Applied Toxicology 14(5): 351-356.

Khare, P., M. Sonane, Y. Nagar, N. Moin, S. Ali, K. C. Gupta and A. Satish (2015). "Size dependent toxicity of zinc oxide nano-particles in soil nematode Caenorhabditis elegans." Nanotoxicology 9(4): 423-432.

Khare, P., M. Sonane, R. Pandey, S. Ali, K. C. Gupta and A. Satish (2011). "Adverse effects of TiO_2 and ZnO nanoparticles in soil nematode, Caenorhabditis elegans." Journal of Biomedical Nanotechnology 7(1): 116-117.

Khatoon, I., P. Vajpayee, G. Singh, A. K. Pandey, A. Dhawan, K. Gupta and R. Shanker (2011). "Determination of internalization of chromium oxide nano-particles in Escherichia coli by flow cytometry." Journal of Biomedical Nanotechnology 7(1): 168-169.

Khatri, D. K. and A. R. Juvekar (2016). "Abrogation of locomotor impairment in a rotenone-induced Drosophila melanogaster and zebrafish model of Parkinson's disease by ellagic acid and curcumin." International Journal of Nutrition, Pharmacology, Neurological Diseases 6(2): 90.

Khillare, P. S. and S. Sarkar (2012). "Airborne inhalable metals in residential areas of Delhi, India: distribution, source apportionment and health risks." Atmospheric Pollution Research 3(1): 46-54.

Kirkland, D., P. Kasper, L. Müller, R. Corvi and G. Speit (2008). "Recommended lists of genotoxic and non-genotoxic chemicals for assessment of the performance of new or improved genotoxicity tests: a follow-up to an ECVAM workshop." Mutation Research/Genetic Toxicology and Environmental Mutagenesis 653(1-2): 99-108.

Kirtikar, K. and B. Basu (1987). "Indian Medicinal Plants. International Book Distributors, Dehradun." Volume I-IV.

Kohli, E., H. G. Raj, R. Kumari, V. Rohil, N. K. Kaushik, A. K. Prasad and V. S. Parmar (2002). "Comparison of the prevention of aflatoxin B1-induced genotoxicity by quercetin and quercetin pentaacetate." Bioorganic and Medicinal Chemistry Letters 12(18): 2579-2582.

Koner, B., B. Banerjee and A. Ray (1997). "Effects of *in-vivo* generation of oxygen free radicals on immune responsiveness in rabbits." Immunology Letters 59(3): 127-131.

Koner, B., B. Banerjee and A. Ray (1998). "Organochlorine pesticide-induced oxidative stress and immune suppression in rats." Indian Journal of Experimental Biology 36(4): 395-398.

Kori, R. K., R. S. Thakur, R. Kumar and R. S. Yadav (2018). "Assessment of Adverse Health Effects Among Chronic Pesticide-Exposed Farm Workers in Sagar District of Madhya Pradesh, India." International Journal of Nutrition, Pharmacology, Neurological Diseases 8(4): 153.

Kornhauser, A., W. Warner and L. Lambert (1996). Cellular and molecular events following ultraviolet irradiation of skin, Taylor & Francis, Washington: 189-220.

Krishnan, A., R. Sonawane and D. Karnad (2007). "Captopril in the treatment of cardiovascular manifestations of Indian red scorpion (Mesobuthus tamulus concanesis Pocock) envenomation." JAPI 55: 22-26.

Kuhad, A. and K. Chopra (2009). "Attenuation of diabetic nephropathy by tocotrienol: involvement of NFkB signaling pathway." Life Sciences 84(9-10): 296-301.

Kuhad, A., S. Pilkhwal, S. Sharma, N. Tirkey and K. Chopra (2007). "Effect of curcumin on inflammation and oxidative stress in cisplatin-induced experimental nephrotoxicity." Journal of Agricultural and Food Chemistry 55(25): 10150-10155.

Kulkarni, G. (2007). "Prevention and control of silicosis: A national challenge." Indian Journal of Occupational and Environmental Medicine 11(3): 95.

Kulkarni, J. and A. Khanna (2006). "Functional hepatocyte-like cells derived from mouse embryonic stem cells: a novel *in vitro* hepatotoxicity model for drug screening." Toxicology *In Vitro* 20(6): 1014-1022.

Kulkarni, M., M. Zaheeruddin, N. Shenoy and H. Vani (2006). "Fetal valproate syndrome." The Indian Journal of Pediatrics 73(10): 937-939.

Kulkarni, P. and C. Venkataraman (2000). "Atmospheric polycyclic aromatic hydrocarbons in Mumbai, India." Atmospheric Environment 34(17): 2785-2790.

Kumar, A. (2011). "Past, present and future of pharmacovigilance in India." Systematic Reviews in Pharmacy 2(1): 55-55.

Kumar, A., I. Ahmad, S. Shukla, B. K. Singh, D. K. Patel, H. P. Pandey and C. Singh (2010). "Effect of zinc and paraquat co-exposure on neurodegeneration: modulation of oxidative stress and expression of metallothioneins, toxicant responsive and transporter genes in rats." Free Radical Research 44(8): 950-965.

Kumar, A., A. Baroth, I. Soni, P. Bhatnagar and P. John (2006). "Organochlorine pesticide residues in milk and blood of women from Anupgarh, Rajasthan, India." Environmental Monitoring and Assessment 116(1-3): 1-7.

Kumar, A., F. Husain, M. Das and S. Khanna (1992). "An out-break of epidemic dropsy in the Barabanki District of Uttar Pradesh, India: a limited trial for the scope of antioxidants in the management of symptoms." Biomedical and Environmental Sciences: BES 5(3): 251.

Kumar, A., P. Misra, R. Mehotra, Y. Govil and G. Rana (1991). "Hepatotoxicity of rifampin and isoniazid." The American Review of Respiratory Disease 143: 1350.

Kumar, A., A. Pandey, S. Singh, R. Shanker and A. Dhawan (2011). "Cellular uptake and mutagenic potential of metal oxide nanoparticles in bacterial cells." Chemosphere 83(8): 1124-1132.

Kumar, A., A. K. Pandey, S. S. Singh, R. Shanker and A. Dhawan (2011). "Cellular response to metal oxide nanoparticles in bacteria." Journal of Biomedical Nanotechnology 7(1): 102-103.

Kumar, A., A. K. Pandey, S. S. Singh, R. Shanker and A. Dhawan (2011). "Cellular uptake and mutagenic potential of metal oxide nanoparticles in bacterial cells." Chemosphere 83(8): 1124-1132.

Kumar, A., A. K. Pandey, S. S. Singh, R. Shanker and A. Dhawan (2011). "Engineered ZnO and TiO₂ nanoparticles induce oxidative stress and DNA damage leading to reduced viability of Escherichia coli." Free Radical Biology and Medicine 51(10): 1872-1881.

Kumar, A., D. Sasmal and N. Sharma (2014). "Deltamethrin induced an apoptogenic signalling pathway in murine thymocytes: exploring the molecular mechanism." Journal of Applied Toxicology 34(12): 1303-1310.

Kumar, A., D. Sasmal and N. Sharma (2015). "Immunomodulatory role of piperine in deltamethrin induced thymic apoptosis and altered immune functions." Environmental Toxicology and Pharmacology 39(2): 504-514.

Kumar, A., A. Sushama, V. Rohil, S. Manral, S. Gangopadhyay, A. K. Prasad, H. G. Raj and V. S. Parmar (2011). "Prevention of benzene-induced genotoxicity in bone marrow and lung cells: superiority of polyphenolic acetates to polyphenols." Archives of Toxicology 85(9): 1141-1150.

Kumar, A. P. and D. Subrahmanyam (2013). "Acute reversible Parkinsonism following accidental exposure to organophosphate insecticide." International Journal of Nutrition, Pharmacology, Neurological Diseases 3(1): 70.

Kumar, A. V., R. Patil and K. Nambi (2001). "Source apportionment of suspended particulate matter at two traffic junctions in Mumbai, India." Atmospheric Environment 35(25): 4245-4251.

Kumar, B. and K. Krishnaswamy (1995). "Detection of sub-clinical lead toxicity in monocasters." Bulletin of Environmental Contamination and Toxicology 54(6): 863-869.

Kumar, B., C. Prasad and K. Krishnaswamy (1992). "Detection of rifampicin-induced nephrotoxicity by N-acetyl-3-D-glucosaminidase activity." The Journal of Tropical Medicine and Hygiene 95(6): 424-427.

Kumar, C. N., C. Andrade and P. Murthy (2009). "A randomized, double-blind comparison of lorazepam and chlordiazepoxide in patients with uncomplicated alcohol withdrawal." Journal of Studies on Alcohol and Drugs 70(3): 467-474.

Kumar, D., S. R. Salian, G. Kalthur, S. Uppangala, S. Kumari, S. Challapalli, S. G. Chandraguthi, H. Krishnamurthy, N. Jain and P. Kumar (2013). "Semen abnormalities, sperm DNA damage and global hypermethylation in health workers occupationally exposed to ionizing radiation." PLoS One 8(7): e69927.

Kumar, J. and S. D'Souza (2010). "An optical microbial biosensor for detection of methyl parathion using Sphingomonas sp. immobilized on microplate as a reusable biocomponent." Biosensors and Bioelectronics 26(4): 1292-1296.

Kumar, K. K., B. U. Devi and P. Neeraja (2017). "Integration of *in silico* approaches to determination of endocrine-disrupting perfluorinated chemicals binding potency with steroidogenic acute regulatory protein." Biochemical and Biophysical Research Communications 491(4): 1007-1014.

Kumar, K. M., M. M. Aruldhas, S. L. Banu, B. Sadasivam, G. Vengatesh, K. M. Ganesh, S. Navaneethabalakrishnan, A. K. Navin, F. M. Michael and S.

Venkatachalam (2017). "Male reproductive toxicity of CrVI: In-utero exposure to CrVI at the critical window of testis differentiation represses the expression of Sertoli cell tight junction proteins and hormone receptors in adult F1 progeny rats." Reproductive Toxicology 69: 84-98.

Kumar, M., P. Dwivedi, A. Sharma, A. Telang, R. Patil and N. Singh (2010). "Immunotoxicity of Ochratoxin and Citrinin in New Zealand White rabbits." World Rabbit Science 16(1).

Kumar, M., P. Dwivedi, A. K. Sharma, M. Sankar, R. D. Patil and N. D. Singh (2014). "Apoptosis and lipid peroxidation in ochratoxin A and citrinin-induced nephrotoxicity in rabbits." Toxicology and Industrial Health 30(1): 90-98.

Kumar, M. R., S. Flora and G. Reddy (2013). "Monoisoamyl 2, 3-dimercaptosuccinic acid attenuates arsenic induced toxicity: behavioral and neurochemical approach." Environmental Toxicology and Pharmacology 36(1): 231-242.

Kumar, N. K. and P. K. Dua (2016). "Status of regulation on traditional medicine formulations and natural products: Whither is India?" Current Science 111(2): 293.

Kumar, P., C. C. Barua, K. Sulakhiya and R. K. Sharma (2017). "Curcumin ameliorates cisplatin-induced nephrotoxicity and potentiates its anticancer activity in SD rats: potential role of curcumin in breast cancer chemotherapy." Frontiers in Pharmacology 8: 132.

Kumar, P., N. B. Bolshette, V. S. Jamdade, N. A. Mundhe, K. K. Thakur, K. K. Saikia and M. Lahkar (2013). "Breast cancer status in India: an overview." Biomedicine and Preventive Nutrition 3(2): 177-183.

Kumar, P., H. Kalonia and A. Kumar (2010). "Cyclosporine A Attenuates 3-Nitropropionic Acid–Induced Huntington-Like Symptoms in Rats: Possible Nitric Oxide Mechanism." International Journal of Toxicology 29(3): 318-325.

Kumar, P., K. S. Prashanth, A. B. Gaikwad, M. Vij, C. C. Barua and B. Bezbaruah (2013). "Disparity in actions of rosiglitazone against cisplatin-induced nephrotoxicity in female Sprague-Dawley rats." Environmental Toxicology and Pharmacology 36(3): 883-890.

Kumar, P., G. Rai and S. Flora (1994). "Immunomodulation following zinc supplementation during chelation of lead in male rats." Biometals 7(1): 41-44.

Kumar, R., A. K. Agarwal and P. K. Seth (1995). "Free radical-generated neurotoxicity of 6-hydroxydopamine." Journal of Neurochemistry 64(4): 1703-1707.

Kumar, R., A. K. Agarwal and P. K. Seth (1996). "Oxidative stress-mediated neurotoxicity of cadmium." Toxicology Letters 89(1): 65-69.

Kumar, R., V. Bhatia, S. Khanal, V. Sreenivas, S. D. Gupta, S. K. Panda and S. K. Acharya (2010). "Antituberculosis therapy–induced acute liver failure: magnitude, profile, prognosis, and predictors of outcome." Hepatology 51(5): 1665-1674.

Kumar, R. and G. Gautam (2006). "Tobacco chewing and male infertility." Indian Journal of Urology 22(2): 161.

Kumar, R., P. Halder, S. K. Sahu, M. Kumar, M. Kumari, K. Jana, Z. Ghosh, P. Sharma, M. Kundu and J. Basu (2012). "Identification of a novel role of

ESAT-6-dependent miR-155 induction during infection of macrophages with *Mycobacterium tuberculosis*." Cellular Microbiology 14(10): 1620-1631.

Kumar, R., J. K. Nagar, H. Kumar, A. S. Kushwah, M. Meena, P. Kumar, N. Raj, M. Singhal and S. Gaur (2007). "Association of indoor and outdoor air pollutant level with respiratory problems among children in an industrial area of Delhi, India." Archives of Environmental and Occupational Health 62(2): 75-80.

Kumar, R., J. K. Nagar, H. Kumar, A. S. Kushwah, M. Meena, P. Kumar, N. Raj, M. Singhal and S. Gaur (2008). "Indoor air pollution and respiratory function of children in Ashok Vihar, Delhi: an exposure-response study." Asia Pacific Journal of Public Health 20(1): 36-48.

Kumar, R., N. Nagpure, B. Kushwaha, S. K. Srivastava and W. Lakra (2010). "Investigation of the genotoxicity of malathion to freshwater teleost fish Channa punctatus (Bloch) using the micronucleus test and comet assay." Archives of Environmental Contamination and Toxicology 58(1): 123-130.

Kumar, R., N. Pant and S. Srivastava (2000). "Chlorinated pesticides and heavy metals in human semen." International Journal of Andrology 23(3): 145-149.

Kumar, R. and R. Prasad (2014). "Smoking cessation: an update." Indian Journal of Chest Diseases and Allied Sciences 56: 161-169.

Kumar, S., P. Kumar, R. selh, R. Dwivedi and P. RAY (1988). "Effect of exposure to toxic gas on the population of Bhopal: Part I-Epidemiological, clinical, radiological & behavioral studies." Indian Journal of Experimental Biology 26: 149-160.

Kumar, S., S. Sahay and M. Sinha (1995). "Bioassay of distillery effluent on common guppy, Lebistes reticulatus (Peter)." Bulletin of Environmental Contamination and Toxicology 54(2): 309-316.

Kumar, S., A. Sharma, G. Singh, A. K. Verma, R. Roy, R. Gupta, A. Misra, A. Tripathi, K. M. Ansari and M. Das (2014). "Allergenic responses of green gram (Vigna radiata L. Millsp) proteins can be vitiated by induction of oral tolerance due to single acute dose in BALB/c mice." Food Research International 57: 130-141.

Kumar, S., V. R. Tripathi and S. K. Garg (2012). "Physicochemical and microbiological assessment of recreational and drinking waters." Environmental Monitoring and Assessment 184(5): 2691-2698.

Kumar, S., A. K. Verma, A. Sharma, D. Kumar, A. Tripathi, B. Chaudhari, M. Das, S. Jain and P. D. Dwivedi (2013). "Phytohemagglutinins augment red kidney bean (Phaseolus vulgaris L.) induced allergic manifestations." Journal of Proteomics 93: 50-64.

Kumar, S., A. K. Verma, A. Sharma, R. Roy, D. Kumar, B. Giridhar, A. Tripathi, B. P. Chaudhari, M. Das and S. Jain (2014). "Phaseolin: A 47.5 kDa protein of red kidney bean (Phaseolus vulgaris L.) plays a pivotal role in hypersensitivity induction." International Immunopharmacology 19(1): 178-190.

Kumar, V., A. K. Gupta, R. K. Shukla, V. K. Tripathi, S. Jahan, A. Pandey, A. Srivastava, M. Agrawal, S. Yadav and V. K. Khanna (2015). "Molecular

Mechanism of Switching of TrkA/p75 NTR Signaling in Monocrotophos Induced Neurotoxicity." Scientific Reports 5: 14038.

Kumar, V., S. Jahan, S. Singh, V. Khanna and A. Pant (2015). "Progress toward the development of *in vitro* model system for chemical-induced developmental neurotoxicity: potential applicability of stem cells." Archives of Toxicology 89(2): 265-267.

Kumaravel, T. and A. N. Jha (2006). "Reliable Comet assay measurements for detecting DNA damage induced by ionising radiation and chemicals." Mutation Research/Genetic Toxicology and Environmental Mutagenesis 605(1-2): 7-16.

Kumari, A. and P. Kakkar (2012). "Lupeol prevents acetaminophen-induced *in vivo* hepatotoxicity by altering the Bax/Bcl-2 and oxidative stress-mediated mitochondrial signaling cascade." Life Sciences 90(15-16): 561-570.

Kumari, D., R. Kumar, S. Sridhara, N. Arora, S. Gaur and B. Singh (2006). "Sensitization to blackgram in patients with bronchial asthma and rhinitis: clinical evaluation and characterization of allergens." Allergy 61(1): 104-110.

Kumari, M., S. S. Khan, S. Pakrashi, A. Mukherjee and N. Chandrasekaran (2011). "Cytogenetic and genotoxic effects of zinc oxide nanoparticles on root cells of Allium cepa." Journal of Hazardous Materials 190(1-3): 613-621.

Kumari, M., A. Mukherjee and N. Chandrasekaran (2009). "Genotoxicity of silver nanoparticles in Allium cepa." Science of the Total Environment 407(19): 5243-5246.

Kumari, R., A. K. Attri, L. I. Panis and B. Gurjar (2013). "Emission estimates of particulate matter and heavy metals from mobile sources in Delhi (India)." Journal of Environmental Science and Engineering 55(2): 127-142.

Kumari, R., S. Subudhi, M. Suar, G. Dhingra, V. Raina, C. Dogra, S. Lal, J. R. van der Meer, C. Holliger and R. Lal (2002). "Cloning and characterization of lin genes responsible for the degradation of hexachlorocyclohexane isomers by Sphingomonas paucimobilis strain B90." Applied Environmental Microbiology 68(12): 6021-6028.

Kumpawat, K. and A. Chatterjee (2003). "The usefulness of cytogenetic parameters, level of p53 protein and endogenous glutathione as intermediate end-points in raw betel-nut genotoxicity." Human and Experimental Toxicology 22(7): 363-371.

Kumudini, N., A. Uma, Y. P. Devi, S. M. Naushad, R. Mridula, R. Borgohain and V. K. Kutala (2014). "Association of Parkinson's disease with altered serum levels of lead and transition metals among South Indian subjects." Indian Journal of Biochemistry and Biophysics 51(2):121-6.

Kundu, M., P. Ghosh, S. Mitra, J. Das, T. Sau, S. Banerjee, J. C. States and A. K. Giri (2011). "Precancerous and non-cancer disease endpoints of chronic arsenic exposure: the level of chromosomal damage and XRCC3 T241M polymorphism." Mutation Research/Fundamental and Molecular Mechanisms of Mutagenesis 706(1-2): 7-12.

Kurmi, O. P., S. Semple, P. Simkhada, W. C. S. Smith and J. G. Ayres (2010). "COPD and chronic bronchitis risk of indoor air pollution from solid fuel: a systematic review and meta-analysis." Thorax 65(3): 221-228.

Kyadarkunte, A., M. Patole and V. Pokharkar (2014). "*In vitro* cytotoxicity and phototoxicity assessment of acylglutamate surfactants using a human keratinocyte cell line." Cosmetics 1(3): 159-170.

LaDou, J., P. Landrigan, J. C. Baila, V. Foa and A. Frank (2001). "A call for an international ban on asbestos." Canadian Medical Association Journal 164(4): 489-490.

Lahon, K., H. M. Shetty, A. Paramel and G. Sharma (2012). "A retrospective study of the metabolic adverse effects of antipsychotics, antidepressants, and mood stabilizers in the psychiatry outpatient clinic of a tertiary care hospital in south India." International Journal of Nutrition, Pharmacology, Neurological Diseases 2(3): 237.

Lakshmana, M. K. and T. R. Raju (1994). "Endosulfan induces small but significant changes in the levels of noradrenaline, dopamine and serotonin in the developing rat brain and deficits in the operant learning performance." Toxicology 91(2): 139-150.

Lakshmanan, J. and G. Padmanaban (1974). "Effect of some "strong" excitants of central neurones on the uptake of L-glutamate and L-aspartate by synaptosomes." Biochemical and Biophysical Research Communications 58(3): 690-698.

Lakshmanan, J. and G. Padmanaban (1974). "Effect of β-N-oxalyl-L-α, β-diamino-propionic acid on glutamate uptake by synaptosomes." Nature 249(5456): 469.

Lakshmanan, J. and G. Padmanaban (1977). "Studies on the tissue and subcellular distribution of beta-N-oxalyl-L-alpha, beta-diaminopropionic acid, the Lathyrus sativus neurotoxin." Journal of Neurochemistry 29(6): 1121-1125.

Lall, S., N. Das, R. Rama, S. Peshin, S. Khattar, K. Gulati and S. Seth (1997). "Cadmium induced nephrotoxicity in rats." Indian Journal of Experimental Biology 35(2): 151-154.

Langston, J. W. (2017). "The MPTP story." Journal of Parkinson's Disease 7(s1): S11-S19.

Lanjewar, D., K. Surve, M. Maheshwari, B. Shenoy and S. Hira (1998). "Toxoplasmosis of the central nervous system in the acquired immunodeficiency syndrome." Indian Journal of Pathology and Microbiology 41(2): 147-151.

Lanjewar, D. N., P. P. Jain and C. R. Shetty (1998). "Profile of central nervous system pathology in patients with AIDS: an autopsy study from India." Aids 12(3): 309-313.

Lata, P., S. Ram, M. Agrawal and R. Shanker (2009). "Enterococci in river Ganga surface waters: propensity of species distribution, dissemination of antimicrobial-resistance and virulence-markers among species along landscape." BMC Microbiology 9(1): 140.

Laxmi Mohanta, V., A. Naz and B. Kumar Mishra (2019). "Distribution of heavy metals in the water, sediments, and fishes from Damodar river basin at steel city, India: a probabilistic risk assessment." Human and Ecological Risk Assessment: An International Journal: 1-24.

Lohani, M., E. Dopp, H.-H. Becker, K. Seth, D. Schiffmann and Q. Rahman (2002). "Smoking enhances asbestos-induced genotoxicity, relative involvement of chromosome 1: a study using multicolor FISH with tandem labeling." Toxicology Letters 136(1): 55-63.

Lohani, M., E. Dopp, D. G. Weiss, D. Schiffmann and Q. Rahman (2000). "Kerosene soot genotoxicity: enhanced effect upon co-exposure with chrysotile asbestos in Syrian hamster embryo fibroblasts." Toxicology Letters 114(1-3): 111-116.

Lohani, M., S. Yadav, D. Schiffmann and Q. Rahman (2003). "Diallylsulfide attenuates asbestos-induced genotoxicity." Toxicology Letters 143(1): 45-50.

Lohiya, N., I. Alam, M. Hussain, S. Khan and A. Ansari (2014). "RISUG: an intravasal injectable male contraceptive." The Indian Journal of Medical Research 140 (Suppl 1): S63.

Ma, K., H. A. Salama, R. Sivaraja and V. Rb (2012). "Detection of bisphenol-A in various environment samples collected from Tamil Nadu, India by solid-phase extraction and GC analysis." 'Advances in Bioresearch 4(1): 59- 64.

Mackensen, F. and H. Billing (2009). "Tubulointerstitial nephritis and uveitis syndrome." Current Opinion in Ophthalmology 20(6): 525-531.

Mahadevaswami, M., U. Jadaramkunti, M. Hiremath and B. Kaliwal (2000). "Effect of mancozeb on ovarian compensatory hypertrophy and biochemical constituents in hemicastrated albino rat." Reproductive Toxicology 14(2): 127-134.

Mahadevaswami, M. and B. Kaliwal (2002). "Effect of dimethoate administration schedules on compensatory ovarian hypertrophy, follicular dynamics, and estrous cycle in hemicastrated mice." Journal of Basic and Clinical Physiology and Pharmacology 13(3): 225-248.

Mahajan, S. and J. Shah (2016). "A mixed toxidrome presenting with bilateral ptosis with normal pupils: The first case in the literature." Journal of Family Medicine and Primary Care 5(3): 682.

Mahapatro, G. and M. Panigrahi (2013). "The case for banning endosulfan." Current Science 104(11): 1476-1479.

Mahata, J., A. Basu, S. Ghoshal, J. Sarkar, A. Roy, G. Poddar, A. Nandy, A. Banerjee, K. Ray and A. Natarajan (2003). "Chromosomal aberrations and sister chromatid exchanges in individuals exposed to arsenic through drinking water in West Bengal, India." Mutation Research/Genetic Toxicology and Environmental Mutagenesis 534(1-2): 133-143.

Mahata, J., M. Chaki, P. Ghosh, L. Das, K. Baidya, K. Ray, A. Natarajan and A. Giri (2004). "Chromosomal aberrations in arsenic-exposed human populations: a review with special reference to a comprehensive study in West Bengal, India." Cytogenetic and Genome Research 104(1-4): 359-364.

Mahato, M., A. K. Sharma and P. Kumar (2013). "Synthesis and characterization of N-ethyl-N'-(3-dimethylaminopropyl)-guanidinyl-polyethylenimine polymers and investigation of their capability to deliver DNA and siRNA in mammalian cells." Colloids and Surfaces B: Biointerfaces 109: 197-203.

Mahboob, M., M. Rahman, K. Danadevi, B. S. Banu and P. Grover (2002). "Detection of DNA damage in mouse peripheral blood leukocytes by the comet assay after oral administration of monocrotophos." Drug and Chemical Toxicology 25(1): 65-74.

Maheshwari, R. K., R. N. Tandon, A.-R. Feuillette, G. Mahouy, G. Badillet and R. M. Friedman (1988). "Interferon inhibits Aspergillus fumigatus growth in mice: an activity against an extracellular infection." Journal of Interferon Research 8(1): 35-44.

Mahimkar, M. B. and R. A. Bhisey (1995). "Occupational exposure to bidi tobacco increases chromosomal aberrations in tobacco processors." Mutation Research/Environmental Mutagenesis and Related Subjects 334(2): 139-144.

Makhija, D. T. and A. G. Jagtap (2014). "Studies on sensitivity of zebrafish as a model organism for Parkinson's disease: comparison with rat model." Journal of Pharmacology and Pharmacotherapeutics 5(1): 39.

Malhotra, K. M., R. Murthy, R. Srivastava and S. V. Chandra (1984). "Concurrent exposure of lead and manganese to iron-deficent rats: Effect on lipid peroxidation and contents of some metals in the brain." Journal of Applied Toxicology 4(1): 22-25.

Malhotra, K. M., G. S. Shukla and S. V. Chandra (1982). "Neurochemical changes in rats coexposed to lead and copper." Archives of Toxicology 49(3-4): 331-336.

Malik, A. and M. Ahmad (1995). "Genotoxicity of some wastewaters in India." Environmental Toxicology and Water Quality 10(4): 287-293.

Malik, A., P. Verma, A. K. Singh and K. P. Singh (2011). "Distribution of polycyclic aromatic hydrocarbons in water and bed sediments of the Gomti River, India." Environmental Monitoring and Assessment 172(1-4): 529-545.

Malik, M., P. Kumar, R. Seth and S. Rishi (2009). "Genotoxic effect of paper mill effluent on chromosomes of fish Channa punctatus." Current World Environment 4(2): 353.

Malik, S., S. Jindal, P. Sharda and N. Banga (1982). "Peak expiratory flow rates of school age girls from Punjab (Second report)." Indian Pediatrics 19(2): 161.

Malik, S., H. Khalique, S. Buch and P. Seth (2011). "A growth factor attenuates HIV-1 Tat and morphine induced damage to human neurons: implication in HIV/AIDS-drug abuse cases." PloS One 6(3): e18116.

Malik, S., R. Saha and P. Seth (2014). "Involvement of extracellular signal-regulated kinase (ERK1/2)-p53-p21 axis in mediating neural stem/progenitor cell cycle arrest in co-morbid HIV-drug abuse exposure." Journal of Neuroimmune Pharmacology 9(3): 340-353.

Malik, S., K. Suchal, J. Bhatia, N. Gamad, A. K. Dinda, Y. K. Gupta and D. S. Arya (2016). "Molecular mechanisms underlying attenuation of cisplatin-induced acute kidney injury by epicatechin gallate." Laboratory Investigation 96(8): 853.

Malik, S., K. Suchal, N. Gamad, A. K. Dinda, D. S. Arya and J. Bhatia (2015). "Telmisartan ameliorates cisplatin-induced nephrotoxicity by inhibiting MAPK mediated inflammation and apoptosis." European Journal of Pharmacology 748: 54-60.

Malikraj, S., T. Senthil and A. Ganguly (2011). "Ergonomic intervention on musculoskeletal problems among welders." International Journal of Advanced Engineering Technology 2(3): 33-35.

Malla, T., C. Senthilkumar, N. Sharma and N. Ganesh (2011). "Chromosome instability among Bhopal gas tragedy survivors." European Journal of Toxicological Sciences 3: 245-249.

Manda, K. and A. Bhatia (2003). "Prophylactic action of melatonin against cyclophosphamide-induced oxidative stress in mice." Cell Biology and Toxicology 19(6): 367-372.

Mandarapu, R., R. Ajumeera, V. Venkatesan and B. M. Prakhya (2014). "Proliferation and T_H1/T_H2 Cytokine Production in Human Peripheral Blood Mononuclear Cells after Treatment with Cypermethrin and Mancozeb *In Vitro*." Journal of Toxicology.

Mani, M. (1993). "Chronic renal failure in India." Nephrology Dialysis Transplantation 8(8): 684-689.

Mani, U., A. Prasad, V. Sureshkumar, P. Kumar, K. Lal, B. Maji and K. Dutta (2004). "Hepatotoxic alterations induced by subchronic exposure of rats to formulated fenvalerate (20% EC) by nose only inhalation." Biomedical and Environmental Sciences 17(3): 309-314.

Manickam, N., A. Bajaj, H. S. Saini and R. Shanker (2012). "Surfactant mediated enhanced biodegradation of hexachlorocyclohexane (HCH) isomers by Sphingomonas sp. NM05." Biodegradation 23(5): 673-682.

Manickam, N., R. Misra and S. Mayilraj (2007). "A novel pathway for the biodegradation of γ-hexachlorocyclohexane by a Xanthomonas sp. strain ICH12." Journal of Applied Microbiology 102(6): 1468-1478.

Manickam, N., A. Pathak, H. Saini, S. Mayilraj and R. Shanker (2010). "Metabolic profiles and phylogenetic diversity of microbial communities from chlorinated pesticides contaminated sites of different geographical habitats of India." Journal of Applied Microbiology 109(4): 1458-1468.

Manickam, N., M. Reddy, H. Saini and R. Shanker (2008). "Isolation of hexachlorocyclohexane-degrading Sphingomonas sp. by dehalogenase assay and characterization of genes involved in γ-HCH degradation." Journal of Applied Microbiology 104(4): 952-960.

Manna, S., D. Bhattacharyya, T. Mandal and S. Dey (2006). "Neuropharmacological effects of deltamethrin in rats." Journal of Veterinary Science 7(2): 133-136.

Manohar, P. R. (2014). "Toxicity of Ayurveda medicines and safety concerns: The need to revive the branch of toxicology in Ayurveda." Ancient Science of Life 34(1): 1.

Maras, J. S., S. Das, S. Sharma, S. M. Shasthry, B. Colsch, C. Junot, R. Moreau and S. K. Sarin (2018). "Baseline urine metabolic phenotype in patients with severe alcoholic hepatitis and its association with outcome." Hepatology Communications 2(6): 628-643.

Marco, G. (1987). "A Summary of Silent Spring." Silent Spring Revisited.

Mascarenhas, S., S. Mutnuri and A. Ganguly (2017). "Deleterious role of trace elements–Silica and lead in the development of chronic kidney disease." Chemosphere 177: 239-249.

Masoud, A., R. Kiran and R. Sandhir (2009). "Impaired mitochondrial functions in organophosphate induced delayed neuropathy in rats." Cellular and Molecular Neurobiology 29(8): 1245-1255.

Masoud, A., R. Kiran and R. Sandhir (2011). "Modulation of dopaminergic system and neurobehavioral functions in delayed neuropathy induced by organophosphates." Toxicology Mechanisms and Methods 21(1): 1-5.

Mathew, S. and G. Kuttan (1997). "Antioxidant activity of Tinospora cordifolia and its usefulness in the amelioration of cyclophosphamide induced toxicity." Journal of Experimental and Clinical Cancer Research: CR 16(4): 407-411.

Mathur, A., S. V. Chandra and S. Tandon (1977). "Comparative toxicity of trivalent and hexavalent chromium to rabbits II. Morphological changes in some organs." Toxicology 8(1): 53-61.

Mathur, A., F. Rizvi and P. Kakkar (2016). "PHLPP2 down regulation influences nuclear Nrf2 stability via Akt-1/Gsk3β/Fyn kinase axis in acetaminophen induced oxidative renal toxicity: Protection accorded by morin." Food and Chemical Toxicology 89: 19-31.

Mathur, A., R. Fatima and P. Kakkar, (2016)."PHLPP2 down regulation influences nuclear Nrf2 stability via Akt-1/Gsk3β/Fyn kinase axis in acetaminophen induced oxidative renal toxicity: Protection accorded by morin". Food and Chemical Toxicology 89:19-31

Maurya, S. K., J. Mishra, S. Abbas and S. Bandyopadhyay (2016). "Cypermethrin stimulates GSK3β-dependent Aβ and p-tau proteins and cognitive loss in young rats: Reduced HB-EGF signaling and downstream neuroinflammation as critical regulators." Molecular Neurobiology 53(2): 968-982.

Maurya, S. K., J. Mishra, V. K. Tripathi, R. Sharma and M. H. Siddiqui (2014). "Cypermethrin induces astrocyte damage: Role of aberrant Ca2+, ROS, JNK, P38, matrix metalloproteinase 2 and migration related reelin protein." Pesticide Biochemistry and Physiology 111: 51-59.

Maurya, S. K., A. Rai, N. K. Rai, S. Deshpande, R. Jain, M. K. R. Mudiam, Y. S. Prabhakar and S. Bandyopadhyay (2011). "Cypermethrin induces astrocyte apoptosis by the disruption of the autocrine/paracrine mode of epidermal growth factor receptor signaling." Toxicological Sciences 125(2): 473-487.

Mazumder, D. G., A. Chakraborty, A. Ghose, J. D. Gupta, D. Chakraborty, S. Dey and N. Chattopadhyay (1988). "Chronic arsenic toxicity from drinking tubewell water in rural West Bengal." Bulletin of the World Health Organization 66(4): 499.

Mazumder, D. G. and U. Dasgupta (2011). "Chronic arsenic toxicity: studies in West Bengal, India." The Kaohsiung Journal of Medical Sciences 27(9): 360-370.

Mazumder, D. N. G., R. Haque, N. Ghosh, B. K. De, A. Santra, D. Chakraborti and A. H. Smith (2000). "Arsenic in drinking water and the prevalence of respiratory effects in West Bengal, India." International Journal of Epidemiology 29(6): 1047-1052.

Mehra, N., G. Kaur, U. Kanga and N. Tandon (2002). "Immunogenetics of autoimmune diseases in Asian Indians." Annals of the New York Academy of Sciences 958(1): 333-336.

Mehra, N. K., N. Kumar, G. Kaur, U. Kanga and N. Tandon (2007). "Biomarkers of susceptibility to type 1 diabetes with special reference to the Indian population." Indian Journal of Medical Research 125(3): 321.

Mehrotra, S., K. Mishra, R. Maurya, R. Srimal and V. Singh (2002). "Immunomodulation by ethanolic extract of Boerhaavia diffusa roots." International Immunopharmacology 2(7): 987-996.

Mehta, A., R. S. Verma and N. Srivastava (2005). "Chlorpyrifos-induced alterations in rat brain acetylcholinesterase, lipid peroxidation and ATPases." Indian Journal of Biochemistry and Biophysics 42(1):54-8.

Mehta, A., R. S. Verma and N. Srivastava (2008). "Chlorpyrifos-induced DNA damage in rat liver and brain." Environmental and Molecular Mutagenesis 49(6): 426-433.

Mehta, R. L., L. Awdishu, A. Davenport, P. T. Murray, E. Macedo, J. Cerda, R. Chakaravarthi, A. L. Holden and S. L. Goldstein (2015). "Phenotype standardization for drug-induced kidney disease." Kidney International 88(2): 226-234.

Mehta, T. Y., L. M. Prajapati, B. Mittal, C. G. Joshi, J. J. Sheth, D. B. Patel, D. M. Dave and R. K. Goyal (2009). "Association of HLA-B* 1502 allele and carbamazepine-induced Stevens-Johnson syndrome among Indians." Indian Journal of Dermatology, Venereology, and Leprology 75(6): 579.

Meshram, B., S. Kondawar, A. Mahajan, R. Mahore and D. Burghate (2014). "Urease immobilized polypyrrole/multi-walled carbon nanotubes composite biosensor for heavy metal ions detection." Journal of the Chinese Advanced Materials Society 2(4): 223-235.

Metgud, D., S. Khatri, M. Mokashi and P. Saha (2008). "An ergonomic study of women workers in a woolen textile factory for identification of health-related problems." Indian Journal of Occupational and Environmental Medicine 12(1): 14.

Mishra, A., P. Dwivedi, A. Verma and P. Ray (1999). "Protein-A Activates Membrane Bound Multicomponent Enzyme Complex, Nadph Oxie in Human Neutrophils®." Immunopharmacology and Immunotoxicology 21(4): 683-694.

Mishra, D. and S. Flora (2008). "Differential oxidative stress and DNA damage in rat brain regions and blood following chronic arsenic exposure." Toxicology and Industrial Health 24(4): 247-256.

Mishra, D., S. K. Tiwari, S. Agarwal, V. P. Sharma and R. K. Chaturvedi (2012). "Prenatal carbofuran exposure inhibits hippocampal neurogenesis and causes learning and memory deficits in offspring." Toxicological Sciences 127(1): 84-100.

Mishra, G., R. Shukla, M. Hasan, S. K. Khanna and M. Das (2009). "Potentiation of neurotoxicity of Lathyrus sativus by manganese: alterations in blood–brain barrier permeability." Toxicology Mechanisms and Methods 19(4): 318-326.

Mishra, G., P. Singh, R. Verma, S. Kumar, S. Srivastav, K. Jha and R. Khosa (2011). "Traditional uses, phytochemistry and pharmacological properties of Moringa oleifera plant: An overview." Der Pharmacia Lettre 3(2): 141-164.

Mishra, J., N. Kaur and A. K. Ganguli (2019). "Selective and sensitive fluorescence recognition of Pb (II) in aqueous medium by organic nanoparticles of a urea linker based tetrapodal receptor: Effect of linker molecules in a sensor on chemosensing." Inorganica Chimica Acta 487: 214-220.

Mishra, K., U. Chauhan and S. Naik (2006). "Effect of lead exposure on serum immunoglobulins and reactive nitrogen and oxygen intermediate." Human and Experimental Toxicology 25(11): 661-665.

Mishra, K., R. Rani, V. Yadav and S. Naik (2010). "Effect of lead exposure on lymphocyte subsets and activation markers." Immunopharmacology and Immunotoxicology 32(3): 446-449.

Mishra, K. and R. C. Sharma (2011). "Assessment of organochlorine pesticides in human milk and risk exposure to infants from North-East India." Science of the Total Environment 409(23): 4939-4949.

Mishra, K. K., S. Dixit, S. K. Purshottam, R. C. Pandey, M. Das and S. K. Khanna (2007). "Exposure assessment to Sudan dyes through consumption of artificially coloured chilli powders in India." International Journal of Food Science and Technology 42(11): 1363-1366.

Mishra, K. P., V. K. Singh, R. Rani, V. S. Yadav, V. Chandran, S. P. Srivastava and P. K. Seth (2003). "Effect of lead exposure on the immune response of some occupationally exposed individuals." Toxicology 188(2-3): 251-259.

Mishra, M., A. Sharma, A. Shukla, R. Kumar, U. Dwivedi and D. K. Chowdhuri (2014). "Genotoxicity of dichlorvos in strains of Drosophila melanogaster defective in DNA repair." Mutation Research/Genetic Toxicology and Environmental Mutagenesis 766: 35-41.

Mishra, M., A. Sharma, A. Shukla, P. Pragya, R. Murthy, D. de Pomerai, U. Dwivedi and D. K. Chowdhuri (2013). "Transcriptomic analysis provides insights on hexavalent chromium induced DNA double strand breaks and their possible repair in midgut cells of Drosophila melanogaster larvae." Mutation Research/ Fundamental and Molecular Mechanisms of Mutagenesis 747: 28-39.

Mishra, M., M. Taneja, S. Malik, H. Khalique and P. Seth (2010). "Human immunodeficiency virus type 1 Tat modulates proliferation and differentiation of human neural precursor cells: implication in NeuroAIDS." Journal of Neurovirology 16(5): 355-367.

Mishra, M., S. Vetrivel, N. B. Siddappa, U. Ranga and P. Seth (2008). "Clade-specific differences in neurotoxicity of human immunodeficiency virus-1 B and C Tat of human neurons: Significance of dicysteine C30C31 motif." Annals of Neurology 63(3): 366-376.

Mishra, P., A. Bhargava, N. Pathak, P. Desikan, K. Maudar, S. Varshney, R. Shrivastava and A. Jain (2011). "Molecular surveillance of hepatitis and tuberculosis infections in a cohort exposed to methyl isocyanate." International Journal of Occupational Medicine and Environmental Health 24(1): 94-101.

Mishra, P., S. Dabadghao, G. Modi, P. Desikan, A. Jain, I. Mittra, D. Gupta, C. Chauhan, S. Jain and K. Maudar (2009). "In utero exposure to methyl isocyanate in the Bhopal gas disaster: evidence of persisting hyperactivation of immune system two decades later." Occupational and Environmental Medicine 66(4): 279-279.

Mishra, P., S. Khan, A. Bhargava, H. Panwar, S. Banerjee, S. Jain and K. Maudar (2010). "Regulation of isocyanate-induced apoptosis, oxidative stress, and inflammation in cultured human neutrophils." Cell Biology and Toxicology 26(3): 279-291.

Mishra, P., R. Samarth, N. Pathak, S. Jain, S. Banerjee and K. Maudar (2009). "Bhopal gas tragedy: review of clinical and experimental findings after 25 years." International Journal of Occupational Medicine and Environmental Health 22(3): 193-202.

Mishra, P. K. (2012). "A pragmatic & translational approach of human biomonitoring to methyl isocyanate exposure in Bhopal." The Indian Journal of Medical Research 135(4): 479.

Mishra, P. K., B. Manivannan, N. Pathak, S. Sriram, S. S. Bhande, S. Panneerdoss and N. K. Lohiya (2003). "Status of spermatogenesis and sperm parameters in langur monkeys following long-term vas occlusion with styrene maleic anhydride." Journal of Andrology 24(4): 501-509.

Mishra, P. K., G. V. Raghuram, H. Panwar, D. Jain, H. Pandey and K. K. Maudar (2009). "Mitochondrial oxidative stress elicits chromosomal instability after exposure to isocyanates in human kidney epithelial cells." Free Radical Research 43(8): 718-728.

Mishra, S. K., P. Singh and S. K. Rath (2011). "A study of toxicity and differential gene expression in murine liver following exposure to anti-malarial drugs: amodiaquine and sulphadoxine-pyrimethamine." Malaria Journal 10(1): 109.

Mishra, S.K., P. Singh and S.K. Rath (2013). "Protective Effect of Quercetin on Chloroquine-Induced Oxidative Stress and Hepatotoxicity in Mice". *Malaria Research and Treatment* 141734.

Mishra, V., D. K. Saxena and M. Das (2009). "Effect of argemone oil and argemone alkaloid, sanguinarine on Sertoli–germ cell coculture." Toxicology Letters 186(2): 104-110.

Mishra, V., M. Srivastava and R. Raizada (1993). "Testicular toxicity of thiram in rat: morphological and biochemical evaluations." Industrial Health 31(2): 59-67.

Misra, A., R. Kumar, V. Mishra, B. Chaudhari, S. Raisuddin, M. Das and P. Dwivedi (2011). "Potential allergens of green gram (Vigna radiata L. Millsp) identified as members of cupin superfamily and seed albumin." Clinical and Experimental Allergy 41(8): 1157-1168.

Misra, A., R. Kumar, V. Mishra, B. P. Chaudhari, A. Tripathi, M. Das and P. D. Dwivedi (2010). "Partial characterization of red gram (Cajanus cajan L. Millsp) polypeptides recognized by patients exhibiting rhinitis and bronchial asthma." Food and Chemical Toxicology 48(10): 2725-2736.

Misra, A., R. Prasad, M. Das and P. D. Dwivedi (2008). "Prevalence of legume sensitization in patients with naso-bronchial allergy." Immunopharmacology and Immunotoxicology 30(3): 529-542.

Misra, A., R. Prasad, M. Das and P. D. Dwivedi (2009). "Probing novel allergenic proteins of commonly consumed legumes." Immunopharmacology and Immunotoxicology 31(2): 186-194.

Misra, R., G. S. Babu, R. Ray and R. Hans (2002). "Tubifex: a sensitive model for UV-B-induced phototoxicity." Ecotoxicology and Environmental Safety 52(3): 288-295.

Misra, R., P. Bajpai, P. Joshi and R. Hans (2001). "An unusual photohaemolytic property of riboflavin." Food and Chemical Toxicology 39(1): 11-18.

Misra, R. and P. Joshi (1999). "Phototoxicity evaluation—Tetrahymena thermophila as an alternative model." Indian Journal of Experimental Biology 37: 750-757.

Misra, R., K. Lal, M. Farooq and R. Hans (2005). "Effect of solar UV radiation on earthworm (Metaphire posthuma)." Ecotoxicology and Environmental Safety 62(3): 391-396.

Misra, R., R. Ray and R. Hans (2005). "Effect of UVB radiation on human erythrocytes *in vitro*." Toxicology *In Vitro* 19(3): 433-438.

Misra, R., V. Sundararaman and P. Joshi (1987). "Riboflavin-induced phototoxicity to paramecium." Indian Journal of Experimental Biology 25(3): 194-201.

Misra, S., A. Kumar, C. Ratnasekhar, V. Sharma, M. K. R. Mudiam and K. R. Ram (2014). "Exposure to endosulfan influences sperm competition in Drosophila melanogaster." Scientific Reports 4: 7433.

Misra, S., A. Singh, V. Sharma, M. K. Reddy Mudiam and K. R. Ram (2014). "Identification of Drosophila-based endpoints for the assessment and understanding of xenobiotic-mediated male reproductive adversities." Toxicological Sciences 141(1): 278-291.

Misra, U., S. Bhargava, D. Nag, M. Kidwai and M. Lal (1988). "Occupational phosphine exposure in Indian workers." Toxicology Letters 42(3): 257-263.

Misra, U., D. Nag, P. Nath, W. Khan, B. Gupta and P. Ray (1988). "A clinical study of toxic gas poisoning in Bhopal, India." Indian Journal of Experimental Biology 26(3): 201-204.

Misra, U., V. Sharma and V. Singh (1993). "Clinical aspects of neurolathyrism in Unnao, India." Spinal Cord 31(4): 249.

Misra, V., Q. Rahman and P. Viswanathan (1978). "Biochemical changes in guinea pig lungs due to amosite asbestos." Environmental Research 16(1-3): 55-61.

Mitra, A., V. Murty and U. Luthra (1982). "Sister chromatid exchanges in leukocytes of patients with cancer of cervix uteri." Human Genetics 60(3): 214-215.

Mitra, S., A. Srivastava and S. Khandelwal (2013). "Tributyltin chloride induced testicular toxicity by JNK and p38 activation, redox imbalance and cell death in sertoli-germ cell co-culture." Toxicology 314(1): 39-50.

Mittal, B. V. (1994). "Acute renal failure following poisonous snake bite." Journal of Postgraduate Medicine 40(3): 123.

Mittal, S., V. Kher, S. Gulati, L. K. Agarwal and P. Arora (1997). "Chronic renal failure in India." Renal Failure 19(6): 763-770.

Mittal, S., V. Kumar, N. Dhiman, L. K. S. Chauhan, R. Pasricha and A. K. Pandey (2018). "Author Correction: Physico-chemical properties based differential toxicity of graphene oxide/reduced graphene oxide in human lung cells mediated through oxidative stress." Scientific Reports 8(1): 15860.

Mittal, S. and A. K. Pandey (2014). "Cerium oxide nanoparticles induced toxicity in human lung cells: role of ROS mediated DNA damage and apoptosis." BioMed Research International 2014: 891934

Moghadamnia, A. A. (2012). "An update on toxicology of aluminum phosphide." DARU Journal of Pharmaceutical Sciences 20(1): 25.

Mohan, A., C. Mohan, P. Aggarwal, R. Handa and J. Wali (2002). "Flumazenil in acute benzodiazepine overdose." The Journal of the Association of Physicians of India 50: 1097.

Mohan, D., P. Sitholey and D. Purohit (1993). "Collaborative study on narcotics drugs and psychotropic substances, subcomponent-Drug abuse monitoring system." New Delhi: ICMR.

Mohan, K., N. Pradhan and S. Channabasavanna (1983). "A report of subclinical psychological deterioration (A type of alcoholic dementia)." Indian Journal of Psychiatry 25(3): 243.

Mohanakumar, K. P., D. Muralikrishnan and B. Thomas (2000). "Neuroprotection by sodium salicylate against 1-methyl-4-phenyl-1, 2, 3, 6-tetrahydropyridine-induced neurotoxicity." Brain Research 864(2): 281-290.

Mohankumar, M. N., S. Janani, B. K. Prabhu, P. V. Kumar and R. Jeevanram (2002). "DNA damage and integrity of UV-induced DNA repair in lymphocytes of smokers analysed by the comet assay." Mutation Research/Genetic Toxicology and Environmental Mutagenesis 520(1-2): 179-187.

Mohanraj, R. and P. Azeez (2003). "Polycyclic aromatic hydrocarbons in air and their toxic potency." Resonance 8(9): 20-27.

Mohanraj, R. and P. Azeez (2004). "Health effects of airborne particulate matter and the Indian scenario." Current Science 87(6): 741-748.

Mohanraj, R., G. Solaraj and S. Dhanakumar (2011). "Fine particulate phase PAHs in ambient atmosphere of Chennai metropolitan city, India." Environmental Science and Pollution Research 18(5): 764-771.

Mohan Rao N., S.K. Dave, H.N. Saiyed, P.K. Kulkarni, B.D. Patel and S.K. Kashyap (1993). "A comparison of airways obstruction in silica and asbestos dust exposed workers". Indian Journal of Occupational Health 36: 1–3.

Mohanty, N. K. (2005). "Cancer urinary bladder etiopathology and its management". Health Administrator, 17, 126-131.

Mohanty, R., S. K. Das and M. Patri (2017). "Modulation of benzo [a] pyrene induced anxiolytic-like behavior by retinoic acid in zebrafish: Involvement of oxidative stress and antioxidant defense system." Neurotoxicity Research 31(4): 493-504.

Moitra, S., P. D. Blanc and S. Sahu (2013). "Adverse respiratory effects associated with cadmium exposure in small-scale jewellery workshops in India." Thorax 68(6): 565-570.

Moitra, S., B. B. Brashier and S. Sahu (2014). "Occupational cadmium exposure-associated oxidative stress and erythrocyte fragility among jewelry workers in India." American Journal of Industrial Medicine 57(9): 1064-1072.

Moitra, S., J. Ghosh, J. Firdous, A. Bandyopadhyay, M. Mondal, J. K. Biswas, S. Sahu, S. Bhattacharyya and S. Moitra (2018). "Exposure to heavy metals alters the surface topology of alveolar macrophages and induces respiratory dysfunction among Indian metal arc-welders." Toxicology and Industrial Health 34(12): 908-921.

Mondal, N. K., P. Bhattacharya and M. R. Ray (2011). "Assessment of DNA damage by comet assay and fast halo assay in buccal epithelial cells of Indian women chronically exposed to biomass smoke." International Journal of Hygiene and Environmental Health 214(4): 311-318.

Mondal, S., S. Mukherjee, K. Chaudhuri, S. N. Kabir and P. Kumar Mukhopadhyay (2013). "Prevention of arsenic-mediated reproductive toxicity in adult female rats by high protein diet." Pharmaceutical Biology 51(11): 1363-1371.

Morehouse, W. and M. A. Subramaniam (1986). The Bhopal tragedy: what really happened and what it means for American workers and communities at risk.

Mudawal, A., A. Singh, S. Yadav, M. Mishra, P. K. Singh, L. P. Chandravanshi, J. Mishra, V. K. Khanna, S. Bandyopadhyay and D. Parmar (2015). "Similarities in lindane induced alterations in protein expression profiling in different brain regions with neurodegenerative diseases." Proteomics 15(22): 3875-3882.

Mudiam, M. K. R., R. Jain, S. K. Maurya, H. A. Khan, S. Bandyopadhyay and R. Murthy (2012). "Low density solvent based dispersive liquid–liquid microextraction with gas chromatography–electron capture detection for the determination of cypermethrin in tissues and blood of cypermethrin treated rats." Journal of Chromatography B 895: 65-70.

Mudiam, M. K. R., S. Pathak, K. Gopal and R. Murthy (2012). "Studies on urban drinking water quality in a tropical zone." Environmental Monitoring and Assessment 184(1): 461-469.

Mudiam, M. K. R. and C. Ratnasekhar (2013). "Ultra sound assisted one step rapid derivatization and dispersive liquid–liquid microextraction followed by gas chromatography–mass spectrometric determination of amino acids in complex matrices." Journal of Chromatography a 1291: 10-18.

Mujtaba, S. F., A. Dwivedi, M. K. R. Mudiam, D. Ali, N. Yadav and R. S. Ray (2011). "Production of ROS by Photosensitized Anthracene Under Sunlight and UV-R at Ambient Environmental Intensities." Photochemistry and Photobiology 87(5): 1067-1076.

Mujtaba, S. F., A. Dwivedi, N. Yadav, R. Ray and G. Singh (2013). "Singlet oxygen mediated apoptosis by anthrone involving lysosomes and mitochondria at ambient UV exposure." Journal of Hazardous Materials 252: 258-271.

Mukherjee, A., K. Agarwal, M. A. Aguilar and A. Sharma (1991). "Anticlastogenic activity β-carotene against cyclophoshamide in mice *in vivo*." Mutation Research Letters 263(1): 41-46.

Mukherjee, A. and A. Giri (1991). "Sister chromatid exchange induced by 'pan masala'(a betel quid ingredient) in male mice *in vivo*." Food and Chemical Toxicology 29(6): 401-403.

Mukherjee, A., H. Rajmohan, S. Dave, B. Rajan, Y. Kakde and S. Raghavendra Rao (1992). "An environmental survey in chrysotile asbestos milling processes in India." American Journal of Industrial Medicine 22(4): 543-551.

Mukherjee, A. K., B. P. Chattopadhyay, S. K. Bhattacharya and H. N. Saiyed (2004). "Airborne endotoxin and its relationship to pulmonary function among workers in an Indian jute mill." Archives of Environmental Health: An International Journal 59(4): 202-208.

Mukherjee, A. K., R. R. Rajmohan, S. K. Dave, B. K. Rajan, Y. Kakde and S. R. Rao (1996). "Pollution and its control in asbestos milling processes in India." Industrial Health 34(1): 35-43.

Mukherjee, P., M. Dutta, P. Datta, A. Dasgupta, R. Pradhan, M. Pradhan, M. Kundu, J. Basu and P. Chakrabarti (2007). "The RD1-encoded antigen Rv3872 of Mycobacterium tuberculosis as a potential candidate for serodiagnosis of tuberculosis." Clinical Microbiology and Infection 13(2): 146-152.

Mukherjee, P., S. Vishnubhatla, D. Amarapurkar, K. Das, A. Sood, Y. Chawla, C. Eapen, P. Boddu, V. Thomas and S. Varshney (2017). "Etiology and mode of presentation of chronic liver diseases in India: A multi centric study." PloS One 12(10): e0187033-e0187033.

Mukherjee, S., S. Sau, D. Madhuri, V. S. Bollu, K. Madhusudana, B. Sreedhar, R. Banerjee and C. R. Patra (2016). "Green synthesis and characterization of monodispersed gold nanoparticles: toxicity study, delivery of doxorubicin and its bio-distribution in mouse model." Journal of Biomedical Nanotechnology 12(1): 165-181.

Mukherjee, S. C., M. M. Rahman, U. K. Chowdhury, M. K. Sengupta, D. Lodh, C. R. Chanda, K. C. Saha and D. Chakraborti (2003). "Neuropathy in arsenic toxicity from groundwater arsenic contamination in West Bengal, India." Journal of Environmental Science and Health, Part A 38(1): 165-183.

Mukhopadhyay, I., D. K. Chowdhuri, M. Bajpayee and A. Dhawan (2004). "Evaluation of *in vivo* genotoxicity of cypermethrin in Drosophila melanogaster using the alkaline Comet assay." Mutagenesis 19(2): 85-90.

Mukhopadhyay, I., A. Nazir, K. Mahmood, D. Saxena, M. Das, S. Khanna and D. K. Chowdhuri (2002). "Toxicity of argemone oil: Effect on hsp70expression and tissue damage in transgenic Drosophila melanogaster (hsp70-lacZ) Bg 9." Cell Biology and Toxicology 18(1): 1-11.

Mukhopadhyay, I., D. K. Saxena and D. K. Chowdhuri (2003). "Hazardous effects of effluent from the chrome plating industry: 70 kDa heat shock protein expression as a marker of cellular damage in transgenic Drosophila melanogaster (hsp70-lacZ)." Environmental Health Perspectives 111(16): 1926-1932.

Mukhopadhyay, I., H. R. Siddique, V. K. Bajpai, D. K. Saxena and D. K. Chowdhuri (2006). "Synthetic pyrethroid cypermethrin induced cellular damage in reproductive tissues of Drosophila melanogaster: Hsp70 as a marker of cellular damage." Archives of Environmental Contamination and Toxicology 51(4): 673-680.

Mukhtar, H., R. Dixit and P. K. Seth (1981). "Reduction in cutaneous and hepatic glutathione contents, glutathione S-transferase and aryl hydrocarbon hydroxylase activities following topical application of acrylamide to mouse." Toxicology Letters 9(2): 153-156.

Mundhe, N. A., P. Kumar, S. Ahmed, V. Jamdade, S. Mundhe and M. Lahkar (2015). "Nordihydroguaiaretic acid ameliorates cisplatin induced nephrotoxicity and potentiates its anti-tumor activity in DMBA induced breast cancer in female Sprague–Dawley rats." International Immunopharmacology 28(1): 634-642.

Munshi, S. R. and S. S. Rao (1972). "Antifertility activity of an indigenous plant preparation (ROC-101). Effect on reproduction." Indian Journal of Medical Research 60(7): 1054-1060.

Muntean, A. and M. Lucan (2013). "Immunosuppression in kidney transplantation." Clujul Medical 86(3): 177.

Murali, R., A. Bhalla, D. Singh and S. Singh (2009). "Acute pesticide poisoning: 15 years experience of a large North-West Indian hospital." Clinical Toxicology 47(1): 35-38.

Murali, T., I. N. Rao, M. Keshavan and H. Narayanan (1983). "Thiamine refractory— wernicke—korsakoffs syndrome—a case report." Indian Journal of Psychiatry 25(1): 80.

Murthy, P., N. Manjunatha, B. Subodh, P. K. Chand and V. Benegal (2010). "Substance use and addiction research in India." Indian Journal of Psychiatry 52(Suppl1): S189.

Murthy, P. B. K. and K. Prema (1979). "Sister-chromatid exchanges in oral contraceptive users." Mutation Research/Genetic Toxicology 68(2): 149-152.

Murthy, R., S. Lal, D. Saxena, G. Shukla, M. M. Ali and S. Chandra (1981). "Effect of manganese and copper interaction on behavior and biogenic amines in rats fed a 10% casein diet." Chemico-Biological Interactions 37(3): 299-308.

Murthy, R., R. Srivastava, S. Gupta and S. Chandra (1980). "Manganese induced testicular changes in monkeys." Experimental Pathology 18(4): 240-244.

Murthy, R. C., M. Junaid and D. K. Saxena (1996). "Ovarian dysfunction in mice following chromium (VI) exposure." Toxicology Letters 89(2): 147-154.

Murti, C. K. (1987). "Occupational experience of exposure to mixtures of chemicals." Methods for Assessing the Effects of Mixtures of Chemicals. Chichester: John Wiley and Sons.

Murti, V., T. Seshadri and T. Venkitasubramanian (1964). "Neurotoxic compounds of the seeds of Lathyrus sativus." Phytochemistry 3(1): 73-78.

Murty, V., A. Mitra, A. Sharma, B. Das and U. Luthra (1987). "Mitomycin C induced chromosomal aberrations and sister chromatid exchanges (SCEs) in lymphocytes of patients with precancerous and cancerous lesions of the uterine cervix." Neoplasma 34(1): 101-105.

Mustafa, M., R. Pathak, A. Tripathi, R. S. Ahmed, K. Guleria and B. Banerjee (2010). "Maternal and cord blood levels of aldrin and dieldrin in Delhi population." Environmental Monitoring and Assessment 171(1-4): 633-638.

Mustafa, S. and S. V. Chandra (1971). "Levels of 5-hydroxytryptamine, dopamine and norepinephrine in whole brain of rabbits in chronic manganese toxicity." Journal of Neurochemistry 18(6): 931-933.

Muthu, K. and P. Krishnamoorthy (2012). "Effect of vitamin C and vitamin E on mercuric chloride-induced reproductive toxicity in male rats." Biochemical Pharmacology 1(102): 2167-0501.1000102.

Nada, S. A., E. A. Omara, O. M. Abdel-Salam and H. G. Zahran (2010). "Mushroom insoluble polysaccharides prevent carbon tetrachloride-induced hepatotoxicity in rat." Food and Chemical Toxicology 48(11): 3184-3188.

Nadkarni, K. and A. Nadkarni (1976). "Indian Materia Medica, Popular Prakashan Pvt." Ltd., Bombay 1: 799.

Nag, D., G. Singh and S. Senon (1977). "Epilepsy epidemic due to benzahexachlorine." Tropical and Geographical Medicine 29(3): 229-232.

Nagaraja, T. and T. Desiraju (1993). "Effects of chronic consumption of metanil yellow by developing and adult rats on brain regional levels of noradrenaline, dopamine and serotonin, on acetylcholine esterase activity and on operant conditioning." Food and Chemical Toxicology 31(1): 41-44.

Nagpure, N., R. Srivastava, R. Kumar, A. Dabas, B. Kushwaha and P. Kumar (2015). "Assessment of pollution of river Ganges by tannery effluents using genotoxicity biomarkers in murrel fish, Channa punctatus (Bloch)." Indian Journal of Experimental Biology 53:476-483.

Naha, N. and A. Chowdhury (2005). "Toxic effect of lead on human spermatozoa: A study among pigment factory workers." Indian Journal of Occupational and Environmental Medicine 9(3): 118.

Naidu, M., A. A. Shifow, K. V. Kumar and K. Ratnakar (2000). "Ginkgo biloba extract ameliorates gentamicin-induced nephrotoxicity in rats." Phytomedicine 7(3): 191-197.

Nair, A., P. Dureja and M. Pillai (1992). "Aldrin and dieldrin residues in human fat, milk and blood serum collected from Delhi." Human and Experimental Toxicology 11(1): 43-45.

Naithani, V. and P. Kakkar (2006). "Effect of ecological variation on heavy metal content of some medicinal plants used as herbal tea ingredients in India." Bulletin of Environmental Contamination and Toxicology 76(2): 285-292.

Naithani, V. and P. Kakkar (2006). "Estimation of organochlorine pesticide residues in two popular spices extensively used as herbal tea ingredients in India." Bulletin of Environmental Contamination and Toxicology 76(3): 429-435.

Nalika, N. and S. Parvez (2015). "Mitochondrial dysfunction in titanium dioxide nanoparticle-induced neurotoxicity." Toxicology Mechanisms and Methods 25(5): 355-363.

Nandha, R., K. Sekhri and A. K. Mandal (2013). "To study the clinical efficacy and nephrotoxicity along with the risk factors for acute kidney injury associated with parenteral polymyxin B." Indian Journal of Critical Care Medicine 17(5): 283.

Nandi, A., S. Dey, J. Biswas, P. Jaiswal, S. Naaz, T. Yasmin and B. Bishayi (2015). "Differential induction of inflammatory cytokines and reactive oxygen species in murine peritoneal macrophages and resident fresh bone marrow cells by acute Staphylococcus aureus infection: contribution of toll-like receptor 2 (TLR2)." Inflammation 38(1): 224-244.

Nandi, S. S. and S. V. Dhatrak (2008). "Occupational noise-induced hearing loss in India." Indian Journal of Occupational and Environmental Medicine 12(2): 53.

Naqshbandi, A., M. Khan, S. Rizwan, A. Yusufi and F. Khan (2011). "Studies on the protective effect of fish oil against cisplatin induced hepatotoxicity." Biology and Medicine 3(2): 86-97.

Nath, A. (2002). "Human immunodeficiency virus (HIV) proteins in neuropathogenesis of HIV dementia." The Journal of Infectious Diseases 186(Supplement_2): S193-S198.

Nath, P., R. K. Arun and N. Chanda (2015). "Smart gold nanosensor for easy sensing of lead and copper ions in solution and using paper strips." Rsc Advances 5(84): 69024-69031.

Nath, R., V. Paliwal, R. Prasad and R. Kambadur (1987). Role of metallothionein in metal detoxification and metal tolerance in protein calorie malnutrition and calcium deficient monkeys (Macaca mulatta). Metallothionein II: 631-638.

Nazir, A., I. Mukhopadhyay, D. Saxena and D. K. Chowdhuri (2001). "Chlorpyrifos-induced hsp70 expression and effect on reproductive performance in transgenic Drosophila melanogaster (hsp70-lacZ) Bg 9." Archives of Environmental Contamination and Toxicology 41(4): 443-449.

Nazir, A., I. Mukhopadhyay, D. Saxena and D. K. Chowdhuri (2003). "Evaluation of the no observed adverse effect level of solvent dimethyl sulfoxide in Drosophila melanogaster." Toxicology Mechanisms and Methods 13(2): 147-152.

Nazir, A., D. K. Saxena and D. K. Chowdhuri (2003). "Induction of hsp70 in transgenic Drosophila: biomarker of exposure against phthalimide group of chemicals." BBA-General Subjects 2(1621): 218-225.

Negi, H., S. K. Saikia, R. Kanaujia, S. Jaiswal and R. Pandey (2017). "3β-Hydroxy-urs-12-en-28-oic acid confers protection against ZnO NPs induced adversity in Caenorhabditis elegans." Environmental Toxicology and Pharmacology 53: 105-110.

Nehru, B. and P. Sidhu (2001). "Behavior and neurotoxic consequences of lead on rat brain followed by recovery." Biological Trace Element Research 84(1-3): 113.

Nehru, B. and P. Sidhu (2002). "Neurotoxic effects of differential doses of lead on rat brain followed by recovery." The Journal of Trace Elements in Experimental Medicine: The Official Publication of the International Society for Trace Element Research in Humans 15(3): 131-140.

Nidheesh, T., C. Salim, P. Rajini and P. Suresh (2016). "Antioxidant and neuroprotective potential of chitooligomers in Caenorhabditis elegans exposed to Monocrotophos." Carbohydrate Polymers 135: 138-144.

Nimesh, S., A. Aggarwal, P. Kumar, Y. Singh, K. Gupta and R. Chandra (2007). "Influence of acyl chain length on transfection mediated by acylated PEI nanoparticles." International Journal of Pharmaceutics 337(1-2): 265-274.

Niphadkar, P., S. Patil and M. Bapat (1997). "Chickpea-induced anaphylaxis." Allergy 52(1): 115-116.

Niyogi, T. (1958). "Chronic manganese poisoning." Indian Journal of Industrial Medicine 3: 3-13.

Noel, S., S. Sharma, R. Shankar and S. K. Rath (2008). "Identification of differentially expressed genes after acute exposure to bulaquine (CDRI 80/53) in mice liver." Basic and Clinical Pharmacology and Toxicology 103(6): 522-529.

Noel, S., S. Sharma, R. Shanker and S. K. Rath (2007). "Primaquine-induced differential gene expression analysis in mice liver using DNA microarrays." Toxicology 239(1-2): 96-107.

Nwani, C. D., W. S. Lakra, N. S. Nagpure, R. Kumar, B. Kushwaha and S. K. Srivastava (2010). "Toxicity of the herbicide atrazine: effects on lipid peroxidation and activities of antioxidant enzymes in the freshwater fish Channa punctatus

(Bloch)." International Journal of Environmental Research and Public Health 7(8): 3298-3312.

Ojha, A. and N. Srivastava (2014). "*In vitro* studies on organophosphate pesticides induced oxidative DNA damage in rat lymphocytes." Mutation Research/Genetic Toxicology and Environmental Mutagenesis 761: 10-17.

Ojha, A., S. K. Yaduvanshi and N. Srivastava (2011). "Effect of combined exposure of commonly used organophosphate pesticides on lipid peroxidation and antioxidant enzymes in rat tissues." Pesticide Biochemistry and Physiology 99(2): 148-156.

Pal, A., S. Alam, L. K. Chauhan, P. N. Saxena, M. Kumar, G. N. Ansari, D. Singh and K. M. Ansari (2016). "UVB exposure enhanced the dermal penetration of zinc oxide nanoparticles and induced inflammatory responses through oxidative stress mediated by MAPKs and NF-κB signaling in SKH-1 hairless mouse skin." Toxicology Research 5(4): 1066-1077.

Pal, A., S. Alam, S. Mittal, N. Arjaria, J. Shankar, M. Kumar, D. Singh, A. K. Pandey and K. M. Ansari (2016). "UVB irradiation-enhanced zinc oxide nanoparticles-induced DNA damage and cell death in mouse skin." Mutation Research/Genetic Toxicology and Environmental Mutagenesis 807: 15-24.

Pal, P., D. Bhattacharyay, A. Mukhopadhyay and P. Sarkar (2009). "The detection of mercury, cadium, and arsenic by the deactivation of urease on rhodinized carbon." Environmental Engineering Science 26(1): 25-32.

Palanivel, M., B. Rajkapoor, R. Kumar, J. Einstein, E. Kumar, M. Kumar, K. Kavitha, M. Kumar and B. Jayakar (2008). "Hepatoprotective and antioxidant effect of Pisonia aculeata L. against CCl4-induced hepatic damage in rats." Scientia Pharmaceutica 76(2): 203-216.

Pamanji, R., M. Bethu, B. Yashwanth, S. Leelavathi and J. V. Rao (2015). "Developmental toxic effects of monocrotophos, an organophosphorous pesticide, on zebrafish (Danio rerio) embryos." Environmental Science and Pollution Research 22(10): 7744-7753.

Panda, K. K., V. M. M. Achary, R. Krishnaveni, B. K. Padhi, S. N. Sarangi, S. N. Sahu and B. B. Panda (2011). "*In vitro* biosynthesis and genotoxicity bioassay of silver nanoparticles using plants." Toxicology *In Vitro* 25(5): 1097-1105.

Pandareesh, M., M. Shrivash, H. N. Kumar, K. Misra and M. S. Bharath (2016). "Curcumin monoglucoside shows improved bioavailability and mitigates rotenone induced neurotoxicity in cell and Drosophila models of Parkinson's disease." Neurochemical Research 41(11): 3113-3128.

Pande, J., S. Singh, G. Khilnani, S. Khilnani and R. Tandon (1996). "Risk factors for hepatotoxicity from antituberculosis drugs: a case-control study." Thorax 51(2): 132-136.

Pandey, A. K., M. Bajpayee, D. Parmar, S. K. Rastogi, N. Mathur, P. K. Seth and A. Dhawan (2005). "DNA damage in lymphocytes of rural Indian women exposed to biomass fuel smoke as assessed by the Comet assay." Environmental and Molecular Mutagenesis 45(5): 435-441.

Pandey, A. K., D. Gurbani, M. Bajpayee, D. Parmar, S. Ajmani and A. Dhawan (2009). "*In silico* studies with human DNA topoisomerase-II alpha to unravel the mechanism of *in vitro* genotoxicity of benzene and its metabolites." Mutation Research/Fundamental and Molecular Mechanisms of Mutagenesis 661(1-2): 57-70.

Pandey, J., S. Khan, V. Joseph and R. Kumar (2002). "Aerosol scavenging: Model application and sensitivity analysis in the Indian context." Environmental Monitoring and Assessment 74(2): 105-116.

Pandey, M., M. Varghese, K. M. Sindhu, S. Sreetama, A. Navneet, K. P. Mohanakumar and R. Usha (2008). "Mitochondrial NAD+-linked State 3 respiration and complex-I activity are compromised in the cerebral cortex of 3-nitropropionic acid-induced rat model of Huntington's disease." Journal of Neurochemistry 104(2): 420-434.

Pandey, N. (1986). "Report on 'Immediate and Residual Effects of MIC Gas Exposure on Animals of Bhopal Gas Tragedy'." Indian Veterinary Research Institute, Izatnagar.

Pandey, N., F. Gundevia, A. Prem and P. Ray (1990). "Studies on the genotoxicity of endosulfan, an organochlorine insecticide, in mammalian germ cells." Mutation Research/Genetic Toxicology 242(1): 1-7.

Pandey, P., A. H. Khan, A. K. Verma, K. A. Singh, N. Mathur, G. C. Kisku and S. C. Barman (2012). "Seasonal trends of PM 2.5 and PM 10 in ambient air and their correlation in ambient air of Lucknow City, India." Bulletin of Environmental Contamination and Toxicology 88(2): 265-270.

Pandey, P., D. Patel, A. Khan, S. Barman, R. Murthy and G. Kisku (2013). "Temporal distribution of fine particulates (PM2. 5, PM10), potentially toxic metals, PAHs and Metal-bound carcinogenic risk in the population of Lucknow City, India." Journal of Environmental Science and Health, Part A 48(7): 730-745.

Pandey, P., R. Raizada and L. Srivastava (2010). "Level of organochlorine pesticide residues in dry fruit nuts." Journal of Environmental Biology 31(5): 705-707.

Pandey, R., S. Mehrotra, R. Ray, P. Joshi and R. Hans (2002). "Evaluation of UV-radiation induced singlet oxygen generation potential of selected drugs." Drug and Chemical Toxicology 25(2): 215-225.

Pandey, S. K., C. R. Suri, M. Chaudhry, R. Tiwari and P. Rishi (2012). "A gold nanoparticles based immuno-bioprobe for detection of Vi capsular polysaccharide of Salmonella enterica serovar Typhi." Molecular BioSystems 8(7): 1853-1860.

Pandit, A., T. Sachdeva and P. Bafna (2012). "Drug-induced hepatotoxicity: a review." Journal of Applied Pharmaceutical Science 2(5): 233-243.

Pandit, G., P. Srivastava and A. M. Rao (2001). "Monitoring of indoor volatile organic compounds and polycyclic aromatic hydrocarbons arising from kerosene cooking fuel." Science of the Total Environment 279(1-3): 159-165.

Pandit, S., P. Kumar and D. Chakrabarti (2013). "Ergonomic problems prevalent in handloom units of North East India." International Journal of Scientific and Research Publications 3(1): 1-7.

Pandya, K., S. Khan, R. Krishnamurthy and P. Ray (1989). "Modulation of benzene toxicity by polyinosinic-polycytidilic acid, an interferon inducer." Biochimica et Biophysica Acta (BBA)-General Subjects 992(1): 23-29.

Pandya, K., R. Shanker, A. Gupta, W. Khan and P. Ray (1986). "Modulation of benzene toxicity by an interferon inducer (6MFA)." Toxicology 39(3): 291-305.

Pandya, K., G. Singh and A. Dhasmana (1976). "Urinary excretion of benzanthrone." Toxicology and Applied Pharmacology 38(1): 217-219.

Panigrahi, G., R. Ch, M. Mudiam, V. Vashishtha, S. Raisuddin and M. Das (2015). "Activity-guided chemo toxic profiling of Cassia occidentalis (CO) seeds: detection of toxic compounds in body fluids of CO-exposed patients and experimental rats." Chemical Research in Toxicology 28(6): 1120-1132.

Panigrahi, G. and A. Rao (1982). "Chromosome-breaking ability of arecoline, a major betel-nut alkaloid, in mouse bone-marrow cells *in vivo*." Mutation Research Letters 103(2): 197-204.

Panigrahi, G. and A. Rao (1983). "Influence of caffeine on arecoline-induced SCE in mouse bone-marrow cells *in vivo*." Mutation Research Letters 122(3-4): 347-353.

Panigrahi, G., S. Tiwari, K. M. Ansari, R. K. Chaturvedi, V. K. Khanna, B. P. Chaudhari, V. M. Vashistha, S. Raisuddin and M. Das (2014). "Association between children death and consumption of Cassia occidentalis seeds: Clinical and experimental investigations." Food and Chemical Toxicology 67: 236-248.

Panigrahi, G. K., A. Yadav, P. Mandal, A. Tripathi and M. Das (2016). "Immunomodulatory potential of Rhein, an anthraquinone moiety of Cassia occidentalis seeds." Toxicology Letters 245: 15-23.

Panigrahi, G. K., A. Yadav, A. Srivastava, A. Tripathi, S. Raisuddin and M. Das (2015). "Mechanism of rhein-induced apoptosis in rat primary hepatocytes: beneficial effect of cyclosporine A." Chemical Research in Toxicology 28(6): 1133-1143.

Panigrahi, G. K., A. Yadav, A. Yadav, K. M. Ansari, R. K. Chaturvedi, V. M. Vashistha, S. Raisuddin and M. Das (2014). "Hepatic transcriptional analysis in rats treated with Cassia occidentalis seed: Involvement of oxidative stress and impairment in xenobiotic metabolism as a putative mechanism of toxicity." Toxicology Letters 229(1): 273-283.

Pant, M., P. Garg and P. Seth (2012). "Central Nervous System Infection by HIV-1: Special Emphasis to NeuroAIDS in India." Proceedings of the National Academy of Sciences, India Section B: Biological Sciences 82(1): 81-94.

Pant, N., N. Mathur, A. Banerjee, S. Srivastava and D. Saxena (2004). "Correlation of chlorinated pesticides concentration in semen with seminal vesicle and prostatic markers." Reproductive Toxicology 19(2): 209-214.

Pant, N., M. Shukla, D. K. Patel, Y. Shukla, N. Mathur, Y. K. Gupta and D. K. Saxena (2008). "Correlation of phthalate exposures with semen quality." Toxicology and Applied Pharmacology 231(1): 112-116.

Pant, P., S. K. Guttikunda and R. E. Peltier (2016). "Exposure to particulate matter in India: A synthesis of findings and future directions." Environmental Research 147: 480-496.

Pant, P., A. Shukla, S. D. Kohl, J. C. Chow, J. G. Watson and R. M. Harrison (2015). "Characterization of ambient PM2. 5 at a pollution hotspot in New Delhi, India and inference of sources." Atmospheric Environment 109: 178-189.

Panwar, H., D. Jain, S. Khan, N. Pathak, G. V. Raghuram, A. Bhargava, S. Banerjee and P. K. Mishra (2013). "Imbalance of mitochondrial-nuclear cross talk in isocyanate mediated pulmonary endothelial cell dysfunction." Redox Biology 1(1): 163-171.

Panwar, H., G. V. Raghuram, D. Jain, A. K. Ahirwar, S. Khan, S. K. Jain, N. Pathak, S. Banerjee, K. K. Maudar and P. K. Mishra (2014). "Cell cycle deregulation by methyl isocyanate: implications in liver carcinogenesis." Environmental Toxicology 29(3): 284-297.

Pari, L. and K. Karthikesan (2007). "Protective role of caffeic acid against alcohol-induced biochemical changes in rats." Fundamental and Clinical Pharmacology 21(4): 355-361.

Parihar, Y. S., J. P. Patnaik, B. K. Nema, G. B. Sahoo, I. B. Misra and S. Adhikary (1997). "Coal workers' pneumoconiosis: A study of prevalence in coal mines of eastern Madhya Pradesh and Orissa states of India." Industrial Health 35(4): 467-473.

Parikh, J., V. Gokani, P. Doctor, P. Kulkarni, A. Shah and H. Saiyed (2005). "Acute and chronic health effects due to green tobacco exposure in agricultural workers." American Journal of Industrial Medicine 47(6): 494-499.

Parmar, D., A. Dhawan, M. Dayal and P. K. Seth (1998). "Immunochemical and biochemical evidence for expression of phenobarbital-and 3-methylcholanthrene-inducible isoenzymes of cytochrome P450 in rat brain." International Journal of Toxicology 17(6): 619-630.

Parmar, D., S. P. Srivastava and P. K. Seth (1986). "Effect of di (2-ethylhexyl) phthalate (DEHP) on spermatogenesis in adult rats." Toxicology 42(1): 47-55.

Parmar, D., S. Yadav, M. Dayal, A. Johri, A. Dhawan and P. Seth (2003). "Effect of lindane on hepatic and brain cytochrome P450s and influence of P450 modulation in lindane induced neurotoxicity." Food and Chemical Toxicology 41(8): 1077-1087.

Parmar, S. R., P. H. Vashrambhai and K. Kalia (2010). "Hepatoprotective activity of some plants extract against paracetamol induced hepatotoxicity in rats." Journal of Herbal Medicine and Toxicology 4(2): 101-106.

Parrish, J. (1982). The scope of photomedicine. The Science of Photomedicine: 3-17.

Part, A. (1963). "Protection by Indigenous Drugs against Hepatotoxic Effects of Carbon Tetrachloride – A Long term Study." Acta Pharmacologica et Toxicologica 20: 274-280.

Parthasarathy, R., G. R. Sarma, B. Janardhanam, P. Ramachandran, T. Santha, S. Sivasubramanian, P. Somasundaram and S. Tripathy (1986). "Hepatic toxicity in South Indian patients during treatment of tuberculosis with short-course regimens containing isoniazid, rifampicin and pyrazinamide." Tubercle 67(2): 99-108.

Parveen, A., S. Rizvi, A. Gupta, R. Singh, I. Ahmad, F. Mahdi and A. Mahdi (2012). "NMR-based metabonomics study of sub-acute hepatotoxicity induced by silica nanoparticles in rats after intranasal exposure." Journal of Cellular and Molecular Biology 58:196-203.

Parveen, A., S. H. M. Rizvi, F. Mahdi, S. Tripathi, I. Ahmad, R. K. Shukla, V. K. Khanna, R. Singh, D. K. Patel and A. A. Mahdi (2014). "Silica nanoparticles mediated neuronal cell death in corpus striatum of rat brain: implication of mitochondrial, endoplasmic reticulum and oxidative stress." Journal of Nanoparticle Research 16(11): 2664.

Patel, C. B., P. Vajpayee, G. Singh, A. Jyoti, R. Upadhyay and R. Shanker (2011). "Computation and in-silico validation of a Real-Time PCR array for quantitative detection of fecal coliforms in surface and potable water." Journal of Bioscience and Biotechnology 1: 184-195.

Patel, C. B., P. Vajpayee, G. Singh, R. Upadhyay and R. Shanker (2011). "Contamination of potable water by enterotoxigenic Escherichia coli: qPCR based culture-free detection and quantification." Ecotoxicology and Environmental Safety 74(8): 2292-2298.

Patel, R. K., A. H. Trivedi, R. J. Jaju, S. G. Adhvaryu and D. B. Balar (1994). "Ethanol potentiates the clastogenicity of pan masala — an *in vitro* experience." Carcinogenesis 15(9): 2017-2021.

Patel, S., M. Bajpayee, A. K. Pandey, D. Parmar and A. Dhawan (2007). "*In vitro* induction of cytotoxicity and DNA strand breaks in CHO cells exposed to cypermethrin, pendimethalin and dichlorvos." Toxicology *In Vitro* 21(8): 1409-1418.

Patel, S., A. K. Pandey, M. Bajpayee, D. Parmar and A. Dhawan (2006). "Cypermethrin-induced DNA damage in organs and tissues of the mouse: evidence from the comet assay." Mutation Research/Genetic Toxicology and Environmental Mutagenesis 607(2): 176-183.

Patel, S., D. Parmar, Y. Gupta and M. Singh (2005). "Review Articles - Contribution of genomics, proteomics, and single-nucleotide polymorphism in toxicology research and Indian scenario." Indian Journal of Human Genetics 11(2): 61-75.

Patel, S., K. Singh, S. Singh and M. P. Singh (2008). "Gene expression profiles of mouse striatum in control and maneb+ paraquat-induced Parkinson's disease phenotype: validation of differentially expressed energy metabolizing transcripts." Molecular Biotechnology 40(1): 59-68.

Patel, S., V. Singh, A. Kumar, Y. K. Gupta and M. P. Singh (2006). "Status of antioxidant defense system and expression of toxicant responsive genes in striatum of maneb-and paraquat-induced Parkinson's disease phenotype in mouse: mechanism of neurodegeneration." Brain Research 1081(1): 9-18.

Patel, S., A. Sinha and M. P. Singh (2007). "Identification of differentially expressed proteins in striatum of maneb-and paraquat-induced Parkinson's disease phenotype in mouse." Neurotoxicology and Teratology 29(5): 578-585.

Patel, T. K., P. B. Patel, M. J. Barvaliya and C. Tripathi (2014). "Drug-induced anaphylactic reactions in Indian population: A systematic review." Indian Journal of Critical Care Medicine: 18(12): 796.

Pathak, A., R. Shanker, S. K. Garg and N. Manickam (2011). "Profiling of biodegradation and bacterial 16S rRNA genes in diverse contaminated ecosystems using 60-mer oligonucleotide microarray." Applied Microbiology and Biotechnology 90(5): 1739-1754.

Pathak, M., M. Fareed, V. Bihari, N. Mathur, A. Srivastava, M. Kuddus and K. Nair (2011). "Cholinesterase levels and morbidity in pesticide sprayers in North India." Occupational Medicine 61(7): 512-514.

Pathak, M. A. and P. C. Joshi (1984). "Production of active oxygen species (1O2 and O2÷) by psoralens and ultraviolet radiation (320–400 nm)." Biochimica et Biophysica Acta (BBA)-General Subjects 798(1): 115-126.

Pathak, M. K., M. Fareed, V. Bihari, M. M. K. Reddy, D. K. Patel, N. Mathur, M. Kuddus and C. Nair Kesavachandran (2011). "Nerve conduction studies in sprayers occupationally exposed to mixture of pesticides in a mango plantation at Lucknow, North India." Toxicological and Environmental Chemistry 93(1): 188-196.

Pathak, M. K., M. Fareed, A. K. Srivastava, B. S. Pangtey, V. Bihari, M. Kuddus and C. Kesavachandran (2013). "Seasonal variations in cholinesterase activity, nerve conduction velocity and lung function among sprayers exposed to mixture of pesticides." Environmental Science and Pollution Research 20(10): 7296-7300.

Pathak, N. and S. Khandelwal (2007). "Role of oxidative stress and apoptosis in cadmium induced thymic atrophy and splenomegaly in mice." Toxicology Letters 169(2): 95-108.

Pathak, R., S. G. Suke, R. S. Ahmed, A. Tripathi, K. Guleria, C. Sharma, S. Makhijani, M. Mishra and B. Banerjee (2008). "Endosulfan and other organochlorine pesticide residues in maternal and cord blood in North Indian population." Bulletin of Environmental Contamination and Toxicology 81(2): 216-219.

Pathak, S. and K. Gopal (2008). "Prevalence of bacterial contamination with antibiotic resistant and enterotoxigenic fecal coliforms in treated drinking water." Journal of Toxicology and Environmental Health, Part A 71(7): 427-433.

Pathak, S., N. Kedia-Mokashi, M. Saxena, R. D'Souza, A. Maitra, P. Parte, M. Gill-Sharma and N. Balasinor (2009). "Effect of tamoxifen treatment on global and insulin-like growth factor 2-H19 locus-specific DNA methylation in rat spermatozoa and its association with embryo loss." Fertility and Sterility 91(5): 2253-2263.

Pathak, S. K., S. Basu, K. K. Basu, A. Banerjee, S. Pathak, A. Bhattacharyya, T. Kaisho, M. Kundu and J. Basu (2007). "Direct extracellular interaction between the early secreted antigen ESAT-6 of Mycobacterium tuberculosis and TLR2 inhibits TLR signaling in macrophages." Nature Immunology 8(6): 610.

Patil, A., V. Bhagwat, J. Patil, N. Dongre, J. Ambekar, R. Jailkhani and K. Das (2006). "Effect of lead (Pb) exposure on the activity of superoxide dismutase and catalase in battery manufacturing workers (BMW) of Western Maharashtra (India) with reference to heme biosynthesis." International Journal of Environmental Research and Public Health 3(4): 329-337.

Patil, G., M. I. Khan, D. K. Patel, S. Sultana, R. Prasad and I. Ahmad (2012). "Evaluation of cytotoxic, oxidative stress, proinflammatory and genotoxic responses of micro-and nano-particles of dolomite on human lung epithelial cells A549." Environmental Toxicology and Pharmacology 34(2): 436-445.

Patil, R. S., R. Kumar, R. Menon, M. K. Shah and V. Sethi (2013). "Development of particulate matter speciation profiles for major sources in six cities in India." Atmospheric Research 132: 1-11.

Patil, S. P., P. V. Niphadkar and M. M. Bapat (2001). "Chickpea: a major food allergen in the Indian subcontinent and its clinical and immunochemical correlation." Annals of Allergy, Asthma and Immunology 87(2): 140-145.

Patra, M., N. Bhowmik, B. Bandopadhyay and A. Sharma (2004). "Comparison of mercury, lead and arsenic with respect to genotoxic effects on plant systems and the development of genetic tolerance." Environmental and Experimental Botany 52(3): 199-223.

Patwardhan, B., D. Kalbag, P. Patki and B. Nagsampagi (1990). "Search of immunomodulatory agents: a review." Indian Drugs 28(2): 56-63.

Paul, B. N., A. Prakash, S. Kumar, A. K. Yadav, U. Mani, A. K. Saxena, A. P. Sahu, K. Lal and K. K. Dutta (2002). "Silica induced early fibrogenic reaction in lung of mice ameliorated by Nyctanthes arbortristis extract." Biomedical and Environmental Sciences 15(3): 215-222.

Paul, D. (2017). "Research on heavy metal pollution of river Ganga: A review." Annals of Agrarian Science 15(2): 278-286.

Paul, R. and A. Borah (2015). "The potential physiological crosstalk and interrelationship between two sovereign endogenous amines, melatonin and homocysteine." Life Sciences 139: 97-107.

Paul, R. and A. Borah (2016). "L-DOPA-induced hyperhomocysteinemia in Parkinson's disease: Elephant in the room." Biochimica et Biophysica Acta (BBA)-General Subjects 1860(9): 1989-1997.

Paul, S., N. Banerjee, A. Chatterjee, T. J. Sau, J. K. Das, P. K. Mishra, P. Chakrabarti, A. Bandyopadhyay and A. K. Giri (2014). "Arsenic-induced promoter hypomethylation and over-expression of ERCC2 reduces DNA repair capacity in humans by non-disjunction of the ERCC2–Cdk7 complex." Metallomics 6(4): 864-873.

Paul, S. P. and S. Manoj (2009). "Screening of food additives on model organism Caenorhabditis elegans." Journal of Industrial Pollution Control 25(2): 1-6.

Pavan, M. (2013). "Acute kidney injury following Paraquat poisoning in India." Iranian Journal of Kidney Diseases 7(1).

Pawar, N., P. Gireesh-Babu, S. Sivasubbu and A. Chaudhari (2016). "Transgenic zebrafish biosensor for the detection of cadmium and zinc toxicity." Current Science 111(10): 1697.

Pawar, N. N., P. C. Badgujar, L. P. Sharma, A. G. Telang and K. P. Singh (2017). "Oxidative impairment and histopathological alterations in kidney and brain of mice following subacute lambda-cyhalothrin exposure." Toxicology and Industrial Health 33(3): 277-286.

Philip, J. M., U. K. Aravind and C. T. Aravindakumar (2018). "Emerging contaminants in Indian environmental matrices – A review." Chemosphere 190: 307-326.

Phoon, W. (2000). "Occupational health hazard due to asbestos mining activities global scenario (Seminar, School of Environmental Science, JN Univ; New Delhi, Oct. 2000)."

Poddar, S., P. Mukherjee, G. Talukder and A. Sharma (2000). "Dietary protection by iron against clastogenic effects of short-term exposure to arsenic in mice *in vivo*." Food and Chemical Toxicology 38(8): 735-737.

Ponrasu, T., M. Ganeshkumar and L. Suguna (2012). "Developmental toxicity evaluation of ethanolic extract of Annona squamosa in zebrafish (Danio rerio) embryo". Journal of Pharmacy Research, 5(1), 277-279.

Pooja Jadiya, S. S. Mir. and A. Nazir (2012). "Effect of Various Classes of Pesticides on Expression of Stress Genes in Transgenic C. elegans Model of Parkinson's Disease." CNS and Neurological Disorders-Drug Targets 11(8):1001-5.

Pope, D. P., V. Mishra, L. Thompson, A. R. Siddiqui, E. A. Rehfuess, M. Weber and N. G. Bruce (2010). "Risk of low birth weight and stillbirth associated with indoor air pollution from solid fuel use in developing countries." Epidemiologic Reviews 32(1): 70-81.

Potula, V. and H. Hu (1996). "Relationship of hemoglobin to occupational exposure to motor vehicle exhaust." Toxicology and Industrial Health 12(5): 629-637.

Powers, K. M., D. M. Kay, S. A. Factor, C. P. Zabetian, D. S. Higgins, A. Samii, J. G. Nutt, A. Griffith, B. Leis and J. W. Roberts (2008). "Combined effects of smoking, coffee, and NSAIDs on Parkinson's disease risk." Movement Disorders 23(1): 88-95.

Prabhakar, N., K. Arora, S. K. Arya, P. R. Solanki, M. Iwamoto, H. Singh and B. Malhotra (2008). "Nucleic acid sensor for M. tuberculosis detection based on surface plasmon resonance." Analyst 133(11): 1587-1592.

Prabodh, S., D. Prakash, G. Sudhakar, N. Chowdary, V. Desai and R. Shekhar (2011). "Status of copper and magnesium levels in diabetic nephropathy cases: a case-control study from South India." Biological Trace Element Research 142(1): 29-35.

Pragya, P., A. Shukla, R. Murthy, M. Abdin and D. Kar Chowdhuri (2015). "Characterization of the effect of Cr (VI) on humoral innate immunity using Drosophila melanogaster." Environmental Toxicology 30(11): 1285-1296.

Prakash, J., A. Gupta, O. Kumar, S. Rout, V. Malhotra and P. Srivastava (1996). Acute renal failure in falciparum malaria — increasing prevalence in some areas of India — a need for awareness, Nephrology Dialysis Transplantation 11(12):2414-6.

Prakash, N. and U. Venkatesh (1996). "Human chorionic gonadotrophin (hcG) protects malathion induced plasma luteinizing hormone and testosterone changes in rats." Indian Journal of Pharmacology 28(4): 257.

Prakash, P., S. Royana, P. Sankarsan and S. Rajeev (2017). "The review of small size silver nanoparticle neurotoxicity: A repeat study." Journal of Cytology and Histology 8: 468.

Prakash, S., B. Misra, R. Adsule and G. Barat (1977). "Distribution of β-N-oxalyl-L-α-β diaminopropionic Acid in Different Tissues of Aging Lathyrus sativus Plant." Biochemie Und Physiologie Der Pflanzen 171(4): 369-374.

Prasad, A., N. Pant, S. Srivastava, R. Kumar and S. Srivastava (1995). "Effect of dermal application of hexachlorocyclohexane (HCH) on male reproductive system of rat." Human and Experimental Toxicology 14(6): 484-488.

Prasad, A., K. Singh, A. Saxena, N. Mathur and P. Ray (1987). "Increased macrophage activity in protein A treated tumor regressed animals." Immunopharmacology and Immunotoxicology 9(4): 541-561.

Prasad, M. and S. Kalra (1967). "Mechanism of anti-implantation action of clomiphene." Reproduction 13(1): 59-66.

Prasad, M., M. Mukundan and K. Krishnaswamy (1995). "Micronuclei and carcinogen DNA adducts as intermediate end points in nutrient intervention trial of precancerous lesions in the oral cavity." European Journal of Cancer Part B: Oral Oncology 31(3): 155-159.

Prasad, P., A. K. Tiwari, K. P. Kumar, A. Ammini, A. Gupta, R. Gupta, A. Sharma, A. Rao, R. Nagendra and T. S. Chandra (2006). "Chronic renal insufficiency among Asian Indians with type 2 diabetes: I. Role of RAAS gene polymorphisms." BMC Medical Genetics 7(1): 42.

Prasad, P., A. K. Tiwari, K. P. Kumar, A. Ammini, A. Gupta, R. Gupta and B. Thelma (2007). "Association of TGFβ1, TNFα, CCR2 and CCR5 gene polymorphisms in type-2 diabetes and renal insufficiency among Asian Indians." BMC Medical Genetics 8(1): 20.

Prasad, P., A. K. Tiwari, K. P. Kumar, A. Ammini, A. Gupta, R. Gupta and B. Thelma (2010). "Association analysis of ADPRT1, AKR1B1, RAGE, GFPT2 and PAI-1 gene polymorphisms with chronic renal insufficiency among Asian Indians with type-2 diabetes." BMC Medical Genetics 11(1): 52.

Prasad, R. and R. Kumar (2013). Allergy situation in India: what is being done? Indian Journal of Chest Diseases and Allied Sciences 55(1):7-8.

Prasad, R. and R. Nath (1995). "Cadmium-induced nephrotoxicity in rhesus monkeys (Macaca, mulatta) in relation to protein calorie malnutrition." Toxicology 100(1-3): 89-100.

Prasad, R., S. Verma, G. Agrawal and N. Mathur (2006). "Prediction model for peak expiratory flow in North Indian population." The Indian Journal of Chest Diseases and Allied Sciences 48(2):103-6.

Priyadarshi, A., S. A. Khuder, E. A. Schaub and S. S. Priyadarshi (2001). "Environmental risk factors and Parkinson's disease: a metaanalysis." Environmental Research 86(2): 122-127.

Priyamvada, S., M. Priyadarshini, N. Arivarasu, N. Farooq, S. Khan, S. A. Khan, M. W. Khan and A. Yusufi (2008). "Studies on the protective effect of dietary fish oil on gentamicin-induced nephrotoxicity and oxidative damage in rat kidney." Prostaglandins, Leukotrienes and Essential Fatty Acids 78(6): 369-381.

Punia, S., M. Das, M. Behari, M. Dihana, S. T. Govindappa, U. B. Muthane, B. Thelma and R. C. Juyal (2011). "Leads from xenobiotic metabolism genes for Parkinson's disease among north Indians." Pharmacogenetics and Genomics 21(12): 790-797.

Punia, S., M. Das, M. Behari, B. K. Mishra, A. K. Sahani, S. T. Govindappa, S. Jayaram, U. B. Muthane, B. Thelma and R. C. Juyal (2010). "Role of polymorphisms in dopamine synthesis and metabolism genes and association of DBH haplotypes with Parkinson's disease among North Indians." Pharmacogenetics and Genomics 20(7): 435-441.

Puri, P. and S. Kumar (2016). "Liver involvement in human immunodeficiency virus infection." Indian Journal of Gastroenterology 35(4): 260-273.

Puri, P., P. Sharma, A. Lolusare, V. Sashindran, S. Shrivastava and A. Nagpal (2017). "Liver Function Tests Abnormalities and Hepatitis B Virus & Hepatitis C Virus Co-infection in Human Immunodeficiency Virus (HIV)-infected Patients in India." Journal of Clinical and Experimental Hepatology 7(1): 1-8.

Purushothaman, S., A. Raghunath, V. Dhakshinamoorthy, L. Panneerselvam and E. Perumal (2014). "Acute exposure to titanium dioxide (TiO2) induces oxidative stress in zebrafish gill tissues." Toxicological and Environmental Chemistry 96(6): 890-905.

Qadri, S. A., S. Islam and M. Ahmad (1992). "Mutagenic activity of oxathiolane steroids: structural requirement for the genotoxic activity in Salmonella and E. coli." Mutation Research/Genetic Toxicology 298(1): 53-60.

Qadri, Y. H., A. Swamy and J. Rao (1994). "Species differences in brain acetylcholinesterase response to monocrotophos *in vitro*." Ecotoxicology and Environmental Safety 28(1): 91-98.

Qayyum, S., A. Ara and J. A. Usmani (2012). "Effect of nickel and chromium exposure on buccal cells of electroplaters." Toxicology and Industrial Health 28(1): 74-82.

Quadri, S. A., A. N. Qadri, M. Ahmad and S. Islam (1997). "Aziridinyl steroid-induced lesions in DNA and apoptosis in promyelocytic leukemia cells." IUBMB Life 43(6): 1353-1365.

Qutubuddin, S., S. Hebbal and A. Kumar (2013). "An ergonomic study of work related musculoskeletal disorder risks in Indian Saw Mills." Journal of Mechanical and Civil Engineering 7(5): 7-13.

Rabinovich, G. A., D. Gabrilovich and E. M. Sotomayor (2007). "Immunosuppressive strategies that are mediated by tumor cells." Annual Review of Immunology 25: 267-296.

Raghavan, S. and K. Basavaiah (2005). "Biological monitoring among benzene-exposed workers in Bangalore city, India." Biomarkers 10(5): 336-341.

Raghavender, C. and B. Reddy (2008). "Human and animal disease outbreaks in India due to mycotoxins other than aflatoxins." World Mycotoxin Journal 2(1): 23-30.

Raheja, G. and K. D. Gill (2002). "Calcium homeostasis and dichlorvos induced neurotoxicity in rat brain." Molecular and Cellular Biochemistry 232(1-2): 13-18.

Rahman, A., S. Ahmed, S. M. Vasenwala and M. Athar (2003). "Glyceryl trinitrate, a nitric oxide donor, abrogates ferric nitrilotriacetate-induced oxidative stress and renal damage." Archives of Biochemistry and Biophysics 418(1): 71-79.

Rahman, M., M. Mahboob, K. Danadevi, B. S. Banu and P. Grover (2002). "Assessment of genotoxic effects of chloropyriphos and acephate by the comet assay in mice leucocytes." Mutation Research/Genetic Toxicology and Environmental Mutagenesis 516(1-2): 139-147.

Rahman, Q., E. Dopp, M. Lohani and D. Schiffmann (2000). "Occupational and environmental factors enhancing the genotoxicity of asbestos." Inhalation Toxicology 12(sup3): 157-165.

Rahman, Q., P. Viswanathan and S. Zaidi (1976). "Effect of silicic acid and polyvinyl pyrrolidone on lysosomal ribonuclease of rat lungs." Toxicology and Applied Pharmacology 38(3): 471-478.

Rahman, Z. and V. P. Singh (2018). "Assessment of heavy metal contamination and Hg-resistant bacteria in surface water from different regions of Delhi, India." Saudi Journal of Biological Sciences 25(8): 1687-1695.

Rai, A., S. K. Maurya, P. Khare, A. Srivastava and S. Bandyopadhyay (2010). "Characterization of developmental neurotoxicity of As, Cd, and Pb mixture: synergistic action of metal mixture in glial and neuronal functions." Toxicological Sciences 118(2): 586-601.

Rai, D. K. and B. Sharma (2007). "Carbofuran-induced oxidative stress in mammalian brain." Molecular Biotechnology 37(1): 66.

Rai, N. K., A. Ashok, A. Rai, S. Tripathi, G. K. Nagar, K. Mitra and S. Bandyopadhyay (2013). "Exposure to As, Cd and Pb-mixture impairs myelin and axon development in rat brain, optic nerve and retina." Toxicology and Applied Pharmacology 273(2): 242-258.

Rai, R., A. Singh, T. Upadhyay, S. Patil and H. Nayar (1981). "Biochemical effects of chronic exposure to noise in man." International Archives of Occupational and Environmental Health 48(4): 331-337.

Rai, S., A. K. Singh, A. Srivastava, S. Yadav, M. H. Siddiqui and M. K. R. Mudiam (2016). "Comparative evaluation of QuEChERS method coupled to DLLME extraction for the analysis of multiresidue pesticides in vegetables and fruits by gas chromatography-mass spectrometry." Food Analytical Methods 9(9): 2656-2669.

Rai, V., P. Kakkar, J. Singh, C. Misra, S. Kumar and S. Mehrotra (2008). "Toxic metals and organochlorine pesticides residue in single herbal drugs used in important ayurvedic formulation–'Dashmoola'." Environmental Monitoring and Assessment 143(1-3): 273-277.

Raisuddin, S., K. Singh, S. Zaidi, B. Paul and P. Ray (1993). "Immunosuppressive effects of aflatoxin in growing rats." Mycopathologia 124(3): 189-194.

Raisuddin, S., K. P. Singh, S. I. A. Zaidi and P. K. Ray (1994). "Immunostimulating effects of protein A in immunosurpressed aflatoxin-intoxicated rats." International Journal of Immunopharmacology 16(12): 977-984.

Raisuddin, S., S. Zaidi, K. Singh and P. Ray (1991). "Effect of subchronic aflatoxin exposure on growth and progression of Ehrlich's ascites tumor in mice." Drug and Chemical Toxicology 14(1-2): 185-206.

Raizada, J. and P. Dwivedi (1987). "Chronic ocular lesions in Bhopal gas tragedy." Indian Journal of Ophthalmology 35(5-6): 453-454.

Raj, G. B., M. Patnaik, P. S. Babu, B. Kalakumar, M. Singh and J. Shylaja (2006). "Heavy metal contaminants in water-soil-plant-animal continuum due to pollution of Musi river around Hyderabad in India." The Indian Journal of Animal Sciences 76(2).

Rajaguru, P., S. Suba, M. Palanivel and K. Kalaiselvi (2003). "Genotoxicity of a polluted river system measured using the alkaline comet assay on fish and earthworm tissues." Environmental and Molecular Mutagenesis 41(2): 85-91.

Rajah, T. and Y. Ahuja (1995). "*In vivo* genotoxic effects of smoking and occupational lead exposure in printing press workers." Toxicology Letters 76(1): 71-75.

Rajak, P., M. Dutta and S. Roy (2014). "Effect of acute exposure of acephate on hemocyte abundance in a non-target victim Drosophila melanogaster." Toxicological and Environmental Chemistry 96(5): 768-776.

Rajak, P., S. Sahana and S. Roy (2013). "Acephate-induced shortening of developmental duration and early adult emergence in a nontarget insect Drosophila melanogaster." Toxicological and Environmental Chemistry 95(8): 1369-1379.

Rajakrishna, L., S. K. Unni, M. Subbiah, S. Sadagopan, A. R. Nair, R. Chandrappa, G. Sambasivam and S. K. Sukumaran (2014). "Validation of a human cell based high-throughput genotoxicity assay 'Anthem's Genotoxicity screen'using ECVAM recommended lists of genotoxic and non-genotoxic chemicals." Toxicology *In Vitro* 28(1): 46-53.

Rajapurkar, M. M., G. T. John, A. L. Kirpalani, G. Abraham, S. K. Agarwal, A. F. Almeida, S. Gang, A. Gupta, G. Modi and D. Pahari (2012). "What do we know about chronic kidney disease in India: first report of the Indian CKD registry." BMC Nephrology 13(1): 10.

Rajashekar, K. (2005). Analysis of Pesticide Residues in Milk and Milk Products, Acharya NG Ranga Agricultural University, Rajendranagar, Hyderabad.

Rajesh, S., B. Rajkapoor, R. Senthil Kumar and K. Raju (2009). "Effect of Clausena dentata (Willd.) M. Roem. against paracetamol induced hepatotoxicity in rats." Pakistan Journal of Pharmaceutical Sciences 22(1).

Rajeshwari, A., S. Kavitha, S. A. Alex, D. Kumar, A. Mukherjee, N. Chandrasekaran and A. Mukherjee (2015). "Cytotoxicity of aluminum oxide nanoparticles on Allium cepa root tip—effects of oxidative stress generation and biouptake." Environmental Science and Pollution Research 22(14): 11057-11066.

Rajeswary, S., N. Mathew, M. A. Akbarsha, M. Kalyanasundram and B. Kumaran (2007). "Protective effect of vitamin E against carbendazim-induced testicular toxicity–histopathological evidences and reduced residue levels in testis and serum." Archives of Toxicology 81(11): 813-821.

Rajkapoor, B., Y. Venugopal, J. Anbu, N. Harikrishnan, M. Gobinath and V. Ravichandran (2008). "Protective effect of Phyllanthus polyphyllus on acetaminophen induced hepatotoxicity in rats." Pakistan Journal of Pharmaceutical Sciences 21(1): 57-62.

Rajkumar, P., K. Pattabi, S. Vadivoo, A. Bhome, B. Brashier, P. Bhattacharya and S. M. Mehendale (2017). "A cross-sectional study on prevalence of chronic obstructive pulmonary disease (COPD) in India: rationale and methods." BMJ Open 7(5): e015211.

Raju, P. S., K. Prasad, Y. V. Ramana, N. Balakrishna and K. Murthy (2005). "Influence of socioeconomic status on lung function and prediction equations in Indian children." Pediatric Pulmonology 39(6): 528-536.

Ram, K. and M. Sarin (2011). "Day–night variability of EC, OC, WSOC and inorganic ions in urban environment of Indo-Gangetic Plain: implications to secondary aerosol formation." Atmospheric Environment 45(2): 460-468.

Ram, M. S., D. Neetu, B. Yogesh, B. Anju, P. Dipti, T. Pauline, S. Sharma, S. Sarada, G. Ilavazhagan and D. Kumar (2002). "Cyto-protective and immunomodulating properties of Amla (Emblica officinalis) on lymphocytes: *an in-vitro* study." Journal of Ethnopharmacology 81(1): 5-10.

Ram, S., P. Vajpayee, P. Dwivedi and R. Shanker (2011). "Culture-free detection and enumeration of STEC in water." Ecotoxicology and Environmental Safety 74(4): 551-557.

Ram, S., P. Vajpayee and R. Shanker (2007). "Contamination of potable water distribution systems by multiantimicrobial-resistant enterohemorrhagic Escherichia coli." Environmental Health Perspectives 116(4): 448-452.

Ramachandran, M. (1984). "DDT and HCH residues in the body fat and blood samples from some Delhi hospitals." Indian Journal of Medical Research 80: 590-593.

Ramachandran, P. (1980). "Chemotherapy of tuberculous meningitis with isoniazid plus rifampicin-interim findings in a trial in children." Indian Journal of Tuberculosis 27(2): 54-57.

Ramamoorthy, H., P. Abraham and B. Isaac (2014). "Mitochondrial dysfunction and electron transport chain complex defect in a rat model of tenofovir disoproxil fumarate nephrotoxicity." Journal of Biochemical and Molecular Toxicology 28(6): 246-255.

Ramana, G. V., B. Su, L. Jin, L. Singh, N. Wang, P. Underhill and R. Chakraborty (2001). "Y-chromosome SNP haplotypes suggest evidence of gene flow among caste, tribe, and the migrant Siddi populations of Andhra Pradesh, South India." European Journal of Human Genetics 9(9): 695.

Ramanathan, A. and V. Subramanian (2001). "Present status of asbestos mining and related health problems in India." Industrial Health 39(4): 309-315.

Ramanathan, N. L. and S. Kashyap (1975). "Occupational environment and health in India." Ambio: 60-64.

Ramanathan, R., S. Rupert, S. Selvaraj, J. Satyanesan, R. Vennila and S. Rajagopal (2017). "Role of Human Wharton's Jelly Derived Mesenchymal Stem Cells (WJ-MSCs) for Rescue of D-Galactosamine Induced Acute Liver Injury in Mice." Journal of Clinical and Experimental Hepatology 7(3): 205-214.

Ramanathan, V., S. Sundar, R. Harnish, S. Sharma, J. Seddon, B. Croes, A. Lloyd, S. Tripathi, A. Aggarwal and W. Al Delaimy (2014). "India California Air Pollution Mitigation Program: Options to Reduce Road Transport Pollution in India." Published by The Energy and Resources Institute in Collaboration with the University of California at San Diego and the California Air Resources Board.

Ramasubban, S., A. Majumdar and P. S. Das (2008). "Safety and efficacy of polymyxin B in multidrug resistant Gram-negative severe sepsis and septic shock." Indian Journal of Critical Care Medicine 12(4): 153.

Ramaswamy, S. (1987). "An Overview of the Health Hazards Due to Toxic Exposure in the Indian Work Environment." Defence Science Journal 37(2): 113-131.

Ramchandani, S., M. Das and S. Khanna (1994). "Effect of metanil yellow, orange II and their blend on hepatic xenobiotic metabolizing enzymes in rats." Food and Chemical Toxicology 32(6): 559-563.

Ramesh, A. and P. E. Ravi (2004). "Electron ionization gas chromatography–mass spectrometric determination of residues of thirteen pyrethroid insecticides in whole blood." Journal of Chromatography B 802(2): 371-376.

Ramkishan, A. and F. Khan (2017). "Similar Biologics: Regulatory Prospective in India." Journal of Pharmaceutical Research 16(3): 191-198.

Ramkumar, M., S. Rajasankar, V. V. Gobi, C. Dhanalakshmi, T. Manivasagam, A. J. Thenmozhi, M. M. Essa, A. Kalandar and R. Chidambaram (2017). "Neuroprotective effect of Demethoxycurcumin, a natural derivative of Curcumin on rotenone induced neurotoxicity in SH-SY 5Y Neuroblastoma cells." BMC Complementary and Alternative Medicine 17(1): 217.

Ramteke, P., J. Bhattacharjee, S. Pathak and N. Kalra (1992). "Evaluation of coliforms as indicators of water quality in India." The Journal of Applied Bacteriology 72(4): 352.

Rana, S., S. Attri, K. Vaiphei, R. Pal, A. Attri and K. Singh (2006). "Role of N-acetylcysteine in rifampicin-induced hepatic injury of young rats." World Journal of Gastroenterology: WJG 12(2): 287.

Ranadive, K. J., S. Ranadive, N. Shivapurkar and S. Gothoskar (1979). "Betel quid chewing and oral cancer: experimental studies on hamsters." International Journal of Cancer 24(6): 835-843.

Ranga, U., R. Shankarappa, N. B. Siddappa, L. Ramakrishna, R. Nagendran, M. Mahalingam, A. Mahadevan, N. Jayasuryan, P. Satishchandra and S. K. Shankar (2004). "Tat protein of human immunodeficiency virus type 1 subtype C strains is a defective chemokine." Journal of Virology 78(5): 2586-2590.

Rani, R., A. Sood and R. Goswami (2004). "Molecular basis of predisposition to develop type 1 diabetes mellitus in North Indians." Tissue Antigens 64(2): 145-155.

Rao, C. V., A. Rawat, A. P. Singh, A. Singh and N. Verma (2012). "Hepatoprotective potential of ethanolic extract of Ziziphus oenoplia (L.) Mill roots against antitubercular drugs induced hepatotoxicity in experimental models." Asian Pacific Journal of Tropical Medicine 5(4): 283-288.

Rao, G. and K. Pandya (1978). "Toxicity of petroleum products: Effects on alkaline phosphatase and lipid peroxidation." Environmental Research 16(1-3): 174-178.

Rao, G., A. Saraf, R. Purkait, V. Sharma, R. Jadhav, H. Chandra and S. Sriramachari (1991). "Bhopal gas disaster: Unidentified compounds in the residue of the MIC Tank-610." Journal of Indian Academy of Forensic Sciences 30: 13-18.

Rao, M., S. Chawla and N. Patel (2009). "Melatonin reduction of fluoride-induced nephrotoxicity in mice." Fluoride 42(2): 110.

Rao, M., N. Chinoy, M. Suthar and M. Rajvanshi (2001). "Role of ascorbic acid on mercuric chloride-induced genotoxicity in human blood cultures." Toxicology *In Vitro* 15(6): 649-654.

Rao, M., M. M. Kumar and M. A. Rao (1999). "*In vitro* and *in vivo* effects of phenolic antioxidants against cisplatin-induced nephrotoxicity." The Journal of Biochemistry 125(2): 383-390.

Rao, N., R. Wadia, S. Karve and K. Grant (1982). "Hepatotoxicity of antituberculous drugs." The Journal of the Association of Physicians of India 30(5): 295.

Rao, P. L. and R. Bhattacharya (1996). "The cyanobacterial toxin microcystin-LR induced DNA damage in mouse liver *in vivo*." Toxicology 114(1): 29-36.

Rao, R. P. and B. B. Kaliwal (2002). "Monocrotophos induced dysfunction on estrous cycle and follicular development in mice." Industrial Health 40(3): 237-244.

Rao, R. V., A. Dhawan and N. Sapra (2005). "Opioid maintenance therapy with slow release oral morphine: Experience from India." Journal of Substance Use 10(5): 259-261.

Rao, S. (1978). "Entry of β-oxalyl-1-α, β-diaminopropionic acid, the lathyrus sativus neurotoxin into the central nervous system of the adult rat, chick and the rhesus monkey." Journal of Neurochemistry 30(6): 1467-1470.

Rao, S. (1978). "A sensitive and specific colorimetric method for the determination of α, β-diaminopropionic acid and the Lathyrus sativus neurotoxin." Analytical Biochemistry 86(2): 386-395.

Rao, S., P. Adiga and P. Sarma (1964). "The isolation and characterization of β-N-oxalyl-L-α, β-diaminopropionic acid: a neurotoxin from the seeds of Lathyrus sativus." Biochemistry 3(3): 432-436.

Rao, S., L. Ramachandran and P. Adiga (1963). "The isolation and characterization of l-homoarginine from seeds of Lathyrus sativus." Biochemistry 2(2): 298-300.

Rao, S., P. Sarma, K. Mani, T. R. Rao and S. Sriramachari (1967). "Experimental neurolathyrism in monkeys." Nature 214(5088): 610.

Rastogi, N., A. Singh and R. Satish (2019). "Characteristics of submicron particles coming from a big firecrackers burning event: Implications to atmospheric pollution." Atmospheric Pollution Research 10(2): 629-634.

Rastogi, R., A. Srivastava and B. N. Dhawan (1997). "Effect of Picroliv on impaired hepatic mixed-function oxidase system in carbon tetrachloride-intoxicated rats." Drug Development Research 41(1): 44-47.

Rastogi, S., I. Ahmad, B. Pangtey and N. Mathur (2003). "Effects of occupational exposure on respiratory system in carpet workers." Indian Journal of Occupational and Environmental Medicine 7(1): 19.

Rastogi, S., P. D. Dwivedi, S. K. Khanna and M. Das (2004). "Detection of aflatoxin M1 contamination in milk and infant milk products from Indian markets by ELISA." Food Control 15(4): 287-290.

Rastogi, S., B. Gupta, H. Chandra, N. Mathur, P. Mahendra and T. Husain (1991). "A study of the prevalence of respiratory morbidity among agate workers." International Archives of Occupational and Environmental Health 63(1): 21-26.

Rastogi, S., B. Gupta and N. Mathur (1988). "Pulmonary effects of silica dust in asymptomatic agate workers." Indian Journal of Environmental Protection 8: 244-247.

Rastogi, S., P. Rathee, T. Saxena, N. Mehra and R. Kumar (2003). "BOD analysis of industrial effluents: 5 days to 5 min." Current Applied Physics 3(2-3): 191-194.

Rastogi, S., S. Tripathi and D. Ravishanker (2010). "A study of neurologic symptoms on exposure to organophosphate pesticides in the children of agricultural workers." Indian Journal of Occupational and Environmental Medicine 14(2): 54.

Rastogi, S. K., B. N. Gupta, T. Husain, H. Chandra, N. Mathur, B. S. Pangtey, S. V. Chandra and N. Garg (1991). "A cross-sectional study of pulmonary function among workers exposed to multimetals in the glass bangle industry." American Journal of Industrial Medicine 20(3): 391-399.

Rastogi, S. K., A. Pandey and S. Tripathi (2008). "Occupational health risks among the workers employed in leather tanneries at Kanpur." Indian Journal of Occupational and Environmental Medicine 12(3): 132.

Rathi, P., D. Amarapurkar, N. Borges, G. Koppikar and R. Kalro (1997). "Spectrum of liver diseases in HIV infection." Indian Journal of Gastroenterology: Official Journal of the Indian Society of Gastroenterology 16(3): 94-95.

Rathore, M., P. Bhatnagar, D. Mathur and G. Saxena (2002). "Burden of organochlorine pesticides in blood and its effect on thyroid hormones in women." Science of the Total Environment 295(1-3): 207-215.

Ratnasekhar, C., M. Sonane, A. Satish and M. K. R. Mudiam (2015). "Metabolomics reveals the perturbations in the metabolome of Caenorhabditis elegans exposed to titanium dioxide nanoparticles." Nanotoxicology 9(8): 994-1004.

Ravi, K., V. Paliwal and R. Nath (1984). "Induction of Cd-metallothionein in cadmium exposed monkeys under different nutritional stresses." Toxicology Letters 22(1): 21-26.

Ravindra, K. and S. Mor (2019). "Distribution and health risk assessment of arsenic and selected heavy metals in Groundwater of Chandigarh, India." Environmental Pollution 250:820-830.

Ravindra, P., A. Bhiwgade, S. Kulkarni, P. V. Rataboli and C. Y. Dhume (2010). "Cisplatin induced histological changes in renal tissue of rat." Journal of Cell and Animal Biology 4(7): 108-111.

Ravindranath, V. and K. Pai (1991). "The use of rat brain slices as an *in vitro* model for mechanistic evaluation of neurotoxicity-studies with acrylamide." Neurotoxicology 12(2): 225-234.

Raviraja, A., G. V. Babu, A. Sehgal, R. B. Saper, I. Jayawardene, C. J. Amarasiriwardena and T. Venkatesh (2010). "Three cases of lead toxicity associated with consumption of ayurvedic medicines." Indian Journal of Clinical Biochemistry 25(3): 326-329.

Rawat, A., S. Chaturvedi, A. Singh, A. Guleria, D. Dubey, A. Keshari, V. Raj, A. Rai, A. Prakash and U. Kumar (2018). "Metabolomics approach discriminates toxicity index of pyrazinamide and its metabolic products, pyrazinoic acid and 5-hydroxy pyrazinoic acid." Human and Experimental Toxicology 37(4): 373-389.

Rawat, A., D. Dubey, A. Guleria, U. Kumar, A. K. Keshari, S. Chaturvedi, A. Prakash, S. Saha and D. Kumar (2016). "1H NMR-based serum metabolomics reveals erythromycin-induced liver toxicity in albino Wistar rats." Journal of Pharmacy and Bioallied Sciences 8(4): 327.

Ray, A., A. Bhaduri, N. Srivastava and S. Mazumder (2017). "Identification of novel signature genes attesting arsenic-induced immune alterations in adult zebrafish (Danio rerio)." Journal of Hazardous Materials 321: 121-131.

Ray, A., S. Chatterjee, S. Ghosh, S. Kabir, A. Pakrashi and C. Deb (1991). "Suppressive effect of quinalphos on the activity of accessory sex glands and plasma concentrations of gonadotrophins and testosterone in rats." Archives of Environmental Contamination and Toxicology 21(3): 383-387.

Ray, M., S. Mukherjee, S. Roychoudhury, P. Bhattacharya, M. Banerjee, S. Siddique, S. Chakraborty and T. Lahiri (2006). "Platelet activation, upregulation of

CD11b/CD18 expression on leukocytes and increase in circulating leukocyte-platelet aggregates in Indian women chronically exposed to biomass smoke." Human and Experimental Toxicology 25(11): 627-635.

Ray, M., S. Roychoudhury, S. Mukherjee and T. Lahiri (2007). "Occupational benzene exposure from vehicular sources in India and its effect on hematology, lymphocyte subsets and platelet P-selectin expression." Toxicology and Industrial Health 23(3): 167-175.

Ray, P. and S. Bandyopadhyay (1983). "Inhibition of rat mammary tumor growth by purified protein A - a potential anti-tumor agent." Immunological Communications 12(5): 453-464.

Ray, P. K., S. Bandyopadhyay, M. Dohadwala, P. Canchanapan and J. Mobini (1984). "Antitumor activity with nontoxic doses of protein A." Cancer Immunology, Immunotherapy 18(1): 29-34.

Ray, P. K., M. Dohadwala, S. K. Bandyopadhyay, P. Canchanapan and D. McLaughlin (1985). "Rescue of rats from large dose cyclophosphamide toxicity using protein A." Cancer Chemotherapy and Pharmacology 14(1): 59-62.

Ray, P. K., S. Raychaudhuri and P. Allen (1982). "Mechanism of regression of mammary adenocarcinomas in rats following plasma adsorption over protein A-containing Staphylococcus aureus." Cancer Research 42(12): 4970-4974.

Ray, R., N. Agrawal, R. Misra, M. Farooq and R. Hans (2006). "Radiation-induced *in vitro* phototoxic potential of some fluoroquinolones." Drug and Chemical Toxicology 29(1): 25-38.

Ray, R., N. Agrawal, A. Sharma and R. Hans (2008). "Use of L-929 cell line for phototoxicity assessment." Toxicology *In Vitro* 22(7): 1775-1781.

Ray, R. and A. Chopra (2012). "Monitoring of substance abuse in India – Initiatives & experiences." The Indian Journal of Medical Research 135(6): 806.

Ray, R., S. Mehrotra, S. Prakash and P. Joshi (1996). "Ultraviolet radiation-induced production of superoxide radicals by selected antibiotics." Drug and Chemical Toxicology 19(1-2): 121-130.

Ray, R., S. Mehrotra, U. Shankar, G. S. Babu, P. Joshi and R. Hans (2001). "Evaluation of UV-induced superoxide radical generation potential of some common antibiotics." Drug and Chemical Toxicology 24(2): 191-200.

Ray, R., R. Misra, M. Farooq and R. Hans (2002). "Effect of UV-B radiation on some common antibiotics." Toxicology *In Vitro* 16(2): 123-127.

Ray, R. S., S. F. Mujtaba, A. Dwivedi, N. Yadav, A. Verma, H. N. Kushwaha, S. K. Amar, S. Goel and D. Chopra (2013). "Singlet oxygen mediated DNA damage induced phototoxicity by ketoprofen resulting in mitochondrial depolarization and lysosomal destabilization." Toxicology 314(2-3): 229-237.

Reddy, K., H. Abbas, C. Abel, W. Shier, C. A. F. d. Oliveira and C. Raghavender (2009). "Mycotoxin contamination of commercially important agricultural commodities." Toxin Reviews 28(2-3): 154-168.

Reddy, N. P. and M. Das (2008). "Interaction of sanguinarine alkaloid, isolated from argemone oil, with hepatic cytochrome p450 in rats." Toxicology Mechanisms and Methods 18(8): 635-643.

Reddy, V. D., P. Padmavathi, S. Gopi, M. Paramahamsa and N. C. Varadacharyulu (2010). "Protective effect of Emblica officinalis against alcohol-induced hepatic injury by ameliorating oxidative stress in rats." Indian Journal of Clinical Biochemistry 25(4): 419-424.

Rehana, Z., A. Malik and M. Ahmad (1995). "Mutagenic activity of the Ganges water with special reference to the pesticide pollution in the river between Kachla to Kannauj (UP), India." Mutation Research 343(2-3): 137-144.

Rehana, Z., A. Malik and M. Ahmad (1996). "Genotoxicity of the Ganges water at Narora (UP), India." Mutation Research/Genetic Toxicology 367(4): 187-193.

Rehman, H., A. Mohan, H. Tabassum, F. Ahmad, S. Rahman, S. Parvez and S. Raisuddin (2011). "Deltamethrin Increases Candida albicans infection susceptibility in mice." Scandinavian Journal of Immunology 73(5): 459-464.

Rehman, I., T. Ahmed, P. Praveen, A. Kar and V. Ramanathan (2011). "Black carbon emissions from biomass and fossil fuels in rural India." Atmospheric Chemistry and Physics 11(14): 7289-7299.

Rita, P., P. Reddy and S. V. Reddy (1987). "Monitoring of workers occupationally exposed to pesticides in grape gardens of Andhra Pradesh." Environmental Research 44(1): 1-5.

Rizvi, F., A. Mathur and P. Kakkar (2015). "Morin mitigates acetaminophen-induced liver injury by potentiating Nrf2 regulated survival mechanism through molecular intervention in PHLPP2-Akt-Gsk3β axis." Apoptosis 20(10): 1296-1306.

Rizwan, S., A. Naqshbandi, Z. Farooqui, A. A. Khan and F. Khan (2014). "Protective effect of dietary flaxseed oil on arsenic-induced nephrotoxicity and oxidative damage in rat kidney." Food and Chemical Toxicology 68: 99-107.

Rizwan, S., B. Nongkynrih and S. K. Gupta (2013). "Air pollution in Delhi: its magnitude and effects on health." Indian Journal of Community Medicine: Official Publication of Indian Association of Preventive and Social Medicine 38(1): 4.

Rogerio, A., A. Kanashiro, C. Fontanari, E. Da Silva, Y. M. Lucisano-Valim, E. G. Soares and L. H. Faccioli (2007). "Anti-inflammatory activity of quercetin and isoquercitrin in experimental murine allergic asthma." Inflammation Research 56(10): 402-408.

Rojo, A. I., G. McBean, M. Cindric, J. Egea, M. G. López, P. Rada, N. Zarkovic and A. Cuadrado (2014). "Redox control of microglial function: molecular mechanisms and functional significance." Antioxidants and Redox Signaling 21(12): 1766-1801.

Roy, B., A. Chowdhury, S. Kundu, A. Santra, B. Dey, M. Chakraborty and P. P. Majumder (2001). "Increased risk of antituberculosis drug-induced hepatotoxicity in individuals with glutathione S-transferase M1 'null'mutation." Journal of Gastroenterology and Hepatology 16(9): 1033-1037.

Roy, D. N., V. Nagarajan and C. Gopalan (1962). "Production of neurolathyrism in chicks by the injection of Lathyrus sativus concentrates." Current Science 32(3): 116-118.

Roy, K. and R. N. Das (2013). "QSTR with extended topochemical atom (ETA) indices. Development of predictive classification and regression models for toxicity of ionic liquids towards Daphnia magna." Journal of Hazardous Materials 254: 166-178.

Roy, K., R. N. Das and P. L. Popelier (2014). "Quantitative structure – activity relationship for toxicity of ionic liquids to Daphnia magna: Aromaticity vs. lipophilicity." Chemosphere 112: 120-127.

Roy, S.-S. and S. Ghosh (2018). Effect of Toxic Heavy Metal Containing Industrial Effluent on Selected Life History Traits, Adult Morphology and Global Protein Expression Pattern of Drosophila melanogaster. Proceedings of the Zoological Society, 71:286-293.

Roy, S., A. Kale, K. Dangat, P. Sable, A. Kulkarni and S. Joshi (2012). "Maternal micronutrients (folic acid and vitamin B12) and omega 3 fatty acids: implications for neurodevelopmental risk in the rat offspring." Brain and Development 34(1): 64-71.

Roy, S., P. Sable, A. Khaire, K. Randhir, A. Kale and S. Joshi (2014). "Effect of maternal micronutrients (folic acid and vitamin B12) and omega 3 fatty acids on indices of brain oxidative stress in the offspring." Brain and Development 36(3): 219-227.

Roychoudhury, A. and A. K. Giri (1989). "Effects of certain food dyes on chromosomes of Allium cepa." Mutation Research/Genetic Toxicology 223(3): 313-319.

Rupa, D., P. Reddy and O. Reddi (1989). "Analysis of sister-chromatid exchanges, cell kinetics and mitotic index in lymphocytes of smoking pesticide sprayers." Mutation Research/Genetic Toxicology 223(2): 253-258.

Rupa, D., P. Reddy and O. Reddi (1989). "Chromosomal aberrations in peripheral lymphocytes of cotton field workers exposed to pesticides." Environmental Research 49(1): 1-6.

Rupa, D., P. Reddy and O. Reddi (1990). "Cytogeneticity of quinalphos and methyl parathion in human peripheral lymphocytes." Human and Experimental Toxicology 9(6): 385-387.

Rupa, D., P. Reddy and O. Reddi (1991). "Clastogenic effect of pesticides in peripheral lymphocytes of cotton-field workers." Mutation Research/Genetic Toxicology 261(3): 177-180.

Rupa, D., P. Reddy and O. Reddi (1991). "Reproductive performance in population exposed to pesticides in cotton fields in India." Environmental Research 55(2): 123-128.

Ruwali, M., M. C. Pant, P. P. Shah, B. N. Mishra and D. Parmar (2009). "Polymorphism in cytochrome P450 2A6 and glutathione S-transferase P1 modifies head and neck cancer risk and treatment outcome." Mutation Research/Fundamental and Molecular Mechanisms of Mutagenesis 669(1-2): 36-41.

Sable, P., K. Dangat, A. Kale and S. Joshi (2011). "Altered brain neurotrophins at birth: consequence of imbalance in maternal folic acid and vitamin B12 metabolism." Neuroscience 190: 127-134.

Sable, P., A. Kale, A. Joshi and S. Joshi (2014). "Maternal micronutrient imbalance alters gene expression of BDNF, NGF, TrkB and CREB in the offspring brain at an adult age." International Journal of Developmental Neuroscience 34: 24-32.

Sachdev, S., J. Sachdev and D. Puri (1969). "Morphological study in a case of lathyrism." Journal of the Indian Medical Association 52(7): 320-322.

Sadhu, H. G., B. Amin, D. Parikh, N. Sathawara, U. Mishra, B. Virani, B. Lakkad, V. Shivgotra and S. Patel (2008). "Poisoning of workers working in small lead-based units." Indian Journal of Occupational and Environmental Medicine 12(3): 139.

Saha, A., N. K. Das, A. Hazra, R. C. Gharami, S. N. Chowdhury and P. K. Datta (2012). "Cutaneous adverse drug reaction profile in a tertiary care out patient setting in eastern India." Indian Journal of Pharmacology 44(6): 792.

Saha, B., G. Das, H. Vohra, N. K. Ganguly and G. C. Mishra (1994). "Macrophage–T cell interaction in experimental mycobacterial infection. Selective regulation of co-stimulatory molecules on Mycobacterium-infected macrophages and its implication in the suppression of cell-mediated immune response." European Journal of Immunology 24(11): 2618-2624.

Saha, B., G. Das, H. Vohra, N. K. Ganguly and G. C. Mishra (1995). "Macrophage-T cell interaction in experimental visceral leishmaniasis: failure to express costimulatory molecules on Leishmania-infected macrophages and its implication in the suppression of cell-mediated immunity." European Journal of Immunology 25(9): 2492-2498.

Saha, S. and B. Banerjee (1993). "Effect of sub-chronic lindane exposure on humoral and cell-mediated immune responses in albino rats." Bulletin of Environmental Contamination and Toxicology 51(6): 795-802.

Sahu, D., G. Kannan, R. Vijayaraghavan, T. Anand and F. Khanum (2013). "Nanosized zinc oxide induces toxicity in human lung cells." ISRN Toxicology 2013.

Sahu, R. K., B. Singh, S. A. Saraf, G. Kaithwas and K. Kishor (2014). "Photochemical toxicity of drugs intended for ocular use." Archives of Industrial Hygiene and Toxicology 65(2): 157-166.

Sahu, S., S. Chattopadhyay, K. Basu and G. Paul (2010). "the ergonomic evaluation of work-related musculoskeletal disorders among construction labourers working in unorganized sectors in West Bengal, India." Journal of Human Ergology 39(2): 99-109.

Saigal, S., S. R. Agarwal, H. P. Nandeesh and S. K. Sarin (2001). "Safety of an ofloxacin-based antitubercular regimen for the treatment of tuberculosis in patients with underlying chronic liver disease: A preliminary report." Journal of Gastroenterology and Hepatology 16(9): 1028-1032.

Sailaja, N., M. Chandrasekhar, P. Rekhadevi, M. Mahboob, M. Rahman, S. B. Vuyyuri, K. Danadevi, S. Hussain and P. Grover (2006). "Genotoxic evaluation of workers employed in pesticide production." Mutation Research/Genetic Toxicology and Environmental Mutagenesis 609(1): 74-80.

Sain, M. K. and M. Meena (2016). "Occupational health and ergonomic intervention in Indian small scale industries: a review." International Journal of Recent Advances in Mechanical Engineering 5(1): 13-24.

Sainani, G., V. Rajkondawar, M. Wechalekar and D. Wechale-Kar (1972). "Epidemic dropsy in Chandrapur (Maharashtra)." Journal of the Association of Physicians of India 20(4): 301-306.

Saini, R., M. Yousuf, G. Allaqaband and S. Kaul (1984). "Silicosis in stone-cutters in Kashmir." Journal of the Indian Medical Association 82(6): 198-201.

Saini, S., N. Nair and M. R. Saini (2013). "Embryotoxic and teratogenic effects of nickel in Swiss albino mice during organogenetic period." BioMed Research International 701439.

Saiyed, H., A. Dewan, V. Bhatnagar, U. Shenoy, R. Shenoy, H. Rajmohan, K. Patel, R. Kashyap, P. Kulkarni and B. Rajan (2003). "Effect of endosulfan on male reproductive development." Environmental Health Perspectives 111(16): 1958-1962.

Saiyed, H., D. Parikh, N. Ghodasara, Y. Sharma, G. Patel, S. Chatterjee and B. Chatterjee (1985). "Silicosis in slate pencil workers: I. An environmental and medical study." American Journal of Industrial Medicine 8(2): 127-133.

Saiyed, H., H. Sadhu, V. Bhatnagar, A. Dewan, K. Venkaiah and S. Kashyap (1992). "Cardiac toxicity following short-term exposure to methomyl in spraymen and rabbits." Human and Experimental Toxicology 11(2): 93-97.

Saiyed, H. N. and R. R. Tiwari (2004). "Occupational health research in India." Industrial Health 42(2): 141-148.

Saleem, T. M., C. M. Chetty, S. Ramkanth, V. Rajan, K. M. Kumar and K. Gauthaman (2010). "Hepatoprotective herbs – a review." International Journal of Research in Pharmaceutical Sciences 1(1): 1-5.

Salian, S., T. Doshi and G. Vanage (2009). "Perinatal exposure of rats to Bisphenol A affects the fertility of male offspring." Life Sciences 85(21-22): 742-752.

Salim, C. and P. Rajini (2014). "Glucose feeding during development aggravates the toxicity of the organophosphorus insecticide Monocrotophos in the nematode, Caenorhabditis elegans." Physiology and Behavior 131: 142-148.

Sandhir, R. and K. D. Gill (1994). "Effect of lead on the biological activity of calmodulin in rat brain." Experimental and Molecular Pathology 61(1): 69-75.

Sandhya, P., S. Mohandass and P. Varalakshmi (1995). "Role of DL α-lipoic acid in gentamicin induced nephrotoxicity." Molecular and Cellular Biochemistry 145(1): 11-17.

Sangeetha Vijayan, P., P. Rekha, U. Dinesh and A. Arun (2016). "Biochemical and histopathological responses of the Swiss albino mice treated with uranyl nitrate and its recovery." Renal Failure 38(5): 770-775.

Sanghi, R., M. K. Pillai, T. Jayalekshmi and A. Nair (2003). "Organochlorine and organophosphorus pesticide residues in breast milk from Bhopal, Madhya Pradesh, India." Human and Experimental Toxicology 22(2): 73-76.

Sankararamakrishnan, N., A. K. Sharma and R. Sanghi (2005). "Organochlorine and organophosphorous pesticide residues in ground water and surface waters of Kanpur, Uttar Pradesh, India." Environment International 31(1): 113-120.

Sankhwar, M. L., R. S. Yadav, R. K. Shukla, A. B. Pant, D. Singh, D. Parmar and V. K. Khanna (2012). "Impaired cholinergic mechanisms following exposure to monocrotophos in young rats." Human and Experimental Toxicology 31(6): 606-616.

Sankhwar, M. L., R. S. Yadav, R. K. Shukla, D. Singh, R. W. Ansari, A. B. Pant, D. Parmar and V. K. Khanna (2016). "Monocrotophos induced oxidative stress and alterations in brain dopamine and serotonin receptors in young rats." Toxicology and Industrial Health 32(3): 422-436.

Santra, A., J. G. Das, B. De, B. Roy and D. M. Guha (1999). "Hepatic manifestations in chronic arsenic toxicity." Indian Journal of Gastroenterology: Official Journal of the Indian Society of Gastroenterology 18(4): 152-155.

Santra, M., S. K. Das, G. Talukder and A. Sharma (2002). "Induction of micronuclei by zinc in human leukocytes." Biological Trace Element Research 88(2): 139-144.

Saradha, B., S. Vaithinathan and P. Mathur (2008). "Single exposure to low dose of lindane causes transient decrease in testicular steroidogenesis in adult male Wistar rats." Toxicology 244(2-3): 190-197.

Sarangi, S., T. Zaidi, R. Pal, D. Katgara, V. Gadag, S. Mulay and D. Varma (2010). "Effects of exposure of parents to toxic gases in Bhopal on the offspring." American Journal of Industrial Medicine 53(8): 836-841.

Sarasin, A. (2003). "An overview of the mechanisms of mutagenesis and carcinogenesis." Mutation Research/Reviews in Mutation Research 544(2-3): 99-106.

Saraswathy, S. and C. Shyamala Devi (2001). "Modulating effect of Liv. 100, an ayurvedic formulation on antituberculosis drug-induced alterations in rat liver microsomes." Phytotherapy Research 15(6): 501-505.

Saravanan, K. S., K. M. Sindhu and K. P. Mohanakumar (2005). "Acute intranigral infusion of rotenone in rats causes progressive biochemical lesions in the striatum similar to Parkinson's disease." Brain Research 1049(2): 147-155.

Saravanan, K. S., K. M. Sindhu, K. S. Senthilkumar and K. P. Mohanakumar (2006). "L-deprenyl protects against rotenone-induced, oxidative stress-mediated dopaminergic neurodegeneration in rats." Neurochemistry International 49(1): 28-40.

Sarda, P., S. Sharma, A. Mohan, G. Makharia, A. Jayaswal, R. Pandey and S. Singh (2009). "Role of acute viral hepatitis as a confounding factor in antituberculosis treatment induced hepatotoxicity." Indian Journal of Medical Research 129(1): 64.

Sargaonkar, A. and V. Deshpande (2003). "Development of an overall index of pollution for surface water based on a general classification scheme in Indian context." Environmental Monitoring and Assessment 89(1): 43-67.

Sarin, S., G. Sachdev, R. Jiloha, A. Bhatt and G. Munjal (1988). "Pattern of psychiatric morbidity and alcohol dependence in patients with alcoholic liver disease." Digestive Diseases and Sciences 33(4): 443-448.

Sarkar, J. and A. Kumar (2016). "Thermo-responsive polymer aided spheroid culture in cryogel based platform for high throughput drug screening." Analyst 141(8): 2553-2567.

Sarkar, R., K. Mohanakumar and M. Chowdhury (2000). "Effects of an organophosphate pesticide, quinalphos, on the hypothalamo-pituitary-gonadal axis in adult male rats." Journal of Reproduction and Fertility 118(1): 29-38.

Sarkar, S. (1948). "Isolation from argemone oil of dihydrosanguinarine and sanguinarine: toxicity of sanguinarine." Nature 162(4111): 265.

Sarkar, S., S. Mukherjee, A. Chattopadhyay and S. Bhattacharya (2014). "Low dose of arsenic trioxide triggers oxidative stress in zebrafish brain: expression of antioxidant genes." Ecotoxicology and Environmental Safety 107: 1-8.

Sarma, G. R., C. Immanuel, S. Kailasam, A. Narayana and P. Venkatesan (1986). "Rifampin-lnduced Release of Hydrazine from Isoniazid: A Possible Cause of Hepatitis during Treatment of Tuberculosis with Regimens Containing Isoniazid and Rifampin." American Review of Respiratory Disease 133(6): 1072-1075.

Satapathy, P., C. Salim, M. Naidu and P. Rajini (2016). "Attenuation of dopaminergic neuronal dysfunction in Caenorhabditis elegans by Hydrophilic Form of Curcumin." Neurochemistry and Neuropharmacology 2(111): 2.

Satheesh, C., A. Sharma, P. Dwivedi, K. Prasanna, R. Patil and S. Rahul (2005). "Immunosuppressive effect of Ochratoxin A in Wistar rats." Journal of Animal and Veterinary Advances 4(6): 603-609.

Satsangi, P. G., S. Yadav, A. S. Pipal and N. Kumbhar (2014). "Characteristics of trace metals in fine (PM2. 5) and inhalable (PM10) particles and its health risk assessment along with *in-silico* approach in indoor environment of India." Atmospheric Environment 92: 384-393.

Saxena, A., B. Paul, M. Sinha, K. Dutta, S. Das and P. Ray (1991). "A study on the B cell activity in protein deficient rats exposed to methyl isocyanate vapour." Immunopharmacology and Immunotoxicology 13(3): 413-424.

Saxena, A., K. Singh, S. Nagle, B. Gupta, P. Ray, R. Srivastav, S. Tewari and R. Singh (1988). "Effect of exposure to toxic gas on the population of Bhopal: Part IV-- Immunological and chromosomal studies." Indian Journal of Experimental Biology 26(3): 173-176.

Saxena, D., R. Murthy, V. Jain and S. Chandra (1990). "Fetoplacental-maternal uptake of hexavalent chromium administered orally in rats and mice." Bulletin of Environmental Contamination and Toxicology 45(3): 430-435.

Saxena, D., R. Murthy, C. Singh and S. Chandra (1989). "Zinc protects testicular injury induced by concurrent exposure to cadmium and lead in rats." Research Communications in Chemical Pathology and Pharmacology 64(2): 317-329.

Saxena, D., C. Singh, R. Murthy, N. Mathur and S. V. Chandra (1994). "Blood and placental lead levels in an Indian city: a preliminary report." Archives of Environmental Health: An International Journal 49(2): 106-110.

Saxena, D. K., R. C. Murthy, B. Lal, R. S. Srivastava and S. V. Chandra (1990). "Effect of hexavalent chromium on testicular maturation in the rat." Reproductive Toxicology 4(3): 223-228.

Saxena, K. (1967). "The acute effect of manganese chloride on the central nervous system of rats. A preliminary report." Indian Journal of Industrial Medicine 13(2): 66-72.

Saxena, M., T. Seth and P. Mahajan (1980). "Organo chlorine pesticides in human placenta and accompanying fluid." International Journal of Environmental Analytical Chemistry 7(3): 245-251.

Saxena, M., M. Siddiqui, A. Bhargava, C. K. Murti and D. Kutty (1981). "Placental transfer of pesticides in humans." Archives of Toxicology 48(2-3): 127-134.

Selvaraj, K. K., G. Sundaramoorthy, P. K. Ravichandran, G. K. Girijan, S. Sampath and B. R. Ramaswamy (2015). "Phthalate esters in water and sediments of the Kaveri River, India: environmental levels and ecotoxicological evaluations." Environmental Geochemistry and Health 37(1): 83-96.

Sen, S., G. Talukder and A. Sharma (1986). "Carcinogenic, mutagenic and cytotoxic action of betel quid on mammalian systems." The Nucleus 29: 169-182.

Senapati, V. A., A. K. Jain, G. S. Gupta, A. K. Pandey and A. Dhawan (2015). "Chromium oxide nanoparticle-induced genotoxicity and p53-dependent apoptosis in human lung alveolar cells." Journal of Applied Toxicology 35(10): 1179-1188.

Sengupta, G., S. Bhowmick, A. Hazra, A. Datta and M. Rahaman (2011). "Adverse drug reaction monitoring in psychiatry out-patient department of an Indian teaching hospital." Indian Journal of Pharmacology 43(1): 36.

Sengupta, M. and B. Bishayi (2002). "Effect of lead and arsenic on murine macrophage response." Drug and Chemical Toxicology 25(4): 459-472.

Sengupta, P., R. Banerjee, S. Nath, S. Das and S. Banerjee (2015). "Metals and female reproductive toxicity." Human and Experimental Toxicology 34(7): 679-697.

Sengupta, T. and K. Mohanakumar (2010). "2-Phenylethylamine, a constituent of chocolate and wine, causes mitochondrial complex-I inhibition, generation of hydroxyl radicals and depletion of striatal biogenic amines leading to psycho-motor dysfunctions in Balb/c mice." Neurochemistry International 57(6): 637-646.

Senthilkumar, C. S., S. Akhter, T. M. Malla, N. K. Sah and N. Ganesh (2015). "Increased micronucleus frequency in peripheral blood lymphocytes contributes to cancer risk in the methyl isocyanate-affected population of Bhopal." Asian Pacific Journal of Cancer Prevention 16(10): 4409-4419.

Senthilkumar, C. S., T. Malla, N. Sah and N. Ganesh (2013). "Methyl isocyanate exposure and atypical lymphocytes." International Journal on Occupational and Environmental Medicine 238-167-238.

Senthilkumar, C. S., M. Tahir, N. K. Sah and N. Ganesh (2011). "Cancer morbidity among methyl isocyanate exposed long-term survivors and their offspring: a hospital-based five year descriptive study (2006-2011) and future directions to predict cancer risk in the affected population." Asian Pacific Journal of Cancer Prevention 12(12): 3443-3452.

Senthilkumar, R., M. Sengottuvelan and N. Nalini (2004). "Protective effect of glycine supplementation on the levels of lipid peroxidation and antioxidant enzymes in the erythrocyte of rats with alcohol-induced liver injury." Cell Biochemistry and Function: Cellular Biochemistry and its Modulation by Active Agents or Disease 22(2): 123-128.

Seth, B., A. Yadav, S. Agarwal, S. K. Tiwari and R. K. Chaturvedi (2017). "Inhibition of the transforming growth factor-β/SMAD cascade mitigates the anti-neurogenic effects of the carbamate pesticide carbofuran." Journal of Biological Chemistry 292(47): 19423-19440.

Seth, B., A. Yadav, A. Tandon, J. Shankar and R. K. Chaturvedi (2019). "Carbofuran hampers oligodendrocytes development leading to impaired myelination in the hippocampus of rat brain." Neurotoxicology 70: 161-179.

Seth, K., A. Agrawal, M. Aziz, A. Ahmad, Y. Shukla, N. Mathur and P. Seth (2002). "Induced expression of early response genes/oxidative injury in rat pheochromocytoma (PC12) cell line by 6-hydroxydopamine: implication for Parkinson's disease." Neuroscience Letters 330(1): 89-93.

Seth, P. K., R. Husain, M. Mushtaq and S. V. Chandra (1977). "Effect of manganese on neonatal rat: manganese concentration and enzymatic alterations in brain." Acta Pharmacologica et Toxicologica 40: 553-560.

Sethi, B., M. Sharma, J. Trivedi and H. Singh (1987). "Psychiatric morbidity in patients attending clinics in gas affected areas in Bhopal." Indian Journal of Medical Research 86(Suppl.): 45-50.

Sethi, N., R. Mahar, S. K. Shukla, A. Kumar and N. Sinha (2015). "A novel approach for testing the teratogenic potential of chemicals on the platform of metabolomics: studies employing HR-MAS nuclear magnetic resonance spectroscopy." RSC Advances 5(33): 26027-26039.

Sethi, N., R. Srivastava, R. Singh, G. Bhatia and N. Sinha (1990). "Chronic toxicity of styrene maleic anhydride, a male contraceptive, in rhesus monkeys (Macaca mulatta)." Contraception 42(3): 337-347.

Sett, M. and S. Sahu (2012). "Study on work load and work-related musculoskeletal disorders amongst male jute mill workers of West Bengal, India." Work 42(2): 289-297.

Shadab, G., M. Ahmad and M. Azfer (2006). "Anticlastogenic action of vitamin C against genotoxicity of estrogenic drug diethylstilbestrol (DES) in the human lymphocyte chromosomes." Journal of Environmental Biology 27(1): 85.

Shah, H., M. Patel and N. Shrivastava (2017). "Gene expression study of phase I and II metabolizing enzymes in RPTEC/TERT1 cell line: application in *in vitro* nephrotoxicity prediction." Xenobiotica 47(10): 837-843.

Shah, P. P., A. P. Singh, M. Singh, N. Mathur, B. N. Mishra, M. C. Pant and D. Parmar (2008). "Association of functionally important polymorphisms in cytochrome P4501B1 with lung cancer." Mutation Research/Fundamental and Molecular Mechanisms of Mutagenesis 643(1-2): 4-10.

Shah, P. P., A. P. Singh, M. Singh, N. Mathur, M. C. Pant, B. N. Mishra and D. Parmar (2008). "Interaction of cytochrome P4501A1 genotypes with other risk factors and susceptibility to lung cancer." Mutation Research/Fundamental and Molecular Mechanisms of Mutagenesis 639(1-2): 1-10.

Shahjahan, M., K. Sabitha, M. Jainu and C. S. Devi (2004). "Effect of Solanum trilobatum against carbon tetra chloride induced hepatic damage in albino rats." Indian Journal of Medical Research 120: 194-198.

Shaik, A. and K. Jamil (2008). "A study on the ALAD gene polymorphisms associated with lead exposure." Toxicology and Industrial Health 24(7): 501-506.

Shamanna, S. B., R. R. R. Naik and A. Hamide (2016). "Causes of liver disease and its outcome in HIV-infected individuals." Indian Journal of Gastroenterology 35(4): 310-314.

Shamsi, M., S. Venkatesh, R. Kumar, N. Gupta, N. Malhotra, N. Singh, S. Mittal, S. Arora, D. Arya and P. Talwar (2010). "Antioxidant levels in blood and seminal plasma and their impact on sperm parameters in infertile men." Indian Journal of Biochemistry and Biophysics 47:38-43.

Shamsi, M. B., S. N. Imam and R. Dada (2011). "Sperm DNA integrity assays: diagnostic and prognostic challenges and implications in management of infertility." Journal of Assisted Reproduction and Genetics 28(11): 1073-1085.

Shamsi, M. B., S. Venkatesh, D. Pathak, D. Deka and R. Dada (2011). "Sperm DNA damage and oxidative stress in recurrent spontaneous abortion (RSA)." The Indian Journal of Medical Research 133(5): 550.

Shanker, R., G. Singh, A. Jyoti, P. D. Dwivedi and S. P. Singh (2014). Nanotechnology and detection of microbial pathogens. Animal Biotechnology 525-540.

Shanmugam, G., S. Sampath, K. K. Selvaraj, D. J. Larsson and B. R. Ramaswamy (2014). "Non-steroidal anti-inflammatory drugs in Indian rivers." Environmental Science and Pollution Research 21(2): 921-931.

Sharma, A., A. Kar, M. Kaur, S. M. Ranade, A. Sankaran, S. Misra, K. Rawat and S. Saxena (2010). "Specific replication factors are targeted by different genotoxic agents to inhibit replication." IUBMB life 62(10): 764-775.

Sharma, A., M. Mishra, K. R. Ram, R. Kumar, M. Abdin and D. K. Chowdhuri (2011). "Transcriptome analysis provides insights for understanding the adverse effects of endosulfan in Drosophila melanogaster." Chemosphere 82(3): 370-376.

Sharma, A., M. Mishra, A. Shukla, R. Kumar, M. Abdin and D. K. Chowdhuri (2012). "Organochlorine pesticide, endosulfan induced cellular and organismal response in Drosophila melanogaster." Journal of Hazardous Materials 221: 275-287.

Sharma, A., K. Nain and S. Nanda (1996). "Pneumomediastinum, pneumothorax and subcutaneous emphysema with kerosene oil." The Indian Journal of Chest Diseases and Allied Sciences 38(3): 211.

Sharma, A., B. Sangameswaran, V. Jain and M. Saluja (2012). "Hepatoprotective activity of Adina cordifolia against ethanol induce hepatotoxicity in rats." International Current Pharmaceutical Journal 1(9): 279-284.

Sharma, A., K. Saurabh, S. Yadav, S. K. Jain and D. Parmar (2013). "Expression profiling of selected genes of toxication and detoxication pathways in peripheral blood lymphocytes as a biomarker for predicting toxicity of environmental chemicals." International Journal of Hygiene and Environmental Health 216(6): 645-651.

Sharma, A., A. Shukla, M. Mishra and D. K. Chowdhuri (2011). "Validation and application of Drosophila melanogaster as an *in vivo* model for the detection of double strand breaks by neutral Comet assay." Mutation Research/Genetic Toxicology and Environmental Mutagenesis 721(2): 142-146.

Sharma, A. K., V. Singh, R. Gera, M. P. Purohit and D. Ghosh (2017). "Zinc oxide nanoparticle induces microglial death by NADPH-oxidase-independent reactive oxygen species as well as energy depletion." Molecular Neurobiology 54(8): 6273-6286.

Sharma, B., S. Malhotra, V. Bhatia and M. Rathee (1999). "Epidemic dropsy in India." Postgraduate Medical Journal 75(889): 657-661.

Sharma, B. M., J. Bečanová, M. Scheringer, A. Sharma, G. K. Bharat, P. G. Whitehead, J. Klánová and L. Nizzetto (2019). "Health and ecological risk assessment of emerging contaminants (pharmaceuticals, personal care products, and artificial sweeteners) in surface and groundwater (drinking water) in the Ganges River Basin, India." Science of the Total Environment 646: 1459-1467.

Sharma, D., C. Meena, L. Mittal, G. Yadav and S. Meena (2014). "Aluminium phosphide poisoning." Indian Medical Gazette 9: 333-339.

Sharma, K., R. Singh, S. Barman, D. Mishra, R. Kumar, M. Negi, S. Mandal, G. Kisku, A. Khan and M. Kidwai (2006). "Comparison of trace metals concentration in PM10 of different locations of Lucknow City, India." Bulletin of Environmental Contamination and Toxicology 77(3): 419-426.

Sharma, M., V. N. Kumar, S. K. Katiyar, R. Sharma, B. P. Shukla and B. Sengupta (2004). "Effects of particulate air pollution on the respiratory health of subjects who live in three areas in Kanpur, India." Archives of Environmental Health: An International Journal 59(7): 348-358.

Sharma, M. and S. Maloo (2005). "Assessment of ambient air PM10 and PM2. 5 and characterization of PM10 in the city of Kanpur, India." Atmospheric Environment 39(33): 6015-6026.

Sharma, M., N. Sharma and R. Sharma (2012). "Neuroprotective effect of Zingiber officinale in 3-np-induced huntington disease." IOSR Journal of Pharmacy 2(6): 61-70.

Sharma, N. and A. Kumar (2014). "Mechanism of immunotoxicological effects of tributyltin chloride on murine thymocytes." Cell Biology and Toxicology 30(2): 101-112.

Sharma, P., V. Bihari, S. K. Agarwal, V. Verma, C. N. Kesavachandran, B. S. Pangtey, N. Mathur, K. P. Singh, M. Srivastava and S. K. Goel (2012). "Groundwater Contaminated with Hexavalent Chromium [Cr (VI)]: A Health Survey and Clinical Examination of Community Inhabitants (Kanpur, India)." PLoS One 7(10).

Sharma, P., A. U. Huq and R. Singh (2013). "Cypermethrin induced reproductive toxicity in male Wistar rats: Protective role of Tribulus terrestris." Journal of Environmental Biology 34(5): 857.

Sharma, P., A. U. Huq and R. Singh (2014). "Cypermethrin-induced reproductive toxicity in the rat is prevented by resveratrol." Journal of Human Reproductive Sciences 7(2): 99.

Sharma, P., K. Sablok, V. Bhalla and C. R. Suri (2011). "A novel disposable electrochemical immunosensor for phenyl urea herbicide diuron." Biosensors and Bioelectronics 26(10): 4209-4212.

Sharma, P. and R. Singh (2010). "Protective role of curcumin on lindane induced reproductive toxicity in male Wistar rats." Bulletin of Environmental Contamination and Toxicology 84(4): 378-384.

Sharma, R. (2013). "Birth defects in India: Hidden truth, need for urgent attention." Indian Journal of Human Genetics 19(2): 125.

Sharma, R. and S. Mogra (2013). "Effects of gestational exposure to lead acetate on implantation and neonatal mice." Journal of Cell and Molecular Biology 11(1):47-58.

Sharma, R., S. Singh, G. Singh, A. Khajuria, T. Sidiq, S. Singh, G. Chashoo, S. Pagoch, A. Kaul and A. Saxena (2009). "*In vivo* genotoxicity evaluation of a plant based antiarthritic and anticancer therapeutic agent Boswelic acids in rodents." Phytomedicine 16(12): 1112-1118.

Sharma, R. K., M. Agrawal and F. M. Marshall (2008). "Atmospheric deposition of heavy metals (Cu, Zn, Cd and Pb) in Varanasi city, India." Environmental Monitoring and Assessment 142(1-3): 269-278.

Sharma, R. K., M. Agrawal and F. M. Marshall (2008). "Heavy metal (Cu, Zn, Cd and Pb) contamination of vegetables in urban India: A case study in Varanasi." Environmental Pollution 154(2): 254-263.

Sharma, S., M. Anjaneyulu, S. Kulkarni and K. Chopra (2006). "Resveratrol, a polyphenolic phytoalexin, attenuates diabetic nephropathy in rats." Pharmacology 76(2): 69-75.

Sharma, S., S. K. Kulkarni and K. Chopra (2006). "Curcumin, the active principle of turmeric (Curcuma longa), ameliorates diabetic nephropathy in rats." Clinical and Experimental Pharmacology and Physiology 33(10): 940-945.

Sharma, S., A. K. Nagpal and I. Kaur (2018). "Heavy metal contamination in soil, food crops and associated health risks for residents of Ropar wetland, Punjab, India and its environs." Food Chemistry 255: 15-22.

Sharma, S., N. Nagpure, R. Kumar, S. Pandey, S. K. Srivastava, P. J. Singh and P. Mathur (2007). "Studies on the genotoxicity of endosulfan in different tissues of fresh water fish Mystus vittatus using the comet assay." Archives of Environmental Contamination and Toxicology 53(4): 617-623.

Sharma, S., R. Singh and P. Kakkar (2011). "Modulation of Bax/Bcl-2 and caspases by probiotics during acetaminophen induced apoptosis in primary hepatocytes." Food and Chemical Toxicology 49(4): 770-779.

Sharma, S., V. Venkatesan, B. M. Prakhya and R. Bhonde (2014). "Human mesenchymal stem cells as a novel platform for simultaneous evaluation of cytotoxicity and genotoxicity of pharmaceuticals." Mutagenesis 30(3): 391-399.

Sharma, S. K., A. Balamurugan, P. K. Saha, R. M. Pandey and N. K. Mehra (2002). "Evaluation of clinical and immunogenetic risk factors for the development of hepatotoxicity during antituberculosis treatment." American Journal of Respiratory and Critical Care Medicine 166(7): 916-919.

Sharma, S. K., R. Singla, P. Sarda, A. Mohan, G. Makharia, A. Jayaswal, V. Sreenivas and S. Singh (2010). "Safety of 3 different reintroduction regimens of antituberculosis drugs after development of antituberculosis treatment–induced hepatotoxicity." Clinical Infectious Diseases 50(6): 833-839.

Sharma, V., D. Anderson and A. Dhawan (2011). "Zinc oxide nanoparticles induce oxidative stress and genotoxicity in human liver cells (HepG2)." Journal of Biomedical Nanotechnology 7(1): 98-99.

Sharma, V., D. Anderson and A. Dhawan (2012). "Zinc oxide nanoparticles induce oxidative DNA damage and ROS-triggered mitochondria mediated apoptosis in human liver cells (HepG2)." Apoptosis 17(8): 852-870.

Sharma, V., R. K. Shukla, N. Saxena, D. Parmar, M. Das and A. Dhawan (2009). "DNA damaging potential of zinc oxide nanoparticles in human epidermal cells." Toxicology Letters 185(3): 211-218.

Sharma, V., S. K. Singh, D. Anderson, D. J. Tobin and A. Dhawan (2011). "Zinc oxide nanoparticle induced genotoxicity in primary human epidermal keratinocytes." Journal of Nanoscience and Nanotechnology 11(5): 3782-3788.

Sharma, V. K., A. K. Sharma, G. N. Srivastava and A. Roy (2017). "ToxiM: A toxicity prediction tool for small molecules developed using machine learning and chemoinformatics approaches." Frontiers in Pharmacology 8: 880.

Shashi, A. (2003). "Histopathological investigation of fluoride-induced neurotoxicity in rabbits." Fluoride 36(2): 95-105.

Shashi, A. and N. Sharma (2015). "Cerebral neurodegeneration in experimental fluorosis." International Journal of Basic and Applied Medical Sciences 5(1): 146-151.

Shashi, A., J. Singh and S. Thapar (2002). "Toxic effects of fluoride on rabbit kidney." Fluoride 35(1): 38-50.

Shashikumar, S. and P. Rajini (2010). "Cypermethrin elicited responses in heat shock protein and feeding in Caenorhabditis elegans." Ecotoxicology and Environmental Safety 73(5): 1057-1062.

Sheelendra, B. (2015). "GMO's Foods: Regulatory Mechanism and Challenges in India." Journal of Bioremediation and Biodegredation 6(5): 1.

Shenolikar, I., C. Rukmini, K. Krisnamachari and K. Satayanarayana (1974). "Sanguinarine in the blood and urine of cases of epidemic dropsy." Food and Cosmetics Toxicology 12(5-6): 699-702.

Sheth, S. C., B. J. Northover, N. Tibrewala, U. Warerkar and V. Karande (1960). "IV. Therapy of cirrhosis of liver and liver damage with indigenous drugs — Experimental and clinical studies." Indian Journal of Pediatrics 27(6): 204-211.

Shetty, P. K. (2004). "Socio-ecological implications of pesticide use in India." Economic and Political Weekly: 5261-5267.

Shifow, A., K. Kumar, M. Naidu and K. Ratnakar (2000). "Melatonin, a pineal hormone with antioxidant property, protects against gentamicin-induced nephrotoxicity in rats." Nephron 85(2): 167-174.

Shila, S., M. Subathra, M. A. Devi and C. Panneerselvam (2005). "Arsenic intoxication-induced reduction of glutathione level and of the activity of related enzymes in rat brain regions: reversal by dl-α-lipoic acid." Archives of Toxicology 79(3): 140-146.

Shivarajashankara, Y., A. Shivashankara, S. H. Rao and P. G. Bhat (2001). "Oxidative stress in children with endemic skeletal fluorosis." Fluoride 34(2): 103-107.

Shivashankara, A., Y. S. Shankara, S. H. Rao and P. G. Bhat (2000). "A clinical and biochemical study of chronic fluoride toxicity in children of Kheru Thanda of Gulbarga district, Karnataka, India." Fluoride 33(2): 66-73.

Shobha, N., A. B. Taly, S. Sinha and T. Venkatesh (2009). "Radial neuropathy due to occupational lead exposure: Phenotypic and electrophysiological characteristics of five patients." Annals of Indian Academy of Neurology 12(2): 111.

Shridhar, V., P. Khillare, T. Agarwal and S. Ray (2010). "Metallic species in ambient particulate matter at rural and urban location of Delhi." Journal of Hazardous Materials 175(1-3): 600-607.

Shrivastava, P., K. Vaibhav, R. Tabassum, A. Khan, T. Ishrat, M. M. Khan, A. Ahmad, F. Islam, M. M. Safhi and F. Islam (2013). "Anti-apoptotic and anti-inflammatory effect of Piperine on 6-OHDA induced Parkinson's rat model." The Journal of Nutritional Biochemistry 24(4): 680-687.

Shrivastava, S., A. Jadon, S. Shukla and R. Mathur (2007). "Chelation Therapy and Vanadium: Effect on Reproductive Organs in Rats." Indian Journal of Experimental Biology 45(6):515-23.

Shukla, A., P. Pragya and D. K. Chowdhuri (2011). "A modified alkaline Comet assay for *in vivo* detection of oxidative DNA damage in Drosophila melanogaster." Mutation Research/Genetic Toxicology and Environmental Mutagenesis 726(2): 222-226.

Shukla, A. K., P. Pragya, H. S. Chaouhan, D. Patel, M. Abdin and D. K. Chowdhuri (2014). "A mutation in Drosophila methuselah resists paraquat induced Parkinson-like phenotypes." Neurobiology of Aging 35(10):2419.

Shukla, G. S., R. Srivastava and S. Chandra (1988). "Glutathione status and cadmium neurotoxicity: studies in discrete brain regions of growing rats." Toxicological Sciences 11(1): 229-235.

Shukla, R. K., R. Gupta, P. Srivastava, Y. K. Dhuriya, A. Singh, L. P. Chandravanshi, A. Kumar, M. H. Siddiqui, D. Parmar and A. B. Pant (2016). "Brain cholinergic alterations in rats subjected to repeated immobilization or forced swim stress on lambda-cyhalothrin exposure." Neurochemistry International 93: 51-63.

Shukla, R. K., A. Kumar, A. K. Pandey, S. S. Singh and A. Dhawan (2011). "Titanium dioxide nanoparticles induce oxidative stress-mediated apoptosis in human keratinocyte cells." Journal of Biomedical Nanotechnology 7(1): 100-101.

Shukla, R. K., V. Sharma, A. K. Pandey, S. Singh, S. Sultana and A. Dhawan (2011). "ROS-mediated genotoxicity induced by titanium dioxide nanoparticles in human epidermal cells." Toxicology *In Vitro* 25(1): 231-241.

Shukla, S., R. K. Chaturvedi, K. Seth, N. S. Roy and A. K. Agrawal (2009). "Enhanced survival and function of neural stem cells-derived dopaminergic neurons under influence of olfactory ensheathing cells in parkinsonian rats." Journal of Neurochemistry 109(2): 436-451.

Siddappa, N. B., P. K. Dash, A. Mahadevan, A. Desai, N. Jayasuryan, V. Ravi, P. Satishchandra, S. K. Shankar and U. Ranga (2005). "Identification of unique B/C recombinant strains of HIV-1 in the southern state of Karnataka, India." Aids 19(13): 1426-1429.

Siddique, H., A. Dhawan, D. Saxena and D. Chowdhuri (2003). "D. melanogaster as an *in vivo* model for somatic cell genotoxicity of chemicals by Comet assay." Drosophila Information Service 86: 149-151.

Siddique, H. R., D. K. Chowdhuri, D. Saxena and A. Dhawan (2005). "Validation of Drosophila melanogaster as an *in vivo* model for genotoxicity assessment using modified alkaline Comet assay." Mutagenesis 20(4): 285-290.

Siddique, H. R., S. C. Gupta, A. Dhawan, R. Murthy, D. Saxena and D. K. Chowdhuri (2005). "Genotoxicity of industrial solid waste leachates in Drosophila melanogaster." Environmental and Molecular Mutagenesis 46(3): 189-197.

Siddique, H. R., K. Mitra, V. K. Bajpai, K. R. Ram, D. K. Saxena and D. K. Chowdhuri (2009). "Hazardous effect of tannery solid waste leachates on development and reproduction in Drosophila melanogaster: 70kDa heat shock protein as a marker of cellular damage." Ecotoxicology and Environmental Safety 6(72): 1652-1662.

Siddique, H. R., A. Sharma, S. C. Gupta, R. C. Murthy, A. Dhawan, D. K. Saxena and D. K. Chowdhuri (2008). "DNA damage induced by industrial solid waste leachates in Drosophila melanogaster: a mechanistic approach." Environmental and Molecular Mutagenesis 49(3): 206-216.

Siddique, Y. and M. Afzal (2008). "A review on the genotoxic effects of some synthetic progestins." International Journal of Pharmacology 4(6): 410-430.

Siddique, Y. H. and M. Afzal (2005). "Evaluation of genotoxic potential of norethynodrel in human lymphocytes *in vitro*." Journal of Environmental Biology 26(2): 387-392.

Siddique, Y. H. and M. Afzal (2005). "Protective role of allicin and L-ascorbic acid against the genotoxic damage induced by chlormadinone acetate in cultured human lymphocytes." Indian Journal of Experimental Biology 43(9):769-72.

Siddique, Y. H., G. Ara, T. Beg, M. Faisal, M. Ahmad and M. Afzal (2008). "Antigenotoxic role of Centella asiatica L. extract against cyproterone acetate induced genotoxic damage in cultured human lymphocytes." Toxicology *In Vitro* 22(1): 10-17.

Siddique, Y. H., T. Beg and M. Afzal (2006). "Protective effect of nordihydroguaiaretic acid (NDGA) against norgestrel induced genotoxic damage." Toxicology *In Vitro* 20(2): 227-233.

Siddique, Y. H., T. Beg and M. Afzal (2007). "Anticlastogenic effects of ascorbic acid against the genotoxic damage induced by norethynodrel. Advances in Environmental Biology 1(1): 27-32.

Siddiqui, A., I. Sayeed, K. Zafar and F. Islam (2002). "Argemone oil augmented oxidative stress in discrete areas of rat brain." Bulletin of Environmental Contamination and Toxicology 69(5): 0734-0740.

Siddiqui, A. H. and M. Ahmad (2003). "The Salmonella mutagenicity of industrial, surface and ground water samples of Aligarh region of India." Mutation Research/Genetic Toxicology and Environmental Mutagenesis 541(1-2): 21-29.

Siddiqui, A. H., S. Tabrez and M. Ahmad (2011). "Short-term *in vitro* and *in vivo* genotoxicity testing systems for some water bodies of Northern India." Environmental Monitoring and Assessment 180(1-4): 87-95.

Siddiqui, A. H., S. Tabrez and M. Ahmad (2011). "Validation of plant based bioassays for the toxicity testing of Indian waters." Environmental Monitoring and Assessment 179(1-4): 241-253.

Siddiqui, E. and J. Pandey (2019). "Assessment of heavy metal pollution in water and surface sediment and evaluation of ecological risks associated with sediment contamination in the Ganga River: a basin - scale study." Environmental Science and Pollution Research 26(11):10926-10940.

Siddiqui, M., M. Kashyap, V. Khanna, S. Yadav, A. Al-Khedhairy, J. Musarrat and A. Pant (2010). "Association of dopamine DA-D2 receptor in rotenone-induced cytotoxicity in PC12 ells." Toxicology and Industrial Health 26(8): 533-542.

Siddiqui, M., V. Kumar, M. Kashyap, M. Agarwal, A. Singh, S. Jahan, V. Khanna, A. Al-Khedhairy, J. Musarrat and A. Pant (2012). "Short-term exposure of 4-hydroxynonenal induces mitochondria-mediated apoptosis in PC12 cells." Human and Experimental Toxicology 31(4): 336-345.

Siddiqui, M., M. Rahman, M. Mahboob, F. Anjum and M. Mustafa (1988). "Species differences in brain acetylcholinesterase and neuropathic target esterase response to monocrotophos." Journal of Environmental Science and Health Part B 23(3): 291-299.

Siddiqui, M. and M. Saxena (1985). "Placenta and milk as excretory routes of lipophilic pesticides in women." Human toxicology 4(3): 249-254.

Siddiqui, M., G. Singh, M. Kashyap, V. Khanna, S. Yadav, D. Chandra and A. Pant (2008). "Influence of cytotoxic doses of 4-hydroxynonenal on selected neurotransmitter receptors in PC-12 cells." Toxicology *In Vitro* 22(7): 1681-1688.

Siddiqui, M., S. Srivastava, P. Mehrotra, N. Mathur and I. Tandon (2003). "Persistent chlorinated pesticides and intra-uterine foetal growth retardation: a possible association." International Archives of Occupational and Environmental Health 76(1): 75-80.

Siddiqui, M. A., Q. Saquib, M. Ahamed, N. N. Farshori, J. Ahmad, R. Wahab, S. T. Khan, H. A. Alhadlaq, J. Musarrat and A. A. Al-Khedhairy (2015). "Molybdenum nanoparticles-induced cytotoxicity, oxidative stress, G2/M arrest, and DNA damage in mouse skin fibroblast cells (L929)." Colloids and Surfaces B: Biointerfaces 125: 73-81.

Sidhu, P. and B. Nehru (2003). "Relationship between lead-induced biochemical and behavioral changes with trace element concentrations in rat brain." Biological Trace Element Research 92(3): 245-256.

Sidhu, P. and B. Nehru (2004). "Lead intoxication: histological and oxidative damage in rat cerebrum and cerebellum." The Journal of Trace Elements in Experimental Medicine: The Official Publication of the International Society for Trace Element Research in Humans 17(1): 45-53.

Sidhu, P. and B. Nehru (2005). "Protective effects of selenium to placental lead neurotoxicity in rat pups." Toxicology Mechanisms and Methods 15(6): 419-423.

Sidhu, S. S., O. Goyal, M. Singla, K. Bhatia, R. S. Chhina and A. Sood (2012). "Pentoxifylline in severe alcoholic hepatitis: a prospective, randomised trial." Journal of the Association of Physicians of India 60(8): 20-22.

Sindhu, K. M., R. Banerjee, K. S. Senthilkumar, K. S. Saravanan, B. C. Raju, J. M. Rao and K. P. Mohanakumar (2006). "Rats with unilateral median forebrain bundle, but not striatal or nigral, lesions by the neurotoxins MPP+ or rotenone display differential sensitivity to amphetamine and apomorphine." Pharmacology Biochemistry and Behavior 84(2): 321-329.

Sindhu, K. M., K. S. Saravanan and K. P. Mohanakumar (2005). "Behavioral differences in a rotenone-induced hemiparkinsonian rat model developed following intranigral or median forebrain bundle infusion." Brain Research 1051(1-2): 25-34.

Singh, A., A. Agrahari, R. Singh, S. Yadav, V. Srivastava and D. Parmar (2016). "Imprinting of cerebral cytochrome P450s in offsprings prenatally exposed to cypermethrin augments toxicity on rechallenge." Scientific Reports 6: 37426.

Singh, A., R. Kamal, M. K. R. Mudiam, M. K. Gupta, G. N. V. Satyanarayana, V. Bihari, N. Shukla, A. H. Khan and C. N. Kesavachandran (2016). "Heat and PAHs emissions in indoor kitchen air and its impact on kidney dysfunctions among kitchen workers in Lucknow, North India." PloS One 11(2): e0148641.

Singh, A., A. Mudawal, P. Maurya, R. Jain, S. Nair, R. K. Shukla, S. Yadav, D. Singh, V. K. Khanna and R. K. Chaturvedi (2016). "Prenatal exposure of cypermethrin induces similar alterations in xenobiotic-metabolizing cytochrome P450s and rate-limiting enzymes of neurotransmitter synthesis in brain regions of rat offsprings during postnatal development." Molecular Neurobiology 53(6): 3670-3689.

Singh, A., A. Mudawal, R. K. Shukla, S. Yadav, V. K. Khanna, R. Sethumadhavan and D. Parmar (2015). "Effect of gestational exposure of cypermethrin on postnatal development of brain cytochrome P450 2D1 and 3A1 and neurotransmitter receptors." Molecular Neurobiology 52(1): 741-756.

Singh, A., S. Yadav, V. Srivastava, R. Kumar, D. Singh, R. Sethumadhavan and D. Parmar (2013). "Imprinting of cerebral and hepatic cytochrome P450s in rat offsprings exposed prenatally to low doses of cypermethrin." Molecular Neurobiology 48(1): 128-140.

Singh, A. B. and P. Kumar (2003). "Aeroallergens in clinical practice of allergy in India. An overview." Annals of Agricultural and Environmental Medicine 10(2): 131-136.

Singh, A. K., Y. M. Farag, B. V. Mittal, K. K. Subramanian, S. R. K. Reddy, V. N. Acharya, A. F. Almeida, A. Channakeshavamurthy, H. S. Ballal and P. Gaccione (2013). "Epidemiology and risk factors of chronic kidney disease in India – results from the SEEK (Screening and Early Evaluation of Kidney Disease) study." BMC Nephrology 14(1): 114.

Singh, A. K., M. P. Kashyap, S. Jahan, V. Kumar, V. K. Tripathi, M. A. Siddiqui, S. Yadav, V. K. Khanna, V. Das and S. K. Jain (2012). "Expression and Inducibility of Cytochrome P450s (CYP1A1, 2B6, 2E1, 3A4) in Human Cord Blood CD34+ Stem Cell–Derived Differentiating Neuronal Cells." Toxicological Sciences 129(2): 392-410.

Singh, A. K., M. P. Kashyap, V. Kumar, V. K. Tripathi, D. K. Yadav, F. Khan, S. Jahan, V. K. Khanna, S. Yadav and A. B. Pant (2013). "3-Methylcholanthrene induces neurotoxicity in developing neurons derived from human CD34+ Thy1+ stem cells by activation of aryl hydrocarbon receptor." Neuromolecular Medicine 15(3): 570-592.

Singh, A. K., M. N. Tiwari, A. Dixit, G. Upadhyay, D. K. Patel, D. Singh, O. Prakash and M. P. Singh (2011). "Nigrostriatal proteomics of cypermethrin-induced dopaminergic neurodegeneration: microglial activation-dependent and-independent regulations." Toxicological Sciences 122(2): 526-538.

Singh, A. K., M. N. Tiwari, G. Upadhyay, D. K. Patel, D. Singh, O. Prakash and M. P. Singh (2012). "Long term exposure to cypermethrin induces nigrostriatal dopaminergic neurodegeneration in adult rats: postnatal exposure enhances the susceptibility during adulthood." Neurobiology of Aging 33(2): 404-415.

Singh, B., K. Kapoor, A. Kumar, R. Agarwal and K. Bhilegaonkar (1996). "Prevalence of enteropathogens of zoonotic significance in meat, milk and their products." Journal of Food Science and Technology 33(3): 251-254.

Singh, B., J. Kaur and K. Singh (2014). "Microbial degradation of an organophosphate pesticide, malathion." Critical Reviews in Microbiology 40(2): 146-154.

Singh, B., G. Singh, V. Trajkovic and P. Sharma (2003). "Intracellular expression of Mycobacterium tuberculosis-specific 10-kDa antigen down-regulates macrophage B7· 1 expression and nitric oxide release." Clinical and Experimental Immunology 134(1): 70-77.

Singh, B. K., A. Kumar, I. Ahmad, V. Kumar, D. K. Patel, S. K. Jain and C. Singh (2011). "Oxidative stress in zinc-induced dopaminergic neurodegeneration: implications of superoxide dismutase and heme oxygenase-1." Free Radical Research 45(10): 1207-1222.

Singh, D. and T. Gupta (2016). "Effect through inhalation on human health of PM1 bound polycyclic aromatic hydrocarbons collected from foggy days in northern part of India." Journal of Hazardous Materials 306: 257-268.

Singh, G., A. Kumar and N. Sinha (2012). "Studying significance of apoptosis in mediating tolbutamide-induced teratogenesis *in vitro*." Fundamental and Clinical Pharmacology 26(4): 484-494.

Singh, G., R. Maurya, A. Kumar and N. Sinha (2015). "Role of apoptosis in mediating diclofenac-induced teratogenesis." Toxicology and Industrial Health 31(7): 614.

Singh, G., R. Maurya, A. Kumar and N. Sinha (2015). "Role of apoptosis in mediating diclofenac-induced teratogenesis: An *in vitro* approach." Toxicology and Industrial Health 31(7): 614-623.

Singh, G., N. Saxena, A. Aggarwal and R. Misra (2007). "Cytochrome P450 polymorphism as a predictor of ovarian toxicity to pulse cyclophosphamide in systemic lupus erythematosus." The Journal of Rheumatology 34(4): 731-733.

Singh, G., S. Sharma and S. Zaidi (1967). "Effect of benzanthrone on the skin of mice." Indian Journal of Medical Sciences 21(11): 727.

Singh, G. and N. Sinha (2010). "Involvement of apoptosis in mediating mitomycin C-induced teratogenesis *in vitro*." Toxicology Mechanisms and Methods 20(4): 190-196.

Singh, G., N. Sinha and S. Mahipag G (2009). "Role of apoptosis in mediating salicylic acid-induced teratogenesis *in vitro*." Toxicology Mechanisms and Methods 19(2): 161-168.

Singh, G. and V. Tripathi (1973). "Effect of benzanthrone on the urinary bladder of guinea-pig." Cellular and Molecular Life Sciences 29(6): 683-684.

Singh, G., P. Vajpayee, N. Rani, A. Jyoti, K. C. Gupta and R. Shanker (2012). "Bio-capture of S. Typhimurium from surface water by aptamer for culture-free quantification." Ecotoxicology and Environmental Safety 78: 320-326.

Singh, G. and S. Zaidi (1969). "Preliminary clinical and experimental studies on benzanthrone toxicity." Journal of the Indian Medical Association 52(12): 558.

Singh, H., S. Lata, M. Angadi, S. Bapat, J. Pawar, V. Nema, M. Ghate, S. Sahay and R. Gangakhedkar (2017). "Impact of GSTM1, GSTT1 and GSTP1 gene polymorphism and risk of ARV-associated hepatotoxicity in HIV-infected individuals and its modulation." The Pharmacogenomics Journal 17(1): 53.

Singh, H., S. Lata, T. Dhole and R. R. Gangakhedkar (2019). "Occurrence of CYP2B6 516G> T polymorphism in patients with ARV-associated hepatotoxicity." Molecular Genetics and Genomic Medicine: e598.

Singh, H., S. Lata, V. Nema, D. Samani, M. Ghate and R. R. Gangakhedkar (2017). "CYP 1A1m1 and CYP 2C9* 2 and* 3 polymorphism and risk to develop ARV-associated hepatotoxicity and its severity." Apmis 125(6): 523-535.

Singh, H. O., S. Jadhav, D. Samani and T. Dhole (2019). "Polymorphisms in miRNAs Gene (146a, 149, 196a) and Susceptibility to ARV-associated Hepatotoxicity." Current Genomics 20: 000-000.

Singh, J., H. Lal and G. Kocher (2012). "Musculoskeletal disorder risk assessment in small scale forging industry by using RULA method." International Journal of Engineering and Advanced Technology 1(5): 513-518.

Singh, J., R. K. Reen and F. J. Wiebel (1994). "Piperine, a major ingredient of black and long peppers, protects against AFB1-induced cytotoxicity and micronuclei formation in H4IIEC3 rat hepatoma cells." Cancer Letters 86(2): 195-200.

Singh, J. S., P. Abhilash, H. Singh, R. P. Singh and D. Singh (2011). "Genetically engineered bacteria: an emerging tool for environmental remediation and future research perspectives." Gene 480(1-2): 1-9.

Singh, K., A. Malik, D. Mohan and R. Takroo (2005). "Distribution of persistent organochlorine pesticide residues in Gomti River, India." Bulletin of Environmental Contamination and Toxicology 74(1): 146-154.

Singh, K., A. Saxena, A. Prasad, P. Dwivedi, S. Zaidi and P. Ray (1987). "Effect of protein A on mast cell numbers and macrophage phagocytic activity." Immunopharmacology and Immunotoxicology 9(2-3): 281-297.

Singh, K., A. Saxena, S. Zaidi, P. Dwivedi, S. Srivastava, P. Seth and P. Ray (1988). "Protection against carbon tetrachloride-induced hepatotoxicity by protein A." Journal of Applied Toxicology 8(6): 407-410.

Singh, K., N. Singh, A. Chandy and A. Manigauha (2012). "*In vivo* antioxidant and hepatoprotective activity of methanolic extracts of Daucus carota seeds in experimental animals." Asian Pacific Journal of Tropical Biomedicine 2(5): 385-388.

Singh, K., S. Singh, N. K. Singhal, A. Sharma, D. Parmar and M. P. Singh (2010). "Nicotine-and caffeine-mediated changes in gene expression patterns of MPTP-lesioned mouse striatum: Implications in neuroprotection mechanism." Chemico-biological Interactions 185(2): 81-93.

Singh, K., S. Zaidi, A. Saxena and P. Ray (1990). "Effects of aflatoxin on lymphoid cells of weanling rat." Journal of Applied Toxicology 10(4): 245-250.

Singh, K. P., S. Gupta and N. Basant (2015). "QSTR modeling for predicting aquatic toxicity of pharmacological active compounds in multiple test species for regulatory purpose." Chemosphere 120: 680-689.

Singh, K. P., S. Gupta, A. Kumar and D. Mohan (2014). "Multispecies QSAR modeling for predicting the aquatic toxicity of diverse organic chemicals for regulatory toxicology." Chemical Research in Toxicology 27(5): 741-753.

Singh, K. P., S. Gupta and P. Rai (2013). "Predicting acute aquatic toxicity of structurally diverse chemicals in fish using artificial intelligence approaches." Ecotoxicology and Environmental Safety 95: 221-233.

Singh, K. P., S. Gupta and P. Rai (2013). "Predicting carcinogenicity of diverse chemicals using probabilistic neural network modeling approaches." Toxicology and Applied Pharmacology 272(2): 465-475.

Singh, L. P., A. Bhardwaj and K. K. Deepak (2010). "Occupational exposure in small and medium scale industry with specific reference to heat and noise." Noise and Health 12(46): 37.

Singh, L. P., A. Bhardwaj and K. K. Deepak (2013). "Occupational noise-induced hearing loss in Indian steel industry workers: an exploratory study." Human Factors 55(2): 411-424.

Singh, L. P., A. Bhardwaj and D. K. Kumar (2012). "Prevalence of permanent hearing threshold shift among workers of Indian iron and steel small and medium enterprises: a study." Noise and Health 14(58): 119.

Singh, M., A. J. Khan, P. P. Shah, R. Shukla, V. Khanna and D. Parmar (2008). "Polymorphism in environment responsive genes and association with Parkinson disease." Molecular and Cellular Biochemistry 312(1-2): 131-138.

Singh, M., V. K. Khanna, R. Shukla and D. Parmar (2010). "Association of polymorphism in cytochrome P450 2D6 and N-acetyltransferase-2 with Parkinson's disease." Disease Markers 28(2): 87-93.

Singh, M., P. Sasi, G. Rai, V. H. Gupta, D. Amarapurkar and P. P. Wangikar (2011). "Studies on toxicity of antitubercular drugs namely isoniazid, rifampicin, and pyrazinamide in an *in vitro* model of HepG2 cell line." Medicinal Chemistry Research 20(9): 1611-1615.

Singh, M., P. P. Shah, A. P. Singh, M. Ruwali, N. Mathur, M. C. Pant and D. Parmar (2008). "Association of genetic polymorphisms in glutathione S-transferases and susceptibility to head and neck cancer." Mutation Research/Fundamental and Molecular Mechanisms of Mutagenesis 638(1-2): 184-194.

Singh, M., V. Singh, D. Patel, P. Tandon, J. Gaur, J. R. Behari and S. Yadav (2010). "Face mask application as a tool to diminish the particulate matter mediated heavy metal exposure among citizens of Lucknow, India." Science of the Total Environment 408(23): 5723-5728.

Singh, M. P., M. Mishra, A. Sharma, A. Shukla, M. Mudiam, D. Patel, K. R. Ram and D. K. Chowdhuri (2011). "Genotoxicity and apoptosis in Drosophila melanogaster exposed to benzene, toluene and xylene: attenuation by quercetin and curcumin." Toxicology and Applied Pharmacology 253(1): 14-30.

Singh, N., D. Kumar, K. Lal, S. Raisuddin and A. P. Sahu (2010). "Adverse health effects due to arsenic exposure: modification by dietary supplementation of jaggery in mice." Toxicology and Applied Pharmacology 242(3): 247-255.

Singh, N., D. Kumar, S. Raisuddin and A. P. Sahu (2008). "Genotoxic effects of arsenic: prevention by functional food-jaggery." Cancer Letters 268(2): 325-330.

Singh, N. D., A. K. Sharma, P. Dwivedi, M. Kumar and R. D. Patil (2011). "Immunosuppressive effect of combined citrinin and endosulfan toxicity in pregnant Wistar rats." Veterinarski Arhiv 81(6): 751-763.

Singh, O., Y. Javeri, D. Juneja, M. Gupta, G. Singh and R. Dang (2011). "Profile and outcome of patients with acute toxicity admitted in intensive care unit: Experiences from a major corporate hospital in urban India." Indian Journal of Anaesthesia 55(4): 370.

Singh, P., M. Barjatiya, S. Dhing, R. Bhatnagar, S. Kothari and V. Dhar (2001). "Evidence suggesting that high intake of fluoride provokes nephrolithiasis in tribal populations." Urological Research 29(4): 238-244.

Singh, P. and D. K. Chowdhuri (2017). "Environmental presence of hexavalent but not trivalent chromium causes neurotoxicity in exposed Drosophila melanogaster." Molecular Neurobiology 54(5): 3368-3387.

Singh, P., P. Lata, S. Patel, A. K. Pandey, S. K. Jain, R. Shanker and A. Dhawan (2011). "Expression profiling of toxicity pathway genes by real-time PCR array in cypermethrin-exposed mouse brain." Toxicology Mechanisms and Methods 21(3): 193-199.

Singh, P. and V. Sharma (2016). "Integrated plastic waste management: environmental and improved health approaches." Procedia Environmental Sciences 35: 692-700.

Singh, P., L. Singh, S. C. Mondal, S. Kumar and I. N. Singh (2014). "Erythromycin -induced genotoxicity and hepatotoxicity in mice pups treated during prenatal and postnatal period." Fundamental and Clinical Pharmacology 28(5): 519-529.

Singh, P. K., M. K. Singh, R. S. Yadav, R. K. Dixit, A. Mehrotra and R. Nath (2017). "Attenuation of Lead-Induced Neurotoxicity by Omega-3 Fatty Acid in Rats." Annals of Neurosciences 24(4): 221-232.

Singh, R. D., R. Tiwari, H. Khan, A. Kumar and V. Srivastava (2015). "Arsenic exposure causes epigenetic dysregulation of IL-8 expression leading to proneoplastic changes in kidney cells." Toxicology Letters 237(1): 1-10.

Singh, R. P., M. Das, R. Khanna and S. K. Khanna (2000). "Evaluation of dermal irritancy potential of benzanthrone-derived dye analogs: structure activity relationship." Skin Pharmacology and Physiology 13(3-4): 165-173.

Singh, R. P., R. Khanna, J. L. Kaw, S. K. Khanna and M. Das (2003). "Comparative effect of benzanthrone and 3-bromobenzanthrone on hepatic xenobiotic metabolism and anti-oxidative defense system in guinea pigs." Archives of Toxicology 77(2): 94-99.

Singh, R. P., C. M. Shafeeque, S. K. Sharma, N. K. Pandey, R. Singh, J. Mohan, G. Kolluri, M. Saxena, B. Sharma and K. V. Sastry (2015). "Bisphenol A reduces fertilizing ability and motility by compromising mitochondrial function of sperm." Environmental Toxicology and Chemistry 34(7): 1617-1622.

Singh, S. and R. Arora (2010). "Ergonomic intervention for preventing musculoskeletal disorders among farm women." Journal of Agricultural Sciences 1(2): 61-71.

Singh, S., D. Chaudhry, D. Behera, D. Gupta and S. Jindal (2001). "Aggressive atropinisation and continuous pralidoxime (2-PAM) infusion in patients with severe organophosphate poisoning: experience of a northwest Indian hospital." Human and Experimental Toxicology 20(1): 15-18.

Singh, S., G. Chowdhary and G. Purohit (2006). "Assessment of impact of high particulate concentration on peak expiratory flow rate of lungs of sand stone quarry workers." International Journal of Environmental Research and Public Health 3(4): 355-359.

Singh, S., J. Dilawari, R. Vashist, H. Malhotra and B. Sharma (1985). "Aluminium phosphide ingestion." British Medical Journal (Clinical research ed.) 290(6475): 1110-1111.

Singh, S., V. Kumar, P. Singh, B. D. Banerjee, R. S. Rautela, S. S. Grover, D. S. Rawat, S. T. Pasha, S. K. Jain and A. Rai (2012). "Influence of CYP2C9, GSTM1, GSTT1 and NAT2 genetic polymorphisms on DNA damage in workers occupationally exposed to organophosphate pesticides." Mutation Research/Genetic Toxicology and Environmental Mutagenesis 741(1-2): 101-108.

Singh, S., V. Kumar, P. Singh, S. Thakur, B. D. Banerjee, R. S. Rautela, S. S. Grover, D. S. Rawat, S. T. Pasha and S. K. Jain (2011). "Genetic polymorphisms of GSTM1, GSTT1 and GSTP1 and susceptibility to DNA damage in workers occupationally exposed to organophosphate pesticides." Mutation Research/Genetic Toxicology and Environmental Mutagenesis 725(1-2): 36-42.

Singh, S., V. Kumar, S. Thakur, B. D. Banerjee, S. Chandna, R. S. Rautela, S. S. Grover, D. S. Rawat, S. T. Pasha and S. K. Jain (2011). "DNA damage and cholinesterase activity in occupational workers exposed to pesticides." Environmental Toxicology and Pharmacology 31(2): 278-285.

Singh, S., V. Kumar, S. Thakur, B. D. Banerjee, R. S. Rautela, S. S. Grover, D. S. Rawat, S. T. Pasha, S. K. Jain and R. L. Ichhpujani (2011). "Paraoxonase-1 genetic polymorphisms and susceptibility to DNA damage in workers occupationally exposed to organophosphate pesticides." Toxicology and Applied Pharmacology 252(2): 130-137.

Singh, S., K. Mukherjee, K. Gill and S. Flora (2009). "Lead-induced peripheral neuropathy following Ayurvedic medication." Indian Journal of Medical Sciences 63(9):408-410.

Singh, S. and R. Pandey (1989). "Gonadal toxicity of short term chronic endosulfan exposure to male rats." Indian Journal of Experimental Biology 27(4): 341-346.

Singh, S. and R. Pandey (1990). "Effect of sub-chronic endosulfan exposures on plasma gonadotrophins, testosterone, testicular testosterone and enzymes of androgen biosynthesis in rat." Indian Journal of Experimental Biology 28(10): 953-956.

Singh, S. and N. Sharma (2000). "Neurological syndromes following organophosphate poisoning." Neurology India 48(4): 308.

Singh, S., G. S. Shukla, R. Srivastava and S. V. Chandra (1979). "The interaction between ethanol and manganese in rat brain." Archives of Toxicology 41(4): 307-316.

Singh, S., K. Singh, S. P. Gupta, D. K. Patel, V. K. Singh, R. K. Singh and M. P. Singh (2009). "Effect of caffeine on the expression of cytochrome P450 1A2, adenosine A2A receptor and dopamine transporter in control and 1-methyl 4-phenyl 1, 2, 3, 6-tetrahydropyridine treated mouse striatum." Brain Research 1283: 115-126.

Singh, S., K. Singh, D. K. Patel, C. Singh, C. Nath, V. K. Singh, R. K. Singh and M. P. Singh (2009). "The expression of CYP2D22, an ortholog of human CYP2D6, in mouse striatum and its modulation in 1-methyl 4-Phenyl-1, 2, 3, 6-tetrahydropyridine-induced Parkinson's disease phenotype and nicotine-mediated neuroprotection." Rejuvenation Research 12(3): 185-198.

Singh, S., K. Singh, S. Patel, D. K. Patel, C. Singh, C. Nath and M. P. Singh (2008). "Nicotine and caffeine-mediated modulation in the expression of toxicant responsive genes and vesicular monoamine transporter-2 in 1-methyl 4-phenyl-1, 2, 3, 6-tetrahydropyridine-induced Parkinson's disease phenotype in mouse." Brain Research 1207: 193-206.

Singh, S. N. and R. D. Tripathi (2007). Environmental bioremediation technologies, Springer Science and Business Media.

Singh, S. P., N. Dwivedi, K. S. R. Raju, I. Taneja and M. Wahajuddin (2016). "Validation of a Rapid and Sensitive UPLC–MS-MS Method Coupled with Protein Precipitation for the Simultaneous Determination of Seven Pyrethroids in 100 μL of Rat Plasma by Using Ammonium Adduct as Precursor Ion." Journal of Analytical Toxicology 40(3): 213-221.

Singh, T., M. Singh and L. Singh (2002). "Teratogenic effect of maternal hypoglycaemia: a study on newborn albino rats." Journal of the Anatomical Society of India 51: 216-219.

Singh, U. S., D. K. Saxena, C. Singh, R. C. Murthy and S. V. Chandra (1991). "Lead-induced fetal nephrotoxicity in iron-deficient rats." Reproductive Toxicology 5(3): 211-217.

Singh, V., C. George, L. Singh and B. Gupta (1983). "Immunomodulatory activity of 6MFA, an interferon inducing antiviral substance from Aspergillus ochraceous ATCC 28706." Indian J. Parasitol 7: 225.

Singh, V., C. George, N. Singh, S. Agarwal and B. Gupta (1983). "Combined treatment of mice with Panax ginseng extract and interferon inducer." Planta Medica 47(04): 234-236.

Singh, V., S. Mitra, A. K. Sharma, R. Gera and D. Ghosh (2014). "Isolation and characterization of microglia from adult mouse brain: selected applications for ex vivo evaluation of immunotoxicological alterations following *in vivo* xenobiotic exposure." Chemical Research in Toxicology 27(5): 895-903.

Singh, V., N. Rastogi, A. Sinha, A. Kumar, N. Mathur and M. P. Singh (2007). "A study on the association of cytochrome-P450 1A1 polymorphism and breast cancer risk in north Indian women." Breast Cancer Research and Treatment 101(1): 73-81.

Singh, V., A. K. Sharma, R. L. Narasimhan, A. Bhalla, N. Sharma and R. Sharma (2014). "Granulocyte colony-stimulating factor in severe alcoholic hepatitis: a randomized pilot study." The American Journal of Gastroenterology 109(9): 1417.

Singh, V. K., M. K. Reddy, C. Kesavachandran, S. Rastogi and M. Siddiqui (2007). "Biomonitoring of organochlorines, glutathione, lipid peroxidation and cholinesterase activity among pesticide sprayers in mango orchards." Clinica Chimica Acta 377(1-2): 268-272.

Singhal, N. K., A. K. Chauhan, S. K. Jain, R. Shanker, C. Singh and M. P. Singh (2013). "Silymarin-and melatonin-mediated changes in the expression of selected genes in pesticides-induced Parkinsonism." Molecular and Cellular Biochemistry 384(1-2): 47-58.

Singhal, N. K., G. Srivastava, D. K. Patel, S. K. Jain and M. P. Singh (2011). "Melatonin or silymarin reduces maneb-and paraquat-induced Parkinson's disease phenotype in the mouse." Journal of Pineal Research 50(2): 97-109.

Singla, N., D. Gupta, N. Birbian and J. Singh (2014). "Association of NAT2, GST and CYP2E1 polymorphisms and anti-tuberculosis drug-induced hepatotoxicity." Tuberculosis 94(3): 293-298.

Singla, R., S. K. Sharma, A. Mohan, G. Makharia, V. Sreenivas, B. Jha, S. Kumar, P. Sarda and S. Singh (2010). "Evaluation of risk factors for antituberculosis treatment induced hepatotoxicity." Indian Journal of Medical Research 132(1): 81-87.

Sinha, A. and A. Rao (1985). "Induction of shape abnormality and unscheduled DNA synthesis by arecoline in the germ cells of mice." Mutation Research/Genetic Toxicology 158(3): 189-192.

Sinha, A. and A. Rao (1985). "Transplacental micronucleus inducing ability of arecoline, a betel nut alkaloid, in mice." Mutation Research/Genetic Toxicology 158(3): 193-194.

Sinha, A., N. Srivastava, S. Singh, A. K. Singh, S. Bhushan, R. Shukla and M. P. Singh (2009). "Identification of differentially displayed proteins in cerebrospinal fluid of

Parkinson's disease patients: a proteomic approach." Clinica Chimica Acta 400 (1-2): 14-20.

Sinha, A., R. S. Tamboli, B. Seth, A. M. Kanhed, S. K. Tiwari, S. Agarwal, S. Nair, R. Giridhar, R. K. Chaturvedi and M. R. Yadav (2015). "Neuroprotective role of novel triazine derivatives by activating Wnt/β catenin signaling pathway in rodent models of Alzheimer's disease." Molecular Neurobiology 52(1): 638-652.

Sinha, B. K. (1987). "Activation of hydrazine derivatives to free radicals in the perfused rat liver: a spin-trapping study." Biochimica et Biophysica Acta (BBA)-General Subjects 924(2): 261-269.

Sinha, N., N. Adhikari, R. Narayan and D. K. Saxena (1999). "Cytotoxic effect of endosulfan on rat Sertoli-germ cell coculture." Reproductive Toxicology 13(4): 291-294.

Sinha, N., N. Adhikari and D. Saxena (2001). "Effect of endosulfan on the enzymes of polyol pathway in rat Sertoli-germ cell coculture." Bulletin of Environmental Contamination and Toxicology 67(6): 821-827.

Sinha, N., N. Adhikari and D. K. Saxena (2001). "Effect of endosulfan during fetal gonadal differentiation on spermatogenesis in rats." Environmental Toxicology and Pharmacology 10(1-2): 29-32.

Sinha, N., R. Narayan and D. Saxena (1997). "Effect of endosulfan on the testis of growing rats." Bulletin of Environmental Contamination and Toxicology 58(1): 79-86.

Sinha, N., R. Narayan, R. Shanker and D. Saxena (1995). "Endosulfan-induced biochemical changes in the testis of rats." Veterinary and Human Toxicology 37(6): 547-549.

Sinha, S., T. Mathews, G. Arunodaya, N. B. Siddappa, U. Ranga, A. Desai, V. Ravi and A. Taly (2004). "HIV-1 clade-C-associated "ALS"-like disorder: first report from India." Journal of the Neurological Sciences 224(1-2): 97-100.

Sitaramayya, A., N. Nagar and S. V. Chandra (1974). "Effect of manganese on enzymes in rat brain." Acta Pharmacologica et Toxicologica 35(3): 185-190.

Siwach, S., D. Yadav, B. Arora and S. Dalal (1988). "Acute aluminum phosphide poisoning--an epidemiological, clinical and histo-pathological study." The Journal of the Association of Physicians of India 36(10): 594-596.

Sleeman, W. H. (1915). Rambles and recollections of an Indian official, Oxford University Press.

Smith, K. R. and S. Mehta (2003). "The burden of disease from indoor air pollution in developing countries: comparison of estimates." International Journal of Hygiene and Environmental Health 206(4-5): 279-289.

Sodhi, P., B. Poddar and V. Parmar (2001). "Fatal cardiac malformation in fetal valproate syndrome." Indian Journal of Pediatrics 68(10): 989-990.

Sonaje, K., J. Italia, G. Sharma, V. Bhardwaj, K. Tikoo and M. R. Kumar (2007). "Development of biodegradable nanoparticles for oral delivery of ellagic acid and evaluation of their antioxidant efficacy against cyclosporine A-induced nephrotoxicity in rats." Pharmaceutical Research 24(5): 899-908.

Soni, A. K. and P. C. Joshi (1997). "High sensitivity of Tubifex for ultraviolet-B." Biochemical and Biophysical Research Communications 231(3): 818-819.

Sood, N., J. Sachdeva, J. Hans and L. Siddhu (1984). "Study of prevalence of silicosis and other lung diseases and pulmonary function derangements in workers employed in stone crushing in Zirakpur of Patiala District, Punjab and adjoining areas." MD (Med) Thesis, Punjabi University, Patiala.

Sridhar, S. B., S. S. F. Al-Thamer and R. Jabbar (2016). "Monitoring of adverse drug reactions in psychiatry outpatient department of a Secondary Care Hospital of Ras Al Khaimah, UAE." Journal of Basic and Clinical Pharmacy 7(3): 80.

Srimuruganandam, B. and S. S. Nagendra (2012). "Application of positive matrix factorization in characterization of PM10 and PM2. 5 emission sources at urban roadside." Chemosphere 88(1): 120-130.

Srinivas, C., C. Sekar and R. Jayashree (2012). "Photodermatoses in India." Indian Journal of Dermatology, Venereology, and Leprology 78(7): 1.

Srinivasa, J., P. Maxim, J. Urban and A. D'Souza (2015). "Effects of pesticides on male reproductive functions." Iranian Journal of Medical Sciences 30(4): 153-159.

Sriramachari, S. (2004). "The Bhopal gas tragedy: An environmental disaster." Current Science 86(7): 905-920.

Sriramachari, S. (2005). "Bhopal gas tragedy: Scientific challenges and lessons for future." Journal of Loss Prevention in the Process Industries 18(4-6): 264-267.

Sriramachari, S. and H. Chandra (1997). "The lessons of Bhopal [toxic] MIC gas disaster scope for expanding global biomonitoring and environmental specimen banking." Chemosphere 34(9-10): 2237-2250.

Srivastav, A. K., A. Kumar, J. Prakash, D. Singh, P. Jagdale, J. Shankar and M. Kumar (2017). "Genotoxicity evaluation of zinc oxide nanoparticles in Swiss mice after oral administration using chromosomal aberration, micronuclei, semen analysis, and RAPD profile." Toxicology and Industrial Health 33(11): 821-834.

Srivastav, A. K., M. Kumar, N. G. Ansari, A. K. Jain, J. Shankar, N. Arjaria, P. Jagdale and D. Singh (2016). "A comprehensive toxicity study of zinc oxide nanoparticles versus their bulk in Wistar rats: toxicity study of zinc oxide nanoparticles." Human and Experimental Toxicology 35(12): 1286-1304.

Srivastav, A. K., S. F. Mujtaba, A. Dwivedi, S. K. Amar, S. Goyal, A. Verma, H. N. Kushwaha, R. K. Chaturvedi and R. S. Ray (2016). "Photosensitized rose Bengal-induced phototoxicity on human melanoma cell line under natural sunlight exposure." Journal of Photochemistry and Photobiology B: Biology 156: 87-99.

Srivastava, A. (2004). "Source apportionment of ambient VOCS in Mumbai city." Atmospheric Environment 38(39): 6829-6843.

Srivastava, A., B. Gupta, A. Mathur, N. Mathur, P. Mahendra and R. Bharti (1991). "The clinical and biochemical study of pesticide sprayers." Human and Experimental Toxicology 10(4): 279-283.

Srivastava, A., A. Joseph, S. Patil, A. More, R. Dixit and M. Prakash (2005). "Air toxics in ambient air of Delhi." Atmospheric Environment 39(1): 59-71.

Srivastava, A., S. S. Peshin, T. Kaleekal and S. K. Gupta (2005). "An epidemiological study of poisoning cases reported to the national poisons information centre, All India Institute of Medical Sciences, New Delhi." Human and Experimental Toxicology 24(6): 279-285.

Srivastava, A., A. Sharma, S. Yadav, S. J. Flora, U. N. Dwivedi and D. Parmar (2014). "Gene expression profiling of candidate genes in peripheral blood mononuclear cells for predicting toxicity of diesel exhaust particles." Free Radical Biology and Medicine 67: 188-194.

Srivastava, A., V. P. Sharma, R. Tripathi, R. Kumar, D. K. Patel and P. K. Mathur (2010). "Occurrence of phthalic acid esters in Gomti River Sediment, India." Environmental Monitoring and Assessment 169(1-4): 397-406.

Srivastava, A. and T. Shivanandappa (2005). "Hexachlorocyclohexane differentially alters the antioxidant status of the brain regions in rat." Toxicology 214(1-2): 123-130.

Srivastava, A., S. Singh, C. Rajpurohit, P. Srivastava, A. Pandey, D. Kumar, V. Khanna and A. Pant (2018). "Secretome of Differentiated PC12 Cells Restores the Monocrotophos-Induced Damages in Human Mesenchymal Stem Cells and SHSY-5Y Cells: Role of Autophagy and Mitochondrial Dynamics." Neuromolecular Medicine 20(2): 233-251.

Srivastava, A., S. Yadav, A. Sharma, U. Dwivedi, S. Flora and D. Parmar (2012). "Similarities in diesel exhaust particles induced alterations in expression of cytochrome P-450 and glutathione S-transferases in rat lymphocytes and lungs." Xenobiotica 42(7): 624-632.

Srivastava, A. K., S. Rai, M. Srivastava, M. Lohani, M. Mudiam and L. Srivastava (2014). "Determination of 17 organophosphate pesticide residues in mango by modified QuEChERS extraction method using GC-NPD/GC-MS and hazard index estimation in Lucknow, India." PloS One 9(5): e96493.

Srivastava, A. K., P. Trivedi, M. Srivastava, M. Lohani and L. P. Srivastava (2011). "Monitoring of pesticide residues in market basket samples of vegetable from Lucknow City, India: QuEChERS method." Environmental Monitoring and Assessment 176(1-4): 465-472.

Srivastava, G., K. Singh, M. N. Tiwari and M. P. Singh (2010). "Proteomics in Parkinson's disease: current trends, translational snags and future possibilities." Expert Review of Proteomics 7(1): 127-139.

Srivastava, L., R. Budhwar and R. Raizada (2001). "Organochlorine pesticide residues in Indian spices." Bulletin of Environmental Contamination and Toxicology 67(6): 856-862.

Srivastava, L., K. Gupta and R. Raizada (2000). "Organochlorine pesticide residues in herbal ayurvedic preparations." Bulletin of Environmental Contamination and Toxicology 64(4): 502-507.

Srivastava, L., S. Khanna, G. Singh and C. K. Murti (1982). "*In vitro* studies on the biotransformation of metanil yellow." Environmental Research 27(1): 185-189.

Srivastava, L., N. Kumar, K. Gupta and R. Raizada (2006). "Status of HCH residues in Indian medicinal plant materials." Bulletin of Environmental Contamination and Toxicology 76(5): 782-790.

Srivastava, L., R. Misra and P. Joshi (1986). "Photosensitized generation of singlet oxygen and superoxide radicals by selected dyestuffs, food additives and their metabolites." Photobiochemistry and Photobiophysics 11(2): 129-137.

Srivastava, L., R. Misra and P. Joshi (1990). "Photosensitizing potential of benzanthrone." Food and Chemical Toxicology 28(9): 653-658.

Srivastava, L., R. Singh and R. Raizada (1999). "Phototoxicity of quinalphos under sunlight *in vitro* and *in vivo*." Food and Chemical Toxicology 37(2-3): 177-181.

Srivastava, P., R. S. Yadav, L. P. Chandravanshi, R. K. Shukla, Y. K. Dhuriya, L. K. Chauhan, H. N. Dwivedi, A. B. Pant and V. K. Khanna (2014). "Unraveling the mechanism of neuroprotection of curcumin in arsenic induced cholinergic dysfunctions in rats." Toxicology and Applied Pharmacology 279(3): 428-440.

Srivastava, R., A. Farookh, N. Ahmad, M. Misra, S. Hasan and M. Husain (1995). "Reduction of cis-platinum induced nephrotoxicity by zinc histidine complex: the possible implication of nitric oxide." Biochemistry and Molecular Biology International 36(4): 855-862.

Srivastava, R., Q. Rahman, M. Kashyap, A. Singh, G. Jain, S. Jahan, M. Lohani, M. Lantow and A. Pant (2013). "Nano-titanium dioxide induces genotoxicity and apoptosis in human lung cancer cell line, A549." Human and Experimental Toxicology 32(2): 153-166.

Srivastava, R. K., M. Lohani, A. B. Pant and Q. Rahman (2010). "Cyto-genotoxicity of amphibole asbestos fibers in cultured human lung epithelial cell line: role of surface iron." Toxicology and Industrial Health 26(9): 575-582.

Srivastava, R. K., A. B. Pant, M. P. Kashyap, V. Kumar, M. Lohani, L. Jonas and Q. Rahman (2011). "Multi-walled carbon nanotubes induce oxidative stress and apoptosis in human lung cancer cell line-A549." Nanotoxicology 5(2): 195-207.

Srivastava, S., P. Mehrotra, S. Srivastava, I. Tandon and M. Siddiqui (2001). "Blood lead and zinc in pregnant women and their offspring in intrauterine growth retardation cases." Journal of Analytical Toxicology 25(6): 461-465.

Srivastava, S., A. Pant, S. Trivedi and R. Pandey (2016). "Curcumin and β-caryophellene attenuate cadmium quantum dots induced oxidative stress and lethality in Caenorhabditis elegans model system." Environmental Toxicology and Pharmacology 42: 55-62.

Srivastava, S., J. G. Pasipanodya, G. Ramachandran, D. Deshpande, S. Shuford, H. E. Crosswell, K. N. Cirrincione, C. M. Sherman, S. Swaminathan and T. Gumbo (2016). "A long-term co-perfused disseminated tuberculosis-3D liver hollow fiber model for both drug efficacy and hepatotoxicity in babies." EBioMedicine 6: 126-138.

Srivastava, S., M. I. Sabri, A. K. Agrawal and P. K. Seth (1986). "Effect of single and repeated doses of acrylamide and bis-acrylamide on glutathione-S-transferase and dopamine receptors in rat brain." Brain Research 371(2): 319-323.

Srivastava, S. P., P. K. Seth and H. Mukhtar (1983). "7-Ethoxycoumarin O-de-ethylase activity in rat brain microsomes." Biochemical Pharmacology 32(23): 3657-3660.

Sudheer, A. and R. Rengarajan (2012). "Atmospheric mineral dust and trace metals over urban environment in western India during winter." Aerosol and Air Quality Research 12(5): 923-933.

Sugumar, E., I. Kanakasabapathy and P. Abraham (2007). "Normal plasma creatinine level despite histological evidence of damage and increased oxidative stress in the kidneys of cyclophosphamide treated rats." Clinica Chimica Acta; International Journal of Clinical Chemistry 376(1-2): 244.

Sujatha, K., C. Srilatha, Y. Anjaneyulu and P. Amaravathi (2011). "Lead acetate induced nephrotoxicity in wistar albino rats, pathological, immunohistochemical and ultra structural studies." International Journal of Pharma and Bio Sciences 2(2): B459-B469.

Suke, S. G., A. Kumar, R. S. Ahmed, A. Chakraborti, A. Tripathi, P. Mediratta and B. Banerjee (2006). "Protective effect of melatonin against propoxur-induced oxidative stress and suppression of humoral immune response in rats." Indian Journal of Experimental Biology 44:312-315.

Sukhsohale, N. D., U. W. Narlawar and M. S. Phatak (2013). "Indoor air pollution from biomass combustion and its adverse health effects in central India: an exposure-response study." Indian Journal of Community Medicine: Official Publication of Indian Association of Preventive and Social Medicine 38(3): 162.

Sunkaria, A., W. Y. Wani, D. R. Sharma and K. D. Gill (2012). "Dichlorvos exposure results in activation induced apoptotic cell death in primary rat microglia." Chemical Research in Toxicology 25(8): 1762-1770.

Sur, S., V. Tiwari, D. Sinha, M. Z. Kamran, K. D. Dubey, G. Suresh Kumar and V. Tandon (2017). "Naphthalenediimide-Linked Bisbenzimidazole Derivatives as Telomeric G-Quadruplex-Stabilizing Ligands with Improved Anticancer Activity." ACS Omega 2(3): 966-980.

Surathi, P., K. Jhunjhunwala, R. Yadav and P. K. Pal (2016). "Research in Parkinson's disease in India: A review." Annals of Indian Academy of Neurology 19(1): 9.

Susheela, A., A. Kumar, M. Bhatnagar and R. Bahadur (1993). "Prevalence of endemic fluorosis with gastrointestinal manifestations in people living in some north-Indian villages." Fluoride 26(2): 97-104.

Sushma, P., K. Jamil, P. U. Kumar, U. Satyanarayana, M. Ramakrishna and B. Triveni (2015). "Genetic variation in microRNAs and risk of oral Squamous cell carcinoma in South Indian population." Asian Pacific Journal of Cancer Prevention 16(17): 7589-7594.

Tabrez, S. and M. Ahmad (2011). "Mutagenicity of industrial wastewaters collected from two different stations in northern India." Journal of Applied Toxicology 31(8): 783-789.

Tabrez, S., S. Shakil, M. Urooj, G. A. Damanhouri, A. M. Abuzenadah and M. Ahmad (2011). "Genotoxicity testing and biomarker studies on surface waters: an overview of the techniques and their efficacies." Journal of Environmental Science and Health, Part C 29(3): 250-275.

Taksande, A., M. Jain, K. Vilhekar and P. Chaturvedi (2008). "Peak expiratory flow rate of rural school children from Wardha district, Maharashtra in India." World Journal of Pediatrics 4(3): 211.

Talapatra, A. and A. Srivastava (2011). "Ambient Air Non-Methane Volatile Organic Compound (NMVOC) Study Initiatives in India – A Review." Journal of Environmental Protection 2(01): 21.

Tamilselvan, P., K. Langeswaran, S. Vijayaprakash, R. Revathy and M. P. Balasubramanian (2014). "Efficiency of lycopene against reproductive and developmental toxicity of bisphenol A in male Sprague Dawley rats." Biomedicine and Preventive Nutrition 4(4): 491-498.

Tandon, B., S. Acharya and A. Tandon (1996). "Epidemiology of hepatitis B virus infection in India." Gut 38(Suppl 2): S56-S59.

Tandon, D., J. Dewangan, S. Srivastava, V. K. Garg and S. K. Rath (2018). "miRNA genetic variants: As potential diagnostic biomarkers for oral cancer." Pathology-Research and Practice 214(2): 281-289.

Tandon, N., A. Shtauvere-Brameus, W. Hagopian and C. Sanjeevi (2002). "Prevalence of ICA-12 and other autoantibodies in north Indian patients with early-onset diabetes." Annals of the New York Academy of Sciences 958: 214-217.

Tandon, R., D. Saxena, S. Chandra, P. Seth and S. Srivastava (1988). "Testicular effects of acrylonitrile in mice." Toxicology Letters 42(1): 55-63.

Tandon, S., M. Chatterjee, A. Bhargava, V. Shukla and V. Bihari (2001). "Lead poisoning in Indian silver refiners." Science of the Total Environment 281(1-3): 177-182.

Tandon, S., M. Das and S. Khanna (1993). "Biometabolic elimination and organ retention profile of argemone alkaloid, sanguinarine, in rats and guinea pigs." Drug Metabolism and Disposition 21(1): 194-197.

Tandon, S., S. Flora and M. Ashquin (1984). "Vitamin B complex in treatment of cadmium intoxication." Annals of Clinical and Laboratory Science 14(6): 487-492.

Tandon, S., S. Flora and S. Singh (1986). "Chelation in metal intoxication XXI: Chelation in lead intoxication during vitamin B complex deficiency." Bulletin of Environmental Contamination and Toxicology 37(1): 317-325.

Tandon, S. and S. Khandelwal (1982). "Chelation in metal intoxication XII." Archives of Toxicology 50(1): 19-25.

Tandon, S., S. Khandelwal, A. Mathur and M. Ashquin (1984). "Preventive effects of nickel on cadmium hepatotoxicity and nephrotoxicity." Annals of Clinical and Laboratory Science 14(5): 390-396.

Tandon, S. and A. Mathur (1976). "Chelation in metal intoxication. V. Lowering of manganese content in poisoned rat organs." Chemosphere 5(5): 319-325.

Tandon, S. and J. Singh (1975). "Removal of manganese by chelating agents from brain and liver of manganese treated rats: an *in vitro* and an *in vivo* study." Toxicology 5(2): 237-241.

Tang, M. and D. Martino (2013). "Oral immunotherapy and tolerance induction in childhood." Pediatric Allergy and Immunology 24(6): 512-520.

Tanjore, R. R., A. Rangaraju, P. Kerkar, N. Calambur and P. Nallari (2008). "MYBPC3 gene variations in hypertrophic cardiomyopathy patients in India." Canadian Journal of Cardiology 24(2): 127-130.

Tarale, P., S. Sivanesan, A. P. Daiwile, R. Stöger, A. Bafana, P. K. Naoghare, D. Parmar, T. Chakrabarti and K. Kannan (2017). "Global DNA methylation profiling of manganese-exposed human neuroblastoma SH-SY5Y cells reveals epigenetic alterations in Parkinson's disease-associated genes." Archives of Toxicology 91(7): 2629-2641.

Teotia, M., S. Teotia and K. Singh (1998). "Endemic chronic fluoride toxicity and dietary calcium deficiency interaction syndromes of metabolic bone diease and deformities in India: Year 2000." The Indian Journal of Pediatrics 65(3): 371-381.

Tewari, P., P. Mandal, R. Roy, S. Asthana, P. D. Dwivedi, M. Das and A. Tripathi (2017). "A novel function of TLR4 in mediating the immunomodulatory effect of benzanthrone, an environmental pollutant." Toxicology Letters 276: 69-84.

Tewari, P., R. Roy, S. Mishra, P. Mandal, A. Yadav, B. P. Chaudhari, R. K. Chaturvedi, P. D. Dwivedi, A. Tripathi and M. Das (2015). "Benzanthrone induced immunotoxicity via oxidative stress and inflammatory mediators in Balb/c mice." Immunobiology 220(3): 369-381.

Thakur, C. and S. Prasad (1968). "Observations on a recent outbreak of epidemic dropsy." Journal of the Indian Medical Association 50(5): 203-207.

Thakur, D., P. Singh, C. Tripathi, S. Bhadauria and S. Jain (2013). "*In Vitro* Immunotoxicity Testing of Pesticides using Human Cytokine Promoter Based Reporter Cell Lines." Clinical and Experimental Pharmacology 4: 2161-1459.

Thokchom, B. and N. Thacker (2019). Residual Analysis of Pesticides in Surface Water of Nagpur, India: An Approach to Water Pollution Control. Handbook of Research on the Adverse Effects of Pesticide Pollution in Aquatic Ecosystems, IGI Global: 280-300.

Thomas, B. and K. P. Mohanakumar (2004). "Melatonin protects against oxidative stress caused by 1-methyl-4-phenyl-1, 2, 3, 6-tetrahydropyridine in the mouse nigrostriatum." Journal of Pineal Research 36(1): 25-32.

Tikoo, K., I. Y. Ali, J. Gupta and C. Gupta (2009). "5-Azacytidine prevents cisplatin induced nephrotoxicity and potentiates anticancer activity of cisplatin by involving inhibition of metallothionein, pAKT and DNMT1 expression in chemical induced cancer rats." Toxicology Letters 191(2-3): 158-166.

Tikoo, K., D. K. Bhatt, A. B. Gaikwad, V. Sharma and D. G. Kabra (2007). "Differential effects of tannic acid on cisplatin induced nephrotoxicity in rats." FEBS Letters 581(10): 2027-2035.

Tikoo, K., R. Meena, D. Kabra and A. Gaikwad (2008). "Change in post-translational modifications of histone H3, heat-shock protein-27 and MAP kinase p38 expression by curcumin in streptozotocin-induced type I diabetic nephropathy." British Journal of Pharmacology 153(6): 1225-1231.

Tikoo, K., K. Singh, D. Kabra, V. Sharma and A. Gaikwad (2008). "Change in histone H3 phosphorylation, MAP kinase p38, SIR 2 and p53 expression by resveratrol in preventing streptozotocin induced type I diabetic nephropathy." Free Radical Research 42(4): 397-404.

Tiwari, A., P. Pragya, K. R. Ram and D. K. Chowdhuri (2011). "Environmental chemical mediated male reproductive toxicity: Drosophila melanogaster as an alternate animal model." Theriogenology 76(2): 197-216.

Tiwari, A. K., P. Prasad, B. Thelma, K. P. Kumar, A. Ammini, A. Gupta and R. Gupta (2009). "Oxidative stress pathway genes and chronic renal insufficiency in Asian Indians with Type 2 diabetes." Journal of Diabetes and its Complications 23(2): 102-111.

Tiwari, B., N. Manickam, S. Kumari and A. Tiwari (2016). "Biodegradation and dissolution of polyaromatic hydrocarbons by Stenotrophomonas sp." Bioresource Technology 216: 1102-1105.

Tiwari, M., U. Dwivedi and P. Kakkar (2010). "Suppression of oxidative stress and pro-inflammatory mediators by Cymbopogon citratus D. Stapf extract in lipopolysaccharide stimulated murine alveolar macrophages." Food and Chemical Toxicology 10(48): 2913-2919.

Tiwari, M., U. Dwivedi and P. Kakkar (2014). "Tinospora cordifolia extract modulates COX-2, iNOS, ICAM-1, pro-inflammatory cytokines and redox status in murine model of asthma." Journal of Ethnopharmacology 2(153): 326-337.

Tiwari, M. N., S. Agarwal, P. Bhatnagar, N. K. Singhal, S. K. Tiwari, P. Kumar, L. K. S. Chauhan, D. K. Patel, R. K. Chaturvedi and M. P. Singh (2013). "Nicotine-encapsulated poly (lactic-co-glycolic) acid nanoparticles improve neuroprotective efficacy against MPTP-induced parkinsonism." Free Radical Biology and Medicine 65: 704-718.

Tiwari, M. N., A. K. Singh, S. Agrawal, S. P. Gupta, A. Jyoti, R. Shanker, O. Prakash and M. P. Singh (2012). "Cypermethrin alters the expression profile of mRNAs in the adult rat striatum: a putative mechanism of postnatal pre-exposure followed by adulthood re-exposure-enhanced neurodegeneration." Neurotoxicity Research 22(4): 321-334.

Tiwari, M. N., A. K. Singh, I. Ahmad, G. Upadhyay, D. Singh, D. K. Patel, C. Singh, O. Prakash and M. P. Singh (2010). "Effects of cypermethrin on monoamine transporters, xenobiotic metabolizing enzymes and lipid peroxidation in the rat nigrostriatal system." Free Radical Research 44(12): 1416-1424.

Tiwari, R. (2005). "Biomarkers of silicosis: Potential candidates." Indian Journal of Occupational and Environmental Medicine 9(3): 103.

Tiwari, R., R. D. Singh, H. Khan, S. Gangopadhyay, S. Mittal, V. Singh, N. Arjaria, J. Shankar, S. K. Roy and D. Singh (2017). "Oral subchronic exposure to silver nanoparticles causes renal damage through apoptotic impairment and necrotic cell death." Nanotoxicology 11(5): 671-686.

Tiwari, R. R., N. G. Sathwara and H. N. Saiyed (2004). "Serum copper levels among quartz stone crushing workers: a cross sectional study." Indian Journal of Physiology and Pharmacology 48(3): 337-342.

Tiwari, S., A. K. Srivastava, D. S. Bisht, T. Bano, S. Singh, S. Behura, M. K. Srivastava, D. Chate and B. Padmanabhamurty (2009). "Black carbon and chemical characteristics of PM 10 and PM 2.5 at an urban site of North India." Journal of Atmospheric Chemistry 62(3): 193-209.

Tiwari, S. K., S. Agarwal, L. K. S. Chauhan, V. N. Mishra and R. K. Chaturvedi (2015). "Bisphenol-A impairs myelination potential during development in the hippocampus of the rat brain." Molecular Neurobiology 51(3): 1395-1416.

Tiwari, S. K., S. Agarwal, B. Seth, A. Yadav, R. S. Ray, V. N. Mishra and R. K. Chaturvedi (2015). "Inhibitory effects of bisphenol-A on neural stem cells proliferation and differentiation in the rat brain are dependent on Wnt/β-catenin pathway." Molecular Neurobiology 52(3): 1735-1757.

Tiwari, S. K., S. Agarwal, A. Tripathi and R. K. Chaturvedi (2016). "Bisphenol-A mediated inhibition of hippocampal neurogenesis attenuated by curcumin via canonical Wnt pathway." Molecular Neurobiology 53(5): 3010-3029.

Tobit, V., O. Verma, P. Ramteke and R. Ray (2011). "Phototoxic assessment of polycyclic aromatic hydrocarbons by using NIH-3T3 and L-929 cell lines." Journal of AIDS and Clinical Research 2: 123.

Tobit, V., O. Verma, P. Ramteke and R. Ray (2012). "Phototoxic Assesment of Benzanthrone and Anthracene by Using NIH-3t3 and L-929 Cell Lines." Journal of Clinical and Cellular Immunology 3(116): 2.

Tomar, A., S. Vasisth, S. I. Khan, S. Malik, T. C. Nag, D. S. Arya and J. Bhatia (2017). "Galangin ameliorates cisplatin induced nephrotoxicity *in vivo* by modulation of oxidative stress, apoptosis and inflammation through interplay of MAPK signaling cascade." Phytomedicine 34: 154-161.

Tripathi, M., S. K. Khanna and M. Das (2007). "Surveillance on use of synthetic colours in eatables vis a vis Prevention of Food Adulteration Act of India." Food Control 18(3): 211-219.

Tripathi, M., B. K. Singh, C. Mishra, S. Raisuddin and P. Kakkar (2010). "Involvement of mitochondria mediated pathways in hepatoprotection conferred by Fumaria parviflora Lam. extract against nimesulide induced apoptosis *in vitro*." Toxicology *In Vitro* 24(2): 495-508.

Tripathi, R., R. Raghunath, S. Mahapatra and S. Sadasivan (2001). "Blood lead and its effect on Cd, Cu, Zn, Fe and hemoglobin levels of children." Science of the Total Environment 277(1-3): 161-168.

Tripathi, S. and A. K. Srivastav (2010). "Nephrotoxicity induced by long-term oral administration of different doses of chlorpyrifos." Toxicology and Industrial Health 26(7): 439-447.

Tripathi, S. K., N. Gupta, M. Mahato, K. C. Gupta and P. Kumar (2014). "Selective blocking of primary amines in branched polyethylenimine with biocompatible ligand alleviates cytotoxicity and augments gene delivery efficacy in mammalian cells." Colloids and Surfaces B: Biointerfaces 115: 79-85.

Tripathy, N., B. Majhi, L. Dey and C. Das (1988). "Genotoxicity of Rogor studied in the sex-linked recessive lethal test and wing, eye and female germ-line mosaic assays in Drosophila melanogaster." Mutation Research/Genetic Toxicology 206(3): 351-360.

Tripathy, S. P., S. S. Kulkarni, S. D. Jadhav, K. D. Agnihotri, A. J. Jere, S. N. Kurle, S. K. Bhattacharya, K. Singh, S. P. Tripathy and R. S. Paranjape (2005). "Subtype B and subtype C HIV type 1 recombinants in the northeastern state of Manipur, India." AIDS Research and Human Retroviruses 21(2): 152-157.

Tripathy, V., A. Saha and J. Kumar (2017). "Detection of pesticides in popular medicinal herbs: a modified QuEChERS and gas chromatography–mass spectrometry based approach." Journal of Food Science and Technology 54(2): 458-468.

Tripathy, V., A. Saha, D. J. Patel, B. Basak, P. G. Shah and J. Kumar (2016). "Validation of a QuEChERS-based gas chromatographic method for analysis of pesticide residues in Cassia angustifolia (senna)." Journal of Environmental Science and Health, Part B 51(8): 508-518.

Trivedi, A., B. Dave and S. Adhvaryu (1990). "Assessment of genotoxicity of nicotine employing *in vitro* mammalian test system." Cancer Letters 54(1-2): 89-94.

Trivedi, B., D. K. Saxena, R. C. Murthy and S. V. Chandra (1989). "Embryotoxicity and fetotoxicity of orally administered hexavalent chromium in mice." Reproductive Toxicology 3(4): 275-278.

Trivedi, D. and A. Niyogi (1968). "Benzanthrone hazard in dye-factory." Indian Journal of Industrial Medicine 14(1): 13-22.

Trivedi, D. K., K. Ali and G. Beig (2014). "Impact of meteorological parameters on the development of fine and coarse particles over Delhi." Science of the Total Environment 478: 175-183.

Tsuda, S., M. Murakami, N. Matsusaka, K. Kano, K. Taniguchi and Y. F. Sasaki (2001). "DNA damage induced by red food dyes orally administered to pregnant and male mice." Toxicological Sciences 61(1): 92-99.

Tumane, R. G., N. Nath and A. Khan (2019). "Risk assessment in mining-based industrial workers by immunological parameters as copper toxicity markers." Indian Journal of Occupational and Environmental Medicine 23(1): 21.

Upadhyay, G., S. P. Gupta, O. Prakash and M. P. Singh (2010). "Pyrogallol-mediated toxicity and natural antioxidants: triumphs and pitfalls of preclinical findings and their translational limitations." Chemico-biological Interactions 183(3): 333-340.

Upadhyay, G., A. Kumar and M. P. Singh (2007). "Effect of silymarin on pyrogallol- and rifampicin-induced hepatotoxicity in mouse." European Journal of Pharmacology 565(1-3): 190-201.

Upadhyay, G., A. K. Singh, A. Kumar, O. Prakash and M. P. Singh (2008). "Resveratrol modulates pyrogallol-induced changes in hepatic toxicity markers, xenobiotic metabolizing enzymes and oxidative stress." European Journal of Pharmacology 596(1-3): 146-152.

Upadhyay, G., M. N. Tiwari, O. Prakash, A. Jyoti, R. Shanker and M. P. Singh (2010). "Involvement of multiple molecular events in pyrogallol-induced hepatotoxicity and silymarin-mediated protection: Evidence from gene expression profiles." Food and Chemical Toxicology 48(6): 1660-1670.

Upreti, K. K., M. Das and S. K. Khanna (1988). "Biochemical toxicology of argemone alkaloids. III. Effect on lipid peroxidation in different subcellular fractions of the liver." Toxicology Letters 42(3): 301-308.

Upreti, K. K., M. Das and S. K. Khanna (1991). "Biochemical toxicology of argemone oil. I. effect on hepatic cytochrome P-450 and xenobiotic metabolizing enzymes." Journal of Applied Toxicology 11(3): 203-209.

Upreti, K. K., M. Das and S. K. Khanna (1991). "Role of antioxidants and scavengers on argemone oil-induced toxicity in rats." Archives of Environmental Contamination and Toxicology 20(4): 531-537.

Vajpayee, P., I. Khatoon, C. B. Patel, G. Singh, K. C. Gupta and R. Shanker (2011). "Adverse effects of chromium oxide nano-particles on seed germination and growth in Triticum aestivum L." Journal of Biomedical Nanotechnology 7(1): 205-206.

Vajpayee, P., U. Rai, S. Sinha, R. Tripathi and P. Chandra (1995). "Bioremediation of tannery effluent by aquatic macrophytes." Bulletin of Environmental Contamination and Toxicology 55(4): 546-553.

Vallabani, N., S. Mittal, R. K. Shukla, A. K. Pandey, S. R. Dhakate, R. Pasricha and A. Dhawan (2011). "Toxicity of graphene in normal human lung cells (BEAS-2B)." Journal of Biomedical Nanotechnology 7(1): 106-107.

Varadarajan, S., L. Doraiswamy, N. Ayyangar, C. Iyer, A. Khan, A. Lahiri, K. Muzumdar, R. Mashellkar, R. Mitra and O. Nambia (1985). Report on scientific studies on the factors related to Bhopal toxic gas leakage. Report on scientific studies on the factors related to bhopal toxic gas leakage.

Vardhan, K. S., M. P. Rudra and S. Rao (1997). "Inhibition of Tyrosine Aminotransferase by β-N-Oxalyl-l-α, β-Diaminopropionic Acid, the Lathyrus sativus Neurotoxin." Journal of Neurochemistry 68(6): 2477-2484.

Varma, P. (2015). "Prevalence of chronic kidney disease in India - Where are we heading?" Indian Journal of Nephrology 25(3): 133.

Vashishtha, V., A. Kumar, T. J. John and N. Nayak (2007). "Cassia occidentalis poisoning as the probable cause of hepatomyoencephalopathy in children in western Uttar Pradesh." Indian Journal of Medical Research 125(6): 756-762.

Vashishtha, V., N. Nayak, T. J. John and A. Kumar (2007). "Recurrent annual outbreaks of a hepato-myo-encephalopathy syndrome in children in western Uttar Pradesh, India." Indian Journal of Medical Research 125(4): 523.

Vashishtha, V. M., A. Kumar, T. J. John and N. Nayak (2007). "Cassia occidentalis poisoning causes fatal coma in children in western Uttar Pradesh." Indian Pediatrics 44(7): 522.

Vassalotti, J. A., L. A. Stevens and A. S. Levey (2007). "Testing for chronic kidney disease: a position statement from the National Kidney Foundation." American Journal of Kidney Diseases 50(2): 169-180.

Velpandian, T., R. Bankoti, S. Humayun, A. Ravi, S. Kumari and N. Biswas (2006). "Comparative evaluation of possible ocular photochemical toxicity of fluoroquinolones meant for ocular use in experimental models." Indian Journal of Experimental Biology 44:387-391.

Venkatesan, N., C. Ramesh, R. Jayakumar and G. Chandrakasan (1993). "Angiotensin I converting enzyme activity in adriamycin induced nephrosis in rats." Toxicology 85(2-3): 137-148.

Venkatesh, R. and S. Chandramohan (2009)a. "A Study on Current Status: Asbestos Mining and Health Related Problems in India." International Journal of Innovative Research and Development 3(2): 397-401.

Venkatesh, S., A. Riyaz, M. Shamsi, R. Kumar, N. Gupta, S. Mittal, N. Malhotra, R. Sharma, A. Agarwal and R. Dada (2009). "Clinical significance of reactive oxygen species in semen of infertile Indian men." Andrologia 41(4): 251-256.

Verma, A. K., A. K. Keshari, J. Raj, R. Kumari, T. Kumar, V. Sharma, T. B. Singh, S. Srivastava and R. Srivastava (2016). "Prolidase-associated trace elements (Mn, Zn, Co, and Ni) in the patients with Parkinson's disease." Biological Trace Element Research 171(1): 48-53.

Verma, A. K., S. Kumar, A. Tripathi, B. P. Chaudhari, M. Das and P. D. Dwivedi (2012). "Chickpea (Cicer arietinum) proteins induce allergic responses in nasobronchial allergic patients and BALB/c mice." Toxicology Letters 210(1): 24-33.

Verma, A. K., A. Misra, S. Subash, M. Das and P. D. Dwivedi (2011). "Computational allergenicity prediction of transgenic proteins expressed in genetically modified crops." Immunopharmacology and Immunotoxicology 33(3): 410-422.

Verma, K., N. Agrawal, R. Misra, M. Farooq and R. Hans (2008). "Phototoxicity assessment of drugs and cosmetic products using E. coli." Toxicology *In Vitro* 22(1): 249-253.

Verma, N. and A. Bhardwaj (2015). "Biosensor technology for pesticides — a review." Applied Biochemistry and Biotechnology 175(6): 3093-3119.

Verma, N. and M. Singh (2003). "A disposable microbial based biosensor for quality control in milk." Biosensors and Bioelectronics 18(10): 1219-1224.

Verma, N. and M. Singh (2006). "A Bacillus sphaericus based biosensor for monitoring nickel ions in industrial effluents and foods." Journal of Analytical Methods in Chemistry. Journal of Automated Methods and Management in Chemistry: 1–4.

Verma, R. and B. D. Gupta (2015). "Detection of heavy metal ions in contaminated water by surface plasmon resonance based optical fibre sensor using conducting polymer and chitosan." Food Chemistry 166: 568-575.

Verma, R. and B. Mohanty (2009). "Early-life exposure to dimethoate-induced reproductive toxicity: evaluation of effects on pituitary-testicular axis of mice." Toxicological Sciences 112(2): 450-458.

Verma, R., M. Mukerji, D. Grover, B.-R. Chandrika, S. K. Das, S. Kubendran, S. Jain and S. K. Brahmachari (2005). "MLC1 gene is associated with schizophrenia and bipolar disorder in Southern India." Biological Psychiatry 58(1): 16-22.

Verma, R. S. and N. Srivastava (2001). "Chlorpyrifos induced alterations in levels of thiobarbituric acid reactive substances and glutathione in rat brain." Indian Journal of Experimental Biology 39(2) 174-177.

Verma, S. K., G. Raheja and K. D. Gill (2009). "Role of muscarinic signal transduction and CREB phosphorylation in dichlorvos-induced memory deficits in rats: an acetylcholine independent mechanism." Toxicology 256(3): 175-182.

Vij, M., S. Alam, N. Gupta, V. Gotherwal, H. Gautam, K. M. Ansari, D. Santhiya, V. T. Natarajan and M. Ganguli (2017). "Non-invasive Oil-Based Method to Increase Topical Delivery of Nucleic Acids to Skin." Molecular Therapy 25(6): 1342-1352.

Vij, M., R. Grover, V. Gotherwal, N. A. Wani, P. Joshi, H. Gautam, K. Sharma, S. Chandna, R. S. Gokhale and R. Rai (2016). "Bioinspired functionalized melanin nanovariants with a range of properties provide effective color matched photoprotection in skin." Biomacromolecules 17(9): 2912-2919.

Vij, M., P. Natarajan, A. K. Yadav, K. M. Patil, T. Pandey, N. Gupta, D. Santhiya, V. A. Kumar, M. Fernandes and M. Ganguli (2016). "Efficient Cellular Entry of (rxr)-Type Carbamate – Plasmid DNA Complexes and its Implication for Noninvasive Topical DNA Delivery to Skin." Molecular Pharmaceutics 13(6): 1779-1790.

Vijayaprakash, S., K. Langeswaran, A. Jagadeesan, R. Revathy and M. Balasubramanian (2012). "Protective efficacy of Terminalia catappa L. leaves against lead induced nephrotoxicity in experimental rats." International Journal of Pharmacy and Pharmaceutical Sciences: 454-458.

Vimalkumar, K., E. Arun, S. Krishna-Kumar, R. K. Poopal, N. P. Nikhil, A. Subramanian and R. Babu-Rajendran (2018). "Occurrence of triclocarban and benzotriazole ultraviolet stabilizers in water, sediment, and fish from Indian rivers." Science of the Total Environment 625: 1351-1360.

Vinayagamoorthy, N., K. Krishnamurthi, S. S. Devi, P. K. Naoghare, R. Biswas, A. R. Biswas, S. Pramanik, A. R. Shende and T. Chakrabarti (2010). "Genetic polymorphism of CYP2D6* 2 C$\rightarrow$ T 2850, GSTM1, NQO1 genes and their correlation with biomarkers in manganese miners of Central India." Chemosphere 81(10): 1286-1291.

Vipin, A., R. Rao, N. K. Kurrey, A. A. KA and G. Venkateswaran (2017). "Protective effects of phenolics rich extract of ginger against Aflatoxin B1-induced oxidative stress and hepatotoxicity." Biomedicine and Pharmacotherapy 91: 415-424.

Virukalpattigopalratnam, M., T. Singh and A. Ravishankar (2013). "Heptral (ademetionine) in patients with intrahepatic cholestasis in chronic liver disease due to non-alcoholic liver disease: results of a multicentre observational study in India." Journal of the Indian Medical Association 111(12): 856-859.

Viswanathan, P., Q. Rahman, M. Beg and S. Zaidi (1973). "Pulmonary lysosomal enzymes in experimental asbestosis in guinea pigs." Environmental Physiology and Biochemistry 3(120): 62.

Viswanathan, R., M. Boparai, S. Jain and M. Dash (1972). "Pneumoconiosis Survey of Workers in India Ordnance factory in India." Archives of Environmental Health: An International Journal 25(3): 198-204.

Vogel, E. W. and M. J. Nivard (1993). "Performance of 181 chemicals in a Drosophila assay predominantly monitoring interchromosomal mitotic recombination." Mutagenesis 8(1): 57-81.

Vyas, A., V. Kain, Z. Afrasiabi, S. Sitasawad, M. Khetmalas, V. Nivière and S. Padhye (2014). "Novel Mn-SOD mimetics offer superior protection against oxidative damages in Hek293 kidney cells." Journal of Pharmaceutical Sciences and Pharmacology 1(2): 146-153.

Wadia, R. S., S. N. Pujari, S. Kothari, M. Udhar, S. Kulkarni, S. Bhagat and A. Nanivadekar (2001). "Neurological manifestations of HIV disease." The Journal of the Association of Physicians of India 49: 343-348.

Wahajuddin, M., S. P. Singh, I. Taneja, K. S. R. Raju, J. R. Gayen, H. H. Siddiqui and S. K. Singh (2016). "Development and validation of an LC-MS/MS method for simultaneous determination of piperaquine and 97-63, the active metabolite of CDRI 97-78, in rat plasma and its application in interaction study." Drug Testing and Analysis 8(2): 221-227.

Wangikar, P.B., N. Sinha, P. Dwivedi, and A.K. Sharma (2007). "Teratogenic Effects of Ochratoxin A and Aflatoxin B1 Alone and in Combination on Post-Implantation Rat Embryos in Culture". Journal of the Turkish-German Gynecological Association 8(4): 357-364.

Wangikar, P., P. Dwivedi and N. Sinha (2004). "Effect in rats of simultaneous prenatal exposure to ochratoxin A and aflatoxin B1. i. Maternal toxicity and fetal malformations." Birth Effects Research Part B: Developmental and Reproductive Toxicology 71(6): 343-351.

Wangikar P.B., P. Dwivedi, N. Sinha, A.K. Sharma and A.G.Telang (2005). "Effects of aflatoxin B1 on embryo fetal development in rabbits". Food and Chemical Toxicology 43(4): 607-615.

Wanigasuriya, K. P., R. J. Peiris-John and R. Wickremasinghe (2011). "Chronic kidney disease of unknown aetiology in Sri Lanka: is cadmium a likely cause?" BMC Nephrology 12(1): 32.

Weaver, V. M., J. J. Fadrowski and B. G. Jaar (2015). "Global dimensions of chronic kidney disease of unknown etiology (CKDu): a modern era environmental and/or occupational nephropathy?" BMC Nephrology 16(1): 145.

Yadav, A., A. Kumar, P. D. Dwivedi, A. Tripathi and M. Das (2012). "*In vitro* studies on immunotoxic potential of Orange II in splenocytes." Toxicology Letters 208(3): 239-245.

Yadav, A., A. Kumar, A. Tripathi and M. Das (2013). "Sunset yellow FCF, a permitted food dye, alters functional responses of splenocytes at non-cytotoxic dose." Toxicology Letters 217(3): 197-204.

Yadav, A. S. and M. K. Sharma (2008). "Increased frequency of micronucleated exfoliated cells among humans exposed *in vivo* to mobile telephone radiations." Mutation Research/Genetic Toxicology and Environmental Mutagenesis 650(2): 175-180.

Yadav, D., R. Kumar, R. K. Dixit, S. Kant, A. Verma, K. Srivastava, S. Singh and S. Singh (2019). "Association of Nat2 Gene Polymorphism with Antitubercular Drug-induced Hepatotoxicity in the Eastern Uttar Pradesh Population." Cureus 11(4): e4425.

Yadav, J. and P. Chadha (2002). "Genotoxic studies in pan masala chewers: a high cancer risk group." International Journal of Human Genetics 2(2): 107-112.

Yadav, N., A. Dwivedi, S. F. Mujtaba, H. N. Kushwaha, S. K. Singh and R. S. Ray (2013). "Ambient UVA-Induced Expression of p53 and Apoptosis in Human Skin Melanoma A375 Cell Line by Quinine." Photochemistry and Photobiology 89(3): 655-664.

Yadav, N., A. Dwivedi, S. F. Mujtaba, A. Verma, R. Chaturvedi, R. S. Ray and G. Singh (2014). "Photosensitized mefloquine induces ROS-mediated DNA damage and apoptosis in keratinocytes under ambient UVB and sunlight exposure." Cell Biology and Toxicology 30(5): 253-268.

Yadav, R. S., M. L. Sankhwar, R. K. Shukla, R. Chandra, A. B. Pant, F. Islam and V. K. Khanna (2009). "Attenuation of arsenic neurotoxicity by curcumin in rats." Toxicology and Applied Pharmacology 240(3): 367-376.

Yadav, S., A. Dhawan, R. L. Singh, P. K. Seth and D. Parmar (2006). "Expression of constitutive and inducible cytochrome P450 2E1 in rat brain." Molecular and Cellular Biochemistry 286(1-2): 171-180.

Yadav, S., S. P. Gupta, G. Srivastava, P. K. Srivastava and M. P. Singh (2012). "Role of secondary mediators in caffeine-mediated neuroprotection in maneb-and paraquat-induced Parkinson's disease phenotype in the mouse." Neurochemical Research 37(4): 875-884.

Yadav, S., A. Pandey, A. Shukla, S. S. Talwelkar, A. Kumar, A. B. Pant and D. Parmar (2011). "miR-497 and miR-302b regulate ethanol-induced neuronal cell death through BCL2 protein and cyclin D2." Journal of Biological Chemistry 286(43): 37347-37357.

Yadav, S. and P. G. Satsangi (2013). "Characterization of particulate matter and its related metal toxicity in an urban location in South West India." Environmental Monitoring and Assessment 185(9): 7365-7379.

Yadav, S., N. K. Singhal, V. Singh, N. Rastogi, P. K. Srivastava and M. P. Singh (2009). "Association of single nucleotide polymorphisms in CYP1B1 and COMT genes with breast cancer susceptibility in Indian women." Disease Markers 27(5): 203-210.

Yadav, S. K., J. S. Patel, G. Kumar, A. Mukherjee, A. Maharshi, B. K. Sarma, S. Singh and H. B. Singh (2018). "Factors affecting the fate, transport, bioavailability and toxicity of nanoparticles in the agroecosystem." Emerging Trends in Agri-Nanotechnology: Fundamental and Applied Aspects: 118.

Yadav, V. K., S. Prasad, D. K. Patel, A. H. Khan, M. Tripathi and Y. Shukla (2010). "Identification of polycyclic aromatic hydrocarbons in unleaded petrol and diesel exhaust emission." Environmental Monitoring and Assessment 168(1-4): 173-178.

Yamashita, H., K. Takahashi, H. Tanaka, H. Nagai and N. Inagaki (2012). "Overcoming food allergy through acquired tolerance conferred by transfer of Tregs in a murine model." Allergy 67(2): 201-209.

Yugandhar, B., K. Radha Krishna Murthy and S. Sattar (1999). "Insulin administration in severe scorpion envenoming." Journal of Venomous Animals and Toxins 5(2): 200-219.

Yumnamcha T., D. Roy, M. D. Devi and U. Nongthomba (2015). "Evaluation of developmental toxicity and apoptotic induction of the aqueous extract of Millettia pachycarpa using zebrafish as model organism" Toxicological and Environmental Chemistry, 97:10, 1363-1381.

Zafar, K. S., A. Siddiqui, I. Sayeed, M. Ahmad, S. Salim and F. Islam (2003). "Dose-dependent protective effect of selenium in rat model of Parkinson's disease: neurobehavioral and neurochemical evidences." Journal of Neurochemistry 84(3): 438-446.

Zaidi, S. and B. Banerjee (1987). "Enzymatic detoxication of DDT to DDD by rat liver: Effects of some inducers and inhibitors of cytochrome P-450 enzyme system." Bulletin of Environmental Contamination and Toxicology 38(3): 449-455.

Zaidi, S., V. Bhatnagar, B. Banerjee, G. Balakrishnan and M. Shah (1989). "DDT residues in human milk samples from Delhi, India." Bulletin of Environmental Contamination and Toxicology 42(3): 427-430.

Zaidi, S., R. Dogra, R. Shanker and S. Chandra (1973). "Experimental infective manganese pneumoconiosis in guinea pigs." Environmental Research 6(3): 287-297.

Zaidi, S. and J. Kaw (1970). "Effect of general dietary deficiency and protein malnutrition on the fibrogenesis caused by silica dust in rats." Occupational and Environmental Medicine 27(3): 250-259.

Zaidi, S., A. Patel, N. Mehta, K. Patel, R. Takiar and H. Saiyed (2005). "Early biochemical alterations in manganese toxicity: ameliorating effects of magnesium nitrate and vitamins." Industrial Health 43(4): 663-668.

Zaidi, S., S. Raisuddin, K. Singh, A. Jafri, R. Husain, M. Husain, S. Mall, P. Seth and P. Ray (1994). "Acrylamtoe induced immunosuppression in rats and its modulan by 6-MFA, an interferon inducer." Immunopharmacology and Immunotoxicology 16(2): 247-260.

Zaidi, S., R. Shanker and R. Dogra (1971). "Experimental studies on early stages of the development of pulmonary silicosis in pups." Environmental Research 4(3): 243-252.

Zaidi, S., R. Shanker and R. Dogra (1973). "Experimental infective pneumoconiosis: Effect of asbestos dust and Candida albicans infection on the lungs of rhesus monkeys." Environmental Research 6(3): 274-286.

Zaidi, S., K. Singh, Raisuddin, A. Saxena and P. Ray (1990). "Protein A induced abrogation of cyclophosphamide toxicity is associated with concomitant potentiation of immune function of host." Immunopharmacology and Immunotoxicology 12(3): 479-512.

Zaidi, S. H., R. S. Dogra, A. P. Sahu, S. Khanna and R. Shanker (1977). "Experimental infectlve pneumoconiosis: effect of candida albicans and iron ore dust on the lungs of guinea pigs." Industrial Health 15(3-4): 123-129.

Zhou, B.-B. S. and S. J. Elledge (2000). "The DNA damage response: putting checkpoints in perspective." Nature 408(6811): 433.

Index

www.ingramcontent.com/pod-product-compliance
Lightning Source LLC
Chambersburg PA
CBHW070823110726

47973CB00003B/41